KT-102-709

Reader's Digest
HEALTHY BONES, MUSCLES & JOINTS

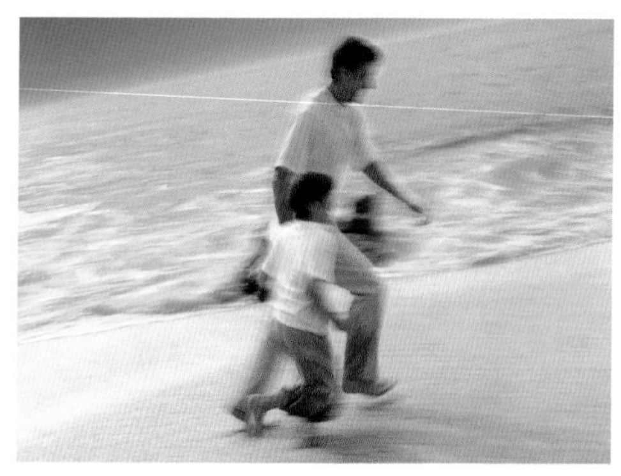

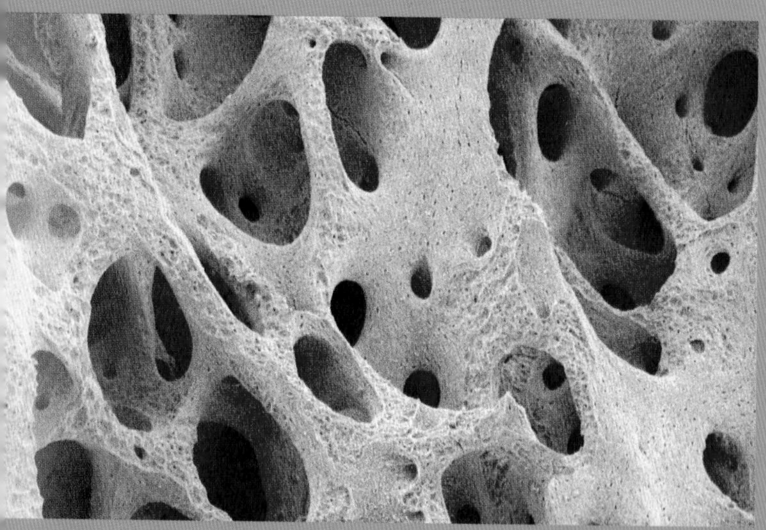

Reader's Digest
HEALTHY BONES,

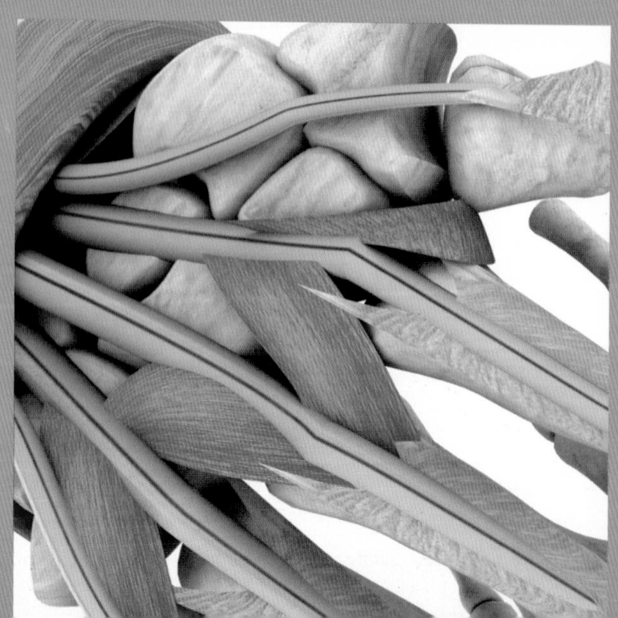

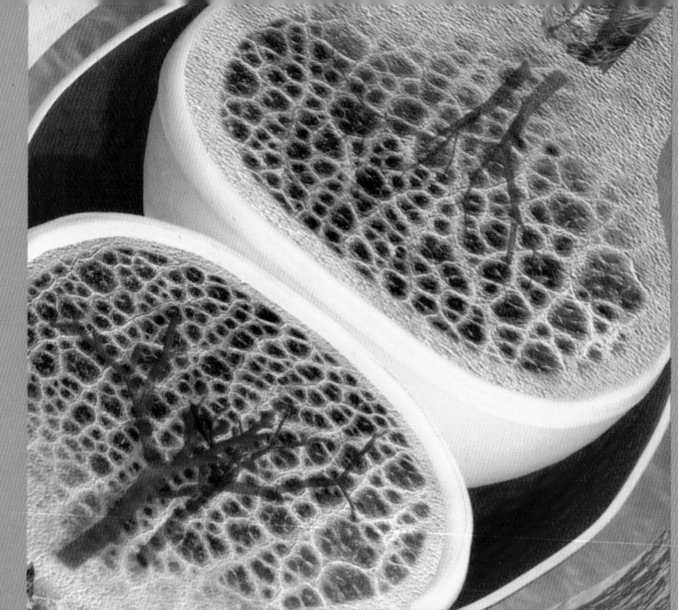

MUSCLES & JOINTS

A lifelong guide to staying active and supple

PUBLISHED BY THE READER'S DIGEST ASSOCIATION LIMITED
LONDON • NEW YORK • SYDNEY • MONTREAL

CONTENTS

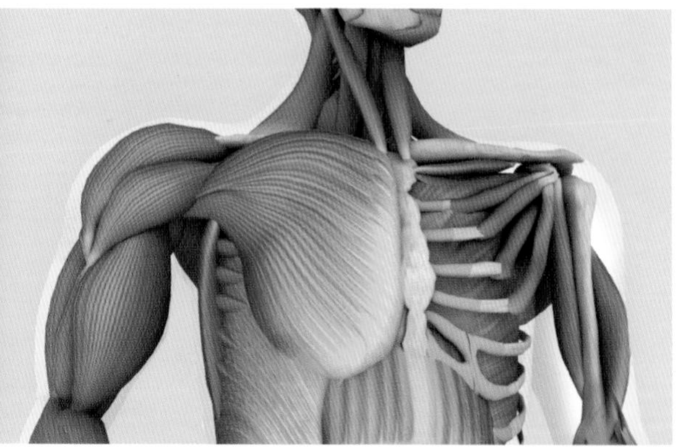

The mechanics of movement 1

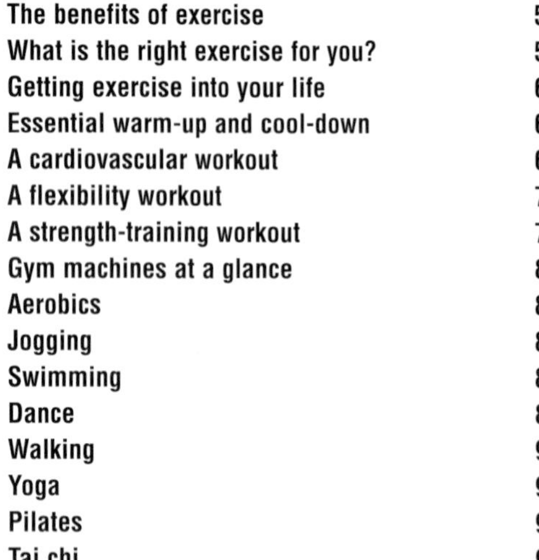

Fit for life 2

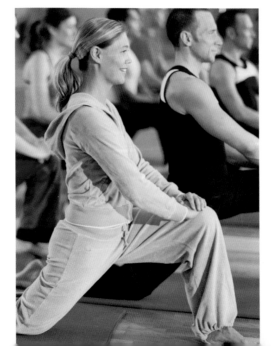

Food facts 3

Early life 4

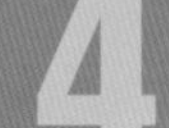

IMPORTANT NOTE TO READERS

While the creators of this work have made every effort to be as accurate and up to date as possible, medical and pharmacological knowledge is constantly changing. Readers are recommended to consult a qualified medical specialist for individual advice. The writers, researchers, editors and the publishers of this work cannot be held liable for any errors and omissions, or actions that may be taken as a consequence of information contained within this work.

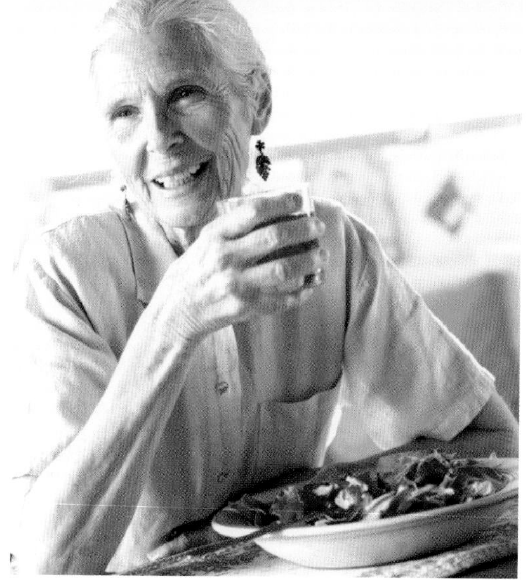

Agile ageing 5

A healthy back and spine 6

Safeguarding your knees 7

Hip health 8

Osteoarthritis 9

Rheumatoid arthritis 10

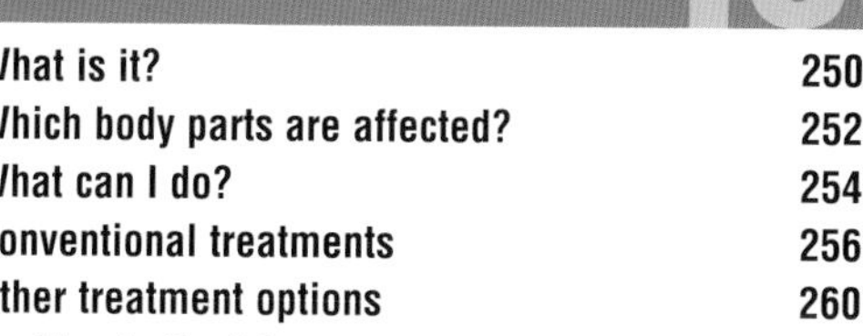

Osteoporosis 11

Directory of disorders 12

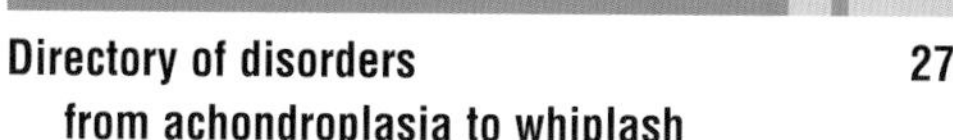

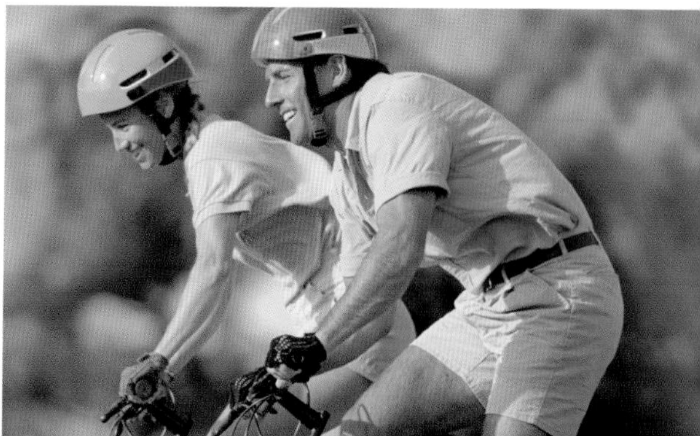

YOUR BUILDING BLOCKS

Bones, muscles and joints are your vital support structure – and looking after them will bring benefits all your life. *Healthy Bones, Muscles & Joints* has been created to give you all the information you need to keep your body's building blocks in peak condition.

This is a book for people who want to ensure that they maintain their strength and flexibility, and also for those with existing problems. Drawing on advice from a wide range of musculoskeletal experts, it presents complex information in a clear, concise way, so you can focus on your own situation, assess your risks, review your options and find the therapies, treatments and lifestyle changes that could help you.

Now is the time to take control and stay active, supple and healthy for life

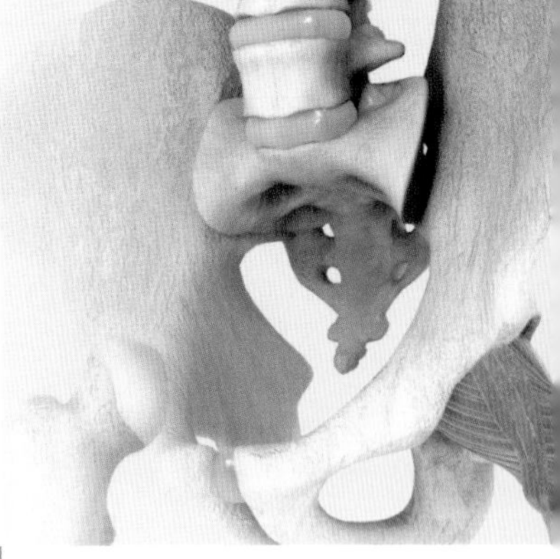

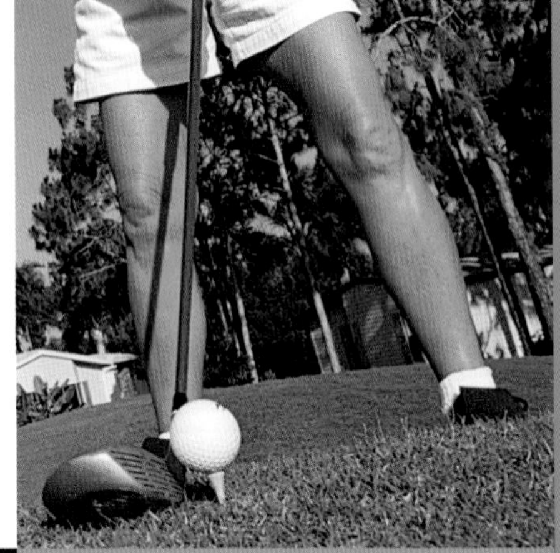

Get moving

Whatever your age or fitness levels, there are certain steps you can take to improve the health of your bones and muscles. Part 2 describes exactly how regular exercise strengthens your bones and muscles. Find out all about:

- The specific benefits of different types of exercise – from dancing to golf – so you can choose what is right for you.
- Basic exercise routines – warm-ups, stretches, exercises that improve flexibility, strengthen your heart, improve muscle tone or increase bone density.
- The best exercises for particular conditions and a range of activities and therapies, including yoga, Pilates and tai chi. All are clearly explained.
- The best ways to incorporate exercise into your daily life and how to build up your routine steadily and safely.

Get up and about and you'll recover from back pain faster

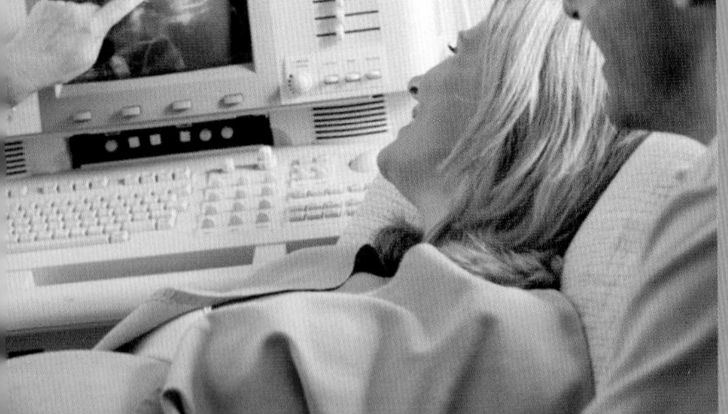

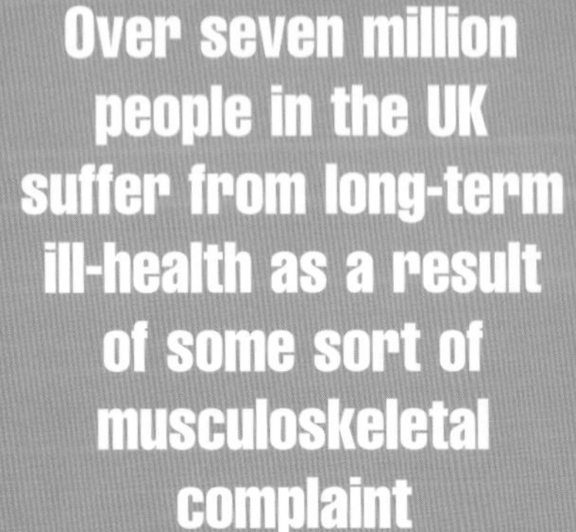

Over seven million people in the UK suffer from long-term ill-health as a result of some sort of musculoskeletal complaint

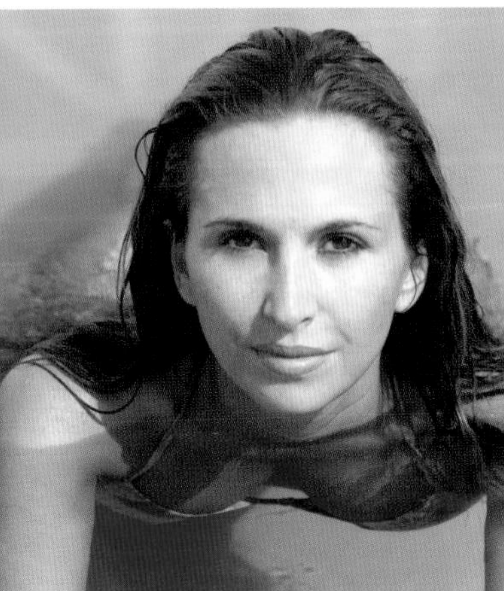

A high vitamin C intake can cut the progression of arthritis

Eating well

Some foods are packed with nutrients that help build and maintain bone and muscle health; in Part 3 you'll discover what they are and how you can adjust your daily diet and make the changes and substitutions to include as many as possible. A clear weight/height chart will also show you whether – for the sake of your bones, muscles and joints – you should be thinking of losing a few pounds. If weight is a problem, you might want to investigate the weight-loss plan – and find out which foods you should enjoy and which to avoid.

A gentle 15-week programme of tai chi has been proven to significantly reduce the risk of falls in people over the age of 70

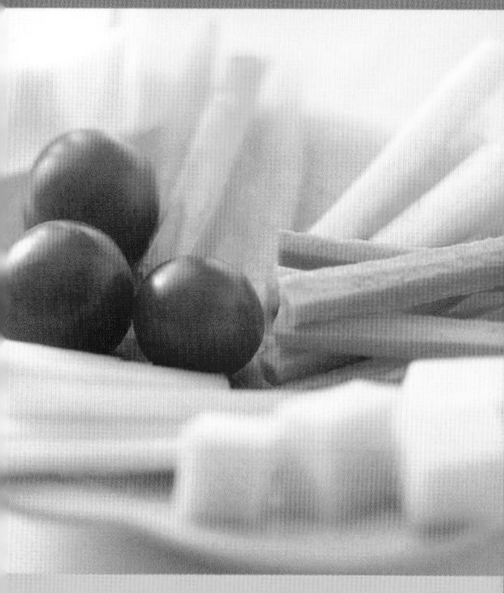

Lifelong care

Bone and joint problems may increase dramatically with age but they are by no means confined to older people.

- Part 4 shows how you can encourage good habits in your children – by helping them to appreciate good food, to take regular exercise and become aware of posture problems – such as slouching or slumping in a chair.
- The new responsibilities and stresses of adulthood can also take their toll. Knowing what can go wrong, how to minimize the effects and keep your bones, muscles and joints strong and healthy can help to avert problems in later life.
- For older people, Part 5 contains plenty of advice on how to improve your health, assess the condition of your bones, muscles and joints and take positive steps to avoid or alleviate possible problems.

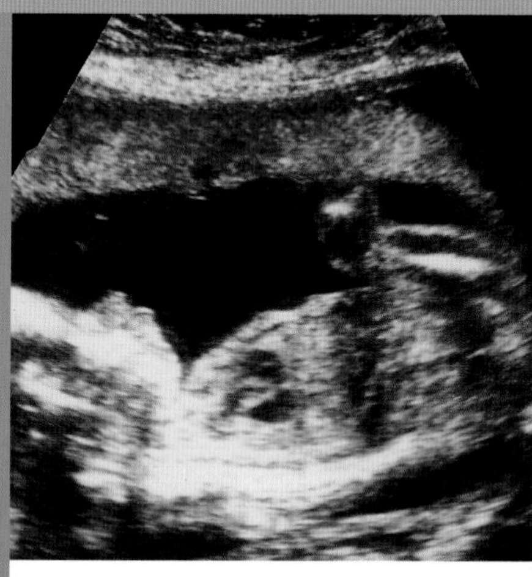

Tackling problems

Later chapters concentrate on particular areas of the body where problems often occur such as the back, knees and hips and the most common disorders, from arthritis to osteoporosis.

Whatever your age, there are steps you can take now to soothe aches and pains and to prevent or mitigate problems in the future.

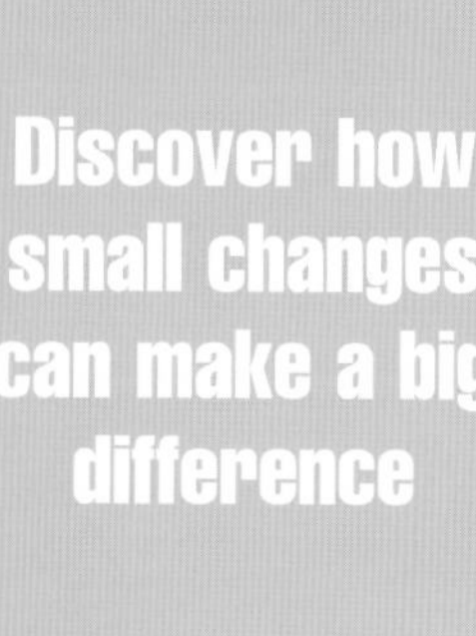

Discover how small changes can make a big difference

Find out which foods to avoid and which foods to enjoy with the weight-loss eating plan

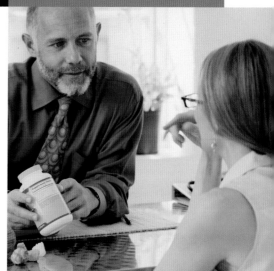

BONES, MUSCLES AND JOINTS FOR LIFE

You don't have to live with aches and pains. Whatever your age or activity level, there are things you can do that will help you – small changes that will make a big difference to your musculoskeletal health. Act now, and you could save yourself a lot of pain and discomfort.

If you lay down the right foundations during childhood and continue to strengthen and exercise your body in later years, you should find that your bones and muscles continue to support and protect you well into old age. Everyday factors can take their toll but the right diet and lifestyle will maximize your bone and muscle health and keep you strong, whatever your age.

This book is all about the simple but effective steps that you can take to maintain the health and vitality of your bones and muscles throughout life. It explains clearly why problems occur and outlines strategies for encouraging and safeguarding bone, joint and muscle health from childhood to old age.

Taking control of your musculoskeletal health means being aware of your body and understanding how it changes: we don't all age at the same rate or experience the same health problems in our daily lives – but during certain periods of your life there are some particular points that could be helpful to bear in mind.

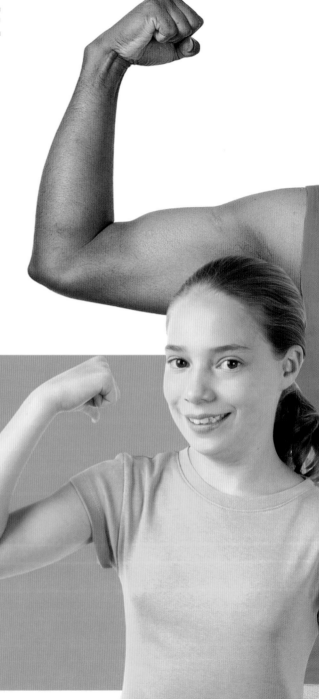

Early Years

■ Start young! Get your children into good eating habits now and they'll thank you for it in later life. Follow the practical advice in this book to help them reach their five-a-day fruit and vegetable intake.

■ Get moving – walk to school, go to the park, clean the car, turn off the TV – anything you can do to get your child moving will benefit their growing bones and muscles and pay big long-term dividends.

■ Make sure that your child wears heavy school bags across both shoulders. Young bodies are still developing and poor postural habits now could lead to muscle imbalances that exacerbate musculoskeletal problems in later life.

■ The bones of the foot are not fully set until around the age of 18, so poorly fitting shoes in childhood and adolescence can significantly increase your child's risk of foot problems in adult life.

■ Most bone mass is laid down before the age of 17, so a calcium-rich diet during childhood and adolescence will protect the skeleton throughout life. Research suggests that for every 5 per cent increase in bone mass during childhood, the risk of later fractures is cut by up to 40 per cent.

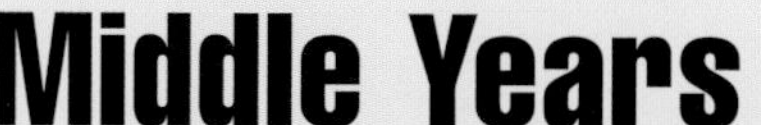

Middle Years

■ Are you eating properly and avoiding the fast food temptations that often come with a busy life? Unhealthy eating patterns can lead to a sluggish digestion and consequent weight gain. Sort your diet out now and you may relieve your joints of a great deal of stress in the future.

■ Around 1.2 million people in the UK suffer from work-related musculoskeletal problems. Avoid repetitive strain injury and protect your back by making sure that your office equipment is set up correctly and you change position regularly.

■ You can improve your bone mineral density by changing from a sedentary to a more active lifestyle in your middle years. Any type of load-bearing exercise will do – and your muscles and joints will benefit from the exercise too.

■ Stop smoking! If you haven't done so before, the best thing you can do for your musculoskeletal health (and for most other aspects of your health and welfare) is to give up now.

Later Years

■ Stay active. Independence and quality of life are directly linked to bone and muscle strength – yet only 10 per cent of people over the age of 65 get the recommended levels of exercise. Both bones and muscles will benefit from weight-bearing exercise at any age.

■ Check your vitamin D levels. If you don't get out and about as much you used to, you may need to take a supplement to compensate for any lack of sunlight.

■ Are you on medications? Drugs such as diuretics can interfere with your absorption of some vitamins and minerals so you may need to increase your intake of bone and muscle-building nutrients to compensate.

■ Work on your core stabilizing muscles – your abdomen, buttocks and lower back – to improve your balance. According to one study, just six months of regular tai chi could halve your risk of damaging falls.

■ Don't forget to stretch. Without regular stretching muscles soon lose their flexibility, making it easier to strain them when performing simple tasks and chores.

HOW HEALTHY ARE YOUR BONES, MUSCLES AND JOINTS?

It is easy to take the good health of your bones, muscles and joints for granted – your musculoskeletal system is very resilient and can put up with a great deal of wear, tear and abuse without complaint. Over time, however, the cumulative effects may start to take their toll. Even if your bones and muscles feel strong and healthy now, you may be storing up problems for the future.

So how can you assess the health of your bones, muscles and joints? It isn't always easy to predict problems before they happen but if you are aware of the factors that put your body at risk you can get a good idea of how much you need to be concerned. And knowing the risk factors now can help you to take steps to improve your musculoskeletal health for the future.

Gender and hormones

Not all of the factors that determine the health of your bones, muscles and joints are completely within your control – in particular, levels of hormones such as oestrogen and testosterone play a significant role in your susceptibility to musculoskeletal problems:

- Lower levels of oestrogen following the menopause mean that women are more susceptible than men to osteoporosis.
- Women are also more vulnerable to many rheumatic joint conditions including rheumatoid arthritis, systemic lupus, fibromylagia or polymyalgia rheumatica.
- Men are more likely to develop gout or ankylosing spondylitis.

DIET AND LIFESTYLE

BONES

- Does your diet contain enough calcium (found in dairy products, green leafy vegetables, baked beans and bony fish)? >>110
- Do you get plenty of sunlight to make vitamin D for healthy bones? Insufficient vitamin D can also affect **muscle** function >>103
- Do you have any history of eating disorders such as anorexia nervosa? >>267
- Do you smoke, or drink an excessive amount of alcohol? This can also affect your **muscles**. >>269
- Do you eat lots of salty foods or drink a lot of soft drinks? >>109

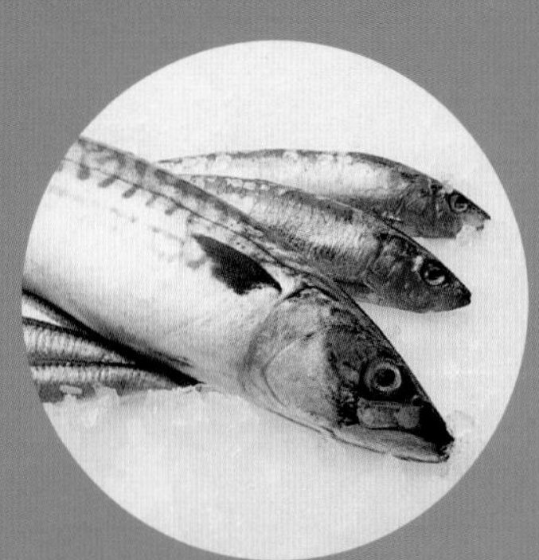

MUSCLES

- Do you eat a balanced diet rich in vitamins and minerals? A healthy diet will also benefit your **bones** and **joints**. >>100
- Do you have a poor posture or spend a lot of time working at a computer, driving, lifting objects or watching television? Poor posture can also affect your **joints**. >>176
- Do you perform tasks involving frequent, repetitive movements? >>132
- Do you get enough sleep?
- Do you drink plenty of water? >>63

JOINTS

- Do you get a good intake of vitamin C and other antioxidants? This can also benefit your **bones** and **muscles** >>100
- Do you eat lots of oily fish or other types of omega-3 containing foods? >>102
- Are you overweight? >>114

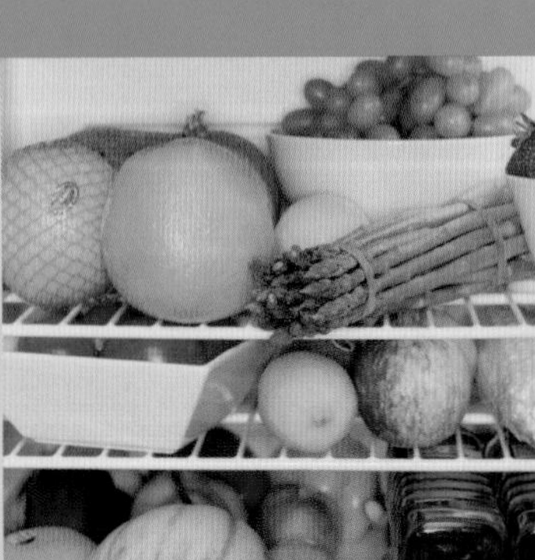

EXERCISE

■ Do you lead a particularly sedentary lifestyle? This can also affect your **muscles** and **joints.** >>271
■ Do you take regular, load-bearing exercise such as running, skipping or weight training to build up bone mass? >>271

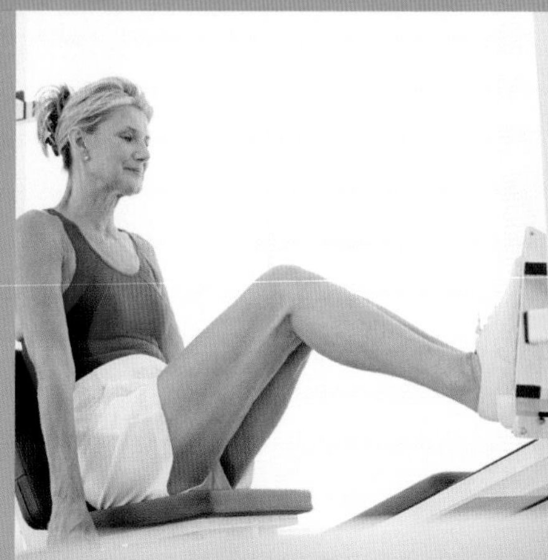

■ Do you warm up properly before exercise to prevent muscle and ligament sprains and strains? >>64
■ Do you stretch your muscles after exercise to prevent tight, inflexible muscles? >>66
■ Do you take regular load-bearing exercise such as weight training to build up muscle mass? >>76
■ Do you perform exercises such as yoga or tai chi that keep your muscles toned and flexible? This can also benefit your **joints** >>92

■ Do you warm up properly before exercise and stretch after exercise to keep your joints flexible? >>66
■ Do you regularly play high-intensity sports or sports that repeatedly place stress on your joints? >>134
■ Do you wear well-fitting, supportive, cushioning trainers? Proper footwear can also help you to avoid **muscle** strains >>48

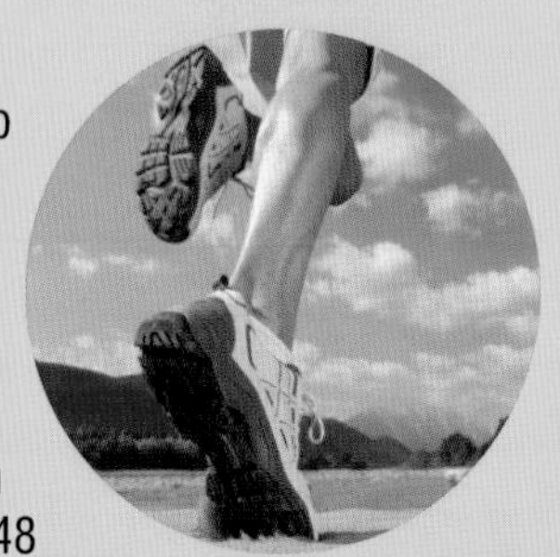

MEDICAL HISTORY

■ Do you have a family history of bone problems such as osteoporosis or have you suffered frequent or unexplained fractures? >>266
■ Do you have a history of bowel disorders such as coeliac disease or of diseases such as diabetes mellitus, kidney or liver disease, or thyroid, endocrine or glandular diseases? >>266
■ Have you ever needed a prolonged period of bed rest? >>190
■ If you are a woman, did you go through the menopause or have a hysterectomy at the age of 45 or younger? >>148
■ If you are a woman, have your periods ever stopped for a period of 12 months or longer, other than during pregnancy? >>148
■ Are you a man who suffers from symptoms of low testosterone such as impotence or loss of libido? >>148

■ Have you recently needed a prolonged period of bed rest or made use of a cast or splint to immobilize a limb? >>190
■ Have you ever needed to take a medication that can cause bone or muscle wasting (such as a corticosteroid, blood thinning drug or seizure drug) for an extended period of time? >>205

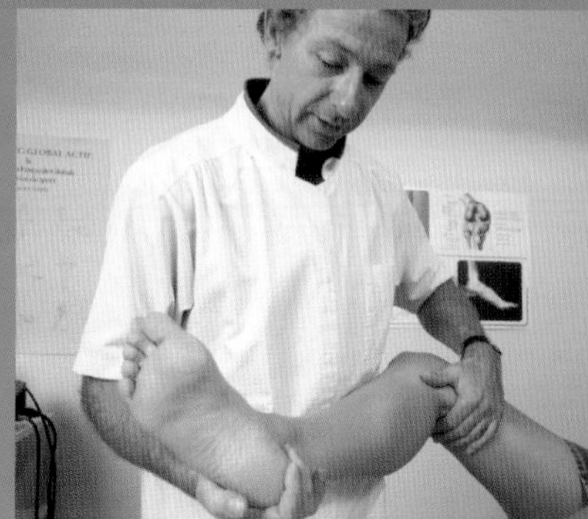

■ Do you have a personal history of joint problems or related rheumatic diseases? >>251
■ Have your joints previously been damaged as a result of injuries, fractures, operations or infections? >>231
■ Do you have any physical abnormality of your joints such as bow legs or knock knees? >>201
■ Do you over-pronate (roll your feet excessively)? >>50

THINGS YOU CAN DO RIGHT NOW TO IMPROVE YOUR ...

You may be surprised at how little effort it takes to make a significant difference to your bone, muscle and joint health. Small changes in your daily routine can add up to big results and, if you already experience problems, can alleviate symptoms and make life easier.

Bones: Beat bone loss

1 Increase your calcium intake A calcium-rich diet (including dairy foods) during childhood and adolescence will protect your bones for life. In later years, a good intake will reduce the effects of bone loss >>102.

2 Try strength-training exercises This type of exercise builds strong bones as well as muscles and can be easily done at home using light weights or your own bodyweight >>76–79.

3 Give up smoking Osteoporosis research has found that smoking leads to greater bone loss and increases the risk of fracture >>269.

4 Avoid fizzy drinks Colas in particular contain phosphoric acid that can take calcium out of the body. It has been estimated that just two cans per day can have an effect.

5 Take a walk in the park Walking is a great low-impact exercise. Aim for a moderate-brisk pace for 30 minutes at least 5 times a week – you'll soon see results >>90–91.

6 Build up your vitamin D levels Vital for calcium absorption, your body can get enough vitamin D to last a year simply by enjoying 15–20 minutes of sunlight a day on your face and arms in the summer months >>102.

7 Watch your alcohol intake Drinking alcohol to excess not only damages the cells that make new bone but also interferes with the production and absorption of vitamin D >>108.

8 Visit a chiropractor Persistent shoulder stiffness or back problems may be due to misaligned vertebrae. A chiropractor may be able to help to realign your spine >>189.

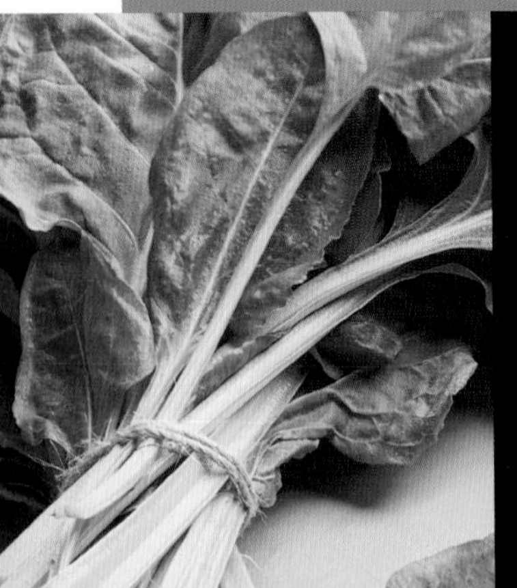

Dark-green leafy vegetables are a good source of magnesium and calcium, both key nutrients for bone and muscle health.

Muscles: Keep your muscles and ligaments in good shape

1 Keep your muscles balanced Every movement you make has an opposite movement: push and pull, raise and lower, twist left and twist right. Exercising opposing muscles equally is the key to good posture, strong physique and lasting mobility >>38–39.

2 Remember RICE This useful mnemonic stands for rest, ice, compression and elevation – these four steps provide essential and effective first-aid treatment for minor soft tissue injuries such as ligament sprains, bruises and impact injuries and muscle tears >>52.

3 Avoid repetitive movements Even very minor stresses and strains on your muscles can cause problems if performed repeatedly. If you need to perform repetitive actions such as moving a computer mouse, try to vary your movements and take plenty of breaks.

4 Take up Pilates Designed to stretch, tone and streamline the core muscles that you use to maintain your posture and stability, Pilates will also help to improve your strength and flexibility and reduce the effects of stress and fatigue on your body >>94–5.

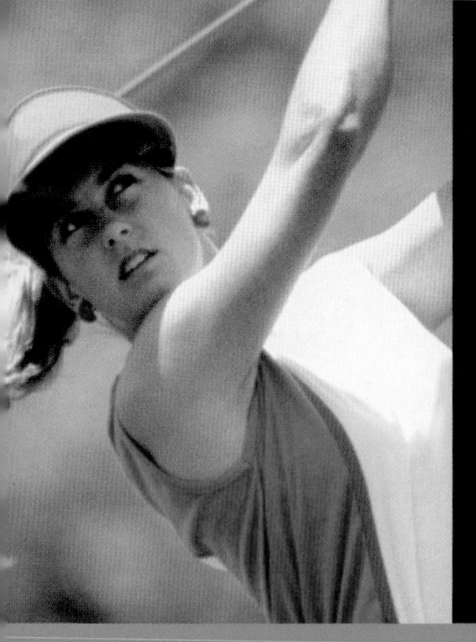

Exercise of any type will build muscle strength, but be sure to warm up and cool down well for long-lasting benefit.

5 Warm up and cool down Warm muscles are less vulnerable to injuries such as strains. It is also important to cool down and stretch following exercise – stretching helps to prevent sore, tight muscles.

6 Have a long soak Warm water will help to ease your aches and pains, and enable your muscles to relax and repair themselves.

7 Watch how you lift Try to bend your knees and not your back. Bending too far too fast, rising awkwardly or twisting badly can all put tremendous strain on your muscles >>179.

8 Keep moving Fidgeting and adjusting your position while at work or play will help your muscles to avoid cramping, can relieve the symptoms of RSI and burns calories >>151.

9 Relax Stress and fatigue can lead to muscle tension and cramps and heighten your chance of tears and sprains. Take some time out to slow down and unwind – a gentle massage will relax muscles, remove painful trigger points and stimulate circulation to speed up healing of minor strains and sprains >>151.

Joints: Keep joint problems at bay

1 Take up tai chi The gentle, controlled movements of tai chi can lessen joint stiffness, improve flexibility and body posture and – by improving balance and coordination – will also reduce the risk of falls and fractures >>96–7.

2 Wear the right shoes Supportive, well-cushioned shoes protect the joints of your ankles hips and knees from impact. Unstable or high-heeled shoes can affect your posture and gait and throw your body out of alignment >>48–9.

3 Set up office equipment correctly A badly positioned computer or an awkward sitting posture while typing can put pressure on the joints in your spine and lead to neck or back ache. Take regular breaks and try to avoid repetitive movements >>132–3.

4 Lose some weight Excess weight puts more stress on your knee and hip joints, the most common candidates for replacement: being just 1kg (2.2lb) overweight can increase your chance of developing osteoarthritis by as much as 10–15 per cent >>200–201.

5 Maintain your muscles Strong muscles help to stop joints being pulled out of position and prevent injuries. But it is not just the size of your muscles that is important: flexible, balanced muscles keep joints supple as well as strong.

6 Eat more fish The essential fatty acid omega-3, most commonly found in oily fish, helps to lubricate joints, decrease inflammation and may even build muscle >>102–3.

7 Review your hobbies It's always good to stay active but some sports and hobbies may lead to joint problems. Try to vary your activities or use protective equipment where appropriate: cycling puts less pressure on your joints than running, for example, and knee pads can protect your knees while gardening >>200–201.

8 Visit the podiatrist A qualified podiatrist can check the joint alignment in your feet, knees and hips, as well as your posture >>53.

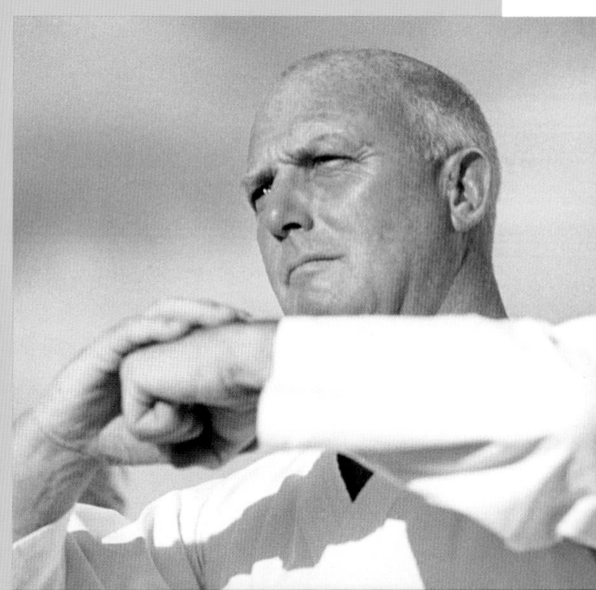

Apart from its musculoskeletal benefits, tai chi (see above) is also calming – perfect exercise for stress reduction.

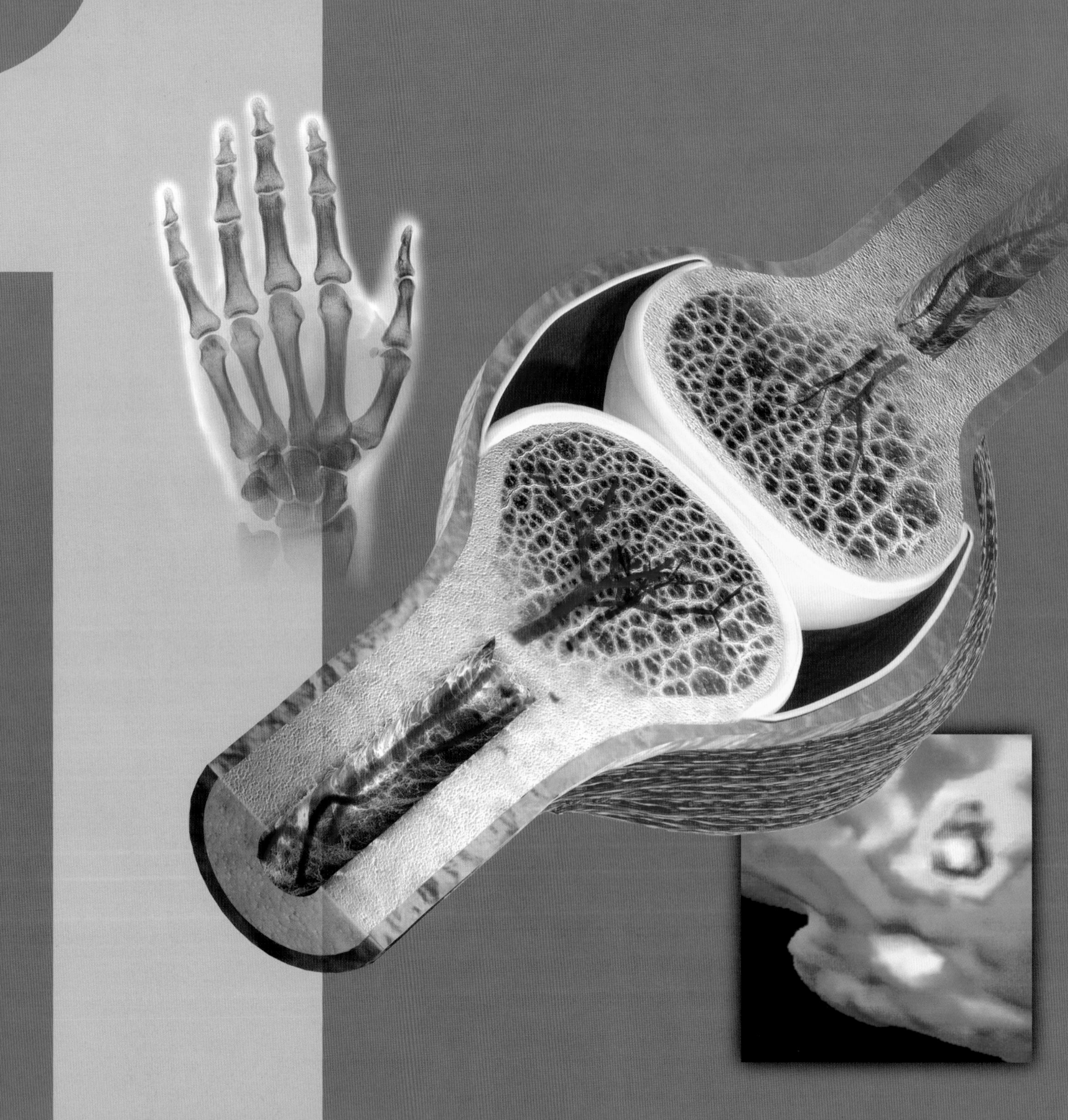

THE MECHANICS OF MOVEMENT

The musculoskeletal system is a miracle of bioengineering. It gives support and strength to your body, protects your vital organs and provides an extraordinary range of movement. Find out how your bones, muscles and joints work, how they support each other and work together so effortlessly, and what part good balance and posture play in their correct function.

1 THE MECHANICS OF MOVEMENT
Neck and skull

Your skull and neck contain and protect the most vital and sensitive organs of your body – the brain and the spinal cord. But your head is much more than simply a protective case for your brain – the bones and muscles of your face, neck and skull help you to move, turn and nod; chew and swallow; look, listen, breathe and talk; and communicate using a huge variety of subtle facial expressions.

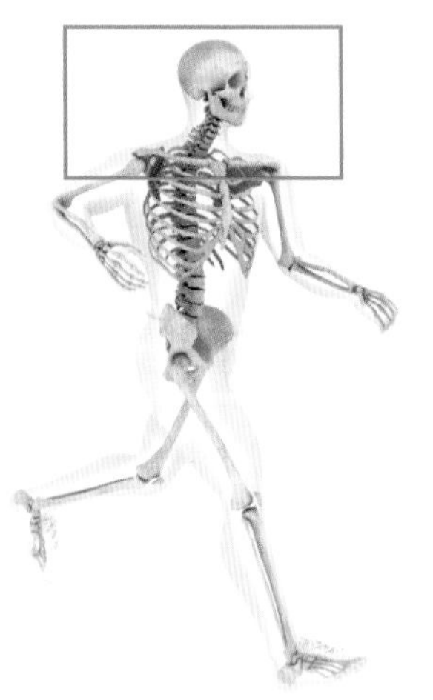

The bones of your skull protect the delicate tissues of your brain from external forces and form the structure and framework of your face.

The skull bones are divided into two main groups: the eight bones forming the cranial vault protect and support your brain while 14 facial bones make up the framework of your face and house your eyes, ears and mouth. Three tiny bones called ossicles conduct sound waves between your ear drum and inner ear – one of these, the malleus, is just 8mm (⅓in) long.

Air-filled cavities called sinuses and a honeycomb of air-filled pockets in the mastoid process (the bony projection behind the ear) lighten the weight of the skull. Small holes in the cranium's tough shell allow blood vessels and nerves to pass through to structures on the surface of the skull. The spinal cord passes out of the head through a hole at the base of the skull and down the vertebrae in the neck. At the front of the neck a group of bones and cartilage rings support the trachea and larynx, the tubes that form your throat.

THE NASAL CAVITY

The nasal cavity is divided by a bone and cartilage septum. Bony protrusions known as conchae interrupt the flow of incoming air so that it bounces around the cavity, depositing dust and germs in the mucus lining. Draining into the cavity are several air-filled chambers (sinuses) lined with mucus-secreting membranes.

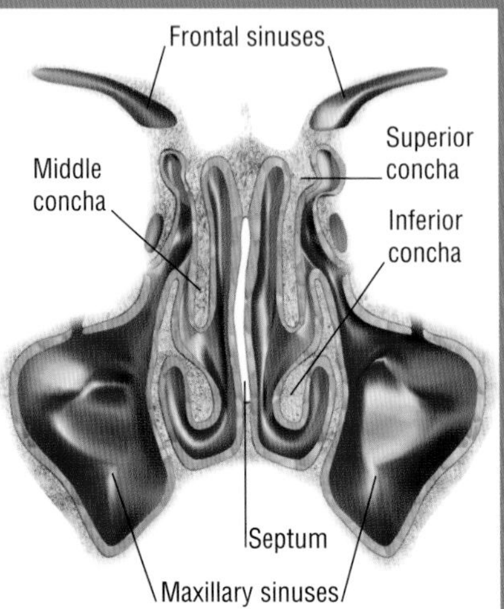

SKULL BONES

- **The cranium** is formed of eight bones that enclose and protect the brain. These bones are held together by bands of fibrous tissue called sutures.
- **The facial bones** make up the structures of the face: your jaw bones, your cheeks and the bones around the eyes and nose.

NECK BONES

Your neck contains seven cervical vertebrae, including two specialized vertebrae at the very top of your spine.

- **The atlas** supports the weight of the head and is named after the mythological giant Atlas who carried the world on his shoulders. This vertebra allows you to nod your head
- **The axis** is so named because it forms a pivot joint around which your skull can rotate from side to side.

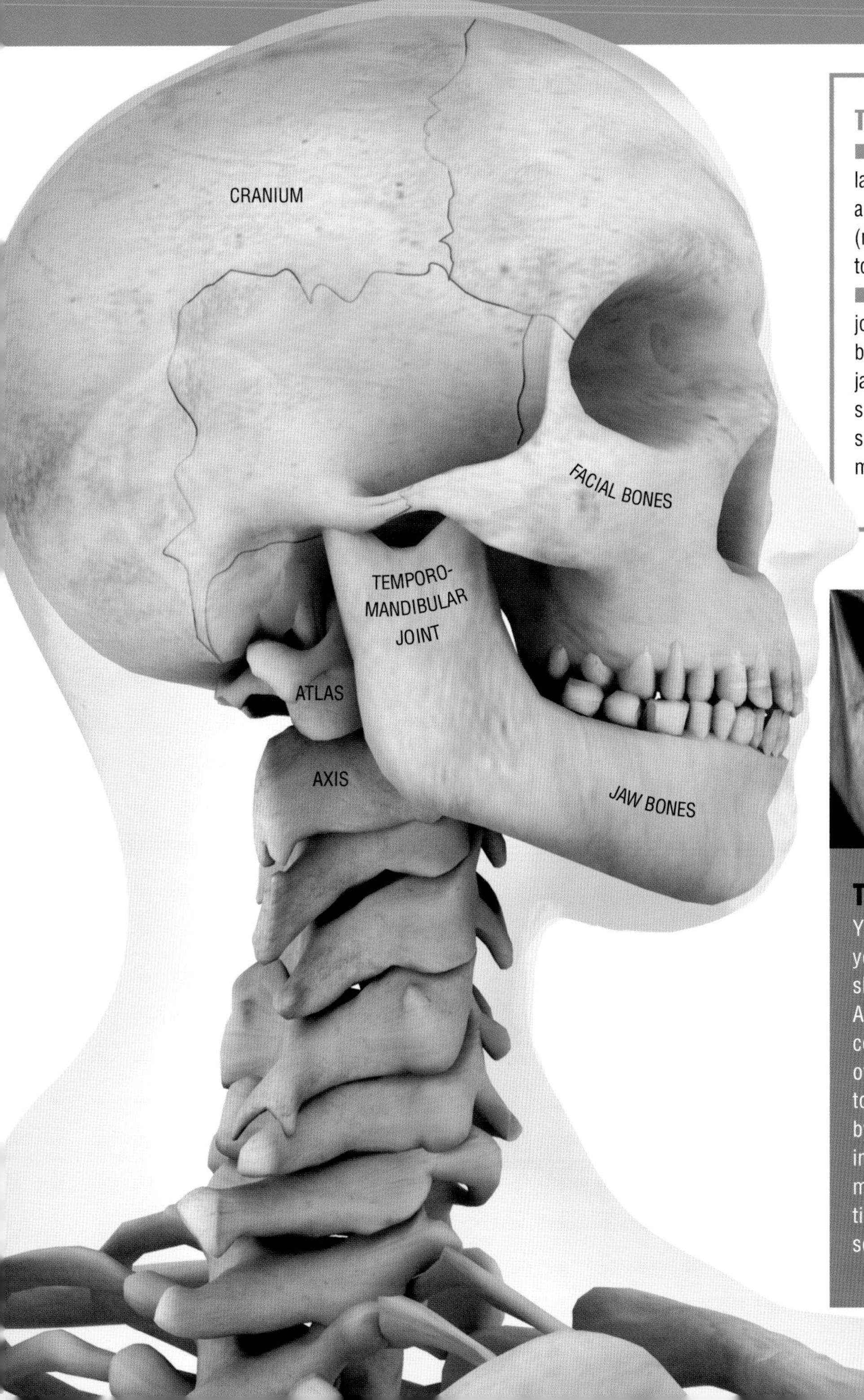

CRANIUM

FACIAL BONES

TEMPORO-MANDIBULAR JOINT

ATLAS

AXIS

JAW BONES

THE JAW

■ **The jaw bones** consist of a large lower jaw bone (mandible) and two upper jaw bones (maxillae). The way your jaws fit together is called occlusion.

■ **The temporomandibular** joints connect the lower jaw bone to the skull and let your jaw open, close and move sideways when chewing and speaking. They are the only moveable joints in your skull.

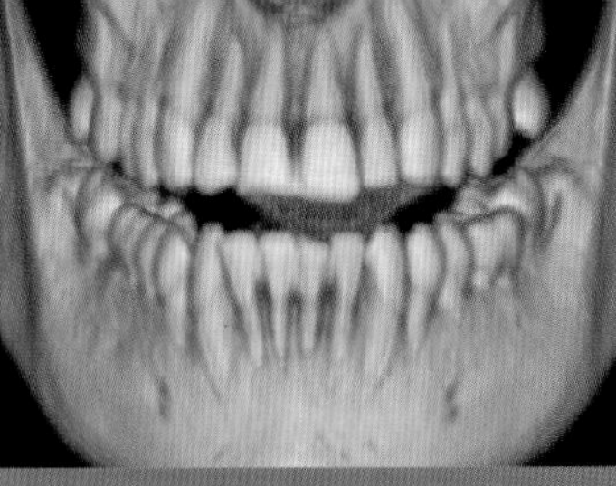

TEETH AND GUMS

Your teeth are fixed in place in your jawbone with fibrous sheets of connective tissue. Above the gum each tooth is covered in a hard outer shell of enamel; below the gum the tooth's outer layer is formed by bone-like cementum. The inside of the tooth contains a more sensitive bone-like tissue called dentine and the soft central pulp cavity.

Head movements

The muscles of the head and neck can be divided into groups of superficial and deeper muscles: your tongue and the muscles that control your jaw allow you to chew and talk; the pharyngeal muscles help you to swallow; your extra-occular muscles let you look almost 180 degrees around you without moving your head. Large muscles in the neck play an essential role in moving and stabilizing your head and a complex and intricate range of muscles control facial expression – many of these are woven directly into the skin of the face so that even a tiny contraction can move the skin to alter your expression.

Some of the smallest muscles in the body are found in the head, including those in the ear and the larynx; these tiny muscles are critical for our sense of hearing and ability to speak. One group of miniature, involuntary muscles forms concentric circles around the pupil of each eye, enabling it to contract and dilate.

MUSCLES OF MASTICATION

Several muscles work the jaw in order to bite, chew and talk.

- **The temporalis and masseter** muscles are powerful muscles along the side of your skull and at the back of your cheek that work together to elevate and retract your jaw.
- **The buccinator** compresses the cheek and moves food from the space inside your cheeks back across your teeth.
- **The platysma** is a thin sheet of muscle positioned between your jaw and collarbone that enables you to open your jaw.

MUSCLES AROUND THE EYE

Each eye is surrounded by six tiny muscles (the extra-occular muscles) that enable it to swivel around in its bony socket by almost 180 degrees. Combined with the rotary muscles of the head this extends your range of vision to 360 degrees.

Eye movements to look in a particular direction are under voluntary control but your ability to focus on an object by changing lens shape and pupil size is involuntary and automatic and depends on tiny muscles inside the eyeball itself.

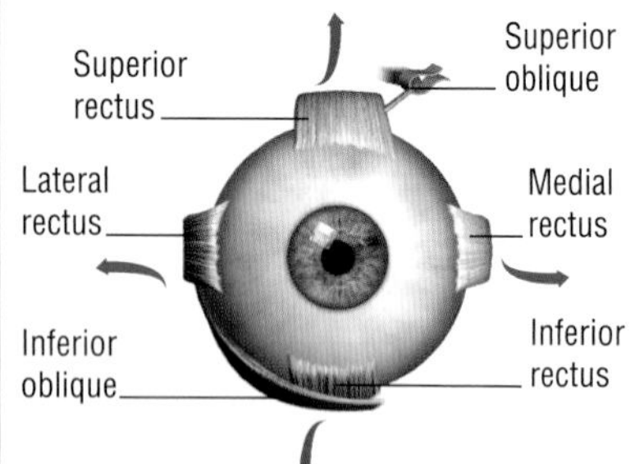

NECK MUSCLES

- **The sternocleidomastoid** muscle extends down the neck to the collarbone and is used to rotate the neck and flex the head. This large muscle is controlled by more than one nerve and specific regions can be made to contract almost independently.

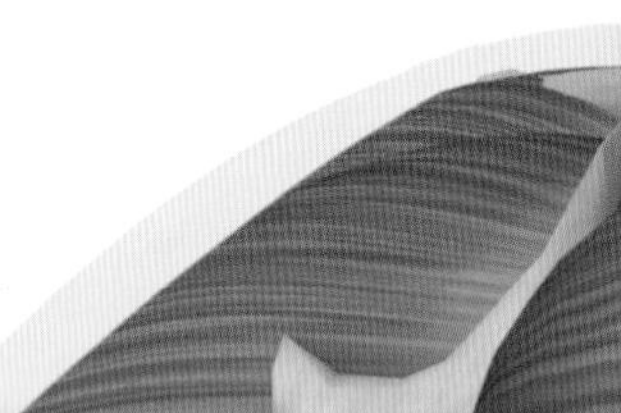

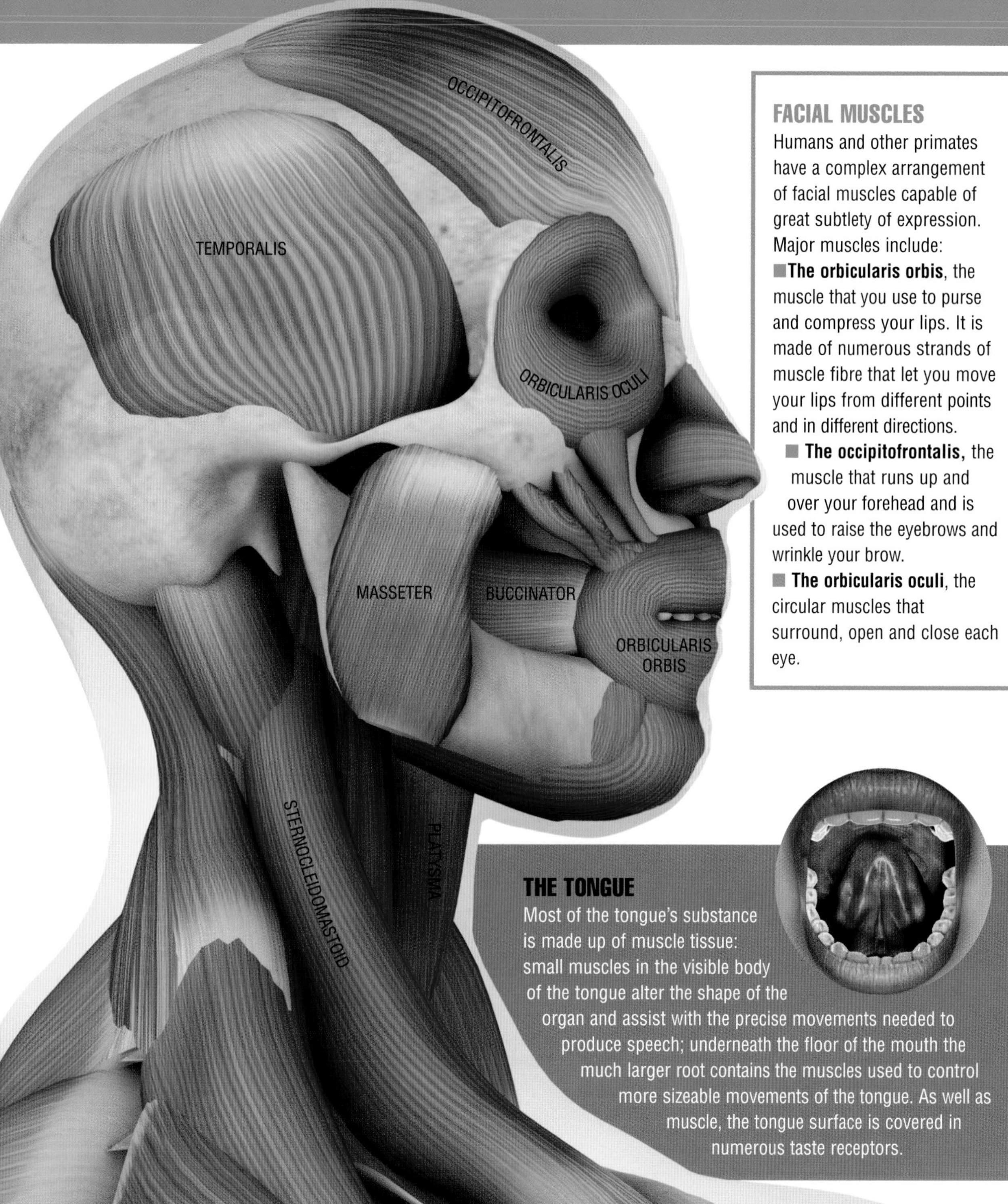

FACIAL MUSCLES

Humans and other primates have a complex arrangement of facial muscles capable of great subtlety of expression. Major muscles include:

- **The orbicularis orbis**, the muscle that you use to purse and compress your lips. It is made of numerous strands of muscle fibre that let you move your lips from different points and in different directions.
- **The occipitofrontalis,** the muscle that runs up and over your forehead and is used to raise the eyebrows and wrinkle your brow.
- **The orbicularis oculi**, the circular muscles that surround, open and close each eye.

THE TONGUE

Most of the tongue's substance is made up of muscle tissue: small muscles in the visible body of the tongue alter the shape of the organ and assist with the precise movements needed to produce speech; underneath the floor of the mouth the much larger root contains the muscles used to control more sizeable movements of the tongue. As well as muscle, the tongue surface is covered in numerous taste receptors.

DID YOU KNOW?

- **In many regions of the world people routinely carry heavy loads balanced on top of their heads. Although strong neck muscles and excellent poise are essential to perform this skill safely, it is surprisingly well suited to the back's natural mechanics. Whereas a heavy rucksack pushes the body's centre of gravity off balance, a load carried directly on top of the head transfers the weight down through the spine's natural curves.**
- **An even more impressive feat is performed by the mountain porters of Nepal who carry large packs from straps across their foreheads. Such techniques require immensely strong neck muscles: a recent Belgian study discovered that it is not uncommon for porters to carry up to 125 per cent of their bodyweight in this way, along steep paths and at high altitudes.**

SPINE AND BACK

Your back is the powerhouse for your entire body, supporting your trunk and involved in every movement you make with your head, arms or legs. The spinal vertebrae and the muscles surrounding them work together to maintain your back's natural curves, to absorb the force of gravity and the weight of your body, and to help your upper body to bend, twist and turn. You back and spine also protect your spinal cord as it travels down from your brain.

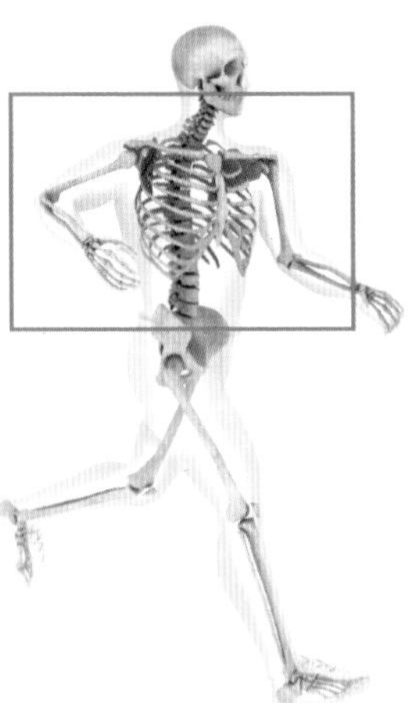

Your central support

Your spinal column is made up of 33 bones – 24 vertebrae in the back and neck and 9 fused vertebrae in the sacrum and the coccyx.

Stacked together, vertebrae form a spinal column that supports your body and encloses and protects the spinal cord. Openings between the vertebrae allow nerves to travel from the spinal cord out to the rest of the body.

Each vertebra is separated from the one below by a pad of cartilage, the intervertebral disc, that acts as a shock absorber and compresses slightly under pressure to produce movement between vertebrae. This gives the column its great flexibility, letting you bend forwards, backwards and sideways, and twist from side to side.

Each portion of the spine is adapted to its function and a healthy spine has four gentle curves along its length: the cervical and lumbar spine in the neck and lower back curve forwards; the thoracic and sacral portions in the upper back and pelvis curve back.

'During very strenuous exercise, the intervertebral discs in your spine can be subjected to forces of several hundred kilos per square metre'

VERTEBRAE

Although the individual vertebrae which make up the spinal column vary slightly in size and shape according to their position, most have certain features in common. Each vertebra has a thick, spherical body; from the back of this body a hollow arch (the neural arch) protrudes. Together these hollows make up the spinal canal through which the spinal cord passes. Bony knobs called processes extend out from the neural arch to form joints with the vertebrae above and below and provide attachment points for your ribs and muscles.

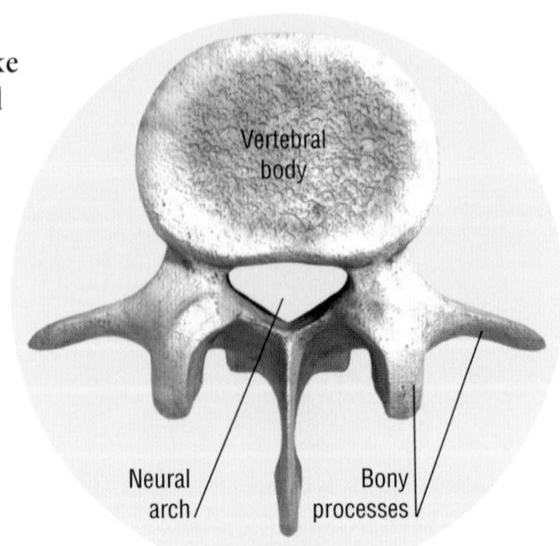

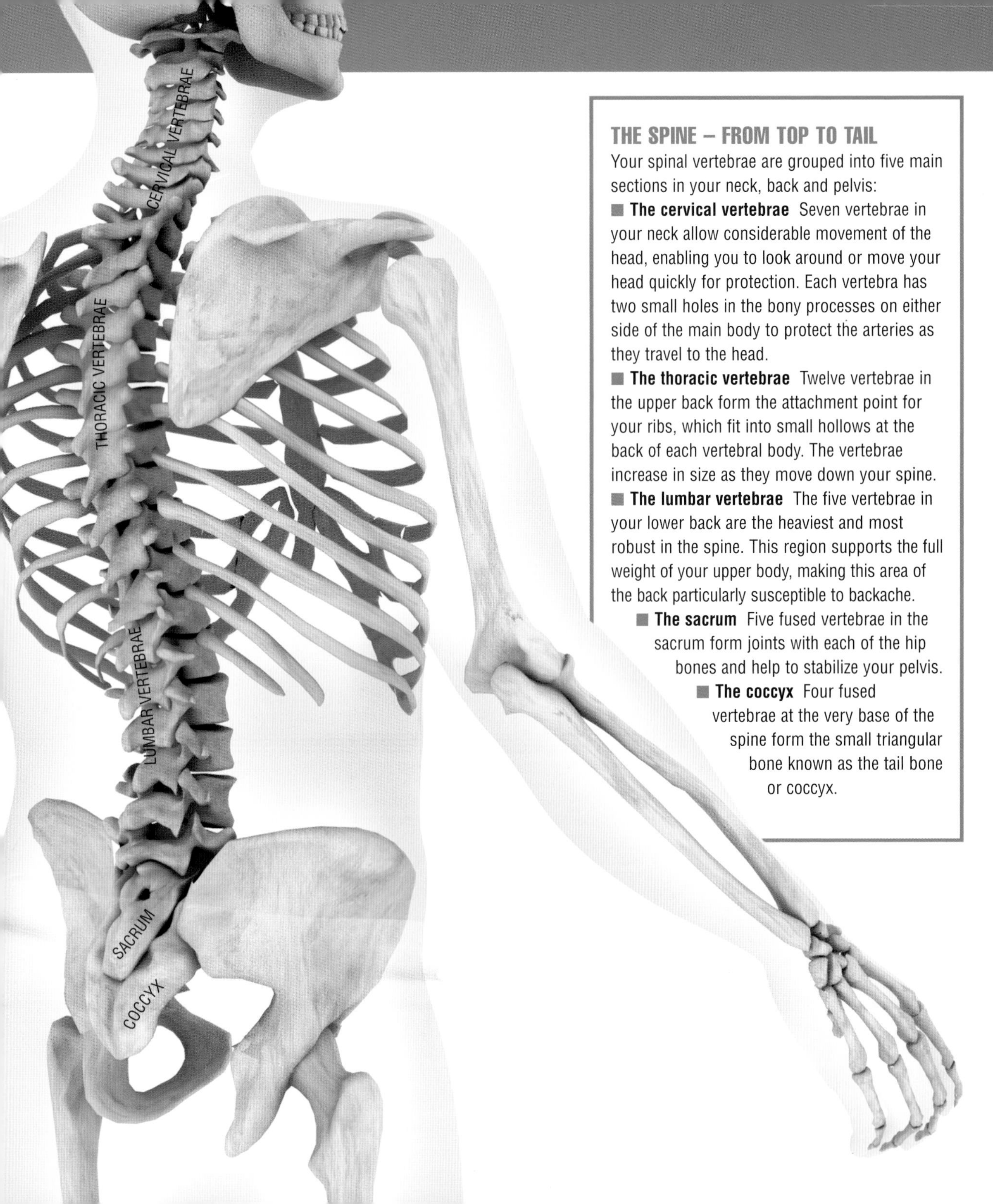

THE SPINE – FROM TOP TO TAIL

Your spinal vertebrae are grouped into five main sections in your neck, back and pelvis:

- **The cervical vertebrae** Seven vertebrae in your neck allow considerable movement of the head, enabling you to look around or move your head quickly for protection. Each vertebra has two small holes in the bony processes on either side of the main body to protect the arteries as they travel to the head.
- **The thoracic vertebrae** Twelve vertebrae in the upper back form the attachment point for your ribs, which fit into small hollows at the back of each vertebral body. The vertebrae increase in size as they move down your spine.
- **The lumbar vertebrae** The five vertebrae in your lower back are the heaviest and most robust in the spine. This region supports the full weight of your upper body, making this area of the back particularly susceptible to backache.
- **The sacrum** Five fused vertebrae in the sacrum form joints with each of the hip bones and help to stabilize your pelvis.
- **The coccyx** Four fused vertebrae at the very base of the spine form the small triangular bone known as the tail bone or coccyx.

Core strength and stability

The most important function of the spinal muscles and ligaments is to keep your body upright, so there are many more extensor (straightening) muscles than there are flexor (bending) muscles. The large abdominal muscles around your stomach do most of the work when you bend forward.

There are three main layers of back muscles, each with a different function. The topmost layer (the trapezius, rhomboid and latissimus dorsi muscles) moves your arm and shoulder girdle and allows sideways movements of the neck. The middle layer comprising the spinal extensor muscles (the erector spinae), are linked to each vertebra all the way up the spine and form the longest and strongest muscle grouping of your body. When the muscles on both sides of the erector spinae contract together your spine straightens; if only one side contracts you will bend towards that side.

The innermost layer (the intervertebral muscles) stabilize and interconnect the vertebrae. To provide further support the vertebrae are bound together by bands of tough connective tissue called ligaments.

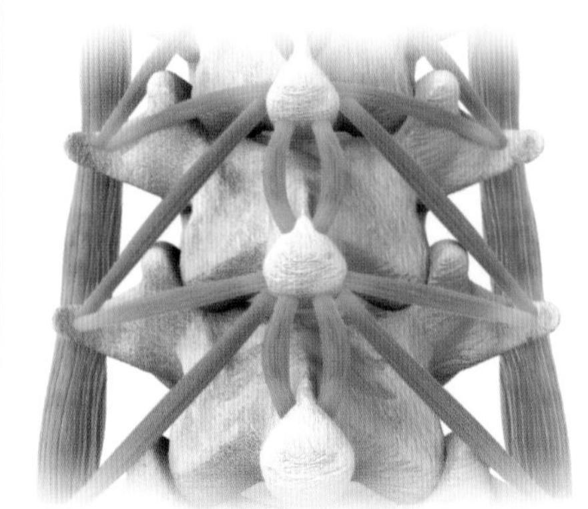

INTERVERTEBRAL MUSCLES
The deepest layer of the spinal muscles are the short muscles that connect individual vertebrae and make delicate adjustments to back position. If injured they can lead to a cycle of pain, muscle spasm and further pain and may put pressure on adjacent spinal nerves.

MUSCLES THAT MOVE THE ARM

- **Latissimus dorsi** The largest muscle in the back, the large, flat latissimus dorsi pulls your arm towards your body and helps to stabilize your back when standing or walking.
- **Infraspinatus** This muscle runs between your upper arm and shoulder blade, beneath the trapezius, and is used to rotate your arm at the shoulder. Together with muscles at the top and front of your shoulder it forms the rotator cuff, a group of muscles that help to keep the joint secure and is a common site for sports injuries.

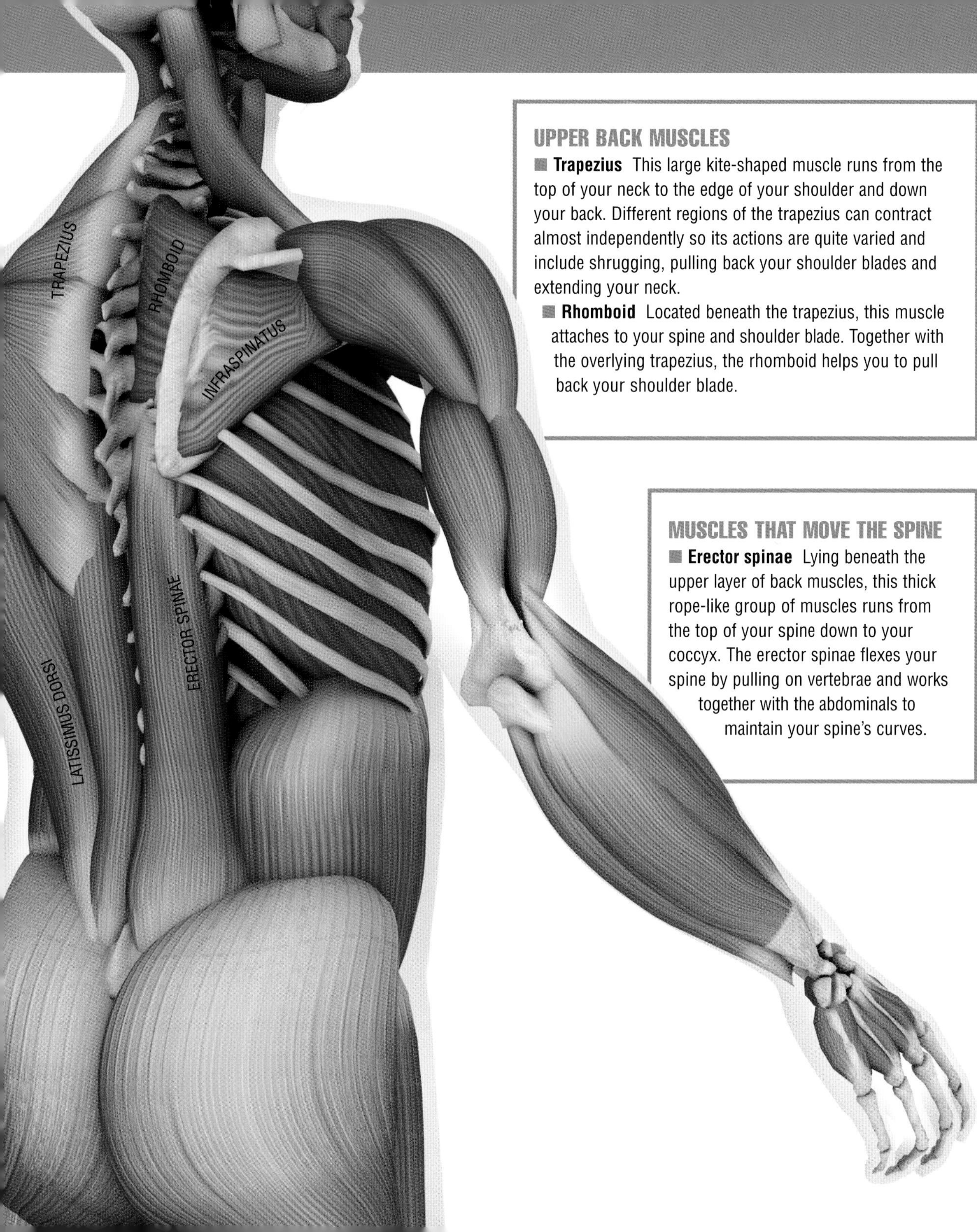

UPPER BACK MUSCLES

■ **Trapezius** This large kite-shaped muscle runs from the top of your neck to the edge of your shoulder and down your back. Different regions of the trapezius can contract almost independently so its actions are quite varied and include shrugging, pulling back your shoulder blades and extending your neck.

■ **Rhomboid** Located beneath the trapezius, this muscle attaches to your spine and shoulder blade. Together with the overlying trapezius, the rhomboid helps you to pull back your shoulder blade.

MUSCLES THAT MOVE THE SPINE

■ **Erector spinae** Lying beneath the upper layer of back muscles, this thick rope-like group of muscles runs from the top of your spine down to your coccyx. The erector spinae flexes your spine by pulling on vertebrae and works together with the abdominals to maintain your spine's curves.

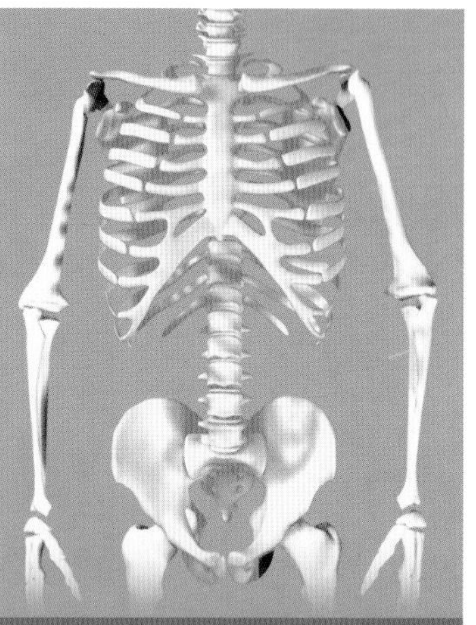

BONE MARROW

All the bones in your body have a central core filled with jelly-like bone marrow but only a few bones – primarily the spine vertebrae, ribs, sternum and pelvis (shown above in pink) – contain red marrow, the type of marrow that produces new blood cells.

Special cells in red marrow called haemopoietic stem cells have the ability to produce many different cell types and are essential to the repair and regeneration of your body's tissues. Marrow stem cells mainly make red and white blood cells – red marrow produces around 3 million new red blood cells every second.

CHEST, RIBS AND STOMACH

The bones of the upper spine, the rib cage and the long, flat sternum form a bony cage that protects and encloses your lungs and heart.

> ‘Around 5 per cent of people are born with one or more extra ribs’

As well as protecting your heart, lungs and other organs from external trauma, the thoracic cage provides an attachment point for the muscles of the thorax such as your pectorals, the large muscles that pull your arms in towards your chest.

Underneath your pectorals, most of the deeper muscles around your chest are involved in breathing, most notably the diaphragm – the major muscle involved in respiration – and the external and internal intercostals, the muscles that connect the ribs. When the diaphragm contracts, the volume of your chest cavity increases and air is drawn into the lungs; when it relaxes, air is forced out. This muscular sheet also forms a partition that separates your chest from your abdomen.

Between your ribs and your pelvis, along the front and side of your abdomen, lie rectus and oblique abdominals. Deep in your pelvis lies a group of specialized muscles called the pelvic floor. These muscles support the organs of the pelvic cavity, flex the joints of the sacrum and coccyx and control the flow of waste from the bladder and rectum.

THE THORACIC CAGE

- **The sternum** is the flat bone along the front of your chest that protects your heart and lungs from front-on impact.
- **The ribs** form the wall of the thoracic cage. The first seven pairs of ribs connect directly to your sternum by costal cartilage and are known as true ribs. The next four ribs connect to your sternum indirectly via cartilage linked to ribs above. The bottom two pairs of ribs have no connection to your sternum and are known as floating ribs.

RIBS

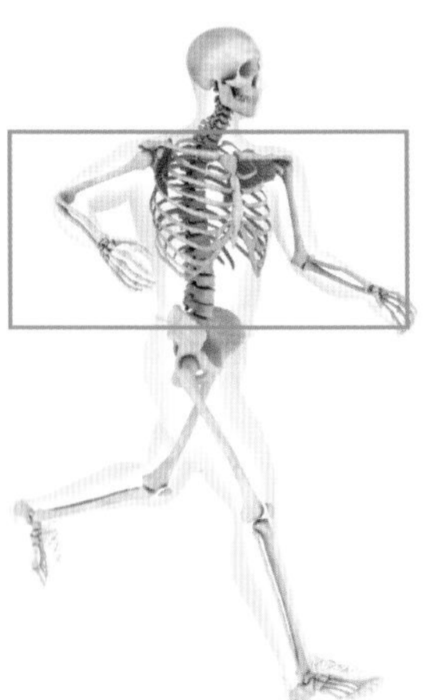

INSIDE THE CHEST

Your heart, the windpipe and the nerve bundles that carry signals to your lungs are enclosed within the thoracic cage in a space between your lungs known as the mediastinum. The diaphragm – a dome-shaped sheet of muscle attached to the sternum (breastbone), spine and ribs – separates the chest from the abdomen.

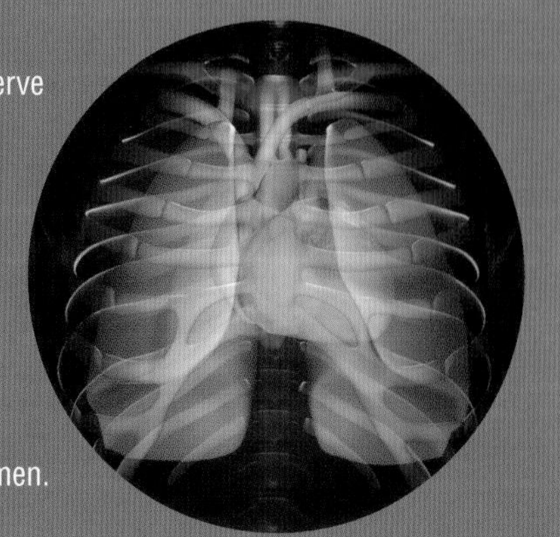

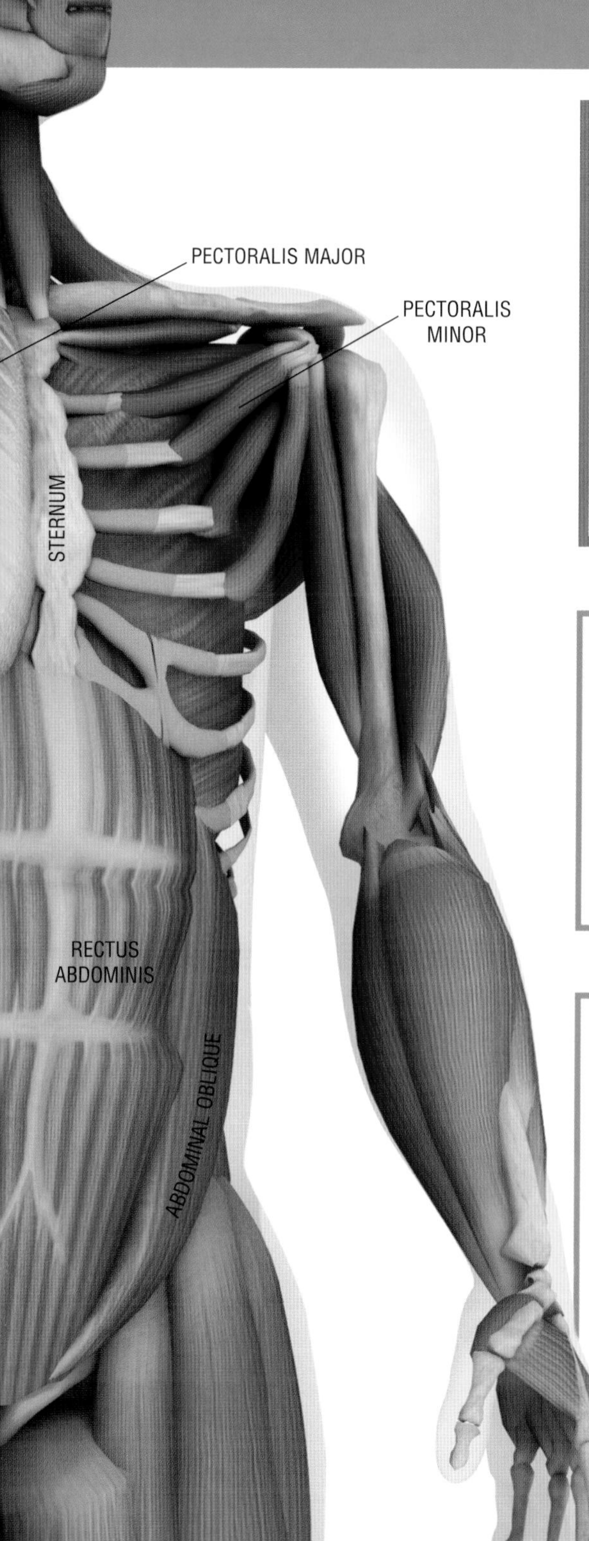

MUSCLES OF RESPIRATION

These muscles increase and decrease lung volume either directly or by moving the bones that surround the lungs. The main force comes from the dome-shaped diaphragm – when this muscle contracts it pulls flat, increasing the size of your chest cavity and lowering pressure inside your lungs. The intercostal muscles attach to and move the ribs and sternum. Various accessory muscles, including the abdominals, assist during heavy or forced breathing.

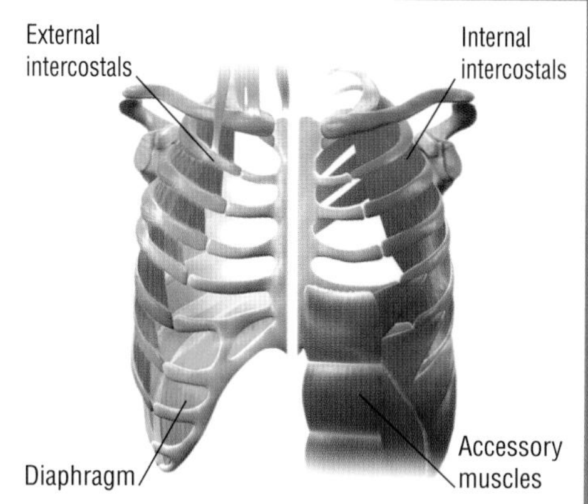

CHEST MUSCLES

- **The pectoralis major**, the large muscle that you can feel along the front of your chest, draws your arms in to your body, helping you to perform hugging and pushing actions.
- **The pectoralis minor** is a deeper, smaller muscle that connects the ribs to your shoulder blade and pulls your shoulder in towards your chest.

STOMACH MUSCLES

Your abdominals support your trunk and lower back, allow you to flex your torso, and regulate internal abdominal pressure.

- **The rectus abdominis**, the muscle along the front of your stomach, is separated into different sections by connective tissue, giving a well-developed stomach its characteristic 'six-pack'. Directly underneath this sits a muscle called the transverse abdominis which helps you to cough or sneeze.
- **The abdominal oblique** muscle runs along the side of your abdomen. This muscle enable you to twist and bend to the side and provides support for your lower back.

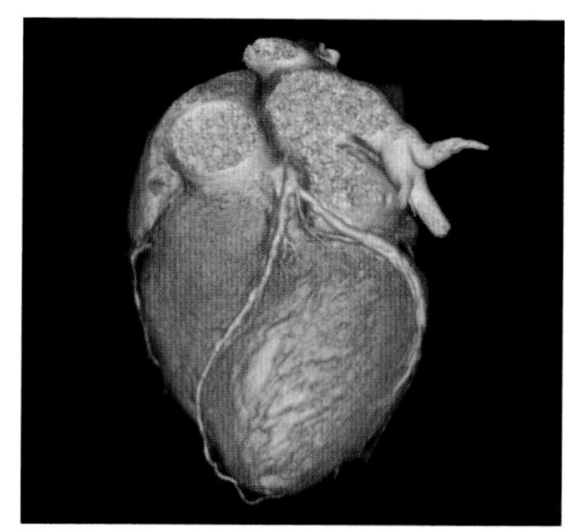

THE HEART

Without doubt the hardest working muscle in your body, your heart pumps around 7200 litres (1600 gallons) of oxygen-rich blood around your body each day, every day, without rest. The muscle fibres contract and relax, in concert, more than once every second – and in times of physical exertion their workload can rise by up to 300 per cent. Each heart beat is generated automatically, triggered by the heart's natural pacemaker, the sinoatrial node.

Shoulder blades to fingertips

Your arms are joined to your trunk at the shoulder by a set of bones called the pectoral girdle. Movements of this girdle (which consists of the collar bone and shoulder blade) stabilize the shoulder joint and form the basis of most arm movements.

COLLAR BONE

The main function of your shoulders is to provide a strong and flexible support for your dextrous, multi-purpose arms. Unlike the pelvic girdle, your shoulder blades are not locked into position by their bony connections but are free to move independently – the only direct link to the rest of the skeleton is via your collar bone. This gives your arms the versatility and wide range of motion needed to handle and manipulate objects effectively.

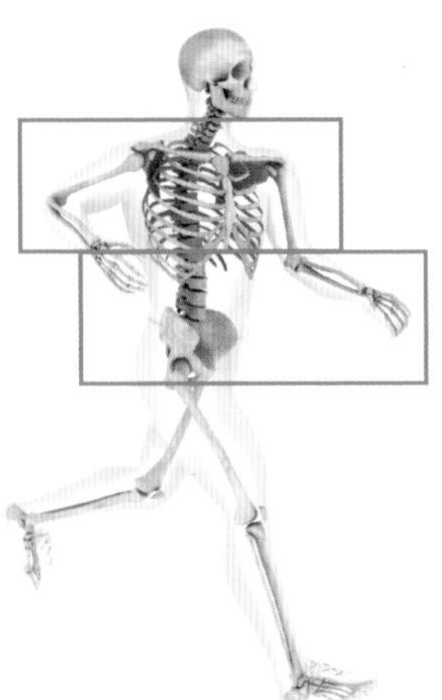

The shoulder joint itself – the point at which the head of the humerus meets the shoulder blade – is a relatively unstable joint. It permits the greatest range of movement of any joint in the body but is easily dislocated and injured.

The bones of the forearm, the radius and ulna, join to the humerus at the elbow and the bones of the hand at the wrist. The elbows and wrists are more stable than the shoulder because they have tighter ligaments and stronger capsules. The joints between individual finger bones are tighter still.

The skeletal structure of your hands is in many ways very similar to that of your feet. The most important difference is that the hands have opposable thumbs that allow you to grip and manipulate objects. The joint at the base of the thumb – the body's only saddle joint – enables it to move in several directions and provides far more mobility than the big toe.

THE ELBOW

This modified hinge joint consists of two linked joints: a small protrusion on the end of the humerus sits in a cavity at the head of the ulna and allows a back-and-forth movement; a second protrusion on the humerus sits in a cavity at the head of the radius and permits a slight rotation of the forearm. The elbow is very stable because the bony surfaces interlock tightly and are surrounded by a thick joint capsule and strong ligaments.

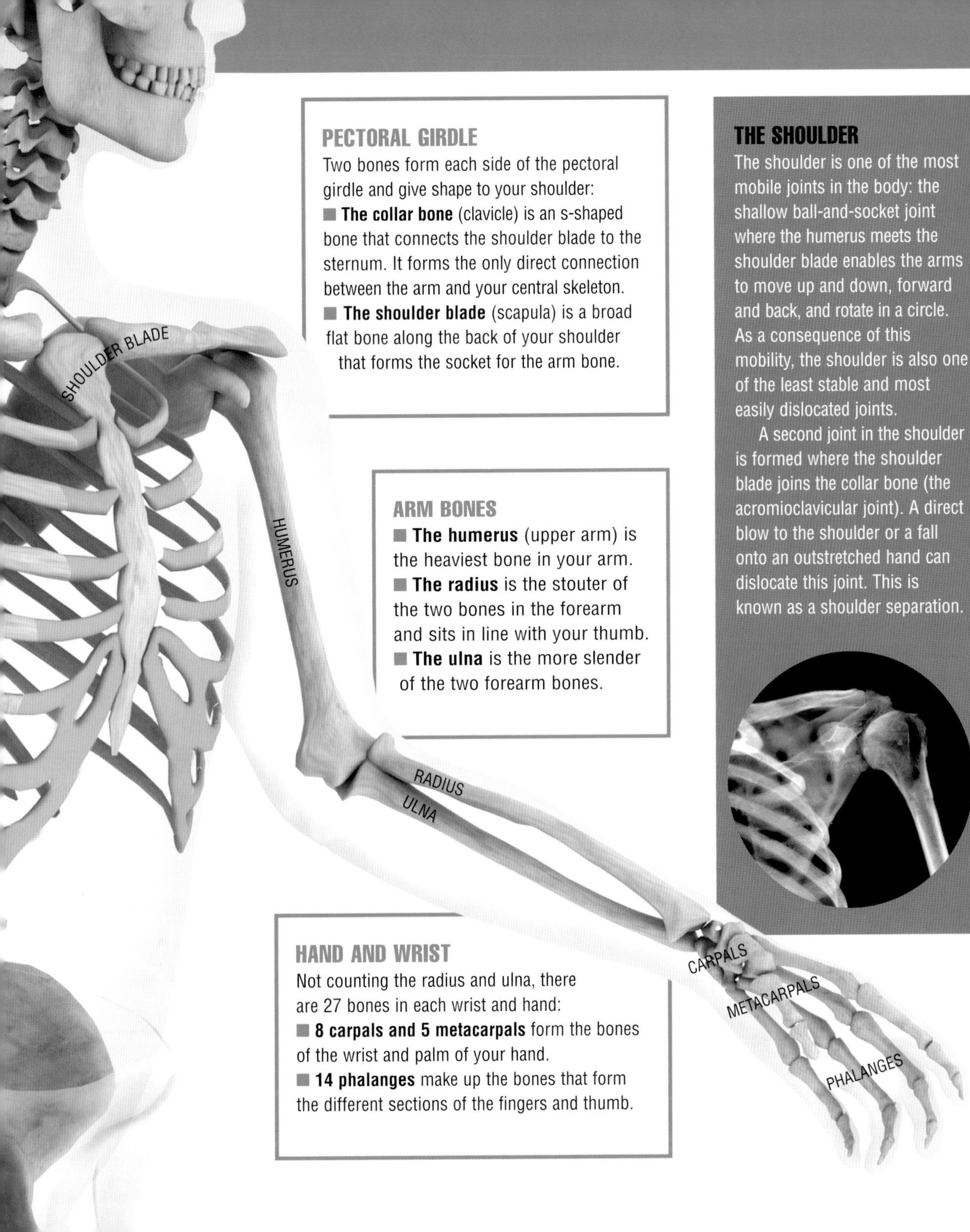

PECTORAL GIRDLE

Two bones form each side of the pectoral girdle and give shape to your shoulder:

- **The collar bone** (clavicle) is an s-shaped bone that connects the shoulder blade to the sternum. It forms the only direct connection between the arm and your central skeleton.
- **The shoulder blade** (scapula) is a broad flat bone along the back of your shoulder that forms the socket for the arm bone.

ARM BONES

- **The humerus** (upper arm) is the heaviest bone in your arm.
- **The radius** is the stouter of the two bones in the forearm and sits in line with your thumb.
- **The ulna** is the more slender of the two forearm bones.

HAND AND WRIST

Not counting the radius and ulna, there are 27 bones in each wrist and hand:

- **8 carpals and 5 metacarpals** form the bones of the wrist and palm of your hand.
- **14 phalanges** make up the bones that form the different sections of the fingers and thumb.

SHOULDER BLADE
HUMERUS
RADIUS
ULNA
CARPALS
METACARPALS
PHALANGES

THE SHOULDER

The shoulder is one of the most mobile joints in the body: the shallow ball-and-socket joint where the humerus meets the shoulder blade enables the arms to move up and down, forward and back, and rotate in a circle. As a consequence of this mobility, the shoulder is also one of the least stable and most easily dislocated joints.

A second joint in the shoulder is formed where the shoulder blade joins the collar bone (the acromioclavicular joint). A direct blow to the shoulder or a fall onto an outstretched hand can dislocate this joint. This is known as a shoulder separation.

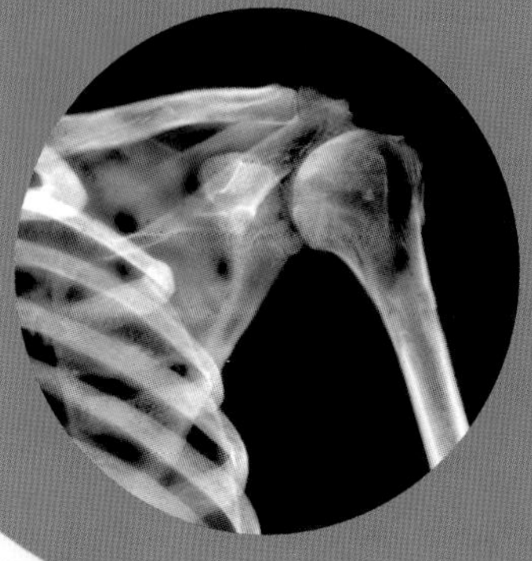

Reaching and gripping

Because the bones of your arm and shoulder blade are only indirectly connected to the main skeleton, the muscles and ligaments around the shoulder play an important structural role, bracing and stabilizing the joint. The muscle connections also act as shock absorbers.

Movements of your arm around the shoulder are controlled by muscles in your shoulder, chest and upper back – primarily the deltoids, pectorals and latissimus dorsi. Muscles in the arms themselves are mostly placed in pairs of flexors (bending muscles) and extensors (straightening muscles): the biceps and triceps provide the most prominent example of this type of pairing; in areas with a wider range of motion, such as the wrist, the relationship between groups of flexors and extensors can be more complex.

Most of the muscles located in the forearm are used to control movements of your hand and wrist. There are many more muscles moving the hands than in any other part of the body because the hands are the most used part of your anatomy.

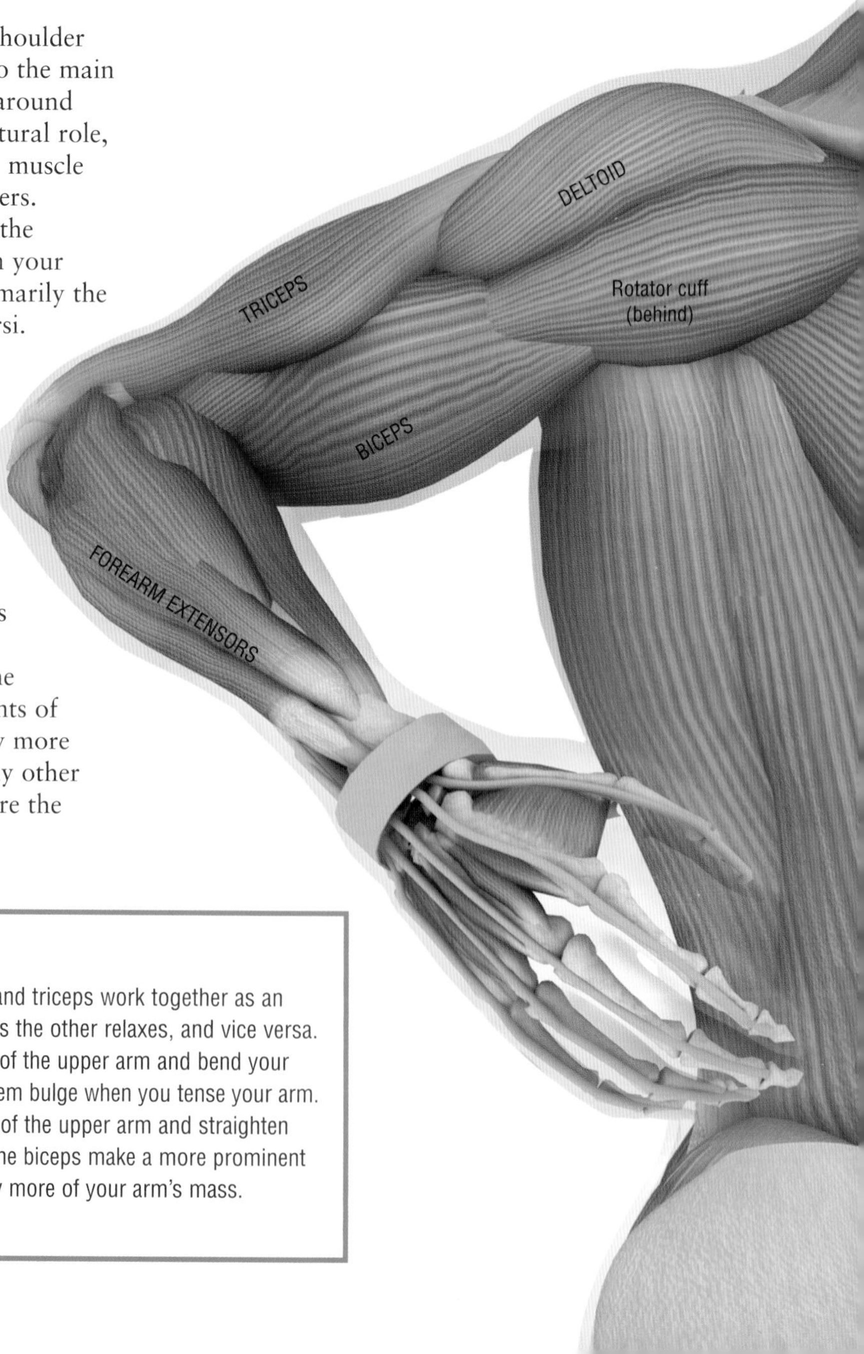

UPPER ARMS

Like many muscles, your biceps and triceps work together as an opposing pair: when one contracts the other relaxes, and vice versa.

■ **The biceps** run along the front of the upper arm and bend your arms at the elbow. You can feel them bulge when you tense your arm.

■ **The triceps** run along the back of the upper arm and straighten your arm at the elbow. Although the biceps make a more prominent bulge, the triceps make up slightly more of your arm's mass.

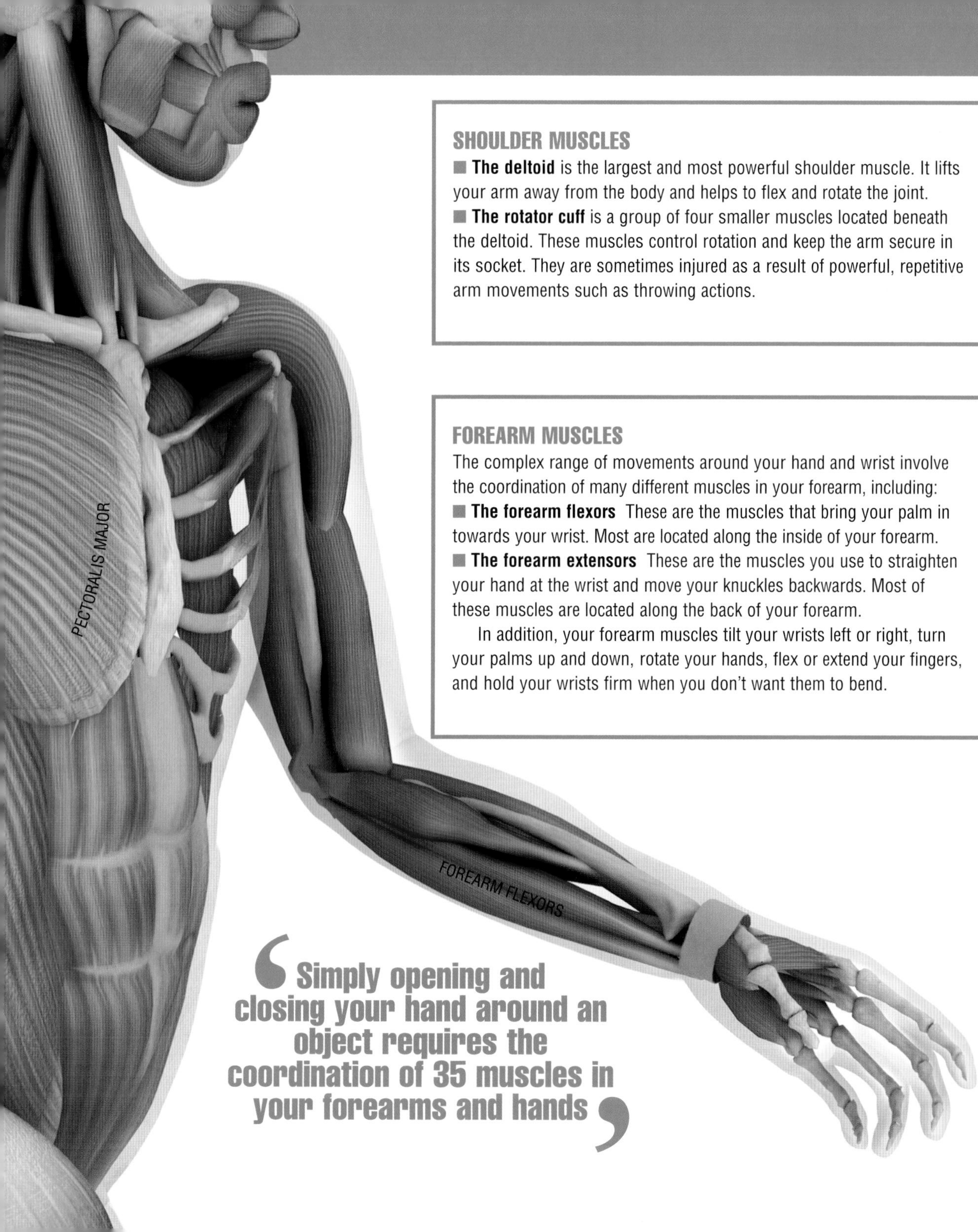

PECTORALIS MAJOR

FOREARM FLEXORS

SHOULDER MUSCLES

- **The deltoid** is the largest and most powerful shoulder muscle. It lifts your arm away from the body and helps to flex and rotate the joint.
- **The rotator cuff** is a group of four smaller muscles located beneath the deltoid. These muscles control rotation and keep the arm secure in its socket. They are sometimes injured as a result of powerful, repetitive arm movements such as throwing actions.

FOREARM MUSCLES

The complex range of movements around your hand and wrist involve the coordination of many different muscles in your forearm, including:

- **The forearm flexors** These are the muscles that bring your palm in towards your wrist. Most are located along the inside of your forearm.
- **The forearm extensors** These are the muscles you use to straighten your hand at the wrist and move your knuckles backwards. Most of these muscles are located along the back of your forearm.

In addition, your forearm muscles tilt your wrists left or right, turn your palms up and down, rotate your hands, flex or extend your fingers, and hold your wrists firm when you don't want them to bend.

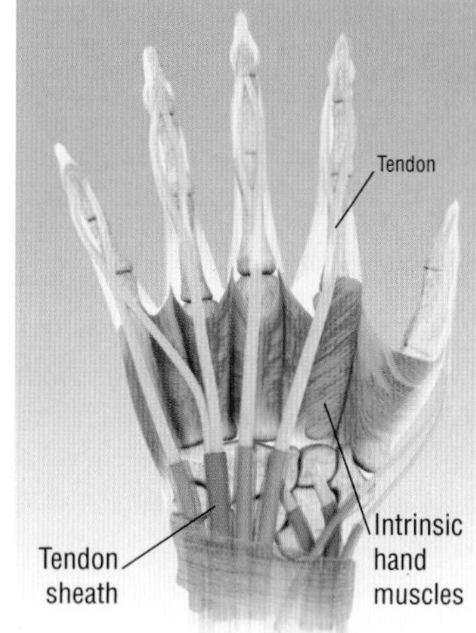

HAND CONTROL

Crude or forceful hand movements are controlled by muscles that run along the forearm – these are known as the extrinsic muscles of the hand. These muscles are connected to the bones of the hand via long tendons – where these tendons pass over the joints of the wrist they are surrounded by lubricated tendon sheaths to reduce friction and are held in place by a band of retaining tissue.

Smaller more delicate hand movements are controlled by intrinsic muscles located within the hand itself. The intrinsic muscles attach directly to the carpal and metacarpal bones of the hand but do not extend significantly past the knuckles. They connect to the fingers via tendons attached to each of the three finger bones (phalanges).

'Simply opening and closing your hand around an object requires the coordination of 35 muscles in your forearms and hands'

LEGS, HIPS AND FEET

Your hips and lower limbs are designed for weight-bearing, balance and locomotion – and their form follows closely from this function. The pelvic girdle is tightly bound to your central skeleton to increase stability and transfer your weight more effectively down to the ground; the bones of your thighs and calves are long and strong; and the muscles in your legs and buttocks are among the most powerful in your body.

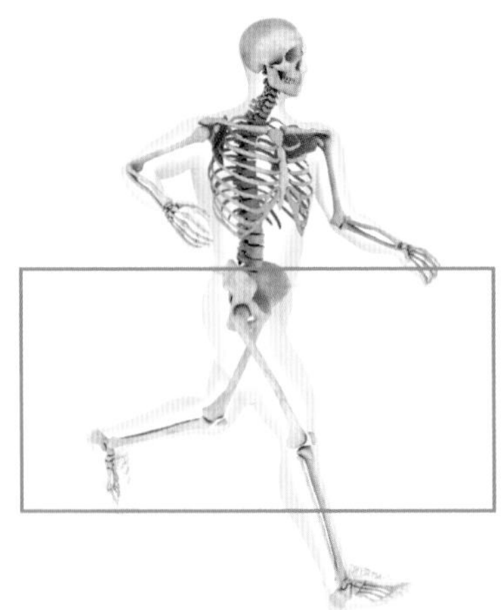

Long, strong, flexible limbs

The long, straight legs of the human body account for almost half the body's height and contain the largest bones and strongest muscles.

The structure of your lower limbs differs so significantly from your upper limbs because of the need to bear the whole weight of your body. Everyday activities such as walking or running can impose a force on your bones, hips, knees and ankles equal to several times your regular body weight. More vigorous activities such as jumping can increase the load on your hips by as much as 12 times your body weight.

To cope with these demands, leg bones are larger and stronger than arm bones; your knees are held in place by strong ligaments and cushioned by thick pads of fibrocartilage while your hip sockets are deeper and more secure than your shoulders. In addition, your feet have a flexible, slightly arched bone structure that absorbs much of the impact from the ground and your weight as you walk.

THE FOOT AND WEIGHT DISTRIBUTION

The bones of your foot are arranged in a similar pattern to those in the hand: the body and heel of the foot contains seven tarsal and five metatarsal bones and the toes, like your fingers, consist of 14 phalangeal bones.

Unlike the hand, the foot is primarily weight bearing and its structure has to reflect this role. In order to distribute the weight of your body evenly over the foot, the bones form an arch. This arch is maintained by the interlocking shape of the bones and the muscles and ligaments of the foot: longitudinal ligaments along the sole of the foot act like the string of a bow to draw the bones at each end together and raise the arch. This structure provides elasticity to absorb the shock of the sudden changes in weight that occur while walking or jumping.

> ‘More than half of the 206 bones inside your body are found in your hands and feet – 52 of these bones are in your feet’

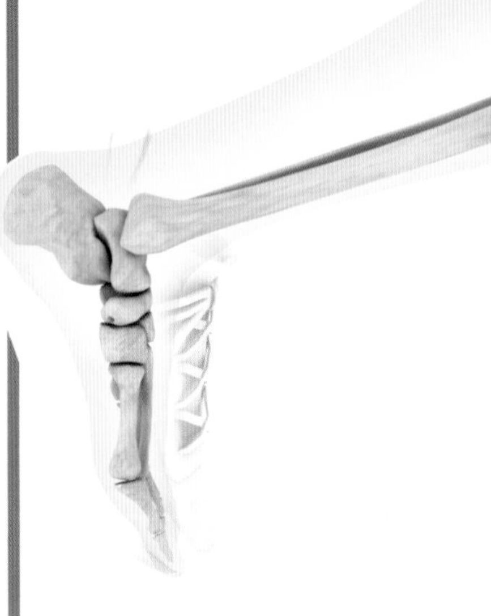

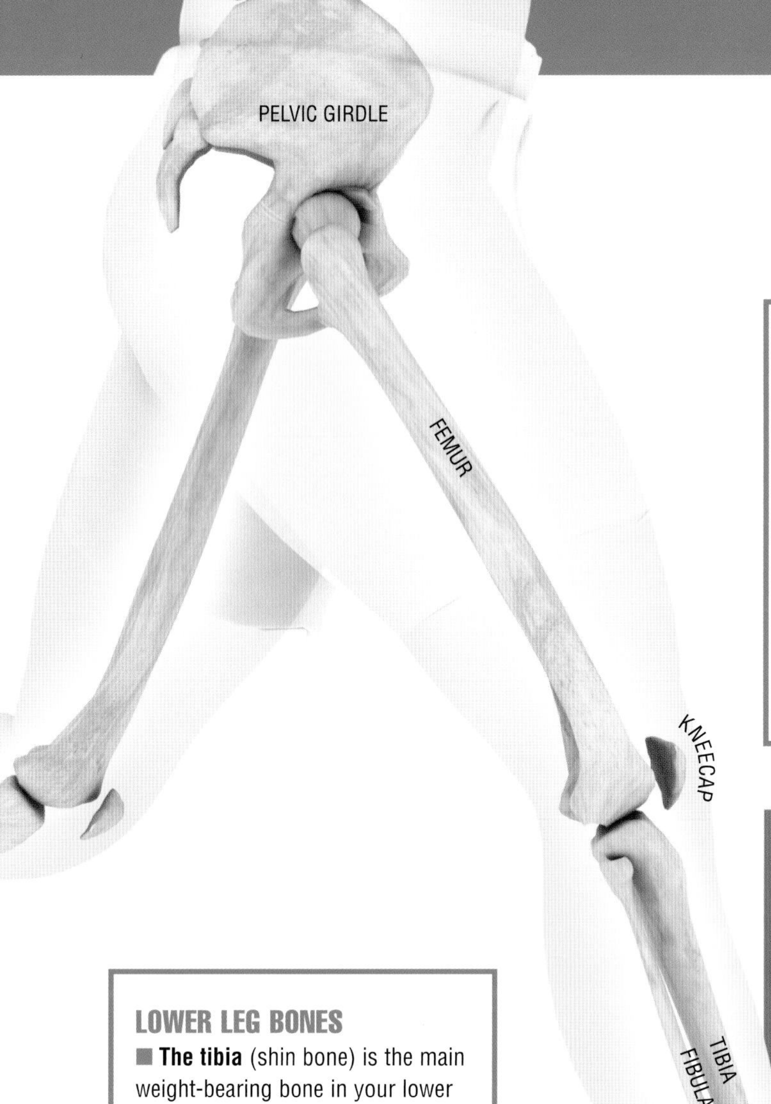

THIGH BONES

■ **The femur** is the longest and strongest bone in your body. It requires a large force – such as a fall from a height or a car accident – to break a healthy femur.

■ **The kneecap** (patella) is a disc-shaped bone embedded into the tendons around your knee to spread the force of any front-on impact. To help you to stand upright it locks back into a groove in your thigh bone when you straighten your leg.

THE ANKLE

The ankle is made up of two main joints: the true ankle joint, formed where the tibia and fibula meet the talus bone, is responsible for the up-and-down motion of the foot; the subtalar joint, where the talus meets the large heel bone, enables side-to-side foot motion.

A sprain occurs when your foot turns further than the ankle ligaments can tolerate, usually as a result of a sudden change in direction or uneven ground. The ligaments along the outside of the ankle are the most commonly sprained.

LOWER LEG BONES

■ **The tibia** (shin bone) is the main weight-bearing bone in your lower leg and the bone that you can feel along the front of your shin. The bony bump on the inside of your ankle is the end of the tibia where it meets the talus bone of your foot.

■ **The fibula**, the smaller bone along the outside of your leg, only carries around 10 per cent of your weight. You can feel the end of the fibula on the outside of your ankle.

Standing, walking and running

The most important function of the muscles around your legs and hips is locomotion – the ability to walk, run, hop, skip or dance. Your muscles not only provide the power to make these movements, they also work hard to maintain your stability as you move.

For this reason the muscles that surround and support your hips are among the strongest in your body: each time you take a step forward your gluteus muscles have to lift the end of your pelvis to prevent your hip dropping and securely transfer your weight from one leg to the other. Your gluteus and hip flexor muscles also move your legs at the hips.

Muscles in your thighs and calves are divided into groups of extensor (straightening) and flexor (bending) muscles: your quadriceps and hamstrings straighten and bend your legs around the knees while your calf muscles flex and extend each foot at the ankle and provide the main thrust required to step forward.

Your feet and toes are moved by muscles stretching via tendons from the calves and by smaller muscles inside the foot itself. To maintain your foot's arches, support your body weight and provide flexibility there are four times as many muscles and ligaments in the foot as there are bones.

BUTTOCK MUSCLES

■ **The gluteus maximus** is a large, powerful muscle that forms the greatest portion of your buttocks. It raises you from sitting to standing and is the primary gluteal muscle employed in cycling, jumping and running actions.

■ **The gluteus medius and minimus** are smaller muscles that lie beneath this muscle and help you to abduct your leg (move it away from your body).

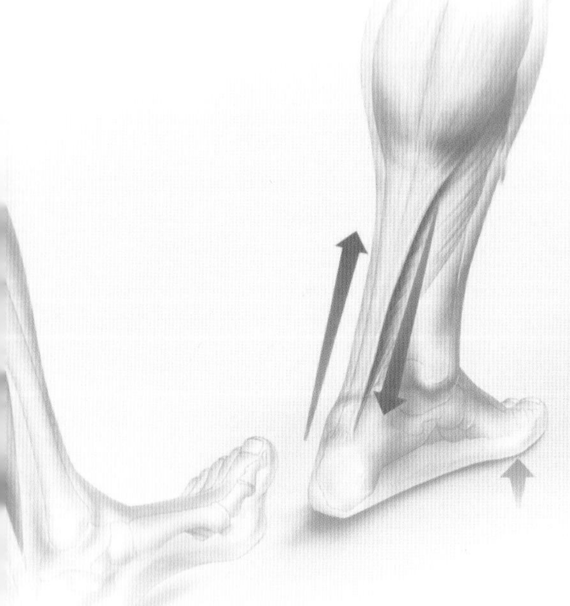

ACHILLES TENDON

The longest and strongest tendon in your body, the Achilles tendon runs along the back of your heel. This tendon connects your calf muscle to your heel bone and pulls the back of your foot up, helping you to stand on your toes, walk, run and jump.

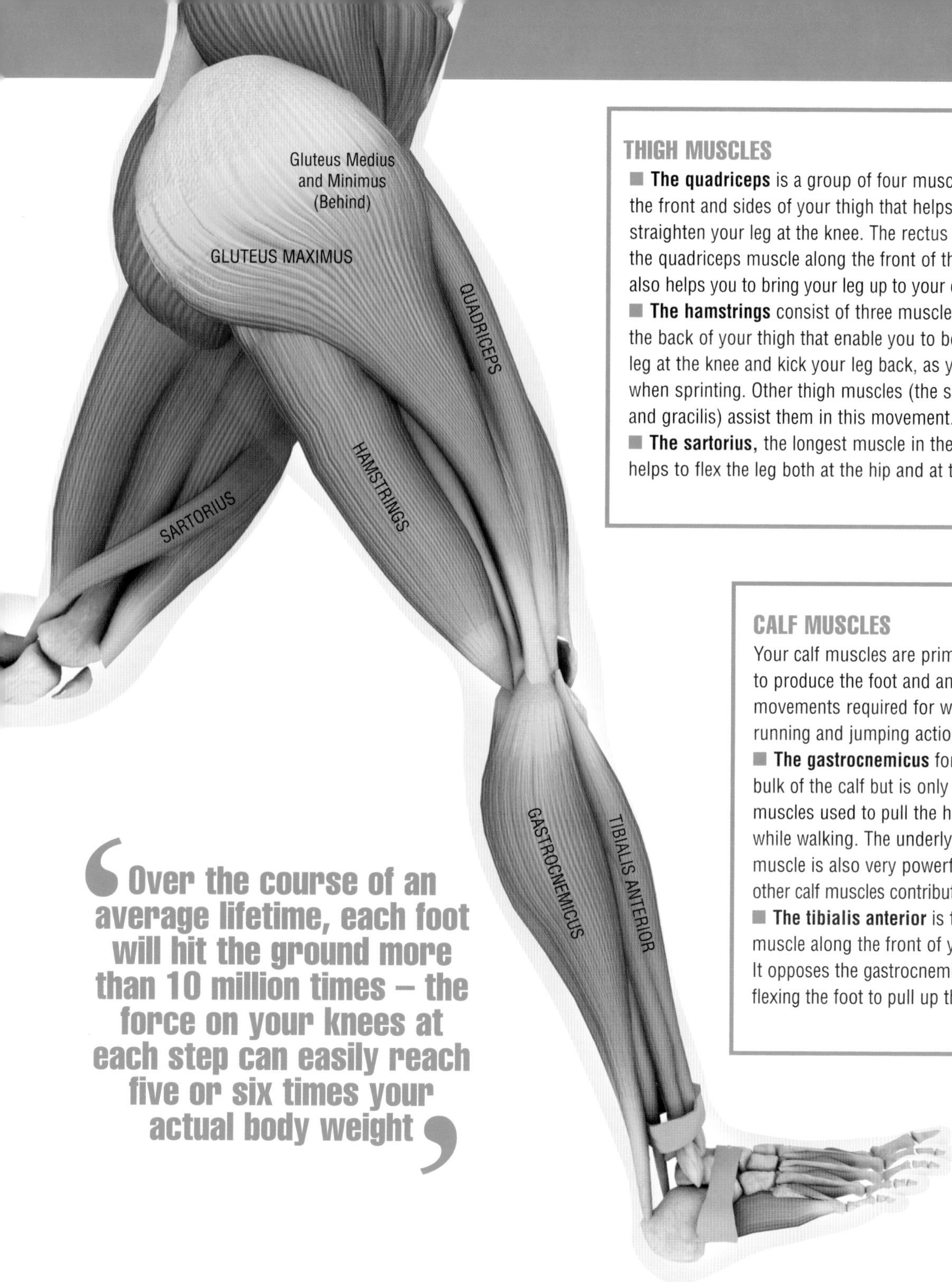

THIGH MUSCLES

- **The quadriceps** is a group of four muscles along the front and sides of your thigh that helps you to straighten your leg at the knee. The rectus femoris, the quadriceps muscle along the front of the thigh, also helps you to bring your leg up to your chest.
- **The hamstrings** consist of three muscles along the back of your thigh that enable you to bend your leg at the knee and kick your leg back, as you do when sprinting. Other thigh muscles (the sartorius and gracilis) assist them in this movement.
- **The sartorius,** the longest muscle in the body, helps to flex the leg both at the hip and at the knee.

CALF MUSCLES

Your calf muscles are primarily used to produce the foot and ankle movements required for walking, running and jumping actions.

- **The gastrocnemicus** forms the bulk of the calf but is only one of the muscles used to pull the heel up while walking. The underlying soleus muscle is also very powerful and other calf muscles contribute too.
- **The tibialis anterior** is the main muscle along the front of your calf. It opposes the gastrocnemicus by flexing the foot to pull up the toes.

‘Over the course of an average lifetime, each foot will hit the ground more than 10 million times – the force on your knees at each step can easily reach five or six times your actual body weight’

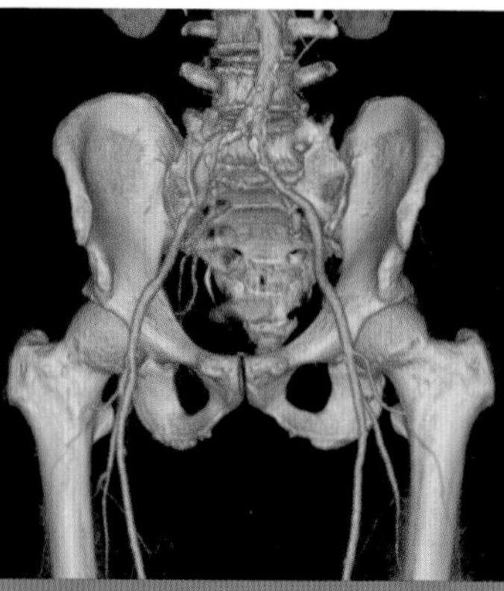

HIPS AND PELVIS

The basin-like bones of the pelvic girdle support and protect your lower abdominal and pelvic organs. They are larger and more dense than those in the thorax because they are involved in weight bearing and locomotion.

The female pelvis is slightly deeper and wider than the average male pelvis (pictured above) and has a larger opening at the centre for the baby to pass through during childbirth.

Most of the muscles attached to the pelvis are used to move your legs at the hips,most notably the gluteus maximus. A group of muscles inside the pelvis – the pelvic floor – support the organs of your pelvic cavity and control the flow of waste from the bladder and rectum.

The structure of bones

The 206 separate bones that make up your skeleton come in all shapes and sizes, ranging from the flat, plate-like bones of your skull to the long, cylindrical bones in your limbs. Their internal structure makes bones light but very strong – human bones are four times stronger than concrete; a 5cm (2in) cube of solid bone could take the weight of an elephant.

What do bones do?

The most obvious functions of your bones are to give your body its basic shape, support your weight and work with your muscles to produce controlled, purposeful movement. Your skull and rib cage also help to protect your brain, heart and lungs from external damage, while the bones of your spine safeguard your spinal cord.

Your bones are also your primary store of calcium, the most abundant mineral in your body. They contain around 99 per cent of all your body's calcium in the form of salts (mostly calcium carbonate and calcium phosphate). As well as being a vital constituent of your bones and teeth, calcium plays an essential part in many chemical processes, including muscle contraction, nerve function and blood clotting.

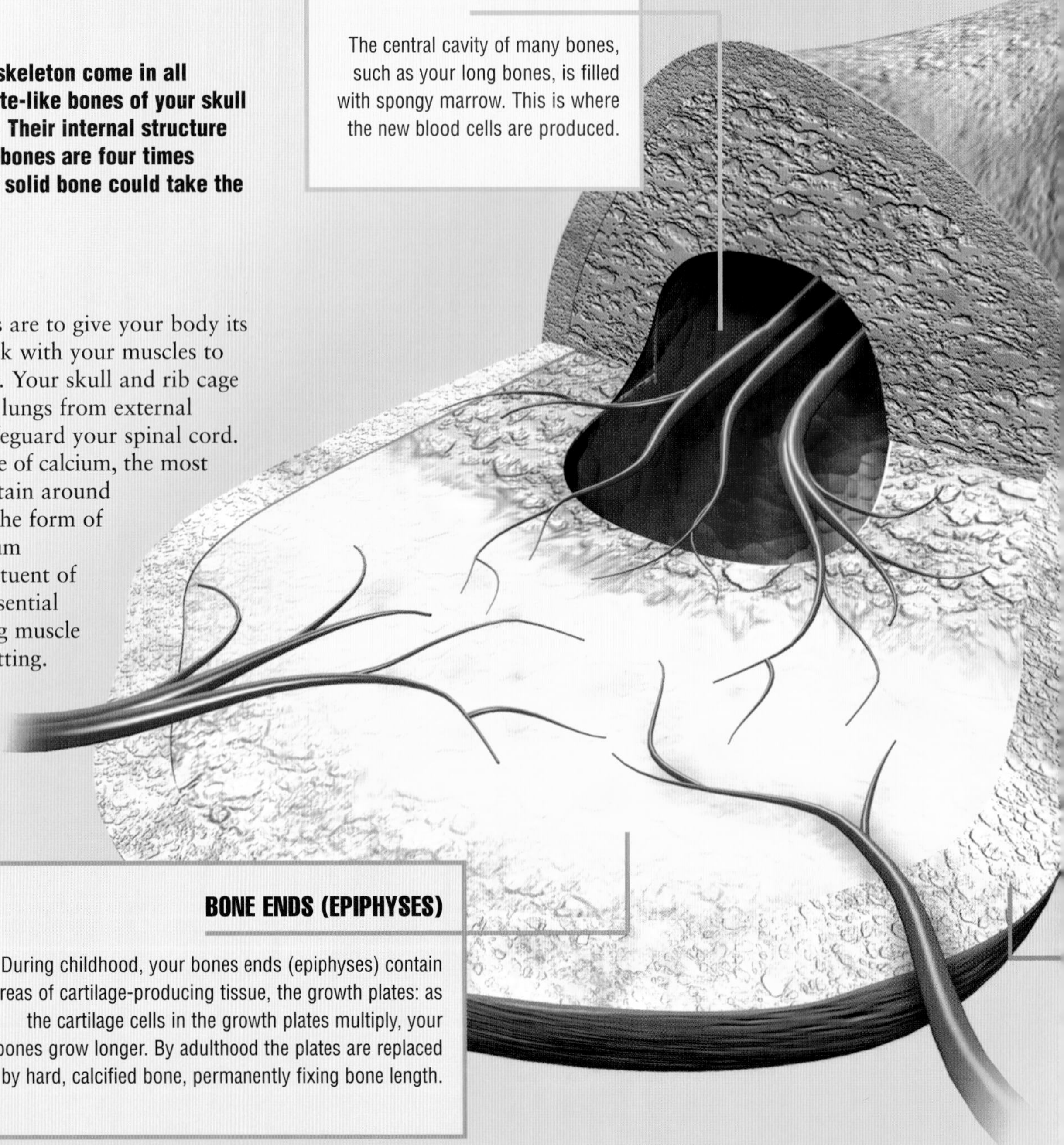

DID YOU KNOW?

- **An unborn baby's skeleton consists mainly of lengths of flexible cartilage. During infancy and childhood this cartilage is replaced by bone.The ends of the bones retain plates of growing cartilage until about 25.**
- **Not all of the cartilage in your body is replaced by bone – some cartilage remains to cushion joint surfaces and is also present in your ears and at the tip of your nose.**

BONE MARROW

The central cavity of many bones, such as your long bones, is filled with spongy marrow. This is where the new blood cells are produced.

BONE ENDS (EPIPHYSES)

During childhood, your bones ends (epiphyses) contain areas of cartilage-producing tissue, the growth plates: as the cartilage cells in the growth plates multiply, your bones grow longer. By adulthood the plates are replaced by hard, calcified bone, permanently fixing bone length.

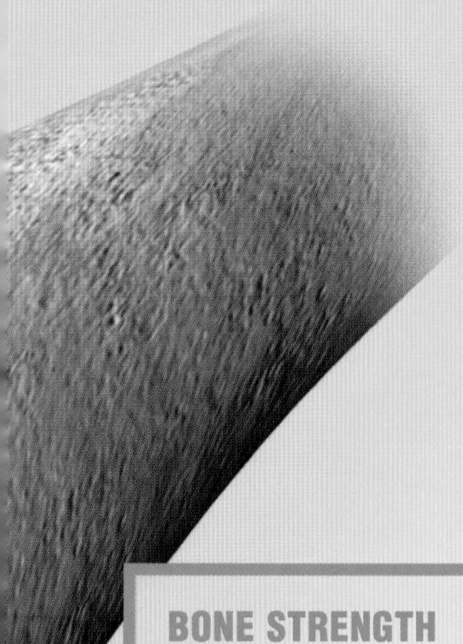

BONE STRENGTH

The crystals of calcium in bone are very strong and able to withstand great compression, but they can also shatter when bent or twisted or if subjected to a sudden impact. Collagen fibres, on the other hand, are very tough and flexible, and can easily tolerate stretching, twisting and bending. It is this combination of hard crystals and flexible collagen that gives bone its great strength.

During clotting, calcium reacts with proteins and other substances to thicken and coagulate the blood, and tiny particles called platelets stick together to plug the damaged blood vessels. Like much of the calcium in your blood, these platelets originate in bones.

Bone marrow

When you are born, your bones contain a jelly-like substance called red marrow. This makes red blood cells to carry oxygen around your body, white blood cells to fight infections and platelets to help your blood to coagulate. By adulthood, yellow marrow (largely fat) will have replaced most of the red marrow in the long bones of your limbs, but your other bones still contain red marrow.

Bone structure

Each of your bones is covered with a fibrous outer membrane, the periosteum. This contains blood vessels to transport nutrients and hormone signals to the inner bone, and nerves to carry information about things such as pain and position.

Beneath the periosteum, the bone itself consists of a dense outer layer of smooth, hard bone called compact bone and inner layers of softer, more porous cancellous bone.

- **Compact bone** consists of cylindrical structures called osteons, each measuring about 0.2mm (1⁄25in) across and about 10mm (2⁄5in) long, which are tightly packed together to form the strong, dense bone. Blood vessels and nerves, connected to the periosteum, occupy the hollow central canals of the osteons.
- **Cancellous bone** lies beneath the compact bone. It consists of a honeycomb of rigid struts (trabeculae) and contains the bone marrow.

COMPACT BONE

The thick, outer layer of compact bone looks solid but consists of numerous cylindrical structures called osteons. Each osteon contains tiny gaps called lacunae and a central canal containing nerves and blood vessels which supply the bone with oxygen and nutrients.

What is bone made of?

The basic material of both compact and cancellous bone is a matrix of collagen (fibres of strong protein) impregnated with calcium salts. The calcium salts give bone its hardness while the collagen fibres give it a degree of resilience. Collagen, a very flexible material, is also found in cartilage, ligaments, tendons and skin, and is the main component of your body's connective tissue, which separates, supports and protects your vital organs.

4 WAYS TO...

Keep your bones strong

1 Eat well Make sure you get plenty of vitamins and minerals and lots of calcium. Good sources of calcium include dairy products and green leafy vegetables >>98–117.

2 Stay strong Take plenty of exercise, particularly bone-loading, weight-bearing exercise to build strong bones >>54–97

3 Stop smoking Chemicals in cigarettes can interfere with calcium absorption and may speed up the ageing process.

4 Drink sensibly Excessive alcohol intake interferes with nutrient absorption and increases bone breakdown.

Bone cells

Although bone is mostly calcium-hardened collagen, it is not simply an inert material. It is an amazing, ever-changing structure created, maintained and constantly renewed by the specialized living cells embedded within it. Each type of bone cell plays its own individual part in the laying down, maintenance and repair of the bone tissue.

- **Osteoblasts** Located near the surfaces of the bones, the bone-forming osteoblast cells produce the collagen matrix that hardens into thin layers of bone when calcium salts crystallize within it.
- **Osteocytes** The osteoblasts eventually trap themselves within the bone they create and are then known as osteocytes. The main function of osteocytes, the most numerous type of bone cell, is to maintain the bone tissue.
- **Osteoclasts** The osteocytes work in conjunction with cells known as osteoclasts. These large cells use acidity and enzyme action to break down bone tissue. They do this either to release calcium from the bone so that it can be used elsewhere in the body or to remove bone damaged by everyday usage or fractures. Osteocytes and osteoblasts then repair the damage.

DID YOU KNOW?

- **You have 14 bones in your face and 27 bones in each hand. The smallest bone in your body is the stirrup bone in your ear, which is just 2.5mm (1/10in) long.**
- **The longest and strongest bone in your body is your femur (thigh bone) but the hardest bone in your body is your jawbone.**

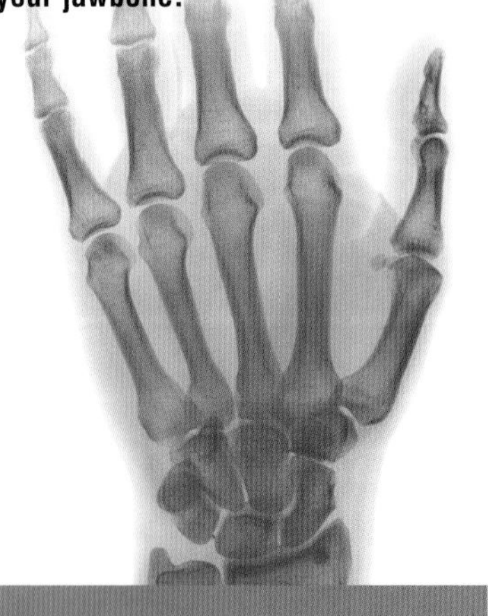

HOW BROKEN BONES HEAL

When a bone breaks, it can take from six weeks to several months for the two broken ends to reunite completely.

1 **When the fracture first occurs, broken blood vessels cause bleeding around the site of the break.**

2 **The damaged blood vessels form a clot, which stops the bleeding, and a mesh of fibrous tissue replaces the clot.**

3 **Bone-building cells called osteoblasts produce a new area of soft spongy bone, called a callus, on the framework of the fibrous tissue.**

4 **As ossification continues, the callus disappears and the soft tissue starts to develop into hard compact bone.**

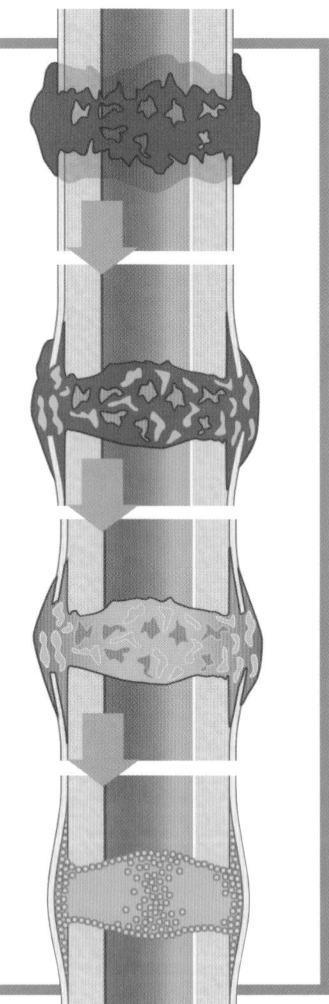

Types of bone

Bones in the human body are classified according to shape:

- **Long bones** are the cylindrical bones found in your arms and legs and the bones of your fingers and toes. They have hollow, tube-like central shafts with solid ends.
- **Short bones** have no central shaft and consist of a hard outer shell of compact bone filled with cancellous bone. The carpal bones of your wrists and the tarsal bones of your ankles are short bones.
- **Flat bones** consist of cancellous bone sandwiched between two layers of compact bone. They include your shoulder blades, the bones in your skull, your breast bone and parts of your pelvis. Your ribs are also flat bones, but they have short sections of long bone at the ends that connect to your spine.
- **Irregular bones** Some bones, such as your vertebrae and the bones in your face, don’t fit into any of these categories so are classified as irregular.
- **Sesamoid bones** are in a class of their own because they are not actually linked to the rest of your skeleton. They are embedded in tendons (the fibrous cords that anchor your muscles to your bones) to reinforce them at points that are subjected to a great deal of friction, such as where they run around the outside of a joint. Most of your sesamoid bones are very small, with the exception of your kneecaps.

The power of muscles

There are around 650 muscles in your body, accounting for between a third and a half of your total body weight. Your muscles not only let you sit, stand, walk and talk, they also pump air in and out of your lungs and your blood around your body, and move and focus your eyes and propel food through your digestive tract.

BODY HEAT

The heat that your muscles generate as a by-product of activity helps to keep your body's internal temperature at about 37°C. When you are resting, about 16 per cent of your body heat comes from your muscles but this increases when you exercise. If you get too cold, your muscles shiver to generate more heat.

Three types of muscle

Muscles are bundles of long, tubular fibres that produce movement by contracting. There are three different types of muscle tissue in your body: cardiac, smooth and skeletal.

Cardiac muscle

This type of muscle forms the large muscles of your heart, which contract to push blood through your arteries and relax to let blood back in from your veins. Cardiac muscle is termed involuntary muscle, because it operates without any conscious control from your brain.

The cardiac muscle cells can each automatically contract and relax, but their actions are synchronized by a group of specialized nerve cells which act as a pacemaker. The pacemaker cells also control the rate at which your heart beats, and increase or decrease your heart rate in response to nerve and hormone signals from other parts of your body. During exercise, for example, when your skeletal muscles are working hard and need an increased blood supply, your heart beats faster to pump more blood around your body.

Smooth muscle

Smooth muscle tissue forms the sheets or layers of muscle within the walls of your blood vessels and your hollow organs, such as your intestines and your bladder. It contracts slowly and rhythmically to move the contents of these organs through your body. Like cardiac muscle, smooth muscle is involuntary muscle because it operates without your conscious control.

Smooth muscle also occurs in other parts of your body. In your eyes, for example, it alters the shape of the lenses so that you can focus. It also alters the size of your pupils to control the amount of light entering your eyes.

Skeletal muscle

The most abundant type of muscle tissue in your body is skeletal muscle, the muscle that moves your body by pulling on your bones and joints. It is also called voluntary muscle, because it operates under your conscious control.

Your skeletal muscles help to keep your bones in position and stop your joints from dislocating, and you use them for almost every body movement you make, from smiling to walking. Even when you are standing still, skeletal muscles are busy maintaining your posture to keep you upright and balanced.

Muscle movements

Skeletal muscle consists of bundles of muscle fibres bound together by tough, silvery-white connective tissue

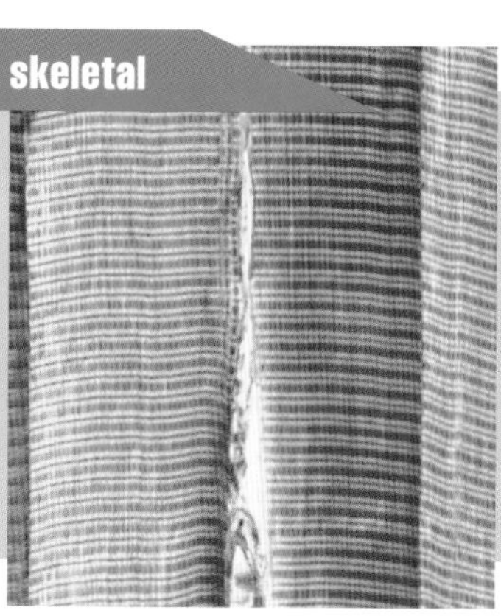

smooth

cardiac

(collagen) that also carries blood vessels and nerves. The connective tissue extends beyond the muscle to form a cord (a tendon) or a sheet (aponeurosis) that links muscle to the bone. Tendon tissue is twice as strong as muscle.

A muscle fibre is a long, slender cell (or a series of cells) that can run the whole length of the muscle – 30–40cm (12–16in) in some leg muscles. Each one is packed with an array of thinner fibres, called myofibrils, that run lengthwise within it. These in turn contain alternating bundles of thick and thin filaments of protein, called myofilaments. The ends of the thin filaments slightly overlap the ends of the thick ones.

When the muscle receives nerve signals telling it to contract, it releases chemicals that make the bundles of thin filaments slide further inside the bundles of thick filaments. This shortens the myofibrils, which in turn shortens the muscle fibres making the muscle contract.

Working in pairs

Because muscles produce movement through contraction, the skeletal muscles can only move bones and limbs by pulling on them. This is why most muscles or groups of muscles work in pairs: one to bend the joint and the other to straighten it.

When you raise your hand to touch your shoulder, for example, the biceps muscle at the front of your upper arm contracts to bend your elbow and pull your forearm upwards. At the same time, the

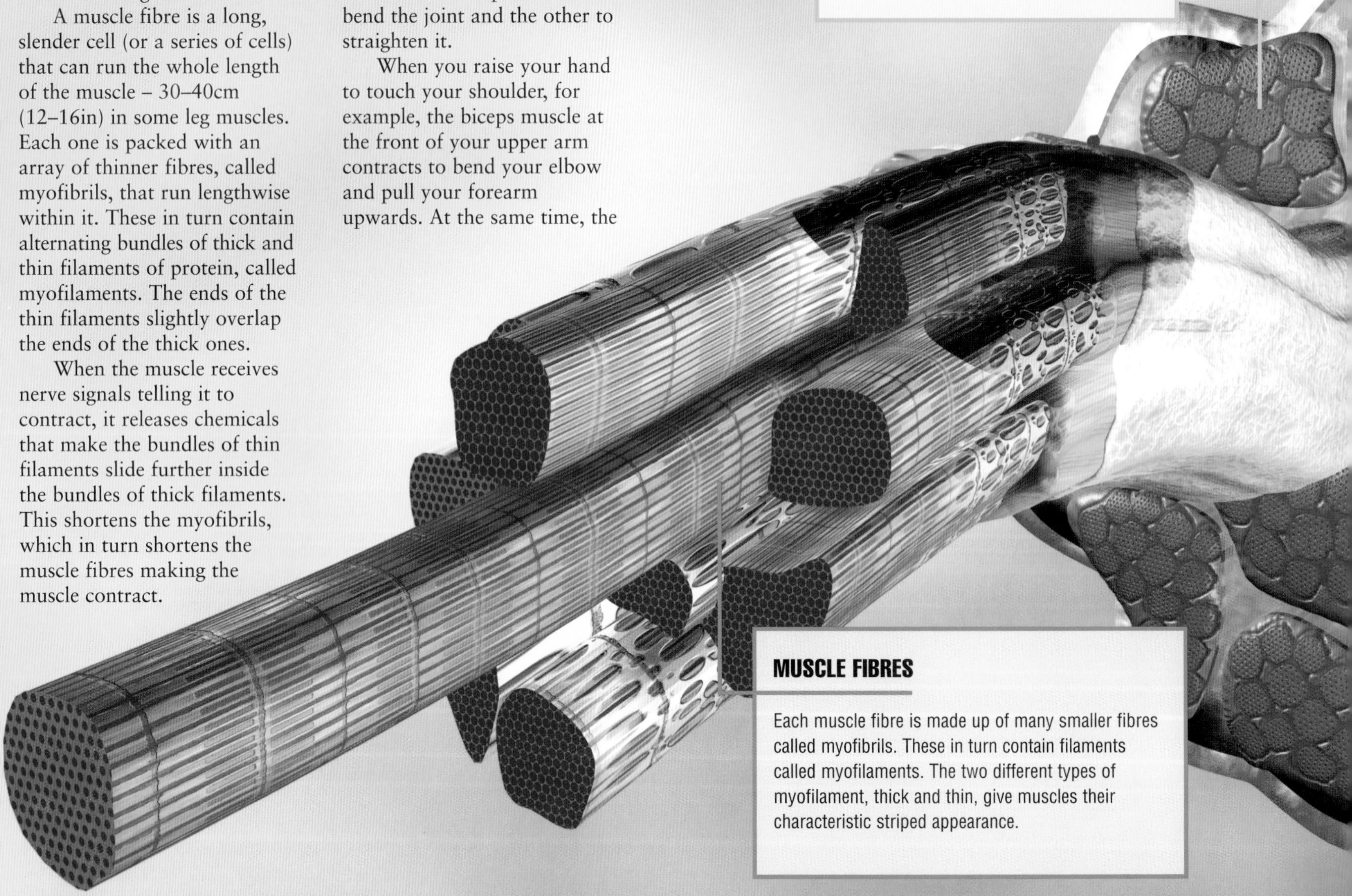

FASCICLES

The muscle fibres are contained in long bundles of muscle called fascicles that are separated from one another by a fibrous tissue called the perimysium.

MUSCLE FIBRES

Each muscle fibre is made up of many smaller fibres called myofibrils. These in turn contain filaments called myofilaments. The two different types of myofilament, thick and thin, give muscles their characteristic striped appearance.

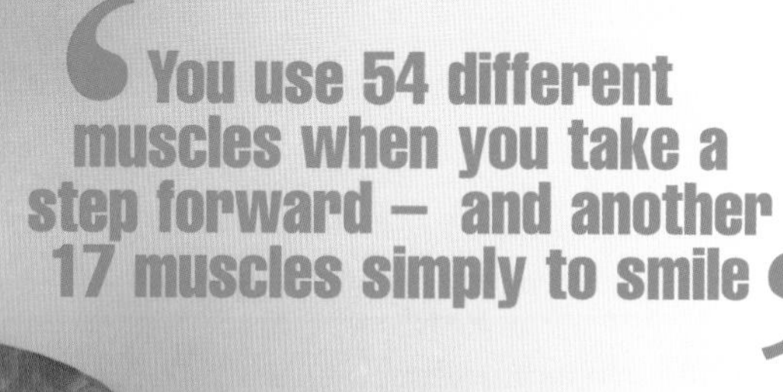

‘You use 54 different muscles when you take a step forward – and another 17 muscles simply to smile’

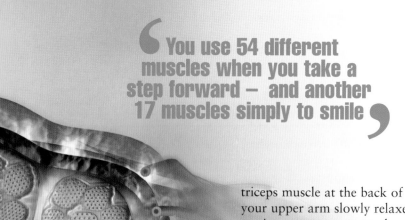

triceps muscle at the back of your upper arm slowly relaxes to give your arm a smooth and controlled movement. When you put your hand down again, the triceps muscle contracts to straighten your arm and the biceps relaxes.

Muscle power

Your muscles get most of the energy that powers them by combining glucose with oxygen. This happens in a biochemical process called aerobic (oxygen-based) respiration, which takes place within the muscle cells. The glucose comes from the food you eat and the oxygen from the air you breathe, and your bloodstream delivers these to your muscles and other cells in your body.

Energy and exercise

When you work your muscles hard, for example when you are exercising, they need a lot more energy than they do when you are resting. Your heart then beats faster and your lungs work harder to keep them supplied with glucose and oxygen.

Sometimes, however, your bloodstream can’t supply all the oxygen and glucose that your muscles need, no matter how hard your heart and lungs are working. This can happen during high-intensity exercise, such as sprinting or uphill cycling. To make up for this shortfall, your muscles get the extra energy they need by drawing on their own reserves of glucose. These reserves take the form of a substance called glycogen, which your body makes from glucose and stores within your muscles and liver.

Your muscles can rapidly change this glycogen back into glucose, then produce energy from it without using oxygen in a process called anaerobic (oxygen-free) respiration.

Anaerobic respiration provides your muscles with a valuable energy boost, but it doesn’t last very long. Fatigue soon sets in when the glycogen runs out and lactic acid – a by-product of anaerobic respiration – builds up in your muscles, making them stiff and painful and often causing cramps. This effect lasts until you slow down or rest. Your bloodstream can then provide all the glucose and oxygen your muscles need and remove the lactic acid from them.

EPIMYSIUM

Each muscle is covered by a layer of fibrous tissue, the epimysium. Blood vessels in this tissue bring in nutrients and remove waste.

DID YOU KNOW?

- **The largest muscle in your body is the gluteus maximus, in your buttocks.The smallest muscle in your body is the stapedius, the muscle that controls the stapes, one of the tiny bones that conduct sound through your middle ear.**
- **The longest muscle in your human body is the sartorius, a muscle in the front of your thigh used to flex at the hip and knee.**
- **When you bite, your jaw muscles can exert a force of up to 91kg (200lb) to bring your teeth together.**

Joints: making connections

Your joints are the points of your body at which two or more bones meet. They give structure and stability to your otherwise rigid skeleton as well as the ability to move, twist and bend your body.

Almost every bone in your body forms a joint with at least one other. The only exceptions to this are the sesamoid bones such as your kneecaps, which are embedded in tendon, and the small, U-shaped hyoid bone, which is located high up in the front of your neck and acts as an anchor point for several important muscles that help you to swallow and speak.

Types of joint

Joints are often classified according to the range of motion that they allow. Some are fixed rigidly and do not permit any movement, some allow a degree of flexibility and others, such as those in your limbs, allow a wide range of motion. The flexibility of the joint is closely related to the structure and type of tissue that holds the joint together:

- **Fibrous joints** are connected by tight bands of connective tissue that don't allow any movement. The bones in your skull are connected by sutures of collagen fibre, for example, while your teeth are connected tightly to your jaw bone by the peridontal ligaments. Fibrous joints are often known as fixed (synarthrotic) joints.
- **Cartilaginous joints** allow limited movement because the bones are connected by slightly more flexible layers or pads of cartilage. These joints provide flexibility rather than a wide range of motion: movement along your spine, for example, is produced by the combined movement of many individual vertebral joints.
- **Synovial joints** allow a wider range of motion. To stop the bones separating, strong, flexible bands or sheets of fibrous ligament hold the joint together. Most of the body's joints are synovial, including those in your limbs, hands and feet – the joints where a lot of movement is required.

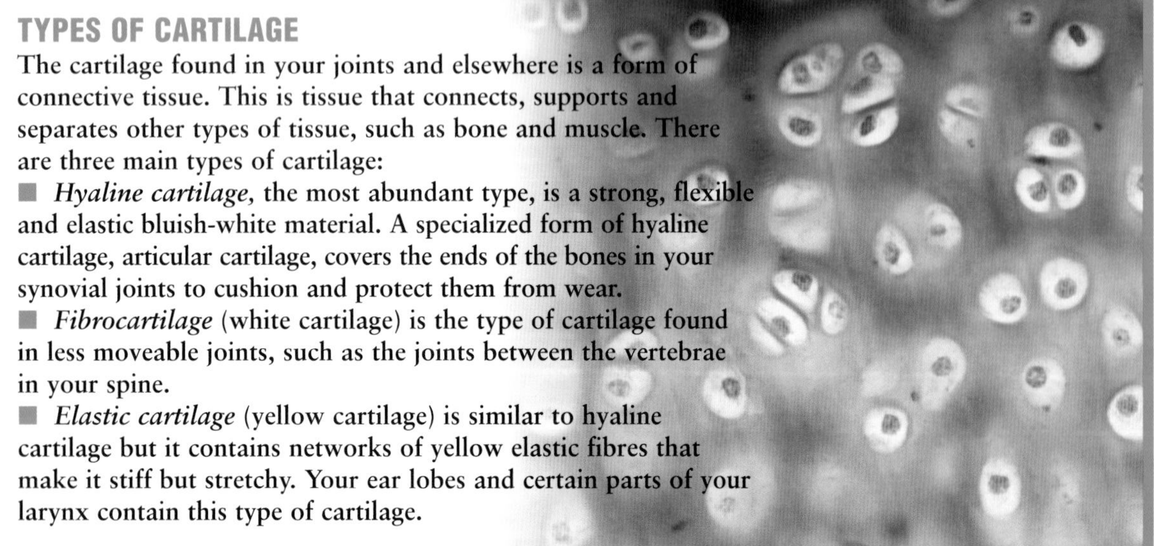

TYPES OF CARTILAGE

The cartilage found in your joints and elsewhere is a form of connective tissue. This is tissue that connects, supports and separates other types of tissue, such as bone and muscle. There are three main types of cartilage:

- *Hyaline cartilage,* the most abundant type, is a strong, flexible and elastic bluish-white material. A specialized form of hyaline cartilage, articular cartilage, covers the ends of the bones in your synovial joints to cushion and protect them from wear.
- *Fibrocartilage* (white cartilage) is the type of cartilage found in less moveable joints, such as the joints between the vertebrae in your spine.
- *Elastic cartilage* (yellow cartilage) is similar to hyaline cartilage but it contains networks of yellow elastic fibres that make it stiff but stretchy. Your ear lobes and certain parts of your larynx contain this type of cartilage.

DID YOU KNOW?

- **Your funny bone isn't really a bone at all: the tingling sensation you get when you knock the inside of your elbow is actually caused by your ulnar nerve, a nerve that passes around the back of your elbow.**
- **The popping sound you get when you 'crack' your knuckles is caused by bubbles in the synovial fluid of your finger joints. The bubbles form as pressure within the fluid drops and then burst. There's no evidence that this leads to arthritis – but it's probably not good to pull your joints repeatedly past their regular range.**

Joint movements

A moveable joint permits one bone to move relative to the other, pulled by muscles attached to the bones by tendons. Your shoulder joint, for example, allows the bone of your upper arm (the humerus) to move relative to your shoulder blade.

Joint flexibility

The range of motion within a synovial joint depends on the structure of the joint, the position of the ligaments and the position and tension of the muscles and tendons around it.

Some people have a much greater than average range of motion in their joints. Although these people are often described as 'double-jointed', they usually just have very long or stretchy tendons or ligaments. Contortionists may have many such joints, letting them twist their bodies into seemingly impossible positions.

Too much joint flexibility can, however, cause problems, since joints that are lax (too loose) are unstable and more easily dislocated.

SYNOVIAL FLUID

The space around the bone ends in a synovial joint contains synovial fluid, a clear, viscous fluid that nourishes the articular cartilage and removes waste. The fluid also lubricates the joint, reducing friction between surfaces, and helps to distribute pressure evenly.

ARTICULAR CARTILAGE

The ends of the bone in a synovial joint are covered in a special type of slippery hyaline cartilage which acts as a shock absorber, helps to reduce friction and protects the bone ends from wear and tear.

JOINT CAPSULE

Each synovial joint is enclosed and protected by a capsule of fibrous collagen and elastin connective tissue. The capsule is lined by a membrane which produces synovial fluid.

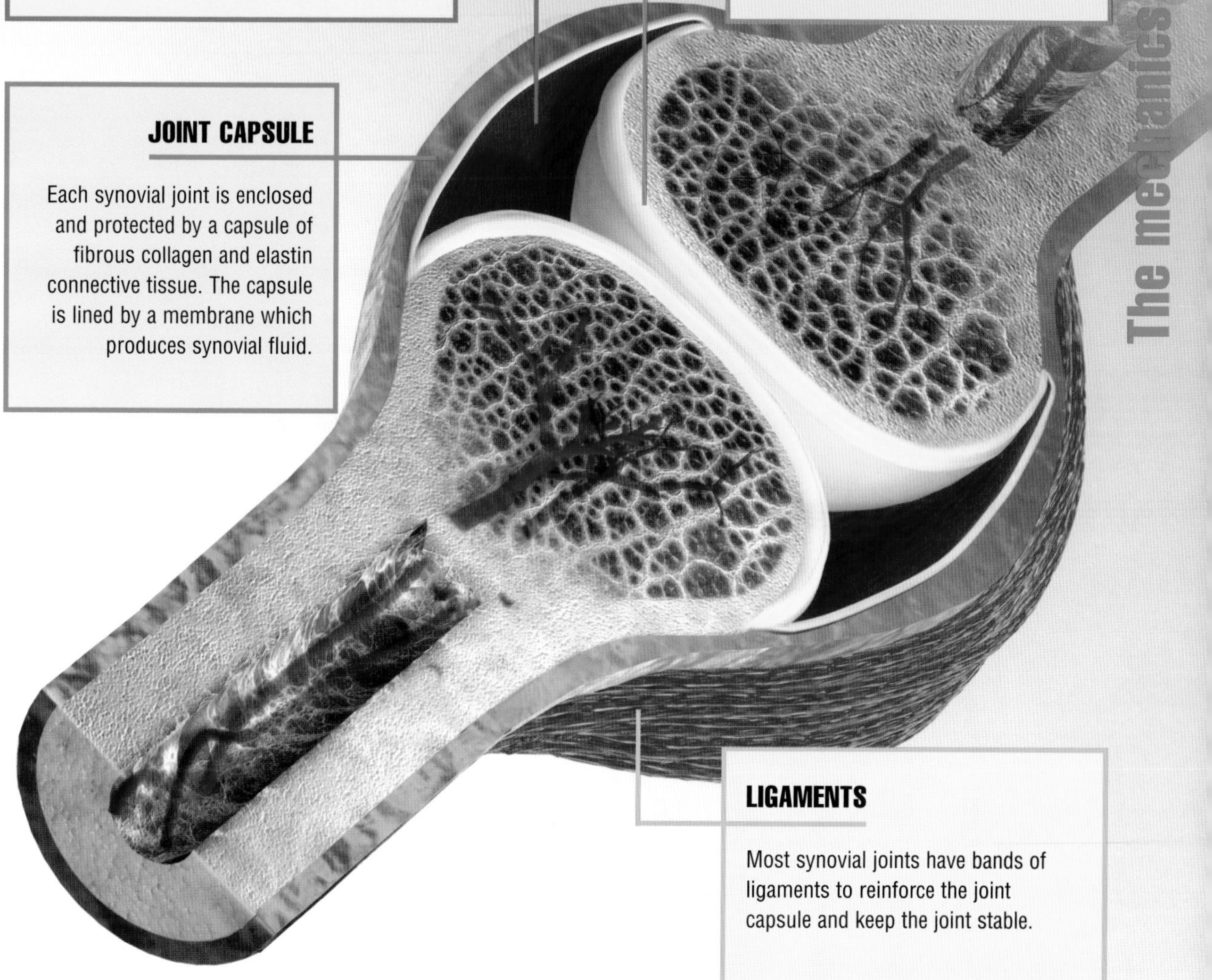

BURSAE

A bursa is a small sac filled with synovial fluid and lined by a synovial membrane. Bursae often form between tissues around synovial joints that are exposed to a lot of friction or pressure, between ligaments or tendons and other tissues, for example, where they help to reduce friction.

LIGAMENTS

Most synovial joints have bands of ligaments to reinforce the joint capsule and keep the joint stable.

Joints: making connections

The human body contains many hundreds of joints. Some of these joints, such as those in your hands and feet, are small and very numerous; a few, such as those in the knees or the shoulders, are far larger. The range and type of motion permitted also varies considerably: even the synovial joints – the joints that allow the greatest degree of movement – vary from highly mobile ball-and-socket joints to those with much more limited motion, such as the small gliding joints in the back of your hand.

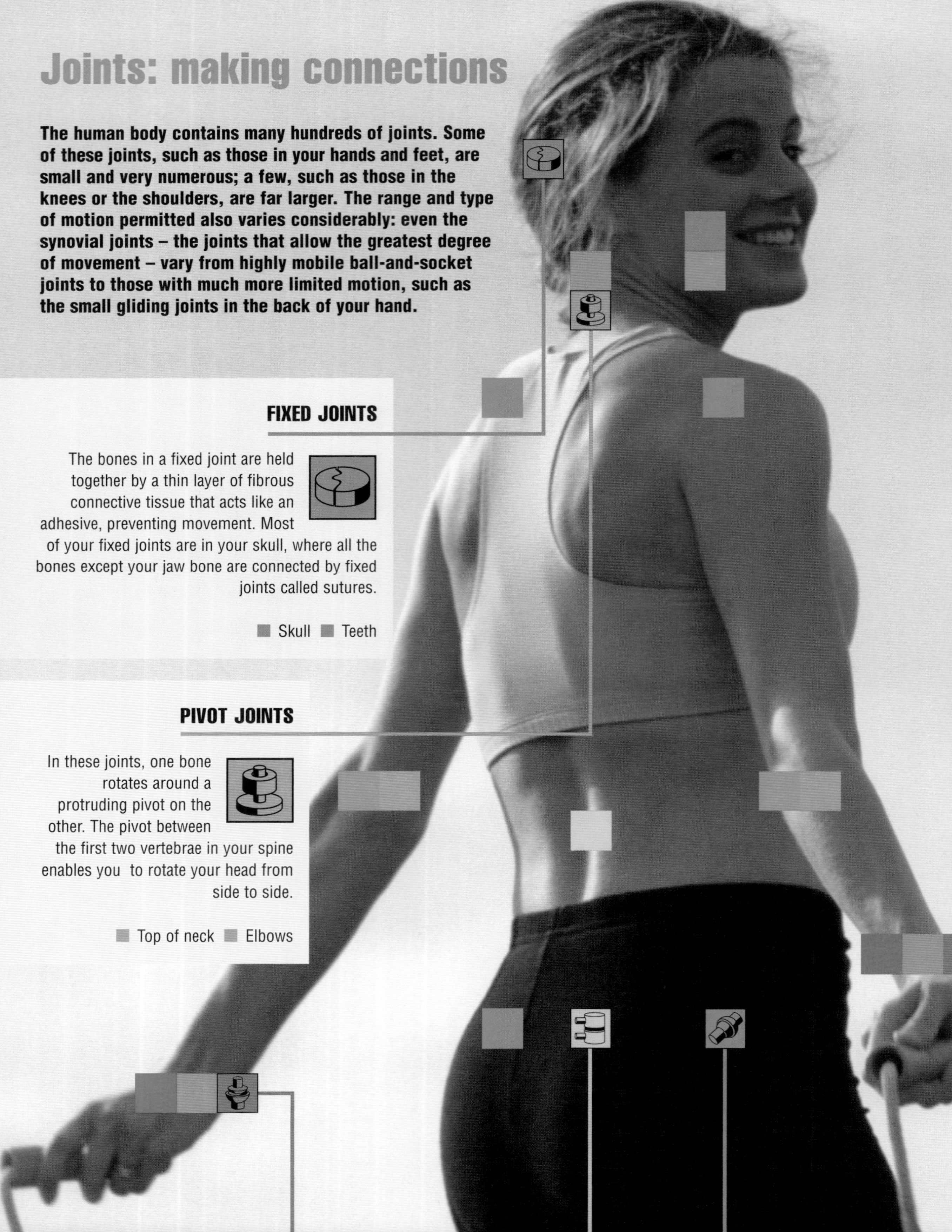

FIXED JOINTS

The bones in a fixed joint are held together by a thin layer of fibrous connective tissue that acts like an adhesive, preventing movement. Most of your fixed joints are in your skull, where all the bones except your jaw bone are connected by fixed joints called sutures.

■ Skull ■ Teeth

PIVOT JOINTS

In these joints, one bone rotates around a protruding pivot on the other. The pivot between the first two vertebrae in your spine enables you to rotate your head from side to side.

■ Top of neck ■ Elbows

SYNOVIAL ELLIPSOIDAL AND SADDLE JOINTS

In an ellipsoidal joint, the oval end of one bone rests in an oval depression in the other. This lets them bend, straighten and rock from side to side. Your body's only saddle joints are at the base of your thumbs: the saddle-shape lets them rock forward and back and from side to side.

■ Hands ■ Wrists ■ Thumbs

INTERVERTEBRAL JOINTS

Tough, fluid-filled fibrocartilage pads lie inbetween the vertebrae in your back. As your muscles pull on your spine, these discs compress at the point that they are placed under pressure, allowing a small degree of movement in that direction.

■ Spine ■ Pelvis

SYNOVIAL HINGE JOINTS

These joints allow a back-and-forth motion, like the opening and closing of a door. The elbows, knees and ankles are the largest hinge joints in the body, but there are many much smaller joints in your fingers and toes. A hinge joint between your skull and your spine lets you nod your head.

■ Elbows ■ Knees ■ Feet and ankles ■ Top of neck ■ Hands ■ Jaw

SYNOVIAL BALL-AND-SOCKET JOINTS

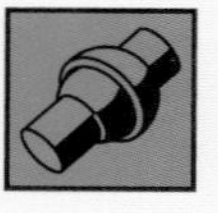

The most mobile joints in your body are the ball-and-socket joints of your shoulders and hips. In these joints, the dome-shaped head of one bone fits inside a similarly shaped cavity in the other bone. This allows the joint to move in all directions.

■ Hips ■ Shoulders

SYNOVIAL GLIDING (PLANE) JOINTS

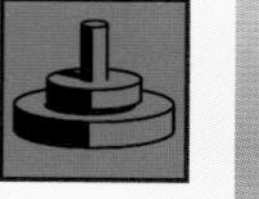

Joints that allow almost-flat bone surfaces to slide over each other are known as plane or gliding joints. Strong ligaments limit the amount of movement in these joints, which include some of the small joints found in your ankles, hands and wrists.

■ Ankles ■ Wrists

Bones, muscles and joints in action

Every movement you make involves a complex interplay of muscle, bone and joint actions: nerve signals from your brain stimulate and synchronize your muscles, which then provide the mechanical power that moves your bones to bend, straighten or rotate your joints.

Making movements

The nerve signals that activate your muscle contractions originate in an area of your brain called the motor cortex. When you decide to move, signals travel to your muscles via your spinal cord and pass along nerve cells called motor neurons, which connect with each muscle fibre at its neuromuscular junction (NMJ).

The nerve signals trigger the release of neurotransmitters, chemicals that bind to receptor sites on the muscle cells. This prompts specialized structures called organelles to release calcium ions which stimulate myofibril contraction (>>38) making your muscles contract. When the muscle action is over, the calcium ions pass back into the cell organelles for reuse.

Flexing and extending

As your muscles contract, they pull on bones producing movement around the joint. Because muscles can only pull, they usually work in opposing pairs; as one muscle contracts, the opposing one relaxes. Then, when you move back in the opposite direction, the contracted muscle relaxes and the relaxed one contracts. You use your bicep to flex your arm at your elbow, for example, and your tricep to extend it again.

Motion control

During every movement you make, your central nervous system (your brain and spinal cord) is continuously processing information to help you on your way.

Specialized nerve endings called proprioceptors monitor the tension and stretching in your muscles and tendons, so that your brain can fine-tune their activity. Sensors inside your joints monitor where the different parts of your body are in relation to one another. At the same time, your brain uses feedback from your eyes and from the balance sensors within your inner ears to help it to maintain your balance.

Muscle tone

Your muscles are in a constant state of partial contraction, which keeps them firm, healthy and ready for action at all times. This is called muscle tone, and it's the only aspect of skeletal muscle activity that you cannot control voluntarily.

Even when a muscle is relaxed, nerve impulses from your brain stimulate groups of muscle fibres within it to contract and keep it toned. If the nerve supply to a muscle or group of muscles is destroyed by injury or illness, it can no longer stimulate the muscle fibres to contract in this way. This will cause the muscle to lose its tone and become flaccid, and eventually it will start to waste away.

TAKING A STEP

1 **As you step forward your calf muscles pull on the tendons attaching them to the foot, flexing the ankle and making your toes point upwards. Your heel bone hits the ground first, absorbing the force of impact.**

2 **The small bones in the middle of your foot form an arch that spreads the weight of your body over the length of your foot as you roll it forward, from heel to toe.**

3 **As your calf muscles contract, pulling on the Achilles tendon, your heel lifts off the ground. At the same time the tendons and muscles along your foot contract, flexing the joints in your toes ready to push off.**

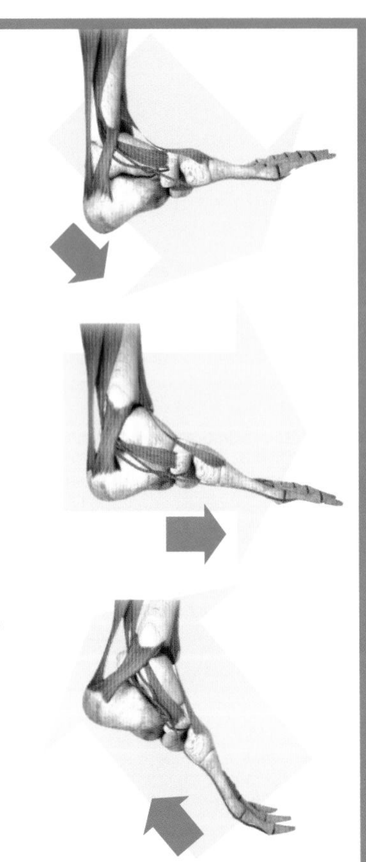

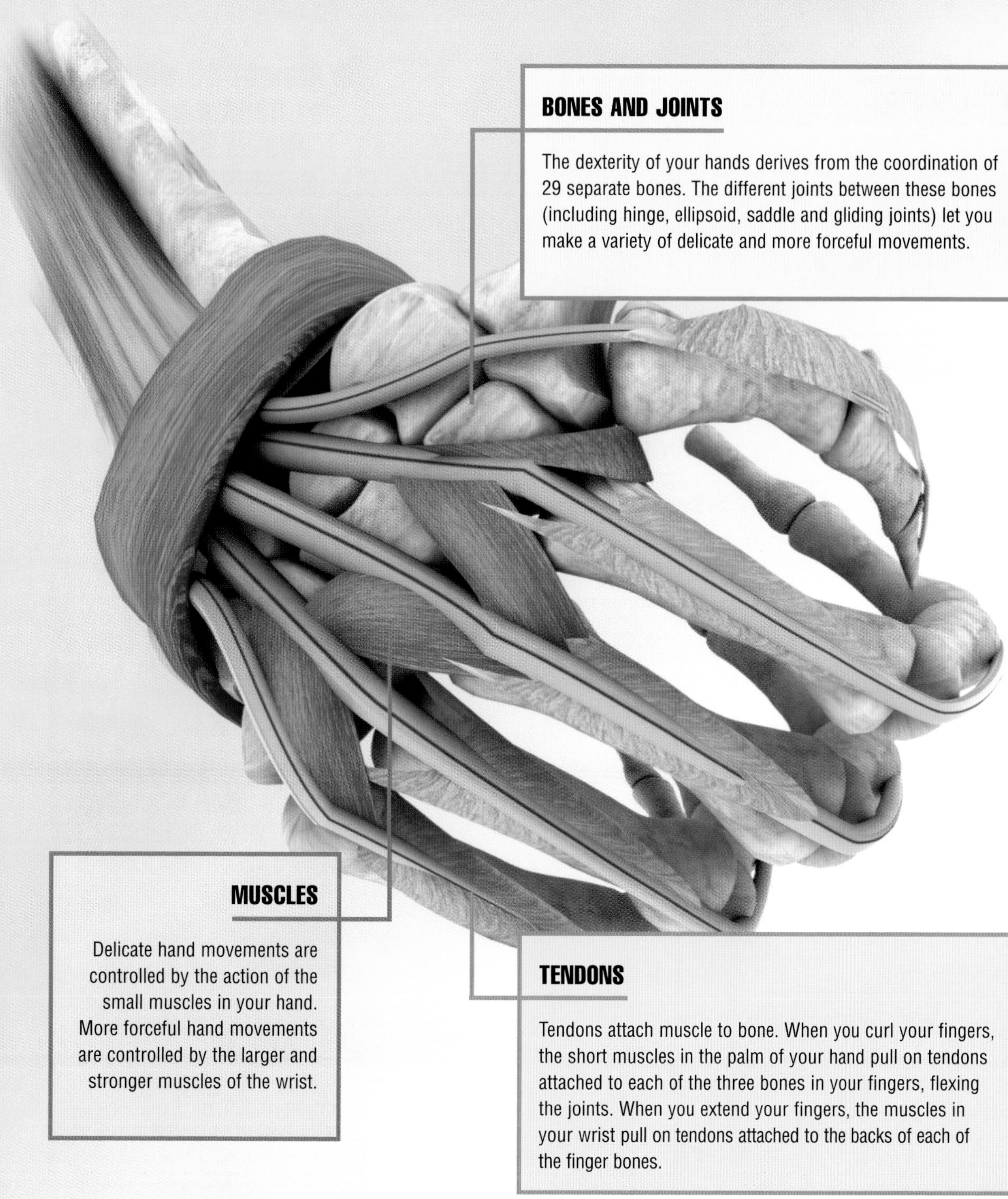

BONES AND JOINTS

The dexterity of your hands derives from the coordination of 29 separate bones. The different joints between these bones (including hinge, ellipsoid, saddle and gliding joints) let you make a variety of delicate and more forceful movements.

MUSCLES

Delicate hand movements are controlled by the action of the small muscles in your hand. More forceful hand movements are controlled by the larger and stronger muscles of the wrist.

TENDONS

Tendons attach muscle to bone. When you curl your fingers, the short muscles in the palm of your hand pull on tendons attached to each of the three bones in your fingers, flexing the joints. When you extend your fingers, the muscles in your wrist pull on tendons attached to the backs of each of the finger bones.

INVOLUNTARY MOVEMENTS

Although the skeletal muscles that you use to move your joints are usually under your voluntary control, they can also contract very quickly without any input from your brain. This happens in reflex actions, such as when you automatically pull your hand away from a hot surface. Then, sensory nerves in your hand send signals not to your brain but to motor neurons in your spinal cord, and these inform the muscles of your arm to contract and pull your hand away.

You also have a number of muscles that always operate automatically, without any conscious control. These involuntary muscles include the cardiac muscle that makes your heart beat and the smooth muscles of your intestines and blood vessels.

Balance and posture

Millions of years ago, our early ancestors evolved from four-legged mammals into bipeds, creatures that stood upright and walked on two legs. Standing and walking now comes naturally to us but defying gravity continues to place strain on our bones and joints.

As we learned to hold our bodies upright, what started off as a horizontal structure slung between two sets of legs evolved into a vertical, load-bearing column. Our spines shortened, our thigh bones became angled in towards the knee and our knees evolved the ability to lock into place. We developed a narrow pelvis to align our legs and large muscles along our hips to keep us stable while walking.

Unfortunately, the human spine is still not fully adapted to standing upright. To keep our bodies erect we need a complex array of muscles, tendons and ligaments. These are vulnerable to damage, which can lead to pain and back problems. The first line of defence against such damage is good posture.

Keeping your balance

Your sense of balance relies on the sensory cues that your body can pick up about your environment and your position in space. You have three main sources for this information:

> 'Almost 10 per cent of people over the age of 65 report balance problems'

- **Visual** If you've ever tried walking through a strange room in the dark, you'll know how disorientating it can be to lose the sensory input from your eyes. It is harder to spot obstacles and, if you do start to lose your balance, you may be slower to react.

DETECTING HEAD MOVEMENTS

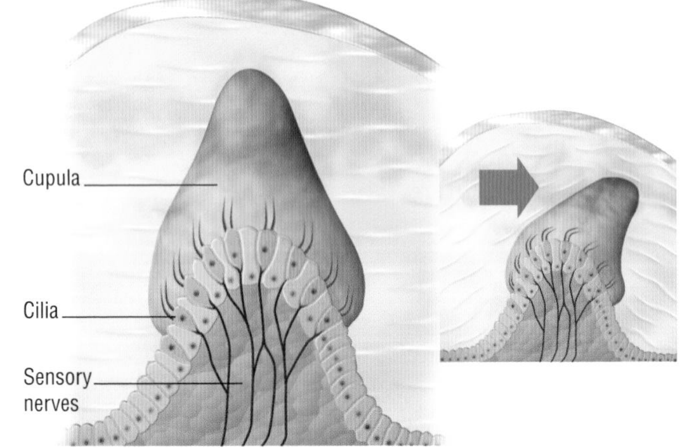

Within each inner ear is a gelatinous mass called a cupula which floats in a electrolyte-rich fluid. As you turn your head the cupula lags slightly behind, making it tug on tiny hairs known as cilia. The movement of the cilia triggers nerve impulses which the brain interprets as head movements.

SENSING THE PULL OF GRAVITY

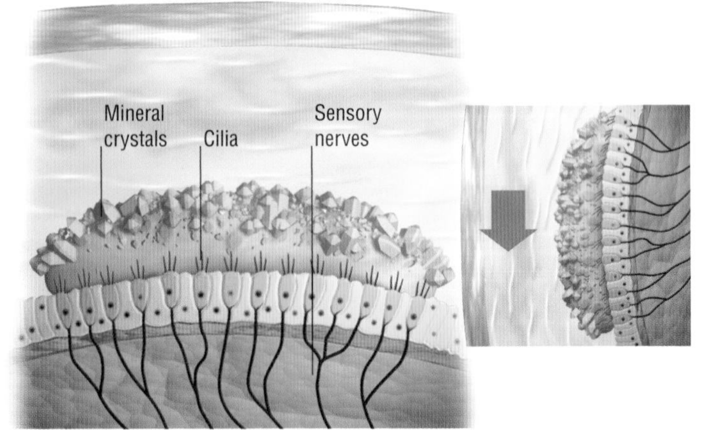

Your inner ears also contain structures called maculae. These consist of millions of tiny mineral crystals attached to cilia. When your head is upright, gravity presses the crystals down against the cilia, triggering nerve impulses. If you tilt your head, the crystals slide to one side, pulling the cilia with them.

THE REFLEX ARC

Your central nervous system processes the information from your proprioceptors and sends signals back to the muscles to make them contract or relax to maintain your body position. This two-way flow of signals is called a reflex arc, and the muscles' responses are called reflex actions. Reflex actions are so automatic that you are unaware that they are happening.

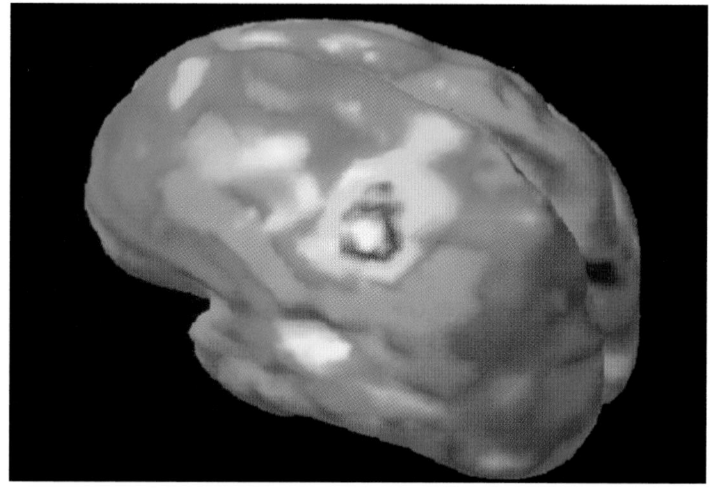

- **Proprioceptive** You have special receptor cells called proprioceptors in the nerve endings of your muscles, joints and ligaments. These provide information about changes in muscle tension, pressure and the movement of your body tissues. Your brain responds to these signals by contracting or relaxing muscles.
- **Vestibular** The inner part of each ear contains a set of three fluid-filled, semicircular canals, set at right angles to each other in the temporal bone at the side of your skull. Each time you move, the fluid in the canals moves and stimulates tiny, hair-like fibres connected to nerve endings.

Signals from these nerve endings tell your brain how much, how fast and in which direction your head and body are moving. Your brain uses this information to control your muscles, which move to keep you balanced.

Another set of sensors, the utricle and the saccule, work in a similar way but respond to gravity rather than movement. They detect the position of your head – whether it is vertical, horizontal or at an angle.

What is good posture?

Good posture is the correct alignment of your bones and joints, especially those of your neck and spine, shoulders, pelvis and legs. If your joints are out of alignment it can lead eventually to damage, pain and disability. The effects of even a slight misalignment over a long period can be considerable. When your posture is correct, however, your muscles and joints keep you upright with a minimum of effort.

Postural muscles

The muscles that you use to maintain your posture include many of the larger muscles of your body (which you also use to move your bones and joints) as well as many smaller muscles called postural muscles.

The postural muscles, such as the muscles that hold your vertebrae in position, are built more for endurance than for strength; their job is to hold and maintain stability rather than create movement. It is thanks to them that the larger muscles can operate your joints effectively and safely. If your posture is poor, your postural muscles are under constant strain and may overstretch.

Posture on the move

Good posture is not static: it is just as important when you are moving as when you are sitting or standing. Professional athletes and dancers go to great lengths to understand and improve the way that their bodies move – but moving effectively is vital for everyone.

DID YOU KNOW?

Not all animals rely on an inner ear for orientation. Some marine invertebrates such as jellyfish and sea anemones have a balance organ called a statocyst. This is a pouch containing a heavy mineralized granule and lined with sensory hairs. As the creature moves, the hairs sense the changing position of the granule, helping it to orient itself.

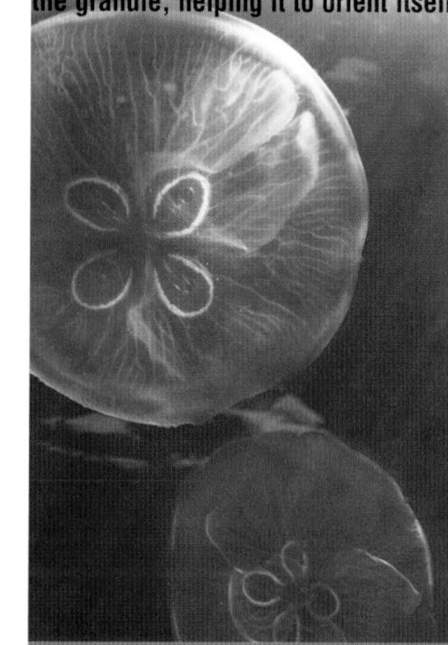

CHOOSING THE RIGHT SHOES

A pair of comfortable, supportive shoes is an essential investment. Inappropriate or ill-fitting shoes may harm your feet, impair your posture and strain the muscles of your legs and back. Good footwear is even more crucial during exercise. Well-designed trainers help you to work out with maximum comfort and minimum risk of injury. They support and cushion your feet and absorb the impact that travels up through your ankles, knees and hips when your feet hit the ground.

Tips for choosing shoes

There are two key factors to consider when buying a pair of shoes: choose a shoe with a solid construction that provides you with all the support you need; and make sure the shoe fits well. Your shoes should match the shape of your feet, fit exactly around the heels without riding down as you walk and leave plenty of room for your toes.

- Feet change in size slightly as you get older. If you are not sure of your exact shoe size, have both feet measured for length and width.
- Feet swell slightly during the day and also when your feet get hot, so buy your shoes towards the end of the day.
- Look for natural materials such as leather that will let your feet breathe.
- Avoid shoes with pointed toes. The toe area should be deep enough to allow your toes to move freely.
- Avoid slip-on shoes. Fastenings such as laces or velcro straps stop your foot slipping forwards or sideways in your shoe.
- Avoid very high heels. The higher the heel the more it affects your gait, pushing your body out of alignment and increasing your risk of knee and back problems.

Choosing the right trainers

You should buy a new pair of trainers after about 100 hours of use – that is, once a year if you do two hour-long sessions per week. There's an enormous range of trainers available, but many are designed as fashion shoes and not as serious sports equipment – to find the right shoe you'll need to consider your foot shape, the way you move, your weight, the surfaces that you intend to run on and the type of activity that you want to perform.

It's usually better to get your shoes from a specialist sports shop, rather than a high street store – especially if you aren't sure which type of trainer is best suited to your needs.

ORTHOTICS

These are devices inserted into shoes to improve foot function and correct abnormal patterns of walking. One of the most common types of insert is the medial post, which is placed under the arch of the foot to prevent over-pronation (>>50–51). Inserts can also be used to help improve body alignment, even up inequalities in leg length or to absorb shock and relieve pressure points. If you feel that you might benefit from orthotics, talk to a podiatrist about getting a pair of custom-made inserts (>>53).

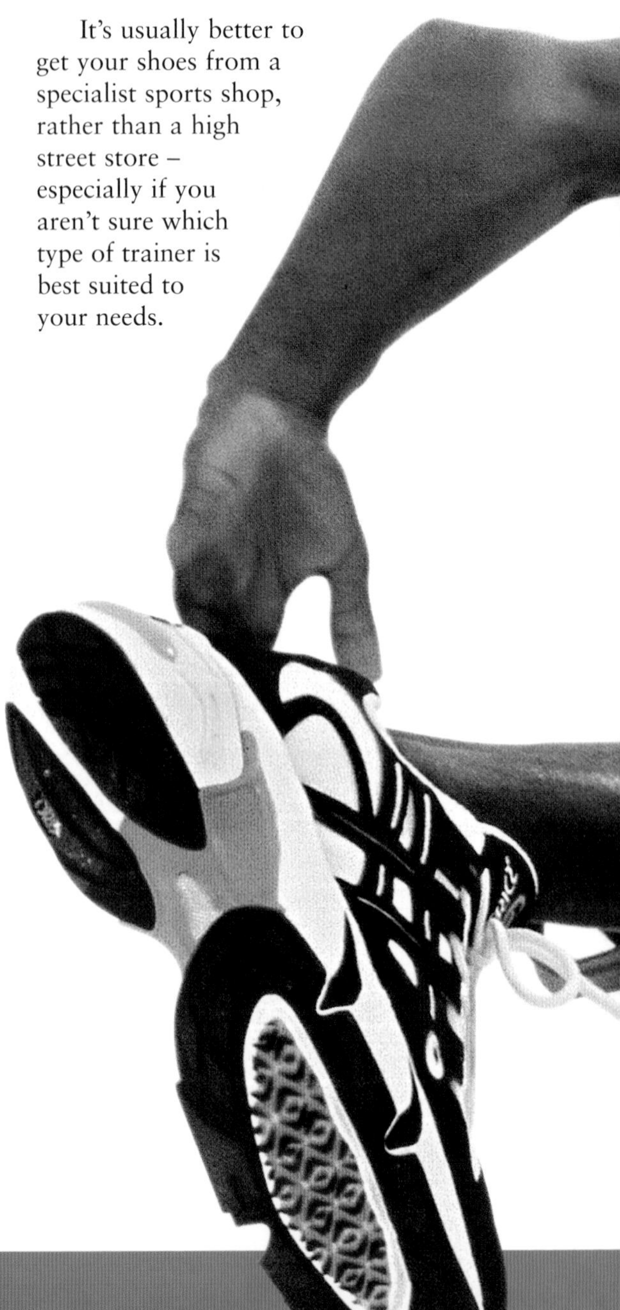

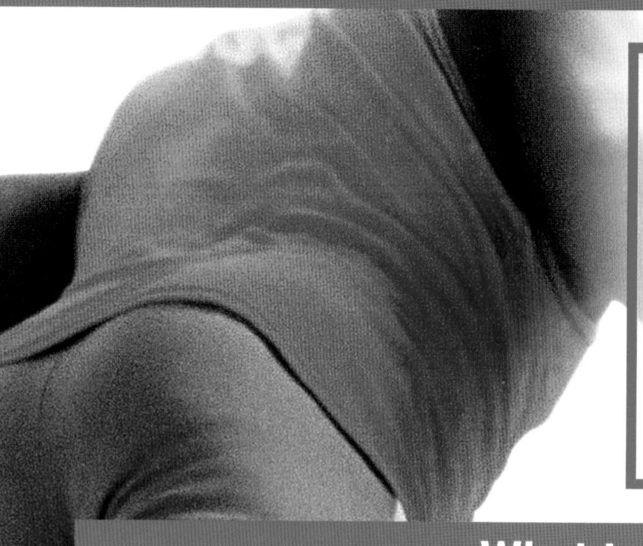

BUYING THE RIGHT RUNNING SHOES

If you are new to running, get advice from a fitness trainer or a specialist sports shop before choosing your shoes. Most manufacturers produce different models to meet the needs of individual runners: there are three basic types of running shoe:

- **Motion control shoes** are relatively rigid, have a straight shape and incorporate a medial post (a support under the arch to prevent the foot rolling inwards). These are designed to counteract excessive rolling and over-pronation >>50-51.
- **Cushioned shoes** have soft midsoles and a more curved shape to encourage roll and are designed for people who under-pronate >>50–51.
- **Stability shoes** offer a compromise. They have some medial support and a semi-curved shape and are suitable for runners with regular pronation.

What type of training shoe do I need?

TYPE OF TRAINER	TYPE OF EXERCISE	WHY IS THE TRAINER APPROPRIATE?
Games shoes	Court games such as tennis, squash or netball that involve sudden sideways movements.	Games shoes should be light and comfortable, with outer soles that grip well and cushioned insoles to absorb the impact when you land. They provide good ankle support to prevent injuries caused by rapid changes of speed and direction.
Cross-trainers	General-purpose activities such as light aerobics and gym work, and occasional walking, jogging or games of tennis or badminton.	Cross-trainers are general-purpose training shoes. They provide a reasonable level of stability, comfort and cushioning and are a good choice if you want to try out a range of activities. However, they lack the proper support and protection offered by sport-specific footwear such as aerobics, walking or running shoes.
Aerobics shoes	Aerobics routines involving sequences of jumping or leaping movements.	Aerobics shoes have soles that grip well to prevent you from slipping, as well as good flexibility and shock absorbency. They also have strong uppers or stabilizing straps to prevent your feet from slipping forwards or sideways within the shoe, and high toe boxes to avoid friction on the tops of your toes and your toenails.
Running shoes	Regular running, running long distances or running over hard ground.	Running shoes should be light but supportive, with plenty of shock-absorbing cushioning and relatively high heels that will prevent excessive strain on your Achilles tendons and calves. Different types of running shoe are available for different runners – see box above for more details.

Maintaining good posture

Poor posture usually involves a distortion in one or more of the three main curves in your spine: the slight forward curve at the base of your neck, the slight backward curve between your shoulders or the forward curve in your lower back.

These curves help your back absorb the force of gravity, and the weight of your body. Any distortion of these, or any sideways curve of your spine (scoliosis), places strain on your vertebrae and on the muscles that support them.

STANDING TALL

- Keep the crown of your head as the highest point
- Tuck in your chin
- Relax your shoulders
- Try to maintain your back's natural curves
- Lift your rib cage
- Pull in your stomach
- Keep your pelvis tucked in
- Keep knees slightly bent
- Breathe evenly

- Do not tilt your head too far forward or back
- Do not arch your back or slouch your body
- Do not tense your body

Risks of poor posture

The long-term effects of poor posture include degeneration of the joints in your spine and lengthening or shortening of the ligaments and muscles of your back. This can lead to musculoskeletal problems ranging from stiffness and poor flexibility to back pain.

When you combine poor posture with lack of regular movement – hours slumped in front of a television or hunched over a computer, for example – you will weaken your back muscles and make yourself even more likely to suffer back problems. Other possible consequences of poor posture include:

- **Headaches** Poor posture while working at a desk or using a computer can also cause your neck and scalp muscles to tense up and this tension can lead to headaches.
- **General health** As well as causing problems for your muscles and joints, a stooped or hunched posture can put pressure on your internal organs. This interferes with their efficiency and function.

Your lungs and digestive system are particularly affected by poor posture: when your chest wall is scrunched up you can only take shallow breaths and pressure on your intestines interferes with your digestion and can lead to constipation.

Walking and running

The way that you walk or run – your gait – is important for your balance and stability as you move. Good gait provides maximum power for minimum effort. The key is to hold your body upright but relaxed, to avoid wasting energy and to keep your balance in check. Leaning too far forward or back while walking or jogging can place unnecessary strain on your hips, knees and spine.

Pronation

When you take a step forward, you should naturally land on the outer edge of your heel,

DID YOU KNOW?

- You use your posture as well as your gestures and facial expressions in order to express your feelings. Good posture makes you look taller, sleeker and more graceful and helps you feel confident. And when your muscles are relaxed, it's almost impossible to feel anxious.
- Good posture also lets you breathe more naturally and efficiently. The key is to keep your body erect without pulling your shoulders too far back or tensing your muscles. People who sit up straight tend to look alert because correct breathing allows the maximum amount of oxygen to reach the brain.

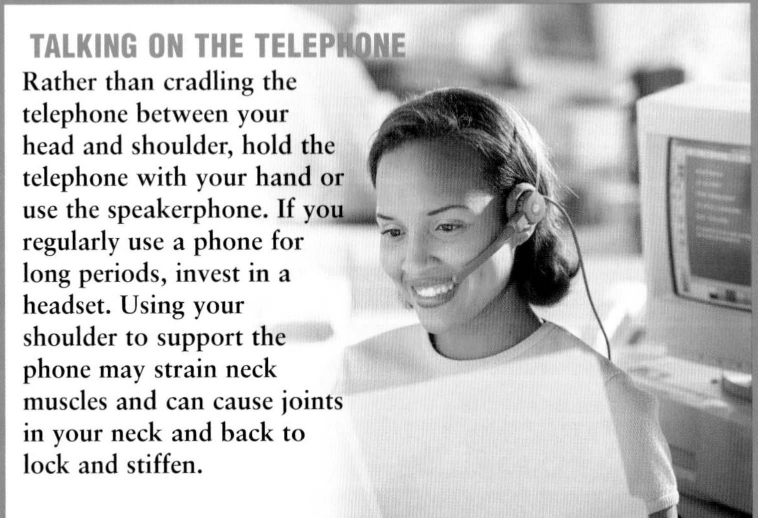

TALKING ON THE TELEPHONE

Rather than cradling the telephone between your head and shoulder, hold the telephone with your hand or use the speakerphone. If you regularly use a phone for long periods, invest in a headset. Using your shoulder to support the phone may strain neck muscles and can cause joints in your neck and back to lock and stiffen.

THE WET TEST

Next time you step out of a bath or shower, check to see what shape footprints your wet feet leave on the floor.

- If the ball, heel and outside edge of your foot leave a mark, but the arch of your foot is not visible, you probably have normal arches.
- If your whole foot, including the arch, leaves a mark, you may have flat feet. Flat feet have a tendency to over-pronate (roll inwards as you walk).
- If the marks left by your heel and the ball of your foot don't join together at all, you may have high arches. People with high arches often under-pronate (do not roll enough).

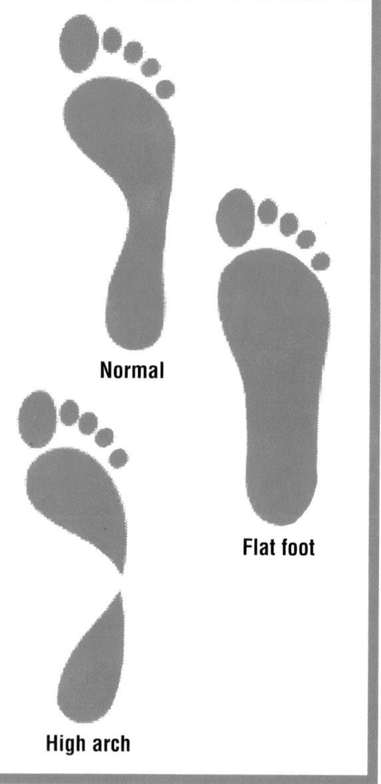

rather than flat on the ground. Your foot then rolls inwards so that the inner edge of the sole takes more of your body weight. This inward roll, known as pronation, helps you to balance and absorbs shock. Without proper pronation, the foot and ankle have problems stabilizing the body. Studies suggest, however, that well over half of the population either under or over-pronate.

- **Over-pronation** Lots of people, particularly people who have very flat or flexible feet, roll their feet too far inwards. This increases the strain on the feet and calves and may contribute to a range of musculoskeletal problems. You may benefit from a special support under the arch known as a medial support.
- **Under-pronation** is most common in people who have very high arches. It is less common than over-pronation, but can be even more harmful for your joints. If you under-pronate, you may benefit from wearing shoes with a soft midsole and curved shape to encourage pronation.

? How well do I walk?

Do any of the following apply to you? If so, you may be rolling your feet too far inwards as you walk and should consider seeing a podiatrist (>>53) or investing in a pair of shoes with good arch support and a firm heel counter.

- [ ] Do you have flat feet? If you are not sure, try the wet test (>>box, left).
- [ ] Check an old pair of shoes. Are the inside edges of your soles particularly worn away?
- [ ] When standing, do your heels lean inwards?
- [ ] When standing, do your knees lean inwards?
- [ ] Do you suffer from knee pain when you are very active which tends to go away when you rest?
- [ ] Do you regularly suffer from problems such as corns, calluses, bunions or ankle sprains?

QUESTIONNAIRE

> ‘Experts estimate that as much as 80 per cent of the population walks with some degree of over-pronation. A much smaller number of people – only a few per cent of the population – under-pronate’

Limiting the damage

However much we try to avoid putting stress on our bodies, the cumulative effects of modern lifestyles take their toll on most of us eventually. The result can be aches, pains, strains and bad backs. Luckily there are lots of ways to limit the effects of poor posture and reduce any symptoms.

Exercise

Strong, well-balanced muscles help to maintain good posture by protecting joints. Poor posture and weak, unbalanced muscles can pull your body out of alignment. Aim for around 45 minutes moderate-intensity exercise three times a week including some weight-bearing exercise and stretching.

Cautious exercise can also relieve pain and reduce damage if problems do occur. Lack of activity, though, makes muscles weaker, slowing recovery time and making re-injury more likely. Certain types of activity may be particularly beneficial:

- **Pilates** Precise, controlled exercises strengthen the body's core stabilizing muscles and improve coordination and muscle balance >>94–95.
- **Alexander Technique** The exercises teach good posture and help to release damaging muscle tensions >>185.
- **Yoga** Gentle, stretching movements improve flexibility; controlled postures encourage body awareness >>92–93.

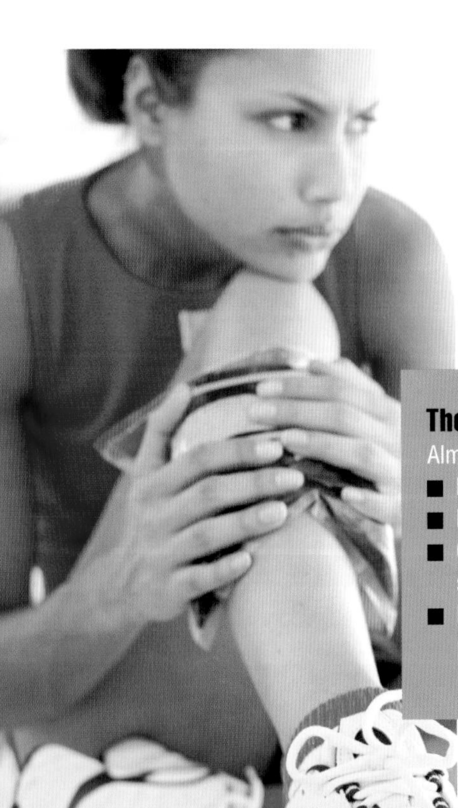

Relaxation

Poor posture places muscles under tension, which can lead to fatigue and further stress. Relaxation techniques such as massage, aromatherapy or even a warm bath can help to release tension from your mind and muscles. Massage is particularly useful as a way to target the painful trigger points and knots in tense muscles that often result from poor posture.

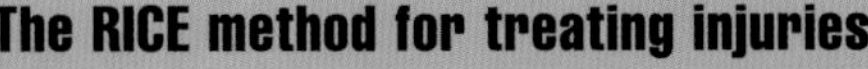

The RICE method for treating injuries

Almost all acute soft-tissue injuries cause less pain and swelling if treated using RICE:

- **Rest** Try to keep the damaged area rested for 2–3 days to give tissues time to recover.
- **Ice** Apply an ice pack immediately after injury to reduce swelling and inflammation.
- **Compression** Wrapping the injured area following injury may also help to reduce swelling and limit movement.
- **Elevation** Keeping the injured area raised can cut swelling by stopping blood from pooling in the injured area.

6 STEPS TO... Give a massage

1 Keep the room warm Maintain a temperature of at least 21°C (70°F) and check there are no draughts. Play some relaxing music.

2 Use massage oil to help prevent friction. Massage with gentle, controlled movements.

3 Check your technique Use the pad of your thumb and rub in small circular motions. Massage the muscles on either side of the spine, rather than the spine itself.

4 Ask the person you are massaging what pressure he or she finds most comfortable. Find out which areas you need to focus on.

5 Find the knots in the muscles and focus on them until you feel them start to loosen.

6 Avoid injured areas Never massage directly over bruises, damaged tissues or varicose veins. Stop the massage if your partner has sudden or unexplained back pain.

Treatments

Acute injuries such as sprains and strains usually respond well to RICE treatment >>box, left.

Painkillers may help in the short term to relieve the pain from both acute injuries and chronic conditions such as back pain. Bear in mind, however, that because painkillers mask the sensation of pain, they do make it easier to cause further damage without realising. Other possible treatments include:

- **Physiotherapy** This can help you to recuperate and relearn good postural habits >>243.
- **Podiatry** A podiatrist can help you to identify and combat any biomechanical problems behind poor posture >>53.

a visit to

THE PODIATRIST (CHIROPODIST)

Podiatrists (also known as chiropodists) diagnose and treat foot and lower limb problems ranging from corns and calluses to arthritis. Podiatrists also analyse gait and posture as it relates to the feet.

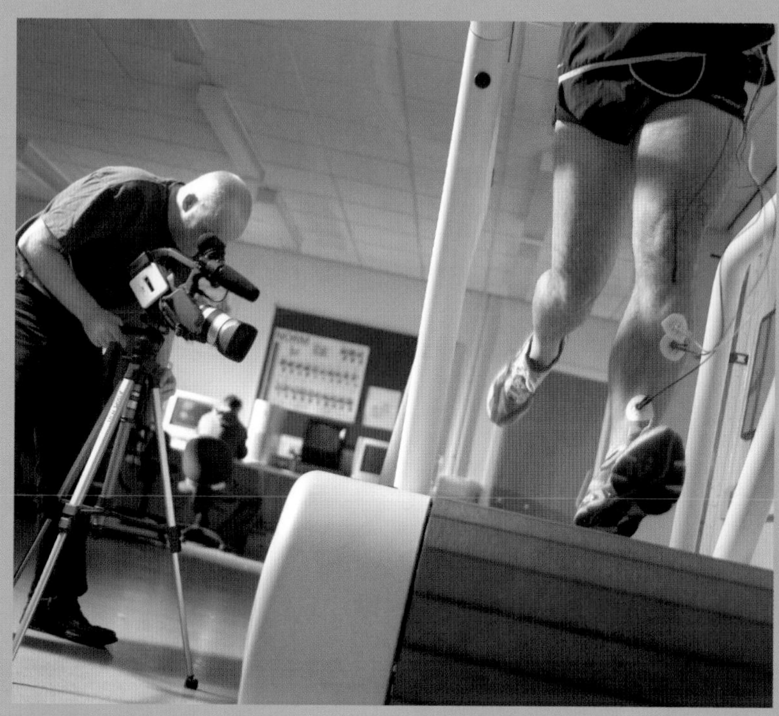

Podiatrists work with people of all ages but play a particularly important role in helping older people to stay mobile and independent. The joints of the foot are small and complex so changes in function due to arthritis or injury can be subtle, which makes the podiatrist's expertise essential.

Podiatrists are also concerned with the mechanics of foot and leg function: factors such as gait, joint alignment and muscle function can affect not only your feet, but also your knees, hips and lower back. A foot that is flatter on one side than the other, for example, can pull you off balance and cause hip pain; a stiff big toe can cause spinal problems.

In most areas of the UK podiatric treatment is available on the NHS – if not, your GP will be able to refer you for private treatment. You can also book private appointments directly. Since July 2003, anyone in the UK calling themselves a chiropodist or podiatrist must be registered with the Health Professions Council (HPC). To ensure professional treatment, you should also check that the podiatrist has completed a degree or diploma in podiatry – look for the letters DPodM or BSc(Podiatry) after the podiatrist's name. Contact the British Chiropody and Podiatry Association if you need a list of practitioners in your area.

Foot care and advice Your podiatrist can offer advice on any aspect of foot care, including foot hygiene, buying properly fitting footwear and common foot problems including infections, circulation problems, bunions, ingrowing toenails, heel pain and arthritis. Podiatrists usually also have experience treating sports injuries such as shin splints, overuse injuries and knee or back pain.

Biomechanical assessment As well as a regular examination, the podiatrist may use X-rays, treadmill gait analysis or pressure-sensitive plates to look at the way that your bones, muscles and other structures are aligned and interact and will consider factors such as stability and posture. Treatments for biomechanical problems range from orthotic inserts to stretching and strengthening exercises or even surgery.

Surgery Most qualified podiatrists are permitted to administer local anaesthetics and are trained in a number of surgical procedures including nail and minor soft tissue surgery. Some podiatrists go on to develop this interest and train as podiatric surgeons. These podiatrists can surgically correct more major foot disorders including joint problems and bone deformities such as hammer toes or heel spurs.

>> **Choosing the right shoes:** page 48 >> **A visit to the physiotherapist:** page 243

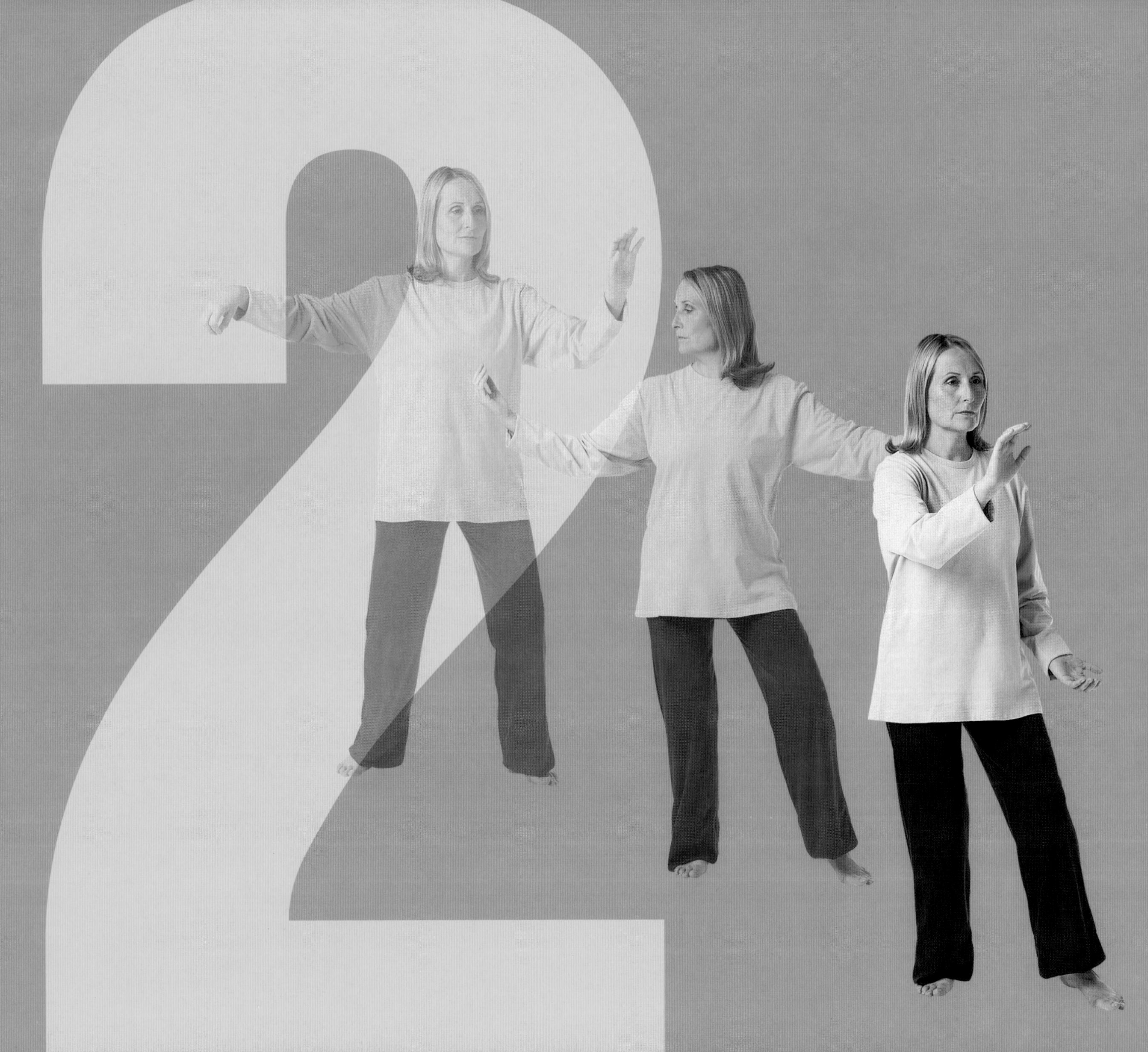
2

FIT FOR LIFE

No matter what age you are, exercise is key to preventing many musculoskeletal problems – building bone, strengthening muscles and increasing joint flexibility. What's more, it helps to promote good balance *and* helps to keep your weight in check. In these pages, you'll find a wealth of options – from strength training to tai chi. All are clearly described so you can easily choose the right exercise for you as you get moving and become truly fit for life.

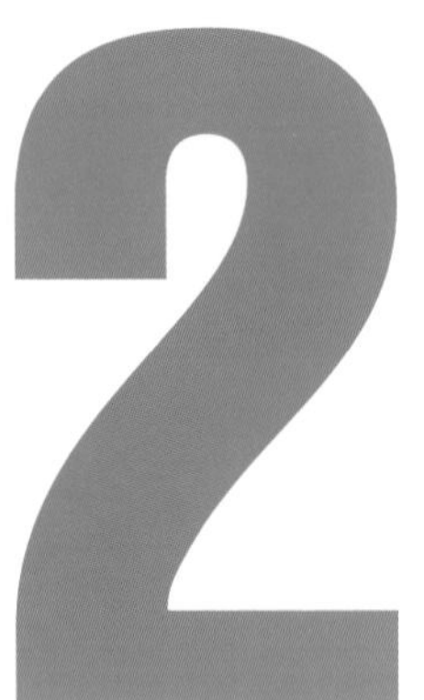

FIT FOR LIFE
The benefits of exercise

Regular exercise is important whatever your age. Frequent activity brings a wide range of benefits for your whole body; it strengthens your muscles, builds and maintains bone density, protects your joints and improves general posture, flexibility and resilience. Exercise is essential to ensure that your mind and body function healthily and happily throughout your life.

Muscle, bone and joint benefits

Regular exercise both maintains and improves the health, strength and resilience of your bones, muscles and joints. Different forms of activity bring different benefits – some improve strength or flexibility, others promote cardiovascular health. Most physical activities bring a combination of these benefits, in varying degrees, but it is useful to understand the main ways in which your body responds to exercise.

Strengthening activities

Movements that place a greater than usual physical load on your body, such as those in weight training or during slow, sustained activities such as yoga, force your bones and muscles to adapt to that stress by growing stronger. Without this type of stimulation your bones and muscles weaken, making it harder to perform everyday activities and increasing your risk of fractures.

Strong muscles also protect your joints. During exercise, muscles not only pull on bones to produce movement, they also work with other muscles to support and stabilize joints. Balanced muscles and stable joints are key to eliminating the poor posture that can place stress on your body.

Most physical activities place some sort of load on your bones and muscles – simply moving your body weight against gravity provides a degree of resistance. Lifting weights is one of the most effective ways to improve musculoskeletal strength, but walking, running and stepping are all weight-bearing activities too. Exercises that involve a sharp impact, such as striking a ball with a racket or landing on the ground after jumping, also put stress on and strengthen your bones and, to some extent, your muscles.

134 Avoiding sports and exercise injuries

158 Exercising with bone and muscle problems

202 Maintaining knee strength through exercise

DID YOU KNOW?

- The human body is designed for constant activity. Astronauts who spend time in a weightless environment (where their bodies don't need to work against gravity) quickly show signs of weakened muscles, high blood pressure and fragile bones – a striking illustration of how inactivity weakens the body.
- During periods of enforced immobilization such as bed rest, up to 25 per cent shrinkage in muscle size can occur in the first 48 hours.

REGULAR EXERCISE

- Improves bone density
- Strengthens your muscles
- Protects your joints
- Strengthens your heart, lungs and circulation
- Bolsters your immunity
- Relieves stress
- Helps weight loss
- Lowers cholesterol

Flexibility and mobility activities

Your body's joints allow a wide range of movements and are supported by a complex arrangement of muscles, tendons and ligaments. For your joints to move freely through their full range of motion, your muscles and other tissues need to stay supple and flexible. Well-balanced muscles also help to maintain good posture.

Unfortunately, many day-to-day activities involve a very limited range of motion and often include long periods spent sitting or bent over. This tightens certain muscles, pulling your body out of alignment. Exercises such as stretching, yoga and Pilates take your joints through their full range of motion, improving your posture and flexibility and reducing your risk of joint injury.

Cardiovascular activities

Any exercise that makes your heart beat faster will help to improve the efficiency with which your heart and lungs supply blood and oxygen to your muscles. As you breathe more deeply you take more oxygen into your lungs; your heart pumps faster and carries oxygen around your body at a greater rate, providing you with energy. Oxygen and nutrients reach your muscles more efficiently and harmful waste products are removed more quickly.

The more you exercise the fitter you become; your heart muscles and the muscles around your lungs grow stronger and your body becomes more proficient at performing this vital process. Improved circulation increases the blood supply to your bones, keeping them healthy and aiding bone mass. Cardiovascular activities such as jogging, brisk walking or aerobics also burn body fat, helping you to lose weight and taking pressure off your joints.

Other benefits

Moderate exercise stimulates your body's immune system by strengthening its response to bacterial infections, viruses and even some forms of cancer. The immune system relies on the efficient circulation of lymph fluid; this fluid helps to remove waste and transports white blood cells to the site of an infection. Since the lymphatic system doesn't have a pump to push it around the body, it relies on muscular activity to help it circulate.

Exercise not only benefits the body; it also works wonders for your mind and emotional well-being. Exercise helps to reduce stress by relaxing tense muscles and releasing chemicals such as endorphins and serotonin, which elevate your mood. This means that exercise can play an important role in pain relief, particularly long-term pain from conditions such as arthritis. Researchers have found that anxiety levels fall most during low-level activities such as walking, yoga and gentle swimming.

WHAT IS THE RIGHT EXERCISE FOR YOU?

TYPE OF EXERCISE	Bone benefits	Muscle benefits	Joint benefits
Cardiovascular workout >> 68		Increases muscle stamina in the active muscles	Improves circulation to the joints
Flexibility workout >> 72		Reduces muscular tension and aids pain relief	Increases range of motion and reduces tightness and pain
Strength-training workout >> 76	Increases bone density	Strengthens and improves muscle tone	Strengthens tendons and ligaments
Aerobics >> 82	Can help to increase bone density	Strengthens and improves muscle tone	Strengthens tendons and ligaments
Jogging >> 84	Increases bone density in the lower body	Increases muscular strength and stamina in the lower body	Strengthens tendons and ligaments in the lower body*
Swimming >> 86		Increases muscle stamina, tone and strength	Increases mobility and improves circulation to the joints
Dance >> 88		Increases muscle stamina and tone	Improves circulation to the joints
Walking >> 90	Can help to increase bone density in the lower body	Increases muscular stamina and tone in the lower body	Increases mobility in the hip, knee and ankle
Skipping		Strengthens and improves muscle tone	Strengthens tendons and ligaments in the lower body*
Golf			
Yoga >> 92	Can help to increase bone density	Improves muscle tone and flexibility	Increases range of motion and reduces tightness and pain
Pilates >> 94		Improves muscle tone and flexibility	Increases range of motion and reduces tightness and pain

CAUTION * If performed excessively, may cause damage to the knees and hips ** If performed excessively or with incorrect form, may impair flexibility

FLEXIBILITY	CARDIOVASCULAR	STRESS	WEIGHT CONTROL
Can help to improve flexibility	Increases lung capacity, strengthens the heart and improves circulation	Releases endorphins and reduces stress	Helps to control weight by raising metabolism and burning calories
Increases flexibility and helps to reduce pain		Reduces stress by relieving muscular tension	
Can improve muscle and joint flexibility**	Increases lung capacity and improves circulation	Releases endorphins and reduces stress	Helps to control weight by burning calories
Can improve muscle and joint flexibility	Increases lung capacity, strengthens the heart and improves circulation	Releases endorphins and reduces stress	Helps to control weight by raising metabolism and burning calories
	Increases lung capacity, strengthens the heart and improves circulation	Releases endorphins and reduces stress	Helps to control weight by raising metabolism and burning calories
Improves joint flexibility	Increases lung capacity, strengthens the heart and improves circulation	Helps reduce stress	Helps to control weight by burning calories
Can help to improve flexibility	Has a mild effect on heart and lung capacity and helps to improve circulation	Relaxes and helps reduce stress	Can help to burn calories
	Has a mild effect on heart and lung capacity and helps to improve circulation	Relaxes and helps reduce stress	Can help to burn calories
	Increases lung capacity, strengthens the heart and improves circulation	Releases endorphins and reduces stress	Helps to control weight by raising metabolism and burning calories
	Helps to improve circulation	Relaxes and helps reduce stress	Can help to burn calories
Increases overall flexibility	Limited cardiovascular effect, except for Ashtanga and Vinyasa yoga	Relaxes and helps reduce stress	Limited effect, with exception of Ashtanga and Vinyasa yoga
Increases overall flexibility		Relaxes and helps reduce stress	Limited effect

Getting exercise into your life

A healthy, active lifestyle is not hard to achieve – it's simply a matter of building some form of recreational activity into your everyday life. Whether you prefer team sports or individual pursuits, the key is to choose an activity that you find convenient, stimulating and enjoyable.

To keep your muscles, bones and joints in good working order you should try to do some form of physical activity every day. You should also take some form of aerobic exercise (that is, something that raises your heart rate, such as brisk walking, cycling or swimming) around three to five times a week. Don't worry if this seems a little daunting at first. It is better to start slowly and work up to this level than adopt an all-or-nothing approach that you won't be able to sustain.

If you currently have a largely inactive lifestyle, start with a little extra activity each day and aim for one or two aerobic-type sessions per week. As you get fitter you will find it easier to do more. Always begin any new exercise programme slowly; this will help you stay motivated and prevent injury.

Make a start!

Exercising with other people is a great way to make new friends and stay motivated. There are many health clubs, sports centres and other organizations that offer regular exercise classes. Your local library will have a list of the sessions in your area.

If you prefer a less organised type of activity, you may enjoy walking, jogging or swimming. A brisk walk is an ideal, low-impact exercise for beginners and older people and swimming provides a gentle aerobic workout without putting too much stress on the joints.

There are also plenty of simple day-to-day changes you can make to improve your bone and muscle health. On short journeys, for example, try walking or cycling instead of taking the car and take 15 minutes out of your day to stretch a little. Whatever type of exercise you choose, there are a few general points worth bearing in mind:

- Choose activities you enjoy and vary them to keep yourself motivated.
- Aim for regular, moderate activity rather than short bursts of exhausting exercise, and set yourself attainable goals.
- Aim to include some form of aerobic exercise, muscle toning and flexibility exercise into your routine.
- Be realistic about your current fitness level – don't try and push yourself too hard or you may injure yourself.
- Leave one or two days' rest between strenuous exercise to give your body time to recover – fatigue and irritability are signs you may be working too hard.
- Find a time of the day that suits you and set aside a regular period each day at that time. If you are a morning person, try

DID YOU KNOW?

- **It is easier than you think to burn off calories: a brisk 20-minute walk can burn up to 100 calories, 20 minutes washing dishes can burn 50 calories.**
- **Small changes add up to big results – walking up two flights of stairs daily instead of taking a lift can burn around 15,000 extra calories over the course of a year.**

?

Do I get enough exercise?

Answer the following questions with a simple yes or no. The more times you tick 'yes', the greater your need to incorporate more regular activity into your daily life. Then, check your resting heart rate against the chart – if your fitness is 'poor' you may need to do more exercise.

YES	NO	
☐	☐	Do you regularly watch more than 3 hours of television a day?
☐	☐	Do you do less than 20 minutes of moderate, physical activity (such as walking, gardening, or golf) per day?
☐	☐	Do you do less than 45 minutes of mid-level activity (such as swimming, aerobics or jogging) twice a week?
☐	☐	Do you get out of breath easily when walking?
☐	☐	Do you prefer to drive short distances (half a mile or so) rather than walking?
☐	☐	Do you get out of breath when climbing your stairs?
☐	☐	Do you have trouble sleeping at night?
☐	☐	Are you overweight?
☐	☐	Do you suffer from non-injury related aches and pains?
☐	☐	Do you often find yourself becoming irritable?
☐	☐	Do you feel you need more exercise? Answer honestly!

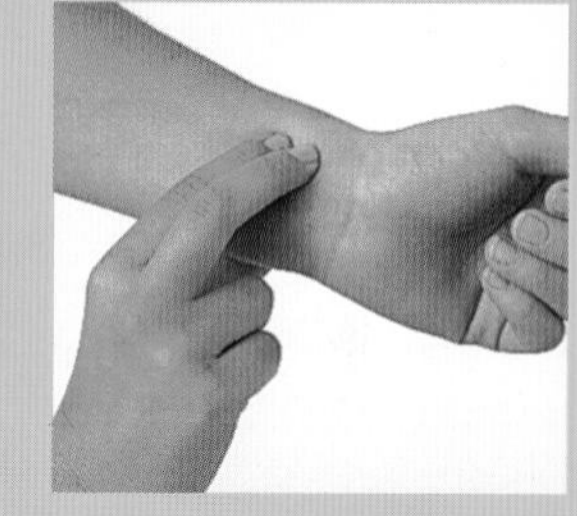

Place the first two fingers of your hand on the inside of your opposite wrist just under the crease and below the large pad at the base of your thumb. Press gently until you can feel your pulse. Start counting the beats with the first beat counting as zero. Count the pulse for 10 seconds, then multiply the number you get by six to get your resting heart rate per minute. Check the chart below to find your approximate fitness level. If you score a 'poor', you may need to do more exercise.

	POOR	REASONABLE	EXCELLENT
Men			
Aged 20–29	Over 84	84–64	Under 64
Aged 30–39	Over 84	84–64	Under 64
Aged 40–49	Over 88	88–66	Under 66
Aged over 50	Over 88	88–68	Under 68
Women			
Aged 20–29	Over 94	94–72	Under 72
Aged 30–39	Over 96	96–72	Under 72
Aged 40–49	Over 98	98–74	Under 74
Aged over 50	Over 102	102–76	Under 76

to set aside some time then; if you have more energy at night, make time for a regular evening work-out.

Exercise your way

The type of exercise you choose will depend on what goals you have set yourself. But you also need to find an exercise that suits your personal likes and interests, your age and the amount of time you have available. No matter how much you know something is good for you, if it becomes a chore you'll soon find plenty of reasons to avoid it. So if the thought of going to the gym fills you with dread, don't go – from yoga and dancing to walking the dog, you are bound to find something that suits you better.

Remember that you lead by example. What your children and grandchildren see and learn from you about keeping active and healthy will affect their behaviour and well-being long into the future.

DID YOU KNOW?

Physical fitness is about more than bulging muscles – it's also about body balance and coordination. An effective exercise programme should encourage good posture and flexibility through stretching as well as increasing muscle strength.

Exercises that simply strengthen your muscles, such as lifting weights, also lead these muscles to contract and tighten, which can cause trapped nerves and increase pressure in your joints. Tight muscles can also pull your body out of alignment, placing strain on other parts of your body. People with tight hamstrings often complain of lower back pain, for example; stretching your hamstrings may help to relieve this pain.

What's the right exercise for me?

Choosing a suitable activity is a personal and a practical matter. Don't take up an exercise simply because you think it is good for you – make sure you enjoy it too. Many people find that alternating between different types of exercise helps them to obtain a wider range of benefits and keeps them motivated. The following questions and answers may help you to decide what is best for you.

Q How can I improve my strength?

A The best way to achieve this is through specific strength-training exercises, such as lifting weights. However, various forms of aerobics training and yoga can also help.

Q How can I lose weight?

A Include aerobic-type exercises to raise your heart rate and burn body fat. Cardiovascular training, skipping, jogging and aerobics are all suitable activities. If you are very overweight, start with a gentle walk or swim – these exercises will not place undue stress on your joints.

Q I haven't done any regular exercise for some time, where should I start?

A If you are very out of condition, start your new exercise programme slowly. Walking and swimming are great ways to start improving your fitness without putting too much stress on your body. Flexibility training is also useful.

Q I hate going to the gym. Is there any type of exercise can I do at home?

A Most forms of exercise are easy to adapt to home training. Good exercises include flexibility training, yoga, Pilates, aerobics, skipping and strength training. All these exercises are discussed in greater detail over the following pages.

Q I've had some problems with my joints – how can I avoid further injury?

A It may be best to stick to a low-impact exercise, such as walking, swimming or gentle cycling, that won't place too much stress on your muscles and joints. Some type of flexibility training, such as yoga or Pilates, may help to prevent further injury.

Q I'm not quite as young as I used to be! What type of exercise should I try?

A Low-impact activities such as walking, swimming, cycling, tai chi and golf are all well suited to older people. Dancing is a fun, sociable way to maintain tone and flexibility.

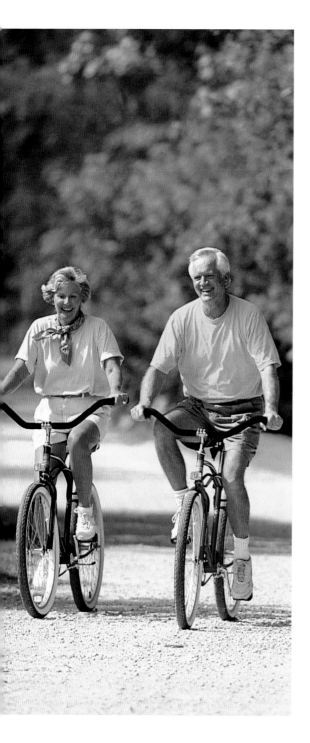

Exercising safely

If you are out of shape or have existing health problems, you should always seek your doctor's advice before embarking on an exercise regime. Bear in mind that you can have too much of a good thing: over-exercising, exercising with an incorrect technique or too much weight loss can harm bone development and cause injuries. To avoid strain, sprains and other injuries, follow these recommendations:

- **Warm up before exercise** This helps to avoid muscle injuries by preparing your body for activity. Stretching is especially important in the morning, when muscles are less flexible and injuries more likely.
- **Cool down after exercise** Rather than stopping abruptly, do a few gentle stretches to keep your muscles flexible and avoid aches and pains later.
- **Exercise within your limits** Build up slowly, pace yourself and listen to your body; pain is a warning sign, so never ignore or try to work through it. Seek medical advice if pain persists after you have stopped exercising.
- **Avoid sudden twisting movements** Movements that cause you to sharply bend or twist your back can place excessive strain on your spine, especially if you are out of condition or have a complaint such as osteoporosis.
- **Stay hydrated** Water is important to maintain your core temperature during exercise and prevent fatigue and muscle cramps. Research suggests that you should rehydrate after activity rather than sipping water continuously during exercise.
- **Wear supportive shoes** Cushioned, flexible soles help to absorb shocks and prevent joint injury. If you have flat feet, choose a 'motion control' or 'stability' shoe that will prevent your foot rolling inwards with each step; choose trail shoes if your activity involves rough terrain. Wear loose, comfortable clothing.

MUSCLE CRAMP

The build-up of chemicals in your muscles after exercise and the loss of salt and water through sweating can cause painful muscle spasms. Stretching and gently massaging the muscle should help to relieve the cramps.

- ***Calf cramps*** **Straighten out your leg and pull your toes towards you to stretch your calf muscle.**
- ***Hamstring cramps*** **Lie down and raise your leg in the air. Straighten your leg and massage the muscles along the back of your thigh.**
- ***Foot cramps*** **Stand on your toes to stretch out the muscles along the soles of your feet.**

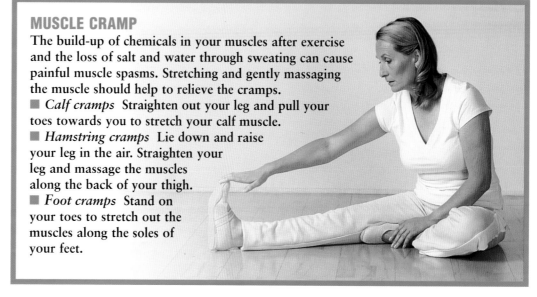

Essential warm-up and cool-down

Warming up before exercise prepares your body for the stress of activity. Likewise, a cooling-down period lets your heart rate and breathing return to pre-exercise levels.

It is also important to stretch after exercise to counteract muscle tightening and reduce the chance of stiffness and sore muscles. Even with a good warm-up and cool-down you may still feel a little muscle soreness a day or so after exercise; you can alleviate any discomfort with a few more gentle exercises.

WARM-UP ROUTINE

Raising your body's temperature and warming your muscles makes them looser and more pliable. It increases blood flow, bringing oxygen and nutrients to the working muscles, and prepares your mind and body for activity.

Your warm-up should consist of gentle physical movements to raise your body temperature. The routine shown here shouldn't take more than 5 minutes: if you are in a hurry and you're not planning anything too strenuous to follow, you can pick just a few exercises – but make sure you include at least 1–2 minutes of side steps or a similar aerobic activity to boost your temperature and elevate your heart rate. If you have the time, you could continue your warm-up with movements specific to the intended activity: if you plan to go running, for example, jog at a slow pace to build up to your normal tempo.

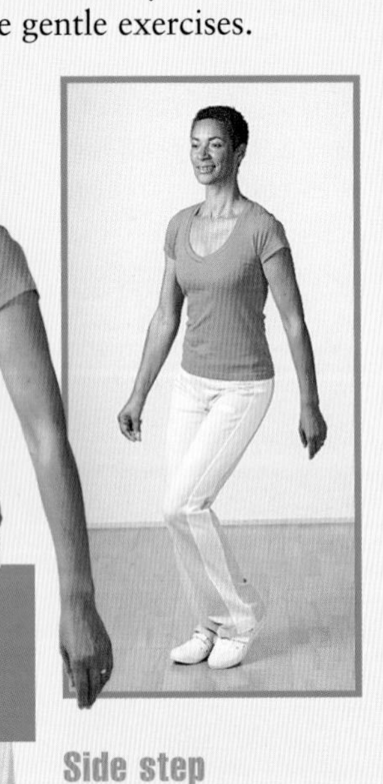

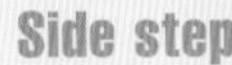

1

Side step

Bring your feet together. As you sway to your right, step your right leg to the side and allow your left leg to follow, so that you are standing with your feet together once more. Repeat the movement over to your left side, with your left leg stepping and your right leg following. Continue stepping in this way for at least 1–2 minutes.

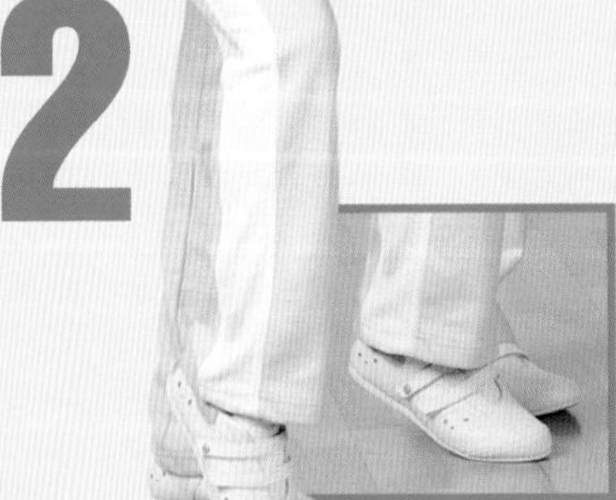

2

Ankle circles

Lift your right foot and place your toes against the floor. Using your toes as a pivot, circle your ankle 10 times in a clockwise direction and 10 times anti-clockwise. Repeat the exercise with your left foot.

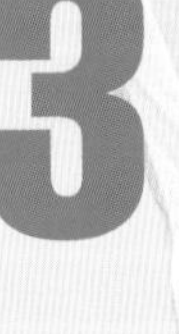

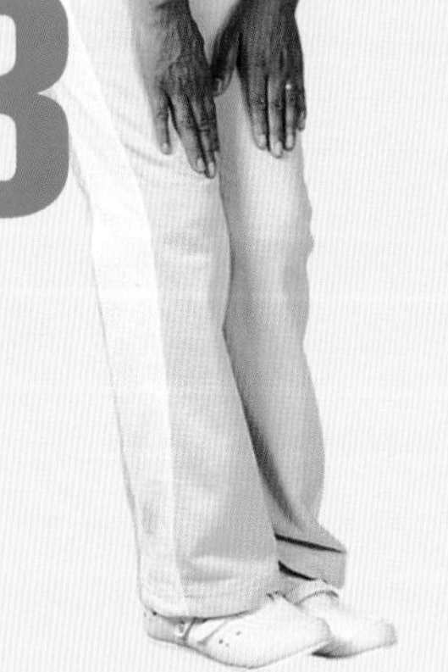

3

Knee circles

Bring your feet together and gently place your hands just above your knees. Bend your knees a little and slowly circle the knees 10 times in one direction, using your hands for support. Repeat 10 times in the opposite direction.

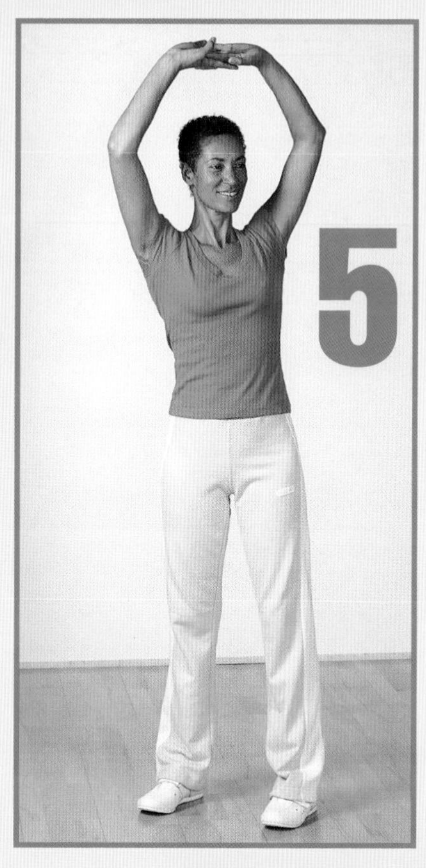

Arm raise and twist

Stand with your feet together, your arms down in front of you and your fingers interlocked. Inhale and raise your arms above your head, turning your palms towards the ceiling. Smoothly twist your torso to face to the right. Try to twist from the waist and keep your feet firmly on the floor. Take three or four normal breaths before twisting to the left.

5

6

Shake

Gently shake your hands, keeping your wrists and fingers loose and breathing normally. Do this about 20 times before moving onto your arms. Keep your hands, elbows and shoulders relaxed and shake your whole arms around 20 times. Finally, let your whole body bounce up and down around 20 times, keeping your limbs as loose and relaxed as possible.

4

Hip circles

Place your hands on your hips. Keep your knees slightly bent and gently circle your hips 10 times to the right and then 10 times to the left. Imagine you are slowly twirling a large hula-hoop around your waist.

CAUTION

Always perform the aerobic warm-up phase before stretching. Your muscles and the connective tissue that surrounds your muscles will not stretch easily while cold, making it easier to injure yourself.

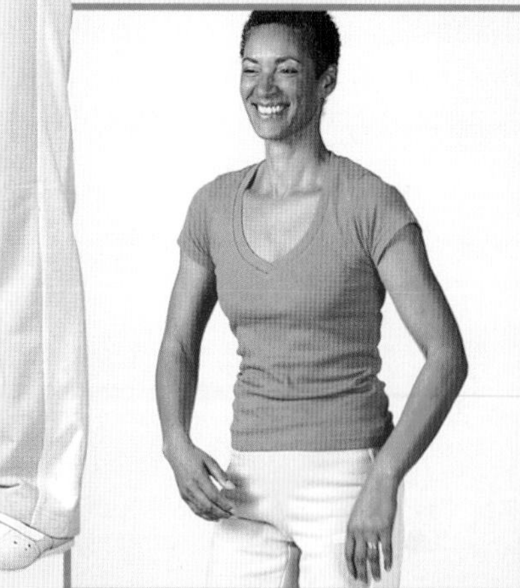

SIMPLE STRETCH ROUTINE

Stretching reduces the risk of injury and stiffness, increases the range of movement in your joints and improves flexibility. You can make stretching the second part of your warm-up routine, if you have time, and you should always stretch after cooling down at the end of your exercise period.

The stretch routine shown here should only take a couple of minutes to perform: you could also add the stretches on pages 74–75 if you have the time. If your exercise routine targets particular muscle groups or areas of the body, try to include some stretches specifically for those areas.

Carry out stretches in a slow and controlled manner and do not hold your breath. Exhale as you move into the stretch and breathe normally as you hold the stretch. Hold each stretch for 15–20 seconds.

Calves

Step your left leg forward and bring your right foot up onto its toes. Bend your knees and place both hands on your left thigh for support. Press your right heel down towards the ground until you feel a slight stretch in your right calf. Hold this stretch for 15–20 seconds, then change legs and repeat. If you wish to increase the stretch, face a wall and use both hands to push against the wall.

Hamstrings

Place your right leg a little way out in front of you. Bend your left leg and place both hands on your left thigh for support. Slowly and without rounding your back, lean forward until you feel a slight stretch at the back of your right leg or behind your right knee. Hold this stretch for 15–20 seconds, then change legs and repeat. If you wish to increase the stretch, place your front leg on a step or low stool.

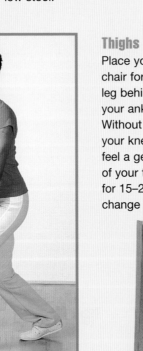

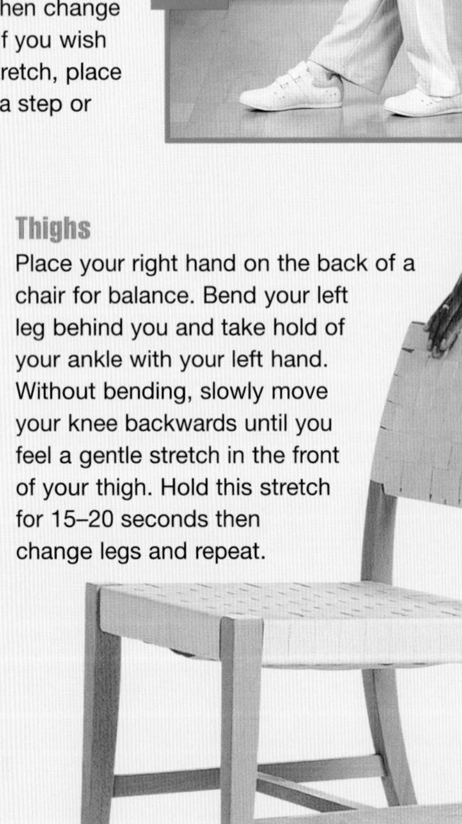

Thighs

Place your right hand on the back of a chair for balance. Bend your left leg behind you and take hold of your ankle with your left hand. Without bending, slowly move your knee backwards until you feel a gentle stretch in the front of your thigh. Hold this stretch for 15–20 seconds then change legs and repeat.

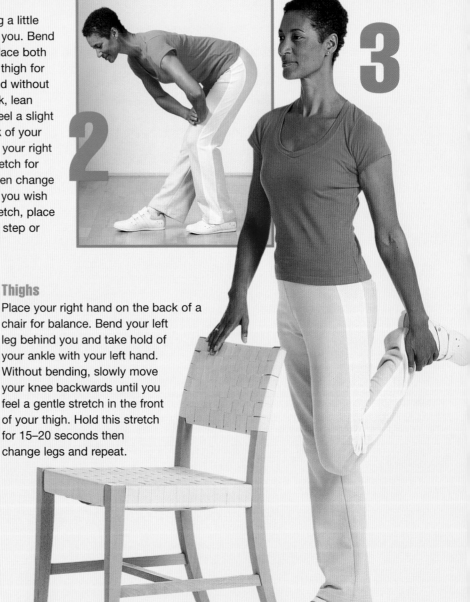

Chest

4

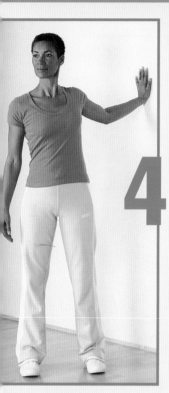

Stand next to a wall. Place your left palm flat against the wall at about shoulder height with your arm slightly bent. Without straining, gently rotate your body to the right until you feel a stretch across your chest. Hold this stretch for 15–20 seconds then change arms and repeat.

Shoulders

5

Cross your left arm in front of your body at shoulder level and place your right hand just behind the elbow. Use your right hand to gently pull your left arm further across your body until you feel a slight stretch at the back of your shoulder. Hold this stretch for 15–20 seconds. Relax both arms for a moment, then change arms and repeat.

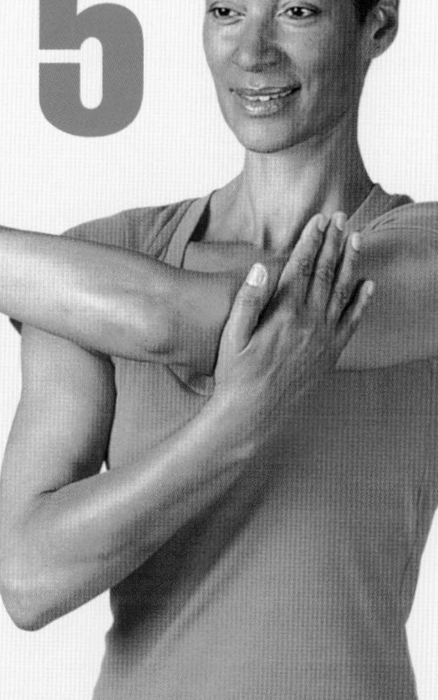

COOL-DOWN ROUTINE

Always cool down for 5–10 minutes after exercise to give your heart rate, temperature and breathing a chance to return gradually to normal. Cooling down properly will help to eliminate waste products in the muscles, such as lactic acid, reducing the potential for muscle soreness. You can cool down in one of two basic ways:

- Continue your chosen exercise at a much lower intensity. If you have just been jogging, for example, spend a few more minutes jogging at a slower pace before gradually slowing to a brisk and then normal walking speed.
- Design your own cool-down routine. This might be made up of light aerobic activity such as walking or cycling for 5–10 minutes, followed by some breathing exercises.

Walking

1

Walk at a brisk pace for a couple of minutes before gradually slowing to a normal walking pace. Continue at normal walking pace until your breathing has returned to a relaxed and comfortable level. If space is a problem, you can walk on the spot.

Breathing

2

Stand with your feet a comfortable distance apart, raise your arms out to the side and then overhead, inhaling deeply as you do. Exhale as you bring your arms back down to your sides. Repeat this for 5 full breaths.

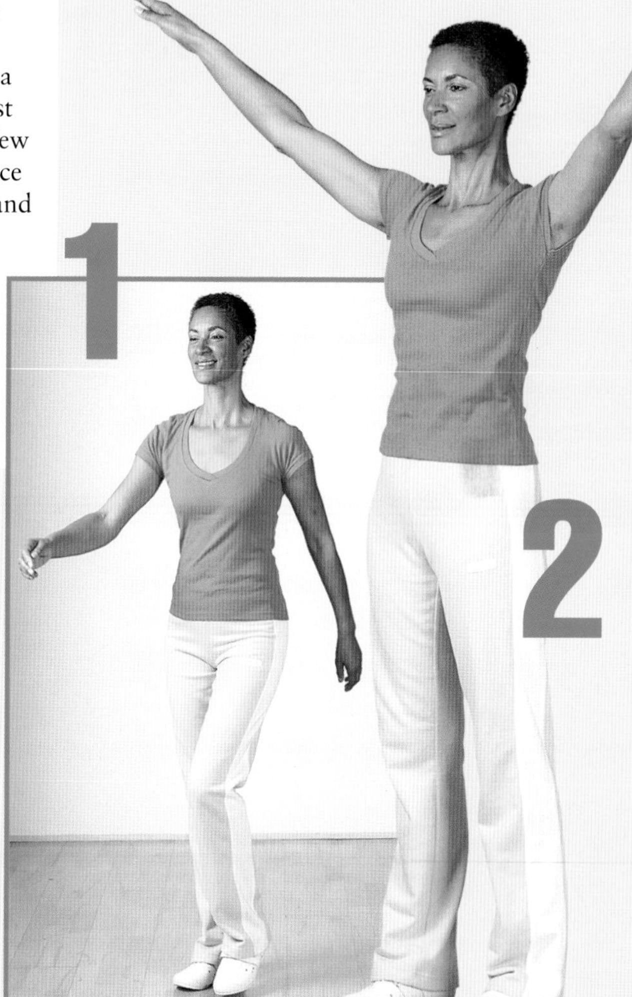

A cardiovascular workout

Regular cardiovascular exercise strengthens your heart and lungs, increasing the efficiency with which your blood vessels supply oxygen and blood to your muscles, and also improves general fitness. It is an excellent way to burn body fat, reducing stress on your bones and muscles, and brings a host of other physical benefits.

What happens?

During cardiovascular exercise your body respires aerobically, meaning 'with oxygen'. Your breathing gets deeper as you take more oxygen into your lungs and your pulse quickens as your heart pumps blood faster and more forcefully around your body. Your blood vessels dilate to allow more oxygenated blood to your muscles and carry waste out of your system.

Bone, joint and muscle benefits

Your heart and the muscles around your lungs, like any other muscles in your body, respond to this type of training by getting stronger. Strong intercostal muscles improve the efficiency with which your lungs transfer oxygen to the blood and a strong heart can pump more blood around the body with each beat. This means your body doesn't need to work as hard to supply your muscles with oxygenated blood, improving your cardiovascular fitness and helping you perform physical tasks more efficiently.

Your body uses the oxygen it takes in during cardiovascular exercise to convert the stored energy in sugars and fats into useable energy; the more exercise you do, the more body fat you burn off. This not only lowers the risk of heart attack, high blood pressure and diabetes, it also reduces the stress on your bones and joints.

Other benefits

Activities such as running and brisk walking help to build bone mineral density in your lower body due to their repetitive impact. This makes bones stronger and less likely to fracture. Rowing helps to build good bone density in the upper body.

In addition to the physical benefits, regular cardio activity releases chemicals called endorphins into your body, which relieve stress and can help to ease pain.

What type of exercise?

Any exercise that raises your heart rate will benefit your cardiovascular system and help you to lose weight, so long as it is performed frequently, for a sufficient duration and at the correct intensity – the FIT principle (see right). Popular cardio activities include running, rowing and cycling, aerobics and gym-based workouts using equipment such as stepping machines.

Because of the range of equipment available, many people prefer to work out at their local gym, but training at home or outside can be equally effective. Running requires no equipment other than a good pair of training shoes; cycling provides excellent cardio benefits and is easy to incorporate into your everyday life; even walking up and down the stairs in your house will give you a fantastic workout.

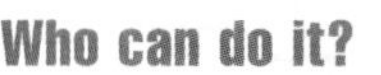

Who can do it?

Cardiovascular training can be demanding and people who lead a

DID YOU KNOW?

- **Your heart beats every second of your life, without rest. During physical exertion your heart's regular workload can rise by up to 300 per cent.**
- **The muscles around your lungs (the diaphragm and intercostal muscles) help you take around 17,000 breaths each day, every day, for life.**
- **The muscular, elastic walls of your arteries and veins drive around 7200 litres (1600 gallons) of blood around your body each day.**

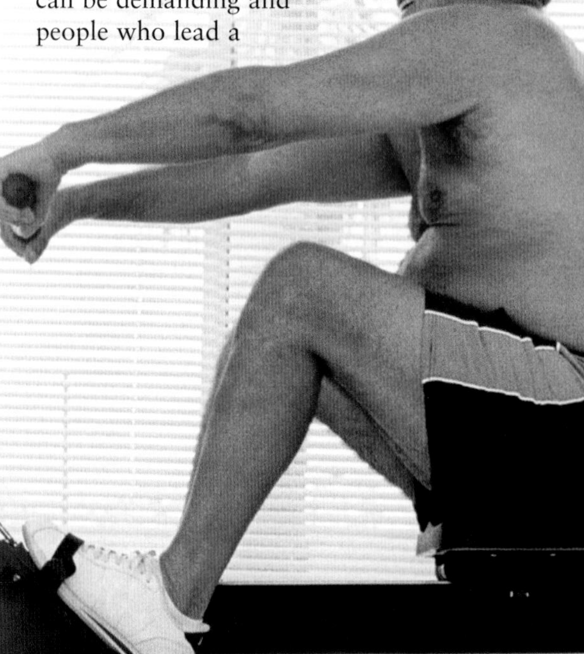

usually sedentary lifestyle or who are overweight should try to build up the intensity and duration of their activity over time. Nonetheless, some form of cardiovascular activity is important for everyone and people who are unfit or overweight will benefit from this type of exercise more than most.

Running can place stress on the joints of the hips and legs and is best avoided by anyone already at risk of joint problems. Rowing, cycling and cross training all provide the benefits of cardiovascular exercise without placing excessive stress on your joints and connective tissues.

The FIT principle

The acronym FIT stands for frequency, intensity and time. The right levels of these elements are key to any cardio programme.

- **Frequency** This is how often you exercise. To achieve a reasonable level of cardiovascular fitness your should work up to exercising three to five times per week. Avoid working out every day – your body needs time to rest and repair.
- **Intensity** If your heart rate does not increase during exercise, you are not working hard enough to receive any cardiovascular benefit from the activity. Work your heart too hard, however, and you may place your health at risk. See the box, right, for advice on finding your target heart rate.
- **Time** This is the duration of the exercise session. Aim for around 10 minutes warm-up, 10–20 minutes of cardiovascular exercise, and a 5–10 minute cool-down period.

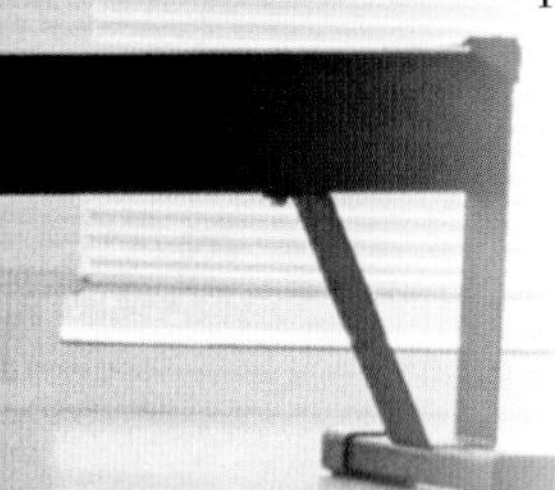

GET YOUR HEART WORKING EFFECTIVELY

To get the most benefit from a cardiovascular regime you need to know your target heart rate and work at an intensity that will keep your heart beating at this rate. To work out your target heart rate, you will first need to know your maximum heart rate (HR max). This is the maximum number of beats per minute that your heart is capable of making. To find your HR max, simply subtract your age from 220. You should aim to work at around 65–90 per cent of your maximum intensity. For most people 75 per cent is a good level at which to operate. To calculate your target active heart rate, therefore, simply take 75 per cent of your HR max.

Try to keep your heart rate around this target level. Many cardio machines have built in pulse monitors so that you can keep track of heart rate as you work out; a slightly more accurate option is a portable heart rate monitor that you strap to your chest – there is now a good range of affordable models on the market. Alternatively, you can also take your heart rate manually: take your pulse after about 5 minutes of activity, count the number of beats over 10 seconds and multiply by 6 to get your heart rate per minute. You can then adapt the intensity of the exercise to get closer to your target rate and check your pulse again. You should soon get a feel for the right level.

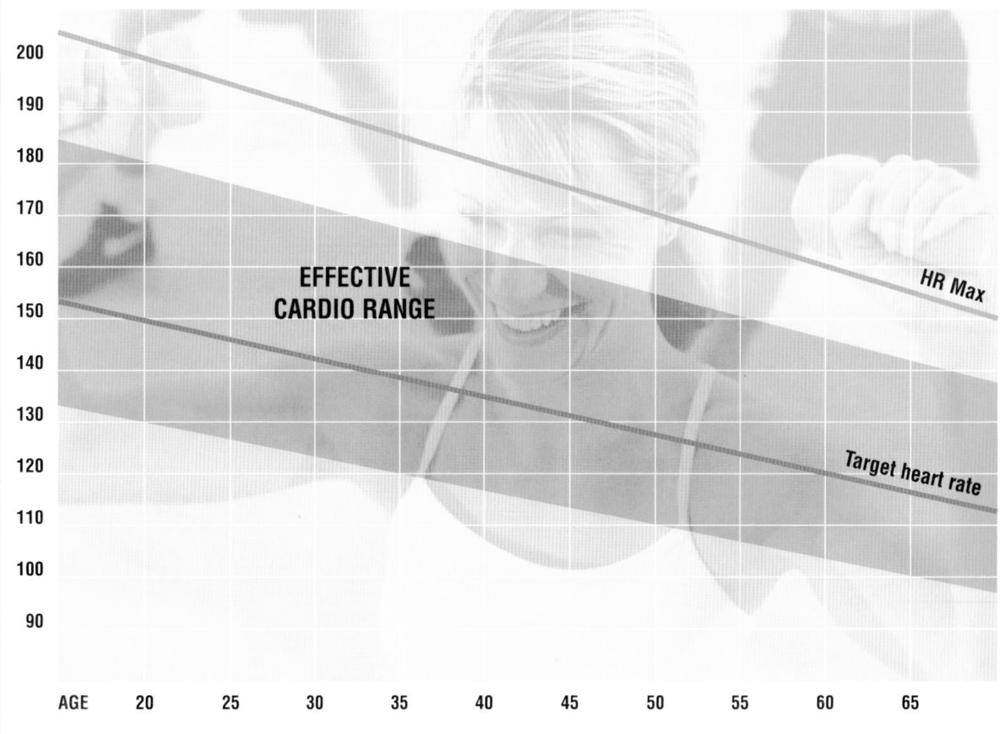

A cardiovascular circuit

Cardiovascular circuits involve performing a series of exercises in quick succession to raise the heart rate while working different areas of the body.

Perform each exercise shown here continuously for 30 seconds, with a short period of rest between each one. This constitutes one circuit. If you are a beginner or are out of shape, perform the circuit with around 30 seconds rest between each exercise. As your fitness increases, slowly decrease the rest periods, first to 25 seconds, then to 20 seconds and finally to 15 seconds. Once you are comfortable with this, perform the complete circuit twice.

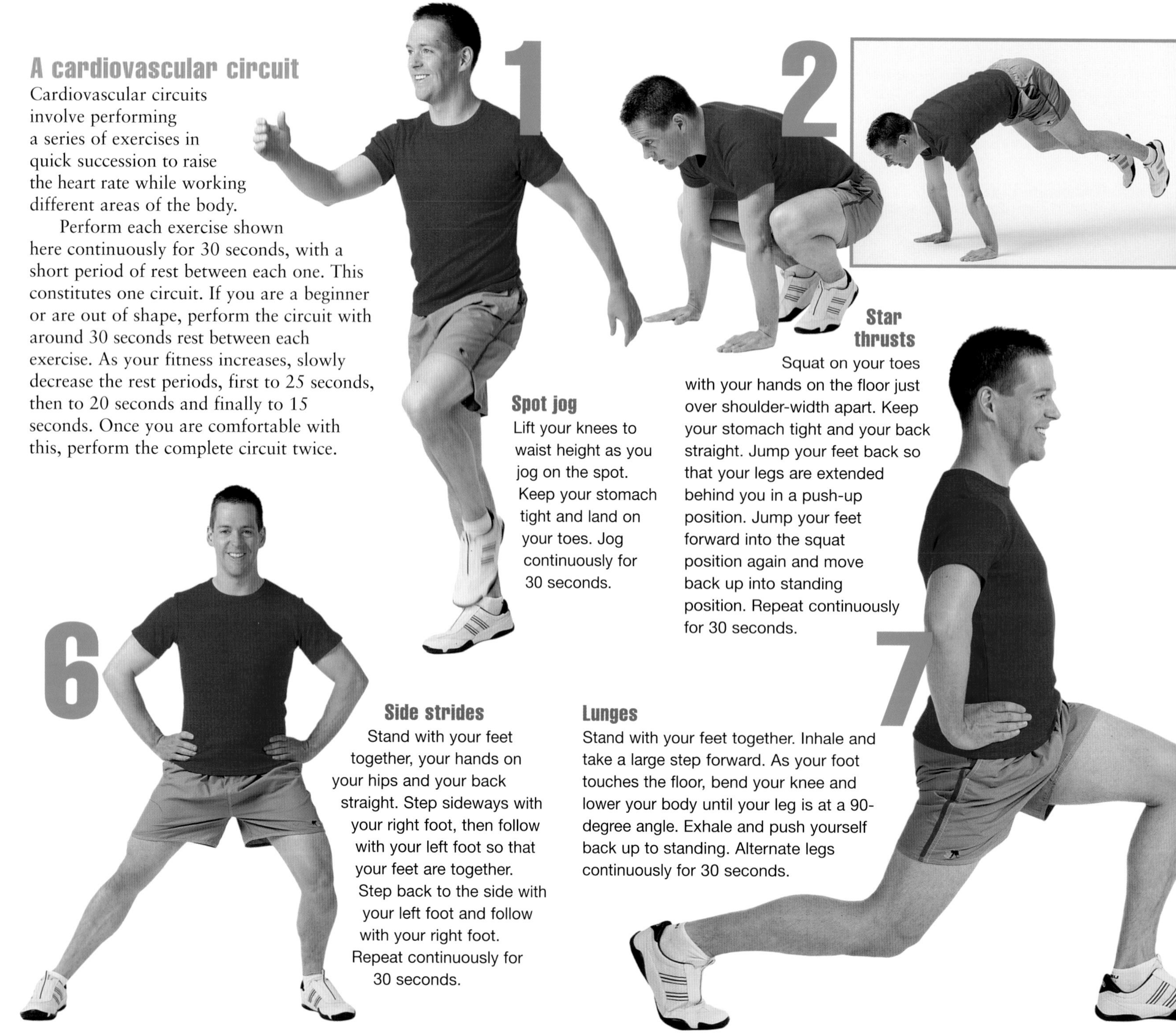

1

Spot jog

Lift your knees to waist height as you jog on the spot. Keep your stomach tight and land on your toes. Jog continuously for 30 seconds.

2

Star thrusts

Squat on your toes with your hands on the floor just over shoulder-width apart. Keep your stomach tight and your back straight. Jump your feet back so that your legs are extended behind you in a push-up position. Jump your feet forward into the squat position again and move back up into standing position. Repeat continuously for 30 seconds.

6

Side strides

Stand with your feet together, your hands on your hips and your back straight. Step sideways with your right foot, then follow with your left foot so that your feet are together. Step back to the side with your left foot and follow with your right foot. Repeat continuously for 30 seconds.

7

Lunges

Stand with your feet together. Inhale and take a large step forward. As your foot touches the floor, bend your knee and lower your body until your leg is at a 90-degree angle. Exhale and push yourself back up to standing. Alternate legs continuously for 30 seconds.

3

Bridges

Lie on your back with your legs bent and your feet flat on the mat. Place your hands flat on the ground beside your body. Exhale as you use your abdominal muscles to push your buttocks up away from the mat, straightening your body. Inhale as you come back onto the mat. Repeat continuously for 30 seconds.

4

Speedball

Bend your arms to 90 degrees and hold them in front of you at chest level. Circle your arms around each other continuously for 15 seconds. Change direction and circle them for another 15 seconds.

5

Star jumps

As you jump up in the air, open your legs wide and move your arms up and out, so that your body forms a star shape. Move down into a squat position as you land, ready to jump again. Repeat continuously for 30 seconds.

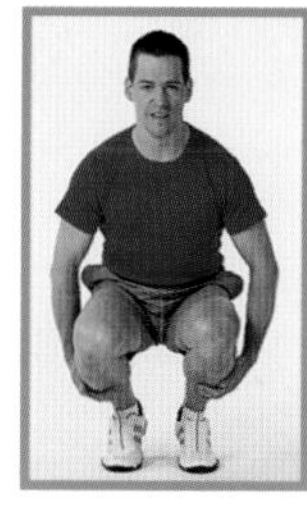

8

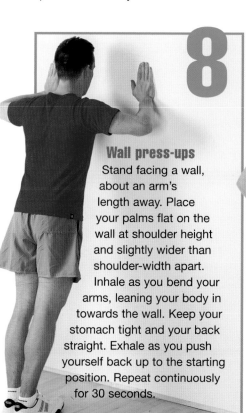

Wall press-ups

Stand facing a wall, about an arm's length away. Place your palms flat on the wall at shoulder height and slightly wider than shoulder-width apart. Inhale as you bend your arms, leaning your body in towards the wall. Keep your stomach tight and your back straight. Exhale as you push yourself back up to the starting position. Repeat continuously for 30 seconds.

9

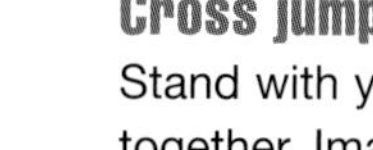

Side jumps

Stand with your feet together. Imagine a straight line on the ground heading away from you. With your feet together and your knees slightly bent, jump from one side of the line to the other. Repeat continuously for 30 seconds.

10

Cross jumps

Stand with your feet together. Imagine you are standing at the centre of a cross with one line extending in front and behind you and the other out to your sides. With your feet together and knees slightly bent, jump forward along the imaginary line then back to the centre point. Jump backwards along the line and then return to the centre. Jump out to the right and return and out to the left and return. Repeat continuously for 30 seconds.

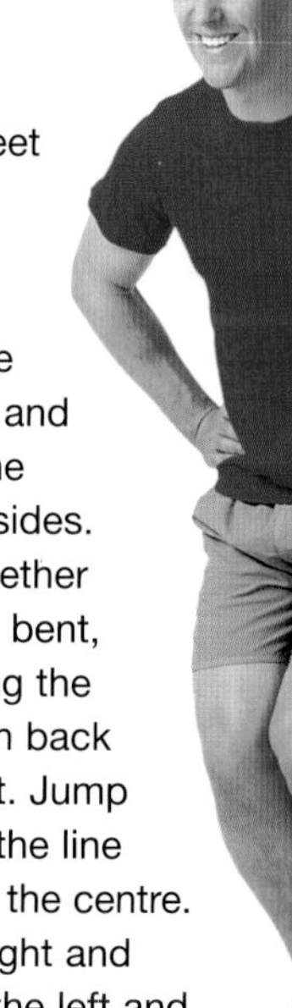

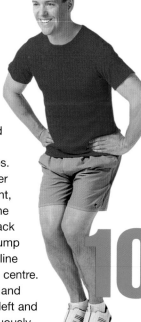

A flexibility workout

Over the years, your muscles start to tighten and the range of motion in your joints grows more restricted. Flexibility exercise will help you to maintain your natural mobility, reducing muscle soreness after other types of exercise and preventing injury to muscles and joints.

Flexibility can be defined as your ability to move a joint through its full range of movement. This aspect of fitness is often overlooked, yet it only takes a few minutes each day to significantly improve your flexibility. Flexibility exercises are easy to perform, require no special equipment and bring benefits for every age group. If you stick to the routine shown below, you will usually start to see improvements within a couple of weeks.

Elements of flexibility

For your flexibility workout to be most effective, it should consist of both mobility exercises and stretching exercises.

- **Mobility exercises** These involve taking your joints through slow, circular ranges of motion. By starting with small rotations and slowly building up to maximum range, you will increase blood flow to your joints, keeping them lubricated and maintaining smooth, healthy joint surfaces.
- **Stretching exercises** Stretching lengthens your muscles, tendons and ligaments, and loosens your joints so that you can move more freely. Tight muscles risk pulling your body out of alignment – stretching counteracts this, improving your posture and making you more supple.

Mobility routine

Always perform these mobility exercises in a slow, controlled manner. Take your joints as far as you can without strain or discomfort, but never go past this point. As your joints become more flexible, your range of motion will improve naturally. Perform each exercise for 20–30 repetitions before moving on to the next.

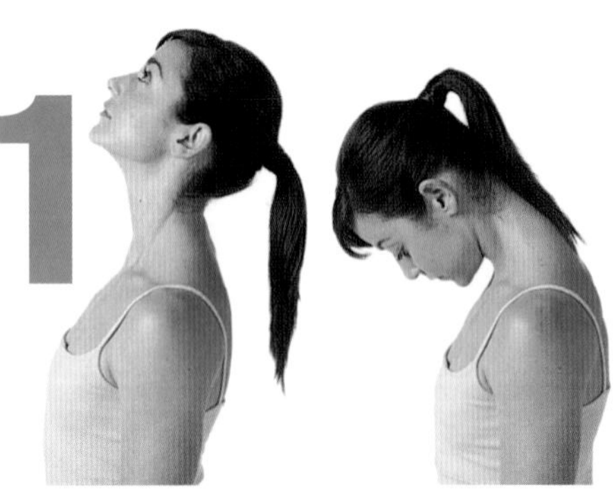

1

Head nod, tilt and turn

Slowly tilt your head back as though you are looking up at the ceiling. Then bring it forward as if you are trying to place your chin on your chest. Then tilt your head over towards your right shoulder as far as is comfortable, and bring it back and over towards your left shoulder. Finally, slowly rotate your head as far round to your right as feels comfortable. Then rotate it back round to your left.

2

Wrist and elbow circles

Keeping your fingers relaxed, circle each wrist in a clockwise direction for 20–30 repetitions, followed by anti-clockwise for 20–30 repetitions. Then hang your arms down by your sides, and, keeping your elbows by your sides and your upper arms as still as possible, circle your lower arms, first clockwise for 20–30 reps, then anti-clockwise for 20–30 reps.

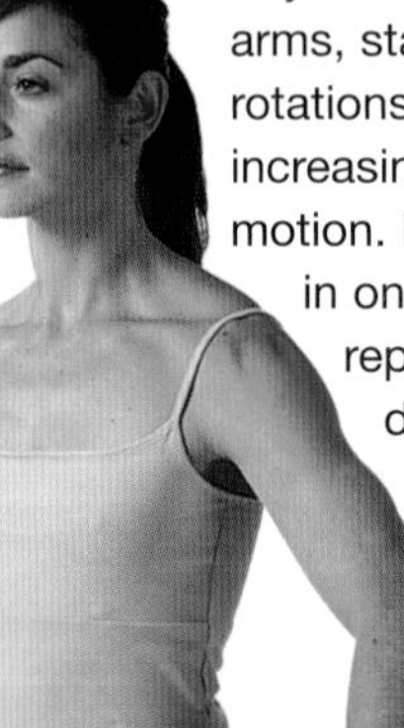

3

Arm circle

Hold your arms straight and slightly out at your sides. Circle your arms, starting with small rotations and slowly increasing the size of the motion. Repeat 20–30 times in one direction and then repeat in the other direction.

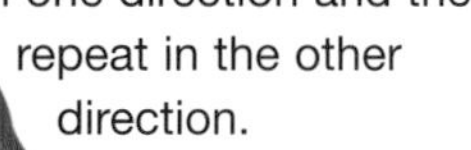

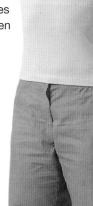

4

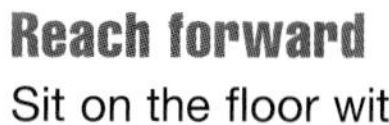

Side bend and stretch up

Lean your body over to your left side. Be careful not to twist your back, bend forward or arch your back. Straighten up and lean over to your right side. Then, reach your hands as far above your head as possible, moving up on to your toes at the same time. Relax back down to a normal standing position and repeat for 20–30 repetitions.

5

Reach forward

Sit on the floor with your legs in front of you and apart. Keep your knees slightly bent. Gently reach forward with both hands as far as is comfortable. Straighten up and repeat 10 times.

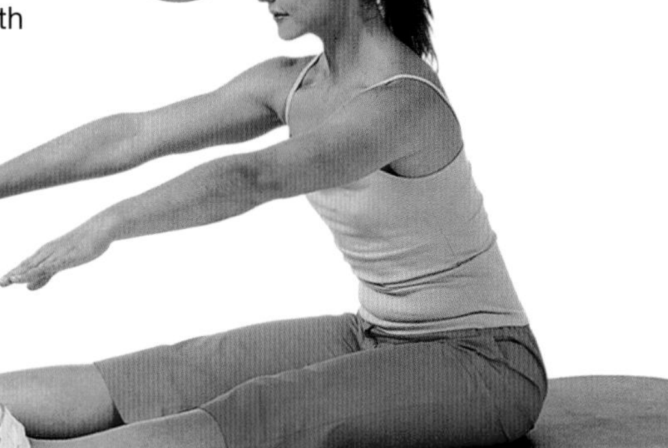

6

Ankle and knee circles

Holding on to a table or a chair for balance, raise your right foot off the ground and slowly circle your ankle, first clockwise for 20–30 repetitions, then anti-clockwise. Repeat with your left ankle.

Then, sitting on a chair, place your hands just above your knees. Straighten your left leg slightly and slowly circle your leg clockwise for 20–30 repetitions, then repeat anti-clockwise. Then repeat with your right leg. Do not force your knees too far: the range of motion in the joint is only a few degrees, so stick to small circles.

7

Hip circle

Stand with your feet shoulder-width apart. Keeping your shoulders as still as possible, rotate your hips clockwise in a wide circle for 20–30 repetitions, then repeat anti-clockwise for 20–30 repetitions.

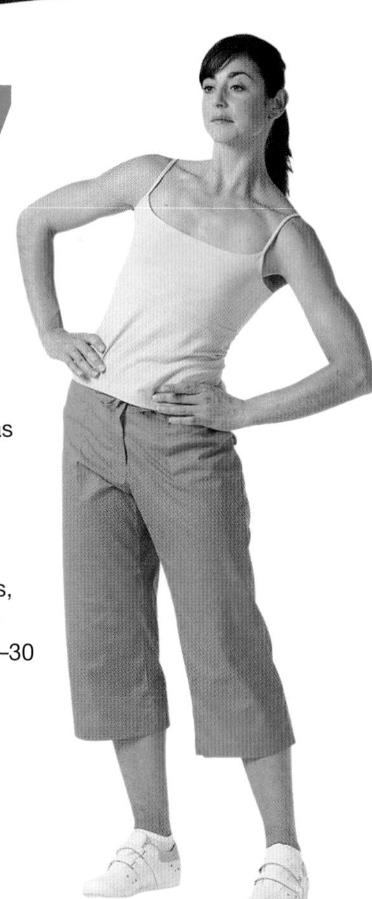

Static stretch routine

A good stretching programme should target all of the major muscle groups. A number of stretches are already covered on pages 66–67. For a full routine, do all the stretches on pages 66–67 a total of three times, together with the following exercises.

These exercises should be performed as static stretches, meaning you should hold each stretch for 15–30 seconds without bouncing. Slowly ease out of the stretch and relax for a few moments before repeating the stretch twice more. Gently exhale as you move into the stretch and breathe normally as you hold the stretch.

Always do your stretch routine after your mobility exercises or other warm-up. Your body responds better to stretching when the muscles and joints are warm.

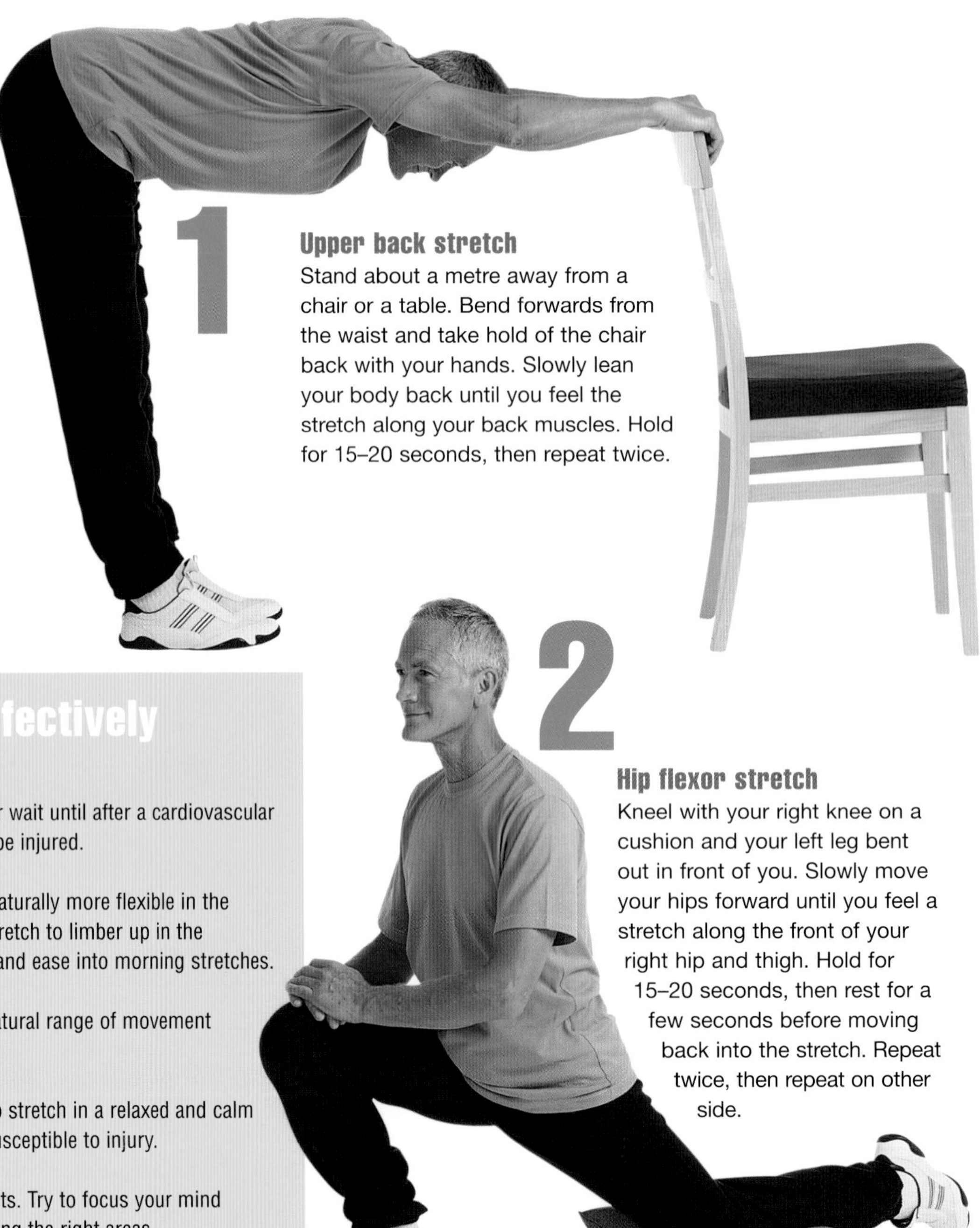

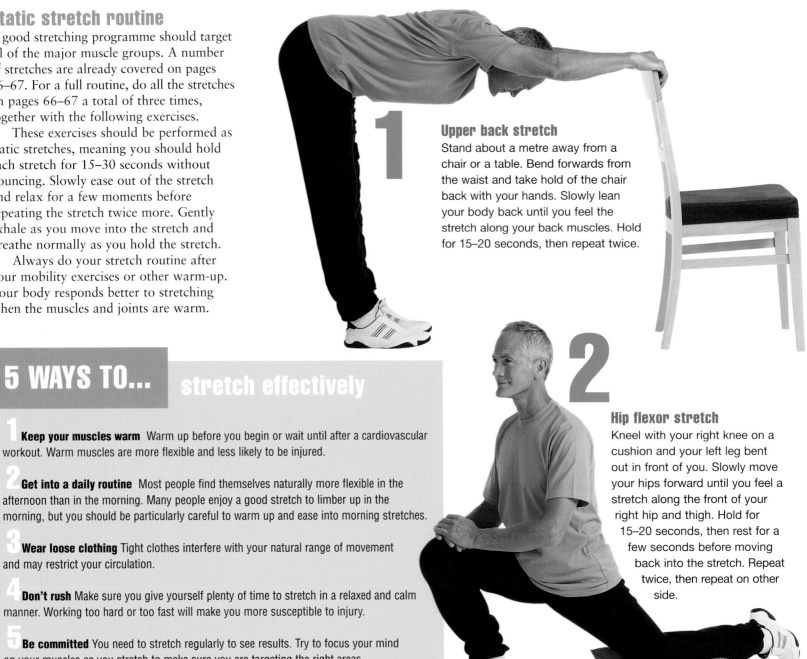

1

Upper back stretch

Stand about a metre away from a chair or a table. Bend forwards from the waist and take hold of the chair back with your hands. Slowly lean your body back until you feel the stretch along your back muscles. Hold for 15–20 seconds, then repeat twice.

2

Hip flexor stretch

Kneel with your right knee on a cushion and your left leg bent out in front of you. Slowly move your hips forward until you feel a stretch along the front of your right hip and thigh. Hold for 15–20 seconds, then rest for a few seconds before moving back into the stretch. Repeat twice, then repeat on other side.

5 WAYS TO... stretch effectively

1 **Keep your muscles warm** Warm up before you begin or wait until after a cardiovascular workout. Warm muscles are more flexible and less likely to be injured.

2 **Get into a daily routine** Most people find themselves naturally more flexible in the afternoon than in the morning. Many people enjoy a good stretch to limber up in the morning, but you should be particularly careful to warm up and ease into morning stretches.

3 **Wear loose clothing** Tight clothes interfere with your natural range of movement and may restrict your circulation.

4 **Don't rush** Make sure you give yourself plenty of time to stretch in a relaxed and calm manner. Working too hard or too fast will make you more susceptible to injury.

5 **Be committed** You need to stretch regularly to see results. Try to focus your mind on your muscles as you stretch to make sure you are targeting the right areas.

3

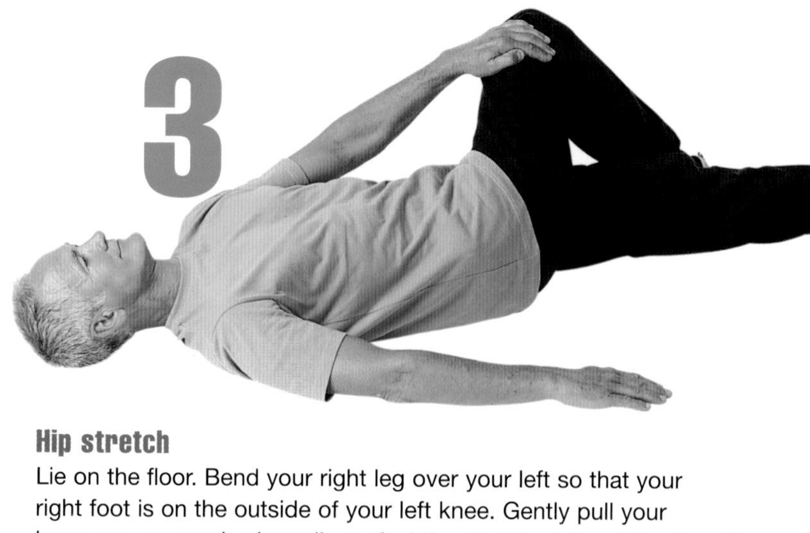

Hip stretch

Lie on the floor. Bend your right leg over your left so that your right foot is on the outside of your left knee. Gently pull your knee across your body until you feel the stretch at the side of your hip or buttock. Hold for 15–20 seconds. Repeat twice, then repeat on other side.

4

Inner leg stretch

Using a chair or table for support, stand with your legs as far apart as you can put them without feeling any stretch. Turn your right foot so that it points out. Hold your body straight and slowly lower yourself by bending your left leg until you feel a stretch along the inside of your right leg. Hold for 15–20 seconds. Repeat twice then change legs.

DID YOU KNOW?

There are many different stretching techniques, though not all are universally accepted as safe.

- ***Static*** **This involves holding a stretch for 15–30 seconds without bouncing. This is the easiest, safest and most commonly practised type of stretch and is unlikely to cause soreness or injury.**
- ***Assisted*** **This is static stretching with a partner who can help you maintain correct form and stretch further. Over-stretching can lead to injury so only try this with an experienced trainer as a partner.**
- ***Dynamic*** **This uses controlled swinging movements to take you to the limit of your range of motion. It can be used as part of a warm-up.**
- ***Muscular Energy Technique (MET)*** **This involves contracting a muscle for several seconds before the stretch so that it stretches further than normal.**
- ***Ballistic*** **This uses the momentum of a swinging motion to force your muscles beyond their normal range of motion. Bouncing your muscles in this way risks over-stretching or even tearing them.**

Spine stretch

Sit on the floor, with the soles of your feet together. Thread your hands between your thighs, under your lower legs, and grasp hold of your feet. Pull your body forward until you can feel the stretch along your spine and hold for 15–20 seconds. Repeat twice.

5

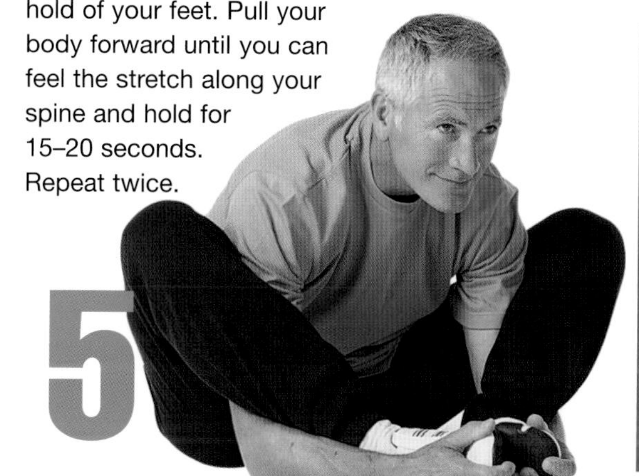

CAUTION

- You should feel only a mild discomfort in your muscle as you stretch. Stop immediately if you feel pain or a stabbing sensation – this may mean you are forcing the stretch too far.
- If you find it hard to breathe in a normal, relaxed manner you may be over-stretching. Move out of the stretch a little until you find a more comfortable, less strained position.

A strength-training workout

On average, adults lose 3 to 5 per cent of their muscle each decade. Strength training reverses this trend by building and maintaining muscle mass and strength. Strong muscles do much more than help you to perform tasks more easily; they also prevent injuries, support and protect your joints and improve your posture.

Each of your muscles consists of many hundreds of muscle fibres enclosed in a sheath of connective tissue. When you place a greater than normal load on your muscles, the extra resistance causes minute tears in these fibres. With rest, your body repairs these tears, increasing the size of the fibres and creating stronger muscles.

Bone and muscle benefits

Weak or unbalanced muscles can pull your body out of alignment; balanced strength training (combined with stretching) will help you to maintain good posture. It will also improve your ligament and cartilage thickness, strengthening your joints and helping ease any pain from rheumatoid arthritis or ostoearthritis.

Strength training also puts stress on your skeleton. Like your muscles, your bones respond to this resistance by increasing in mass. This strengthens your bones, helping to protect against fractures and degenerative conditions such as osteoporosis (>>264–275).

The benefits of lean muscle mass

Although strength training does not burn as many calories as cardiovascular training, it does increase your lean body weight. Each kilo of muscle in your body burns around 75 calories per day just for normal maintenance (during exercise this figure is much higher). Increasing lean muscle mass means you burn more calories all day long, boosting your metabolism and helping weight stay off.

Who can do it?

Everyone can benefit from strength training. Experts used to advise that strength training was not suitable for children, but years of exhaustive studies have found little evidence to substantiate these claims. Moderate strength training helps long-term skeletal and joint development, even in children, and studies show that post-menopausal women suffer fewer hip fractures if they engaged in weight-bearing activity as young girls. The American Academy of Pediatrics now recommends strength training for children.

As with any physical activity, parents should ensure that certain precautions are taken. Children should perform bodyweight exercises rather than using extra weights and should never perform spine-loading exercises (such as squats with a weight held across the shoulders).

At the other end of the spectrum, strength training is equally beneficial for older people, who often suffer from the effects of muscle and bone degeneration. Muscle strength declines by 15 per cent per decade after the age of 50 and 30 per cent per decade after the age of 70 – adding just 1.5kg (3.3lb) of muscle can reverse the effects of almost five years' worth of age-related muscle loss.

How to strength train

You don't need huge weights to make strength training worthwhile – the important thing is to keep your tissues toned, not to build massive muscles. There are two main variations to consider:

- **Bodyweight exercises** are movements performed without additional weight, using your own body mass for resistance. A good example of this is the press-up. Although a little less productive than weighted exercises, bodyweight training is ideal for beginners and can be performed anywhere.
- **Weighted exercises** are movements performed using additional weights such as free weights (barbells and dumb-bells), weight stack machines or a combination of both. Weighted exercises are often more productive than bodyweight exercises

DID YOU KNOW?

- **Many women worry about developing large muscles with strength training, but large muscles require high levels of the male hormone testosterone. Most women have around one tenth of the testosterone levels of men and smaller frames, making it difficult to build large muscles.**
- **Women also tend to have weaker bones and are more susceptible to osteoporosis than men (although men can also develop the disease), making the bone-building benefits of strength training particularly important.**

because you can continuously increase the amount of weight lifted, allowing your muscles to adapt to a higher level.

Which muscles?

When starting strength training you should choose at least one exercise for each major muscle group. This will help to prevent muscle imbalances, such as strong stomach muscles and weak back muscles, that may pull your body out of alignment.

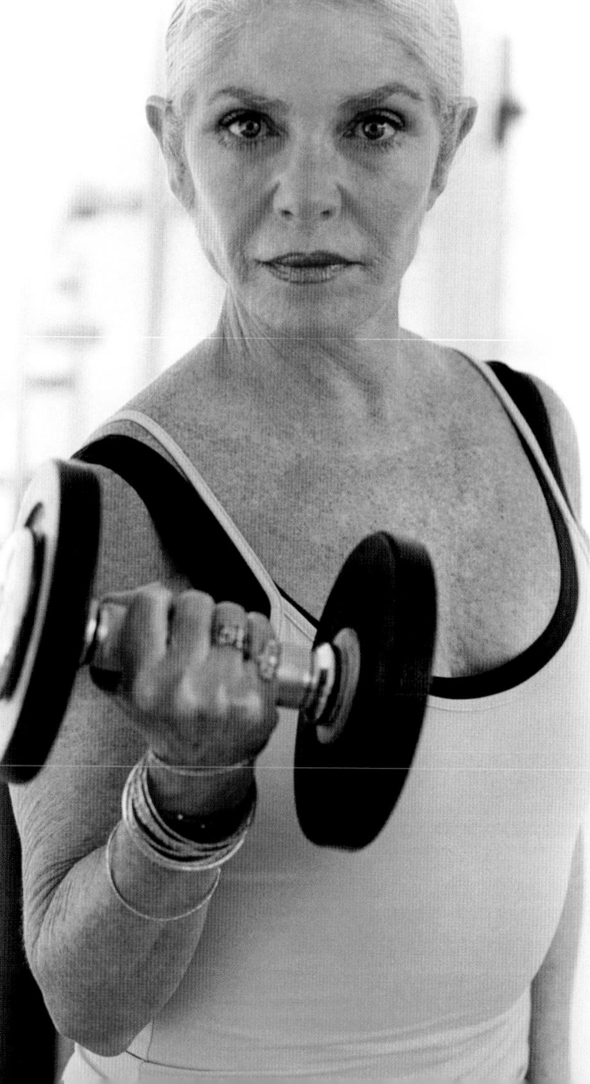

Start with exercises that target the larger muscle groups, such as your leg muscles, and work towards the smaller ones. This allows you to do the most physically demanding moves when you are the least fatigued.

How fast?

Avoid fast, jerky movements that place strain on your muscles and ligaments and never swing or bounce the weights up – this robs your muscles of many of the benefits of training and can lead to injury.

- **Bodyweight exercises** Try to take about 5 seconds for the lifting/pushing/pulling phase and another 5 seconds for the less strenuous lowering/relaxing phase.
- **Weighted exercises** These should be shortened to about 2 seconds for the lifting/pushing phase and 3–4 seconds for the lowering phase.

Breathing

Breathe continuously to supply oxygen to your muscles. Exhale during the most strenuous part of each exercise and inhale during the least strenuous part (the lowering phase). Try not to hold your breath – this can cause your blood pressure to rise.

Sets and reps

After performing a movement, you will need to repeat it a specific number of times. Each repetition of an individual movement is called a rep. A set is a group of reps performed in succession without rest. You should rest for 30–60 seconds between sets.

If you are doing press-ups, for example, and the instructions say to do 3 sets of 10 reps, you should: perform 10 press-ups without stopping; rest for 30–60 seconds and perform another set of 10 press-ups; rest again and perform the third set of 10 press-ups.

Progressions

As your muscles increase in strength, you will need to increase the level at which you work in order to see further results – the 'progressive overload' principle. You can increase the workload by adding more weight, adding to the number of reps and sets of a given exercise, or reducing the rest period in between each set.

- **Bodyweight exercises** As you progress with your training and start to get stronger, slow your movements down. If you slow your speed down to 10 seconds for each phase, you will be working your muscles almost 50 per cent harder. When you can perform the required sets and reps at this speed, try adding an extra rep to each set.
- **Weighted exercises** With these types of exercises, you need to gradually increase the amount of resistance or the number of reps to promote further gains. With each exercise, start with a weight that allows you to do at least 8 reps. Stick with that weight until you have built up to 12 reps then increase the weight by about 5 per cent. This should reduce the number of reps you can do back to around 8, so you can build back up to 12 before increasing the weight again. This way you gradually increase the resistance you are using.

> **‘One group of arthritis sufferers reported a 43 per cent reduction in knee pain after only four months of strength training, according to a report in the *Journal of Rheumatology*.’**

STRENGTH-TRAINING ROUTINE

This routine includes a mixture of weighted and non-weighted exercises but they can all be performed as bodyweight exercises, if you prefer. If you want to try these at home but don't own any free weights, improvise – a bottle of water in each hand works well.

5 WAYS TO...

Train safely

Although strength training is generally very safe, there are a few points you should bear in mind in order to avoid injury:

1 **Get a check-up** Talk to your doctor if you have high blood pressure, heart problems or other conditions. Many gyms and health clubs offer a free health check when you join.

2 **Warm up and stretch** Warm up before training to prevent injury. Stretch after exercise to stop your muscles tightening.

3 **Choose the right weight** Do not aim to lift the heaviest weight possible – a good weight should tire your muscles without affecting your form. As a rule of thumb, women should use weights in the 2–10kg (4–22lb) range and men in the 5–15kg (11–33lb) range.

4 **Take things slowly** Start each exercise in a safe, stable position, focus on good technique and posture, and breathe properly. Do not rush your movement.

5 **Rest your body** Always leave one or two days between workouts. It takes anywhere between 48 and 72 hours for your muscles to grow and recover properly after a workout.

1

Leg press (front of thighs/buttocks)
Stand with your feet shoulder-width apart, your arms by your sides and a dumb-bell in each hand. Do not lock your knees. Inhale as you drop your hips and squat slowly down. Keep your back as straight as possible and do not bend your legs past a 90-degree angle. Exhale as you push back up to your original position, again without locking your knees. ***Three sets of 8 reps***

2

Calf raise (calves)
Stand with your feet shoulder-width apart, arms by your sides and a dumb-bell in each hand. Exhale as you raise your heels off the ground. Inhale as you return your heels slowly back down to the ground. ***Three sets of 8 reps***

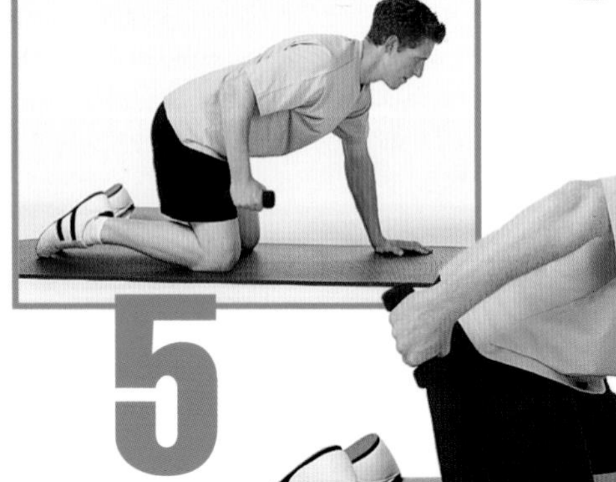

5

Tricep kickback (triceps)
Kneel on all fours with your back straight. Hold a dumb-bell in one hand and bend your arm at the elbow so that your upper arm is in line with the side of your body. Exhale as you straighten your lower arm out behind you. Inhale as you come back into the original position. ***Two sets of 8 reps***

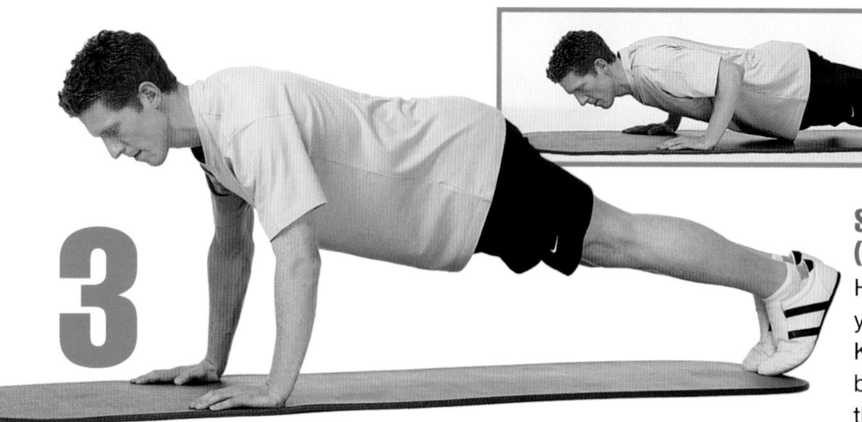

3

Press-up (chest/triceps/shoulders)

Place your palms flat on the floor and slightly wider than shoulder-width apart. Keeping your body straight, come up onto your toes. Slowly bend your arms at the elbows and lower your chest towards the floor. Push back up into the original position. If this is too hard, try it with your knees on the floor. ***Three sets of 8 reps***

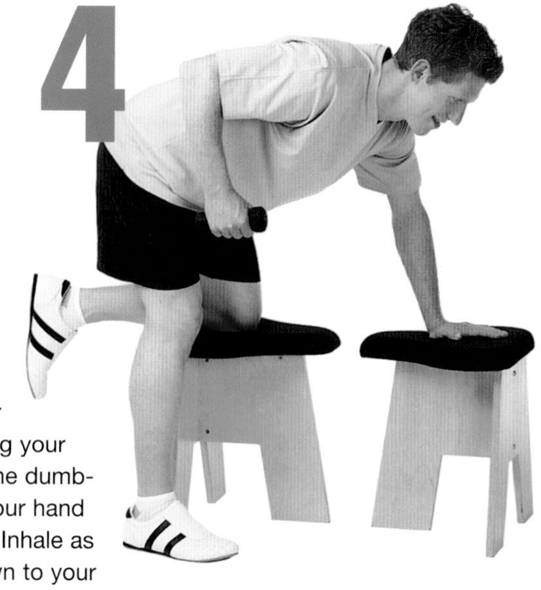

4

Single-arm row (back/biceps)

Hold a dumb-bell in your right hand. Keeping your lower body straight, bend at the hip and place your left hand on a bench for support. Without twisting your spine, exhale and pull the dumb-bell towards you until your hand is level with your chest. Inhale as you lower your arm down to your original position. ***Three sets of 8 reps for both your arms***

6

Lateral raise (shoulders)

Stand with your feet shoulder-width apart, arms by your sides and a dumb-bell in each hand. Keep your arms relaxed and exhale as you raise your arms up and out to your sides. Keep your elbows slightly bent and inhale as you lower your arms back to your sides. ***Two sets of 8 reps***

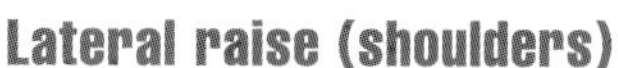

7

Back extension (lower back)

Lie on your front with your hands facing palm up on your buttocks. Look towards the floor just ahead of you. Exhale as you slowly raise your shoulders and upper chest a few centimetres off the mat. Lead the movement with your back and chest, not your head. Inhale as you slowly lower your body back down to the mat. ***Two sets of 8 reps***

8

Abdominal crunch (stomach)

Lie on your back with your legs bent and your feet flat on the floor. Place your hands gently to the sides of your head. Exhale as you curl up and forward in a slow, controlled manner, just far enough to lift your shoulders and upper back from the floor. Do not jerk your body, arch your back or pull on your head or neck. Inhale as you slowly uncurl your body until you come back down onto the floor. ***Three sets of 12 reps***

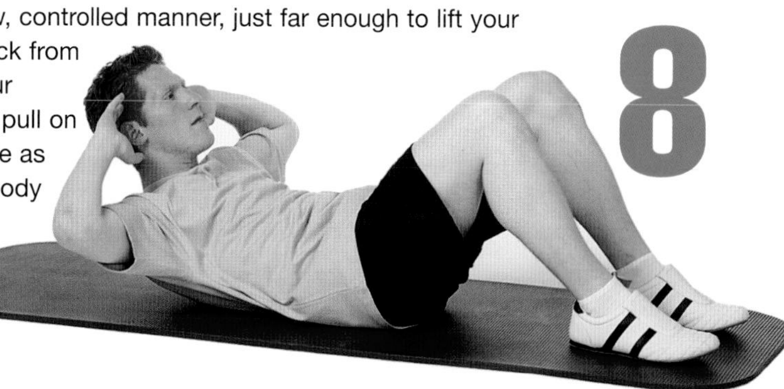

GYM MACHINES AT A GLANCE

The cardio (aerobic) machines at your gym may look very different from one another but they all have the same aim: to work your heart and lungs and burn calories. There is no best cardio machine – used for the right length of time and at the right intensity they all provide a good aerobic workout.

Cardio Machines

NAME	AREA TARGETED	OTHER BENEFITS	SAFETY
1 Cross-trainer	Lungs and heart	Burns fat. Improves muscle tone and bone density in arms and legs.	Provides a safe, low-impact workout.
2 Rowing machine	Lungs and heart	Burns fat. Improves muscle tone and bone density in arms, back and legs.	Keep your back straight and follow directions carefully to avoid straining your back.
3 Stationary bike	Lungs and heart	Burns fat. Improves muscle tone and bone density in legs.	Provides a safe, low-impact workout.
4 Step machine	Lungs and heart	Burns fat. Improves muscle tone and bone density in legs.	Provides a safe, low-impact workout.
5 Treadmill	Lungs and heart	Burns fat. Improves muscle tone and bone density in legs.	Higher impact than exercising on other cardio machines, which can damage joints.

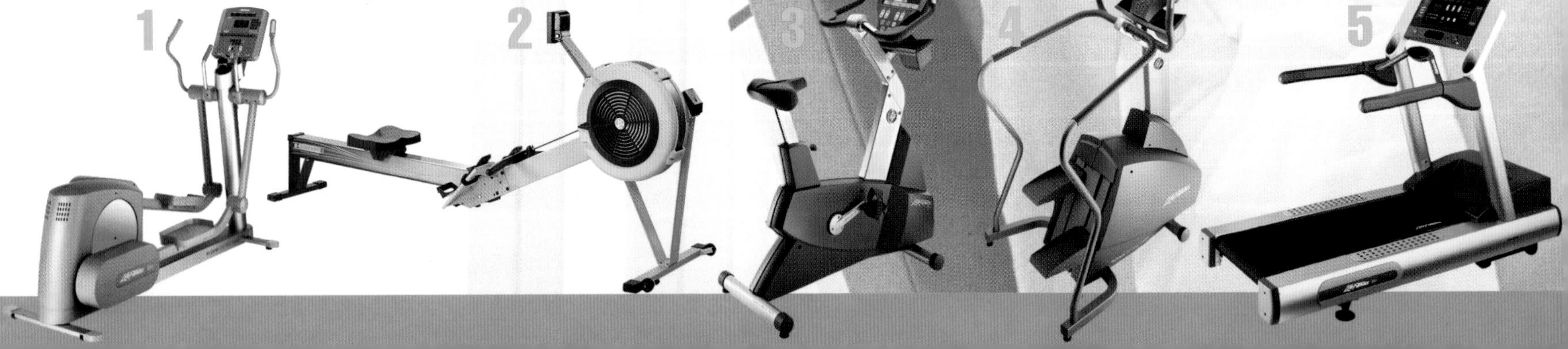

1

2

3

4

5

The weights (resistance) machines are intended to strengthen muscles rather than burn calories. They provide an easy-to-use, controlled alternative to free weights. Different machines target different muscles or muscle groups, so you'll need to use a range of machines each session.

Weights Machines

	NAME	AREA TARGETED	OTHER BENEFITS	SAFETY
1	Lat pulldown	Back	Also strengthens shoulder muscles and biceps. Improves bone density in upper body.	Never pull the bar down behind your neck. This could strain your shoulder ligaments or your rotator cuff muscles.
2	Vertical chest press	Chest	Also strengthens shoulder muscles and triceps. Improves bone density in upper body.	Get advice before using the machine if you have shoulder or elbow problems.
3	Shoulder press	Shoulder	Also strengthens triceps and back muscles. Improves bone density in upper body.	Get advice before using the machine if you have neck, elbow or lower back problems.
4	Triceps extension	Triceps	Also strengthens shoulder and chest muscles. Improves bone density in arms.	Get advice before using the machine if you have any arm problems.
5	Leg press	Buttocks and thighs	Also improves bone density in legs and hips.	Get advice before using the machine if you have any hip or knee problems.

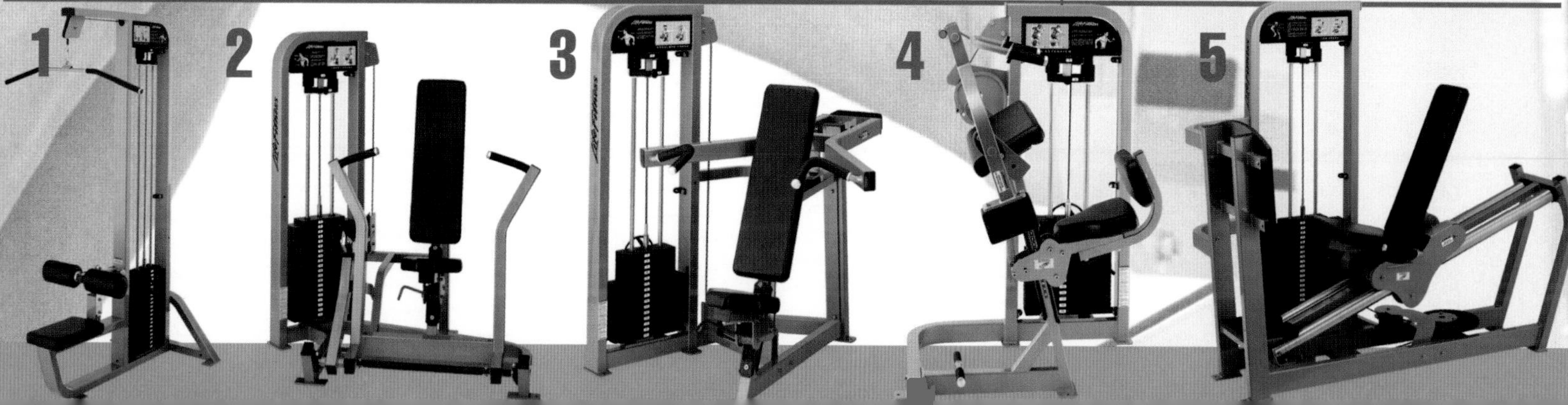

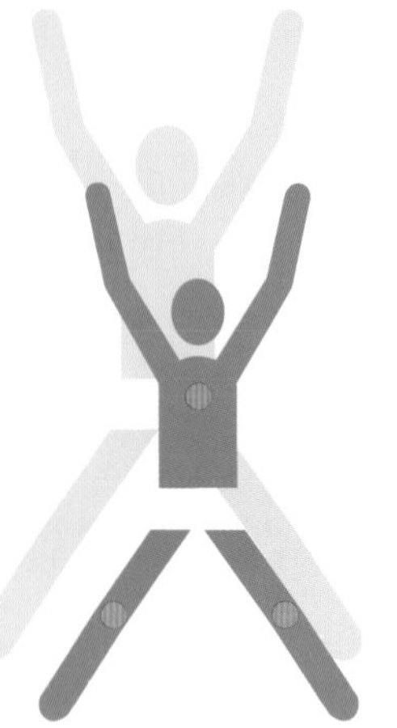

Aerobics

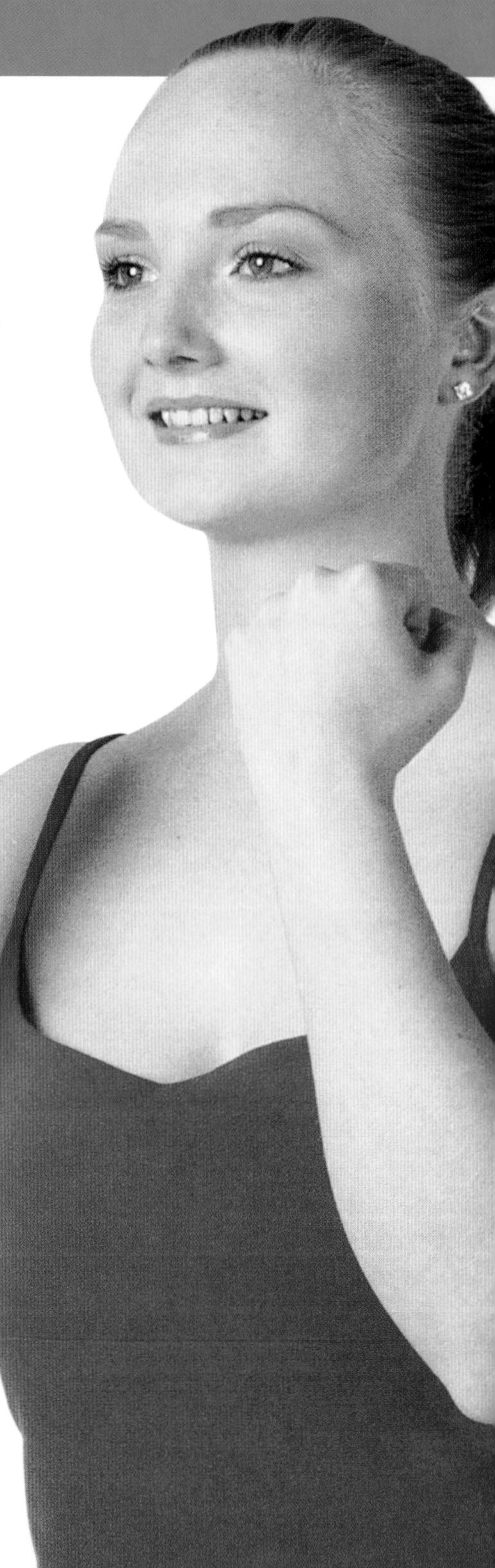

All cardiovascular activity is aerobic – any activity that increases your heart rate and stimulates your circulation also makes you respire aerobically (with oxygen). But while activities such as running, cycling and swimming are all aerobic, the term 'aerobics' is usually reserved for a specific type of workout, often set to music and using choreographed routines.

- **Strengthens heart, lungs and circulation**
- **Helps weight loss**
- **Increases range of motion**
- **Improves bone density in lower body**
- **improves muscle tone in lower body**

SEE ALSO

>>58
>>68
>>70
>>158
>>238

Like any other form of cardiovascular activity, aerobics strengthens your heart and lungs, stimulates your circulation and is excellent for weight loss. In addition to working your cardiovascular system, aerobic exercises also strengthen your muscles – many routines concentrate on the large muscle groups in your lower body (your legs, chest, back and buttocks).

Many forms of aerobics involve relatively high-impact activities such as jumping and jogging. This helps to strengthen the bones in your legs and hips but is not always suitable for people with joint problems. Lower-impact forms of aerobics are easier on the joints while being moderately weight bearing – your bones and muscles still support the weight of your body as you exercise.

Regular aerobics training improves strength, coordination and flexibility, and helps counteract stress by relaxing tense muscles and increasing endorphin production.

What is involved?

There are many different types of aerobics classes available, each with its own particular characteristics. Some classes use a variety of different movements that work your bones and muscles in different ways. Other types of aerobics, such as step aerobics, place greater emphasis on the repetition of a particular movement. Most gyms and health centres have a range of different sessions available, and may feature classes including:

- **Step aerobics** Initially devised by a keen aerobics fan who wanted to continue training despite a knee injury, this lower-impact style is ideal for people with joint pain. Step aerobics uses an elevated step, to provide a vigorous workout without the harsh impact of some other methods of aerobic training.

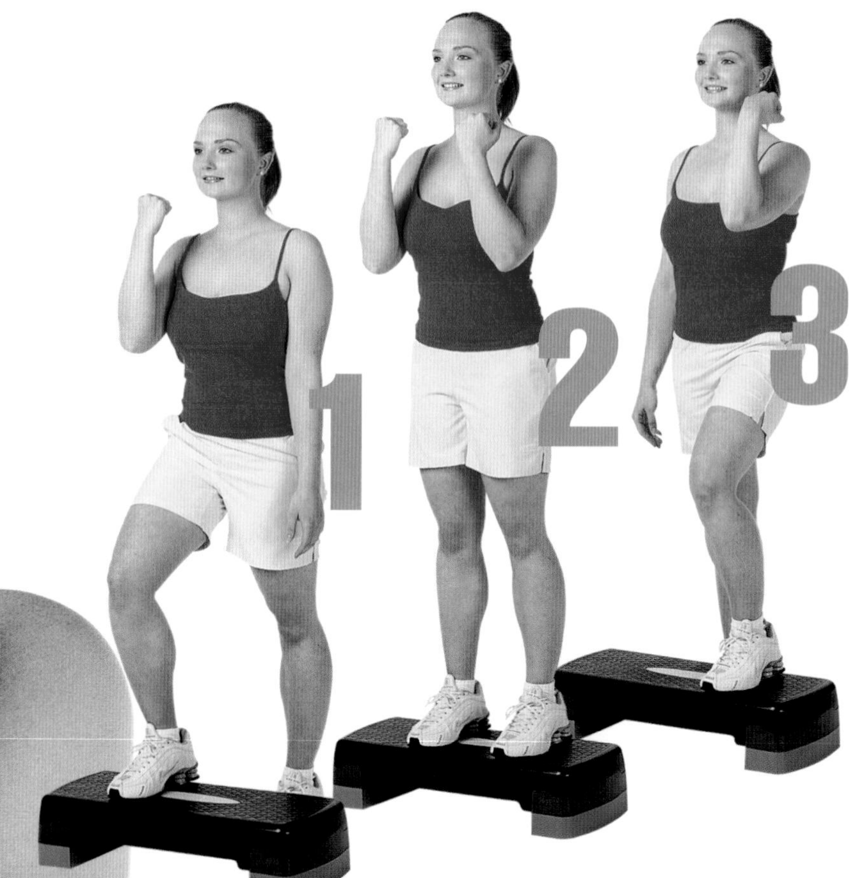

One to try ... the step curl

The stepping action provides a high-intensity but relatively low-impact aerobic exercise. It is good for your bones and works your quadriceps and calves.

1 Stand in front of a step. Place your left foot on top of the step, keeping your knee in line with your foot and using good toe-to-heel contact on the step. As you step up, curl your left arm up towards your left shoulder with your fist lightly clenched.
2 Step up with your right leg and curl up your right arm so that you are standing with both feet on the step and both arms curled towards your shoulders.
3 Step off with your left foot, lifting your toe and heel together. Uncurl your left arm and open your hand.
4 Step off with your right foot and uncurl your right arm.

Repeat the whole sequence, this time leading with the right leg and arm. Continue to step and curl for at least 15 minutes. To increase the intensity you can perform this exercise holding hand weights.

- **Dance aerobics** Music and rhythm can make even the most strenuous and challenging aerobic workout enjoyable. The choreographed dance routines often involve more complex steps than are practised in regular aerobics classes.
- **Circuit aerobics** This involves a series of exercises performed in a specific order and in quick succession to raise the heart rate and test muscles in different ways. Circuit aerobics often incorporates elements of strength and flexibility training but, because these are performed in quick succession and with little rest, they all contribute to the general aerobic workout.
- **Slide aerobics** A slide board is a slippery plastic board with angled rubber bumpers on each end to stop your feet sliding off. The movements, which resemble sliding over a newly waxed floor, provide a high intensity workout. Slide aerobics is often used to get into shape for activities such as skiing.
- **Box aerobics** Sometimes called boxercise, this is a non-contact routine of boxing, chopping and kicking movements, usually performed to music. Box aerobics provides a rigorous, stress-relieving work-out and is a good way to let off steam.

How to work out

You should always work at a pace that is comfortable, steady and allows you to talk normally and without strain. Moderate-intensity exercise is not only efficient but also more enjoyable.

Organized aerobics classes usually last 45 minutes to an hour, but beginners should start with 10–20 minutes and gradually build up. Increase the intensity and duration of exercise only gradually, especially if you are recovering from injury, are elderly or overweight. If in doubt, go slower and continue for a shorter time.

Although fitness can be maintained with as little as two workouts a week, ideally you should try to train three to five times a week. You should start to see improvements in your energy and stamina within a few weeks of regular exercise.

Jogging

Less stressful for the joints than sprinting, jogging is still a useful bone-loading exercise and a very effective way to achieve cardio-vascular fitness and burn calories. However, because jogging is a relatively high-impact activity it is not always suitable for people with knee or ankle problems.

- **Strengthens heart, lungs and circulation**
- **Improves bone density in lower body**
- **Helps weight loss**
- **Improves muscle tone in lower body**

SEE ALSO

>>58
>>194
>>201
>>215
>>234

As you get older, your bones naturally lose mass and become more brittle, which can put you at increased risk from bone disorders such as osteoporosis and fractures, especially of the hip and spine.

What will it do for me?

Jogging is an effective way to build strong muscles and bones in your lower body because the force of impact from each step makes the tissues grow stronger in response.

By the same token, however, the extra strain on muscles and joints from this type of repetitive impact can lead to injuries – knee pain and shin splints are common complaints (>>196–199). Long-term jogging on hard surfaces can play a role in degenerative joint conditions such as osteoarthritis (>>228–247). For this reason, it is vital to wear good running shoes that cushion and support your feet – regular joggers should buy a new pair of running shoes every six months to a year (>>48–49).

Getting started

Always remember to warm up and stretch thoroughly before you start >>64–67. If you have never run before or are very out of shape, take things slowly to begin with. You could start by walking for most of your session and include just 1 minute of jogging. As you become fitter, you can gradually increase the proportion of your session spent jogging.

You will need to breathe a little harder than normal to get more oxygen into your body, but

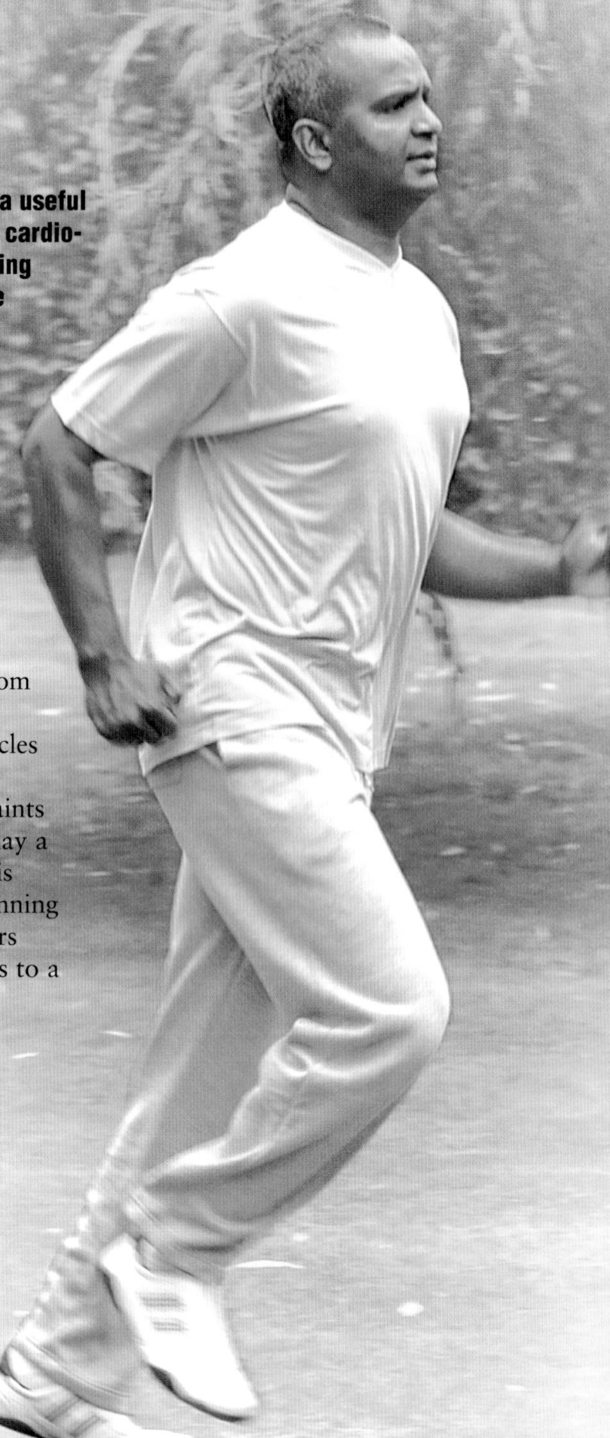

you should still be able to hold a conversation while you jog – this is a sign that you are not overdoing things. If you find yourself getting too out of breath, slow down or walk until you have recovered. When your breathing has returned to a more comfortable level you can start to jog again.

Be realistic

Don't plan to run a marathon in a few months' time if you have only just started training. Concentrate first on good technique and then build up the length and intensity of your runs. Set yourself achievable goals and you are far more likely to stay motivated and feel a real sense of personal achievement.

If you have a history of diabetes, chest pain, angina, asthma, epilepsy, high blood pressure, have had recent surgery or are pregnant, you should consult a doctor before taking up jogging. If you have any joint problems, particularly knee problems, you should avoid jogging on hard surfaces such as asphalt roads or pavements.

DID YOU KNOW?

- **A report in the *American Journal of Public Health* in 2001, based on a health survey and hip X-rays from over 4,000 men, revealed that joggers have on average 8 per cent higher bone density than men who take little or no exercise.**
- **The study also suggested that the more often you jog, the stronger your bones become. Men who jog at least nine times a month have around a 5 per cent higher bone density than men who jog less frequently.**

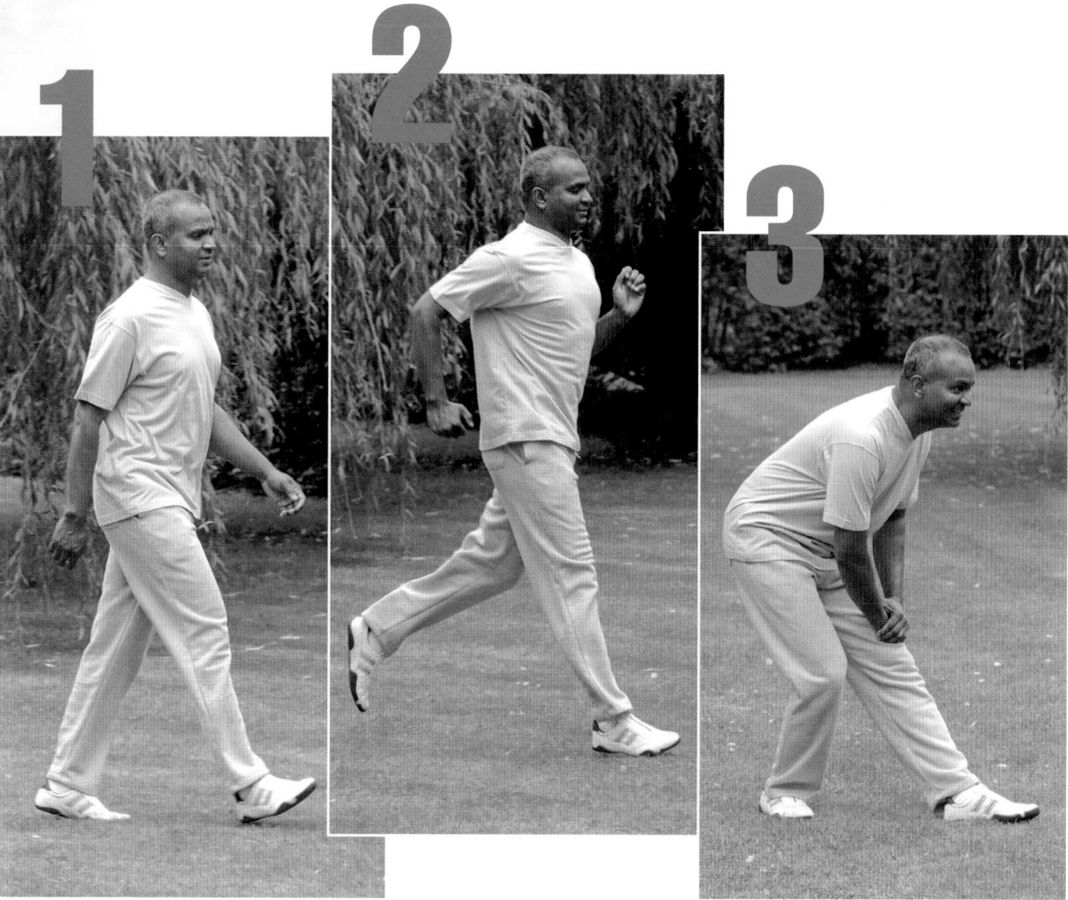

Get it right ... jogging

1 Warm up first with a fast walk, then gradually break into a slow jog until you have found a pace that is comfortable for you.
2 Land on your heels and roll through the foot, pushing off with your toes. Keep your back straight and shoulders open. Keep your arms relaxed and swinging naturally for momentum.
3 At the end of your jogging session, gradually decrease your speed until you reach walking pace. Continue walking until your heart rate and breathing have returned to normal. Stretch your muscles while they are still warm, paying particular attention to your calf muscles.

Continue this run/walk procedure for a total of 10 minutes every two to three days, gradually reducing the time you spend walking and increasing the time you spend jogging. An increase of around 10 per cent of your running time should avoid over-training and injury.

Swimming

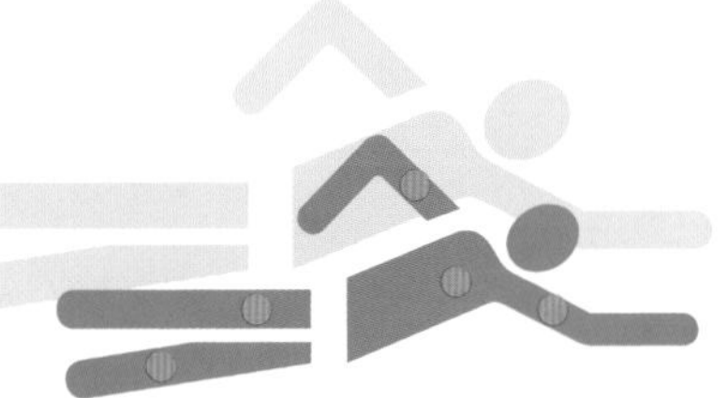

Water-based exercises such as swimming and aquaerobics increase muscle stamina and strength and improve cardiovascular fitness. The buoyancy of water and the support it provides means that the risk of injuring bones, muscle and joints is extremely low.

- **Strengthens heart, lungs and circulation**
- **Helps weight loss**
- **Improves muscle strength**
- **Improves range of motion in knees and shoulders**
- **Low impact**
- **Low risk of injury**

SEE ALSO

>>58
>>159
>>190
>>254

Swimming is ideal for people of all ages and almost all levels of fitness. By using all the major muscle groups, swimming increases strength, stamina and suppleness, as well as offering great cardiovascular benefits. Unlike most land-based activities, swimming uses the arms as well as the legs for propulsion, making it a particularly effective exercise for strengthening the shoulders.

The benefits of water

Water supports your body weight as you swim, reducing the jarring and pounding that can occur during land-based activities. This makes swimming and other water-based exercises particularly useful if you suffer from arthritis, neck and back problems, obesity, or if you are pregnant. Water also provides more resistance to your movements than air, promoting better muscular endurance and tone.

Warm water will soothe and warm your muscles as you swim, letting your joints move through a greater range of motion with less risk of injury and making you less vulnerable to aches and soreness. It is important to get the stroke right, however – keeping your head raised in breast stroke, for instance, can put strain on your neck.

Water and bone health

Although very beneficial for your muscles and joints, aquatic exercises do not place enough of a load on your bones or produce sufficient impact to improve your bone density significantly. It is worth including some form of strengthening exercises in your weekly fitness routine in addition to water-based activities.

If you have osteoporosis or very brittle bones, your doctor may advise you to avoid weight-bearing exercise. In this case, exercise that takes your weight off your bones, such as swimming, may be beneficial. You can work out much harder in water because it cushions you from falls and knocks during exercise.

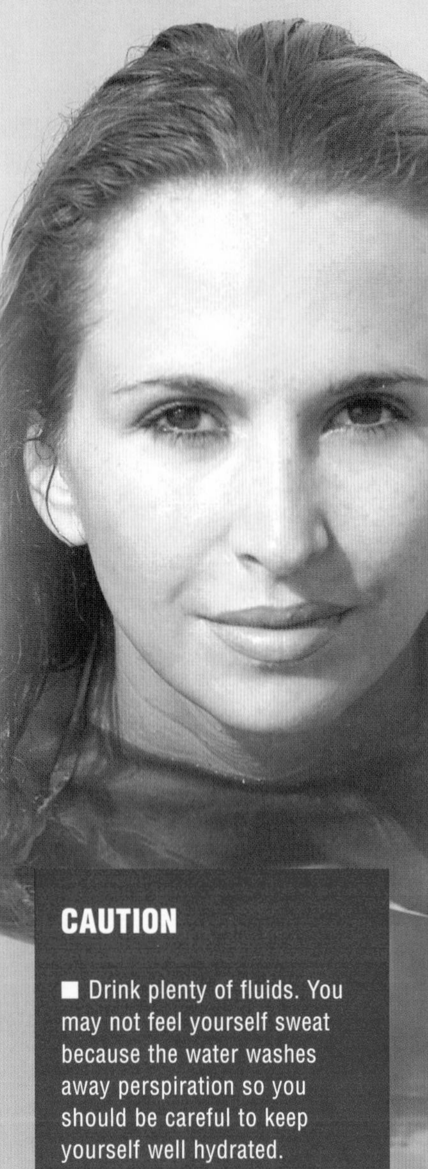

CAUTION

- Drink plenty of fluids. You may not feel yourself sweat because the water washes away perspiration so you should be careful to keep yourself well hydrated.
- Do not forget to warm up – water pressure on your body can initially cause an increase in blood pressure, so you should ease in gently.

Getting started

Swimming can be performed by anyone at their own pace and level. Most public baths and health club pools offer lessons for beginners and more advanced swimmers might enjoy the social element of a club or a class, although swimming is also a good individual pursuit. Most pools sell a range of accessories. If you dislike the feeling of water on your face, consider buying a pair of goggles or a nose clip to keep the water out of your nose. This should help you maintain a better position in the water.

Take advice and make sure you get the stroke corrrect to avoid muscle strains. If you are unfit or out of practice, start by swimming a length and then rest for half a minute. Gradually over subsequent weeks, decrease the intervals until you can swim continuously. Once you feel fit enough, aim for 20–40 minutes of continuous swimming, using a variety of strokes.

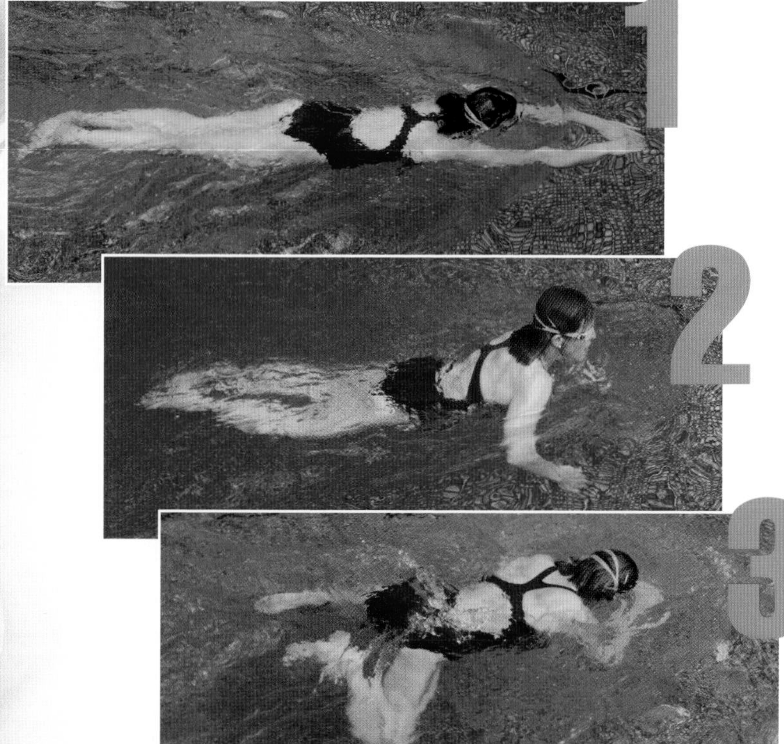

AQUAEROBICS

Water-based aerobics offers an excellent way to improve cardiovascular conditioning and – because of the consistent resistance from the water – can increase strength.

Classes generally include a variety of gentle, rhythmic movements, usually performed standing in waist- or chest-deep water. At waist-level, water supports around 50 per cent of your body weight; chest-deep, it supports 80–90 per cent of your weight. This makes aquaerobics very low-impact. Occasionally exercises are performed in deeper water, often with the aid of a flotation device, for a completely impact-free work-out.

A range of special equipment is also available, including waterproof dumb-bells and webbed resistance gloves, designed to increase the resistance of the water.

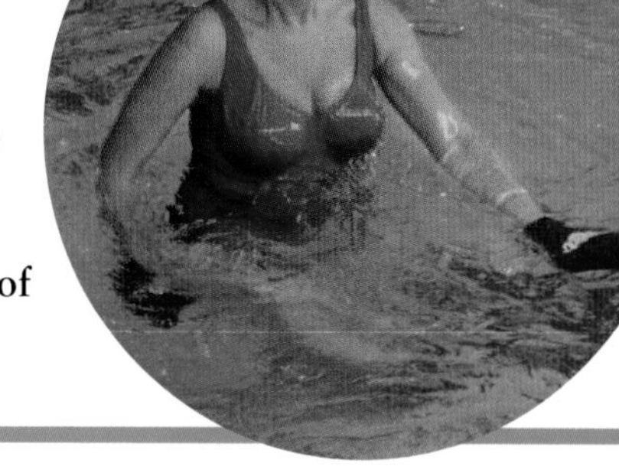

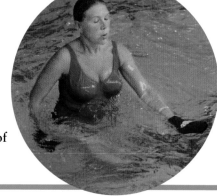

Get it right ... breast stroke

This stroke provides a good overall workout and improves joint mobility. As a leg dominant stroke it particularly tones your lower body.

1 Exhale as you launch into the glide with your arms and legs extended, your face submerged and your eyes looking down towards the floor.
2 Scoop your arms in towards your chest, turn your feet out and draw your heels towards your buttocks. Gently tilt your head to bring your face out of the water and inhale.
3 Bow your head into the water and begin to exhale gently. Thrust your legs back and out, feeling the pressure of the water against the soles of your feet and between your thighs as they close. Extend your arms and legs into the glide with your body as streamlined as possible.

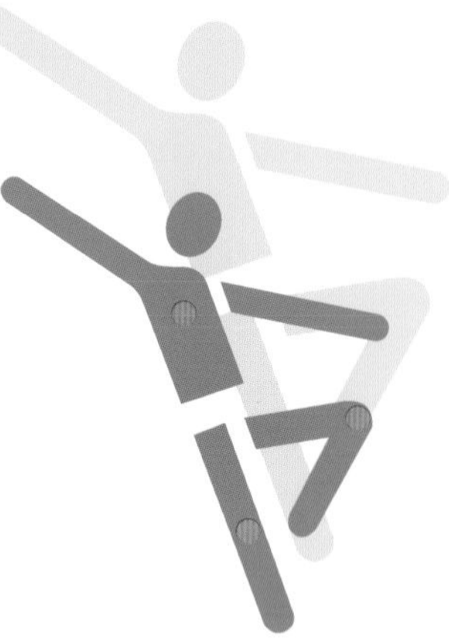

Dance

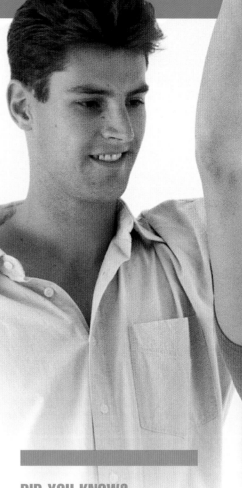

The key to any successful exercise programme is to find an activity that is enjoyable and easy to stick with; many people enjoy dancing because it doesn't really feel like exercise at all. It brings all the physical benefits of any other form of exercise but is also a way to have fun and meet new people.

- **Strengthens heart, lungs and circulation**
- **Helps weight loss**
- **Improves muscle strength in lower body**
- **Improves bone density in lower body**
- **Improves balance and coordination**

SEE ALSO

>>58
>>156
>>214

One of the great advantages of dancing as a form of exercise is the variety. From quick, lively forms of dance such as salsa and swing through to elegant, graceful waltzes or exotic flamenco, you are bound to find a style to suit your taste and ability.

What will it do for me?

The primary physical benefit of dance is that it provides a fun, aerobic workout, helping condition the heart and lungs – dancing can burn as many calories as walking or riding a bike. Many people who find it difficult to summon up the enthusiasm for a step class or a gym session will consider the rhythm and choreography of dance a far more tempting option.

Dancing for any length of time requires strength, balance and coordination, so it is an excellent way to improve poise and stability. This is especially important as we grow older, since good balance helps to safeguard against falls. Another bonus is that the weight-bearing movements strengthen the bones and muscles in your hips and legs.

There are many hundreds of distinct forms of dance originating from all over the world. Different types of dance place emphasis on different sorts of movement and bring their own particular benefits.

- The dips, turns and side-to-side movements found in dances such as jive and salsa are good for the range of motion in your muscles and joints. Belly dancing particularly targets the back and pelvic floor muscles, vital for maintaining your body's stability.
- Poised, graceful techniques such as ballroom dancing and ballet encourage coordination, balance and poise – particularly important qualities in later life to avoid falls and fractures.
- Line dancing provides a gentle cardiovascular workout that brings similar musculoskeletal benefits to step aerobics.

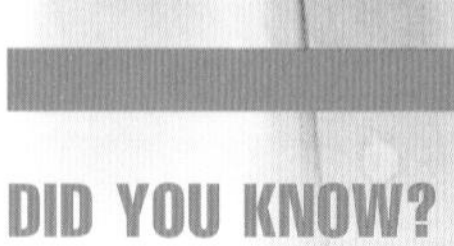

DID YOU KNOW?

According to a report in the *New England Journal of Medicine* (2003), dancing is good for your brain as well as your body. In a comparison of 11 physical activities, dancing was the only one associated with a significant decrease in the incidence of dementia, including Alzheimer's disease. This may be because the activity involves learning and remembering complex steps. The positive social influence of dancing may also play a role.

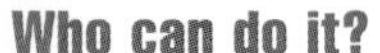

Who can do it?

Dance is suitable for all ages and levels of fitness, although different types of dance require different levels of physical aptitude. Most line dances, for example, have relatively simple step patterns that are easy for beginners to learn; some types of ballroom dancing, in contrast, can take years to master. This doesn't mean that you need a particularly high level of fitness to start ballroom dancing classes – much of the emphasis for beginners is on position and posture.

Energetic types of dance such as jazz and tap may require a good basic level of fitness before you begin. Slower, more graceful dances such as the waltz allow you to exercise at a slightly gentler pace, bringing cardiovascular benefits without being overly strenuous. This makes them particularly suitable for more elderly exercisers, who also benefit from the improvements in balance and stability.

What do I need?

Dancing requires little in the way of special equipment. Some dance classes require special clothing, but you'll usually be best wearing something loose and comfortable that doesn't restrict your movements. Wear well-fitting, cushioned shoes that won't slip underneath you – if trainers aren't suitable, there are light, flexible dance shoes available in many styles. Alternatively, adapt ordinary shoes by fitting stick-on soles for better grip.

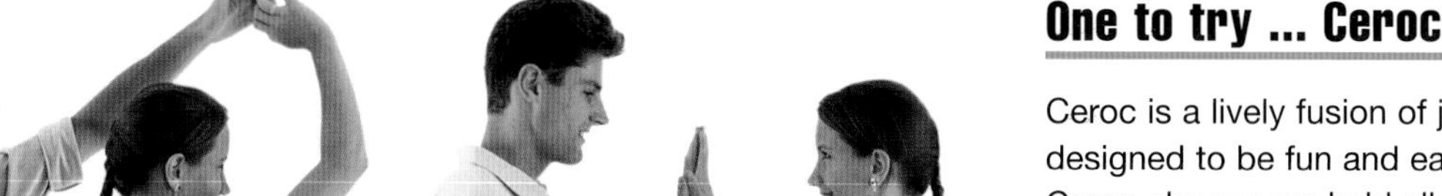

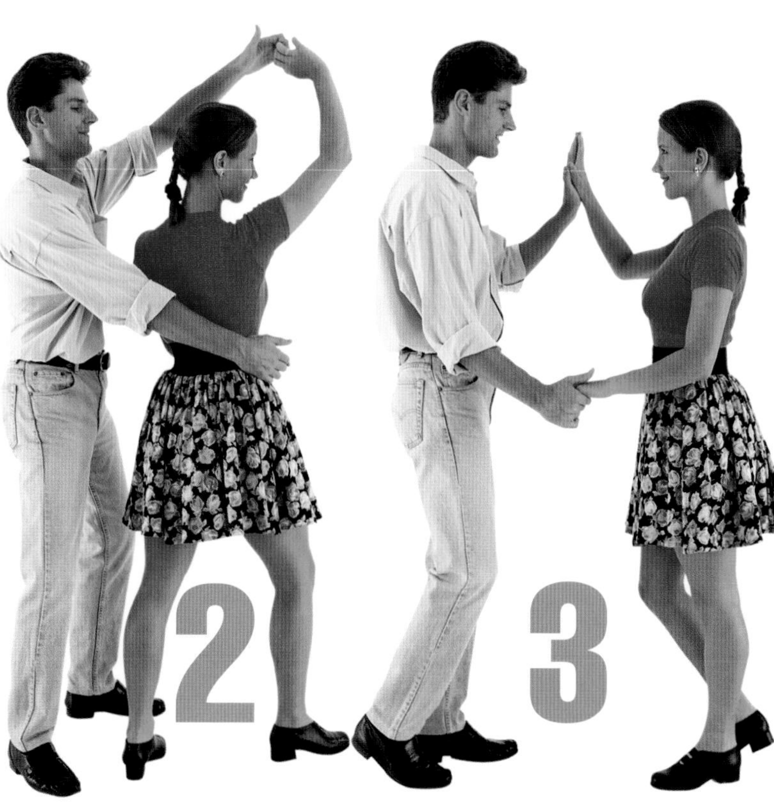

One to try ... Ceroc

Ceroc is a lively fusion of jive and salsa, designed to be fun and easy to pick up. Ceroc classes are held all over the UK, so you're bound to find one near you. The steps shown here come from a move called the basket.

1 On the first beat the gentleman spins the lady half a turn to wrap against his right side, his left hand holding her right at waist level.
2 On the next beat the gentleman raises his left hand and spins the lady a quarter turn as she takes a step forward.
3 On the next beat the lady continues the turn, letting go with her left hand and taking a step back to face the gentleman before taking his right hand with her left.

Walking

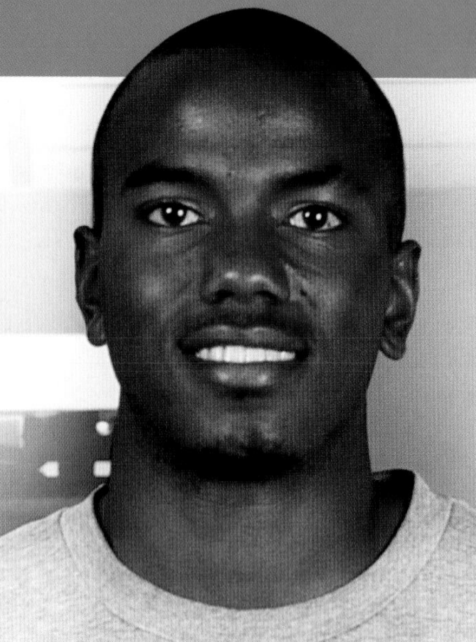

Walking is a great way to increase fitness and improve your general health. It is safe, low-impact and can be enjoyed by almost anyone, yet brings similar benefits to many more strenuous activities. It is also easy to incorporate into your everyday routine.

- **Strengthens heart, lungs and circulation**
- **Improves bone density in lower body**
- **Helps weight loss**
- **Improves muscle tone in lower body**

SEE ALSO

>>58
>>60
>>191
>>215

Walking offers both convenience and variety. Outdoor walking gets you out in the fresh air and lets you explore different areas and types of terrain. Indoor walking on a treadmill provides an all-weather alternative. It is easy to combine with other tasks; you could try walking to work each day, for example, or walking instead of driving to the shops.

Regular walking strengthens your muscles and joints, reducing the likelihood of injury. Stronger bones mean that regular brisk walkers are less likely to suffer fractures. Walking also helps to improve mood and reduce symptoms of depression and anxiety.

Walking at a vigorous pace is beneficial for the heart and lungs and has been shown to reduce mortality rates in both young and old people. It is also an excellent way to lose weight – walking for just one mile can burn up to 100 calories. One study, published in the *Journal of the American Medical Association*, compared the calorie-burning effect of treadmills with a range of other gym machines. It concluded that strenuous walking on a treadmill burns more calories than a similar-intensity workout on any other machine.

How to do it

Organizations such as the British Heart Foundation recommend that you walk at a brisk pace for 30 minutes a day, most days – but even 10 minutes of vigorous walking a day can increase fitness levels. Aim for an intensity that allows you to hold a conversation while walking, without becoming breathless.

A common mistake when walking at a faster pace than normal is to place the foot too far in front. This can lead to jarred ankles and knees and can cause pain along the muscles at the front of the shins. Focus on taking shorter but quicker steps. The power you generate while walking comes from your back leg, so concentrate on pushing off with your back leg and foot on each successive step.

Taking it further

If you are a keen walker you may want to try longer distances or rough terrain. You don't need to walk further or faster to work your muscles harder – walking up hills or on soft surfaces such as sand will also increase the work your muscles need to do.

Walking over uneven ground increases the risk of sprained ankles, particularly if you already have weak joints. To protect against sprains, always wear good hiking shoes – rigid leather boots that come up high on the ankles offer good stability on rough ground. If you carry a pack it should have adjustable, padded straps and, preferably, a hip belt to spread the load.

Nordic walking

This increasingly popular style of walking, developed in Scandinavia, uses two walking poles to up the intensity of the activity. The basic technique is similar to the cross-training machine in a gym: as you stride with your left foot you move the right pole forward, and vice versa. The poles encourage you to increase the length of your stride, so you can burn more calories than during normal walking, and the swinging arm and torso motion means you get more of an upper-body work out. The poles are also a good way to reduce the load on your knees and hips.

STEP OUT WITH A PEDOMETER

Could the humble pedometer be the key to keeping fit? It's certainly a great way to stay motivated: by counting the number of steps you take each day you can check how active you are, how far you've walked and how many calories you've burned – some models even do the calculations for you. So how many steps should you take each day? The ideal, according to the British Heart Foundation, is 10,000 steps (about 5 miles) – you can get much of this total without spending any time on organized exercise, though you should include at least 30 minutes of proper walking a day.

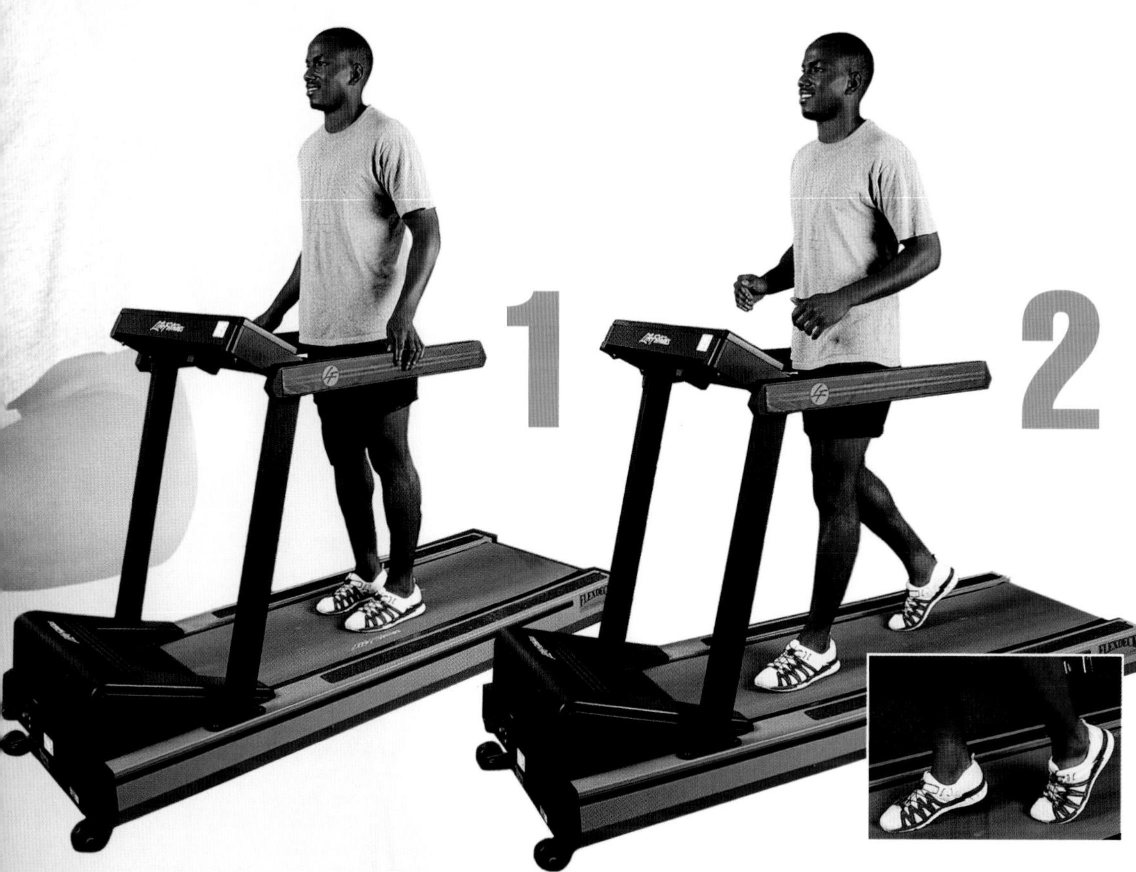

Get it right ... using a treadmill

1 Stand on the treadmill with your head and chin up and your chest lifted. You can touch the rails for balance, but do not grip them.

2 Start the machine slowly. As you walk, roll your foot from heel to ball and push up with your toes as you swing your other leg forward. Keep your arms slightly bent and let them swing naturally.

3 Gradually increase the speed of the belt. You should start to breathe a little harder, but not so hard that you find it difficult to hold a conversation. If you need to hold on to the rails, you are probably working too hard and should slow down.

4 At the end of your session, slowly decrease your speed until you reach a gentle walking pace. Cool down at this speed for 5 minutes.

Yoga

Having evolved in India over many thousands of years, this ancient system of physical and mental therapy is now widely practised in the West as a way to relax and tone the body and improve flexibility. The various techniques and postures of yoga keep joints lubricated and free, relieve stress and increase general well-being.

- Improves flexibility
- Improves body awareness
- Aids posture
- Tones muscles, particularly the core stabilizing muscles
- Increases range of motion
- Low impact

SEE ALSO

>>58
>>154
>>156
>>250
>>255

There are many different types of yoga, each one emphasizing a slightly different aspect of health and fitness. Styles such as Hatha and Iyengar yoga may be beneficial for older practitioners as the slow, gentle movements avoid straining the joints but still tone the body and increase endurance and flexibility. Ashtanga and Vinyasa yoga are generally faster paced and more energetic. Bikram is a particularly challenging style performed in a heated room so that muscles and ligaments can be stretched further without injury.

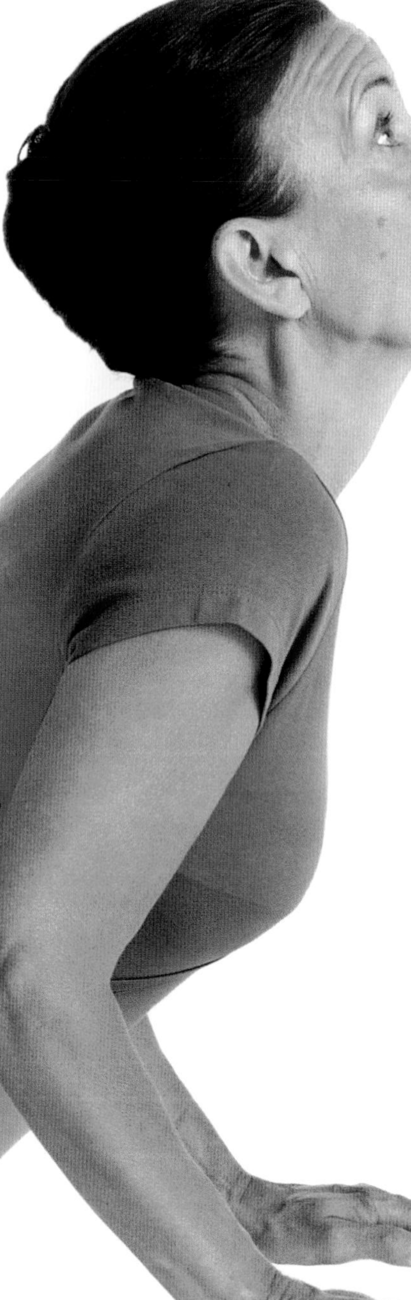

What can it do for me?

Most forms of yoga practice concentrate on three fundamental principles, although different styles place differing degrees of emphasis on each one.

- **Postures** Yoga postures give your muscles and ligaments a slow, gentle stretch, making them healthier, improving circulation and mobility, and reducing pain and stiffness. The postures tone your muscles and improve body awareness.
- **Breathing** Correct breathing throughout your practice focuses your thoughts and helps you concentrate. It also increases the oxygen supply to your muscles, helping eliminate lactic acid in the tissues as well as reducing heart rate.
- **Meditation** Meditation is a method of deep relaxation to help clear your mind from the stresses and worries of everyday life. This reduces anxiety and increases your sense of well-being.

A holistic approach

As well as improving general fitness, yoga is considered therapeutic in its own right – the movements helping to relieve chronic pain from back problems or conditions such as arthritis. Many people also report improvements in ailments ranging from allergies to insomnia.

Yoga's benefits are also preventative. As your muscles and tendons become more flexible, they also become more resistant to injury, even when you are performing other physical activities.

Getting started

Most sport centres and health clubs now run yoga sessions – your local library may well have information about classes in your area. If you prefer to train at home, there are plenty of illustrated books, yoga videos and DVDs available.

Whatever style of yoga you practise, do not push yourself too hard and never try to bounce or force your body into an uncomfortable pose. The emphasis should always be on correct, gentle and fluid positions and movements. Don't worry if you find it hard to complete the full extension of a posture: even if you can only move a few degrees outside your normal range of motion, the posture will still prove beneficial. After just a few weeks of regular practice you should find that your body becomes much more flexible and postures are easier to reach.

DID YOU KNOW?

- **According to a 1994 report in the *Journal of Rheumatology*, a ten-week upper-body yoga programme can significantly reduce symptoms of osteoarthritis in the hand.**
- **Another study in 1998, reported in the *Journal of the American Medical Association*, found that yoga poses improved the symptoms of carpal tunnel syndrome (>>284).**

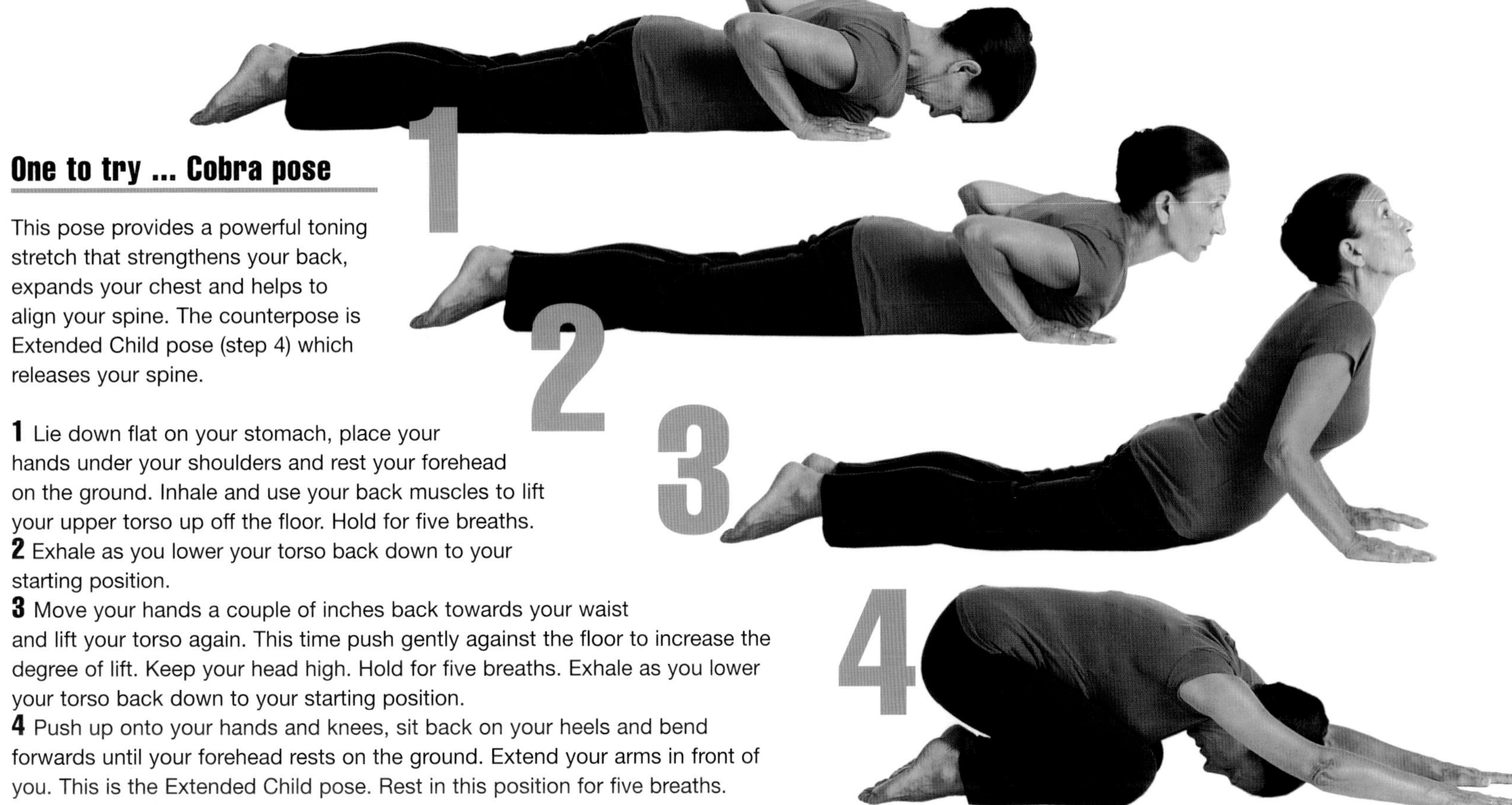

One to try ... Cobra pose

This pose provides a powerful toning stretch that strengthens your back, expands your chest and helps to align your spine. The counterpose is Extended Child pose (step 4) which releases your spine.

1 Lie down flat on your stomach, place your hands under your shoulders and rest your forehead on the ground. Inhale and use your back muscles to lift your upper torso up off the floor. Hold for five breaths.
2 Exhale as you lower your torso back down to your starting position.
3 Move your hands a couple of inches back towards your waist and lift your torso again. This time push gently against the floor to increase the degree of lift. Keep your head high. Hold for five breaths. Exhale as you lower your torso back down to your starting position.
4 Push up onto your hands and knees, sit back on your heels and bend forwards until your forehead rests on the ground. Extend your arms in front of you. This is the Extended Child pose. Rest in this position for five breaths.

Pilates

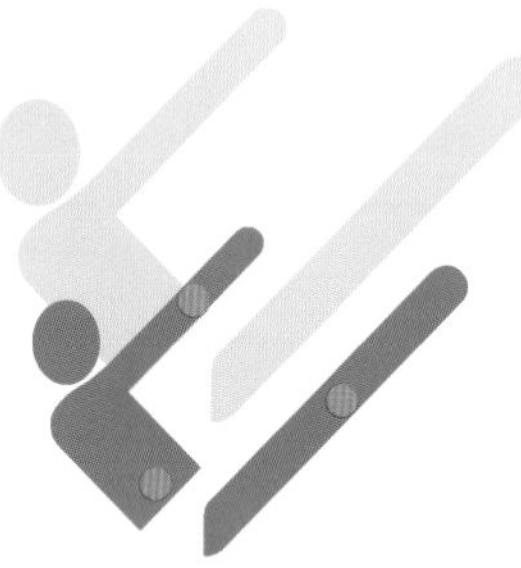

Pilates is a system of slow, controlled exercises intended to strengthen your body's core stabilizing muscles while improving their natural flexibility. It was developed in the early 20th century by an athlete and boxer named Joseph Pilates and has now been used by professional dancers and other athletes for more than 80 years.

- **Improves flexibility**
- **Improves body awareness**
- **Aids posture**
- **Tones muscles, particularly the core stabilizing muscles**
- **Increases range of motion**
- **Low impact**

SEE ALSO

>>58
>>185

Since its founder's day, Pilates has evolved to incorporate many advances in biomechanics, but the emphasis of the exercises remain squarely on good posture and body awareness – which makes it perfect for musculoskeletal fitness.

Whereas exercises such as weight training tend to focus on individual muscles or areas of the body, Pilates provides a more holistic approach – Joseph Pilates defined his method as 'the complete coordination of mind, body and spirit'. Each exercise flows into the next in a smooth, controlled sequence, reflecting the way that your body engages muscles and joints dynamically during movement.

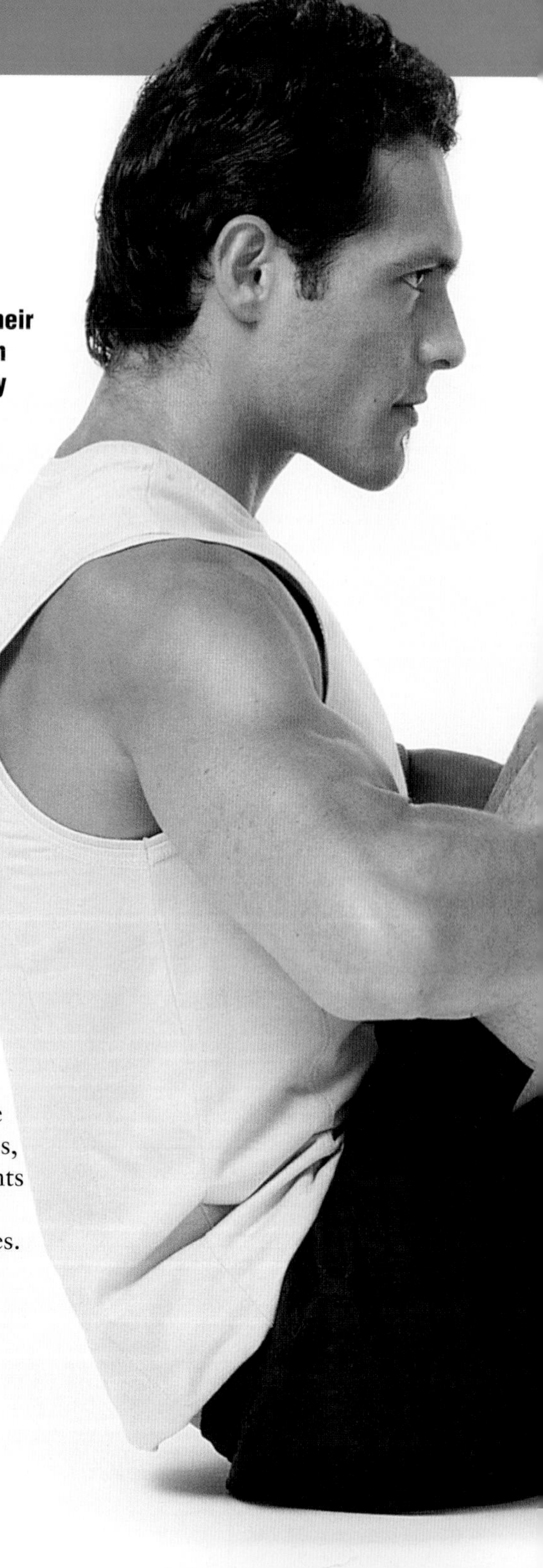

What are the benefits?

The slow, controlled movements condition muscles, helping them to strengthen and elongate in an even, balanced manner. In particular, Pilates concentrates on the abdomen, back and pelvic-girdle region: the core muscles used to stabilize the body. This aids posture and keeps the hips and spine supple.

The exercises use gentle, lengthening motions to increase the body's flexibility, taking pressure off joints and reducing soreness, pain and fatigue. The stretching motions also pump vital nutrients to the muscles and joints, improving joint lubrication.

Pilates is low impact, making it suitable for people of all ages. The lack of bouncing and jarring also makes it ideal for people with joint problems or weak muscles.

The principles of Pilates

- **Centring** The core muscles of your body (the abdominals, buttocks, inner thigh and lower back) form your 'centre' – the fulcrum around which all movements are made.

■ **Precision and control** Instead of casually moving from one position into another, Pilates emphasises the importance of maintaining precise control and coordination as you do so.
■ **Concentration** Good form relies on focus, visualization and muscle awareness – as Pilates wrote, 'it is the mind that controls the body'. Try to notice how your mind controls your muscles.
■ **Flow** Each exercise should flow gracefully and naturally into the next with what Joseph Pilates called 'energetic dynamics'. This reflects the fact that your body's posture is also dynamic, constantly adjusting to counteract forces placed on it. The flowing movements in Pilates reflect the way we use our bodies much better than static poses.
■ **Breathing** Deep, rhythmic breathing is essential to control each exercise and coordinate with the flow of the movement.

Getting started

Plenty of sport centres and health clubs now run Pilates classes. Check in your local library or health centre to find one near you. There are also a number of excellent instruction books, Pilates videos and DVDs available.

In a Pilates mat class (the most common form) the teacher will guide you through a series of mat-based exercises designed to improve your strength, suppleness and body awareness. Most sessions last between 60 and 90 minutes. More technical classes are also available, usually held in a dedicated studio containing a range of specialized equipment. As with most forms of exercise, learning Pilates is an ongoing process. The programme is divided into several levels, with each new level involving slightly more advanced versions of each exercise. As you progress towards more advanced techniques, the benefits of each exercise should increase.

With all Pilates exercises, the emphasis is on quality of movement rather than quantity. This means you can safely practise every day without overstressing your muscles or joints. Joseph Pilates recommended that you do Pilates four times a week, but you should still see improvements with less frequent practice.

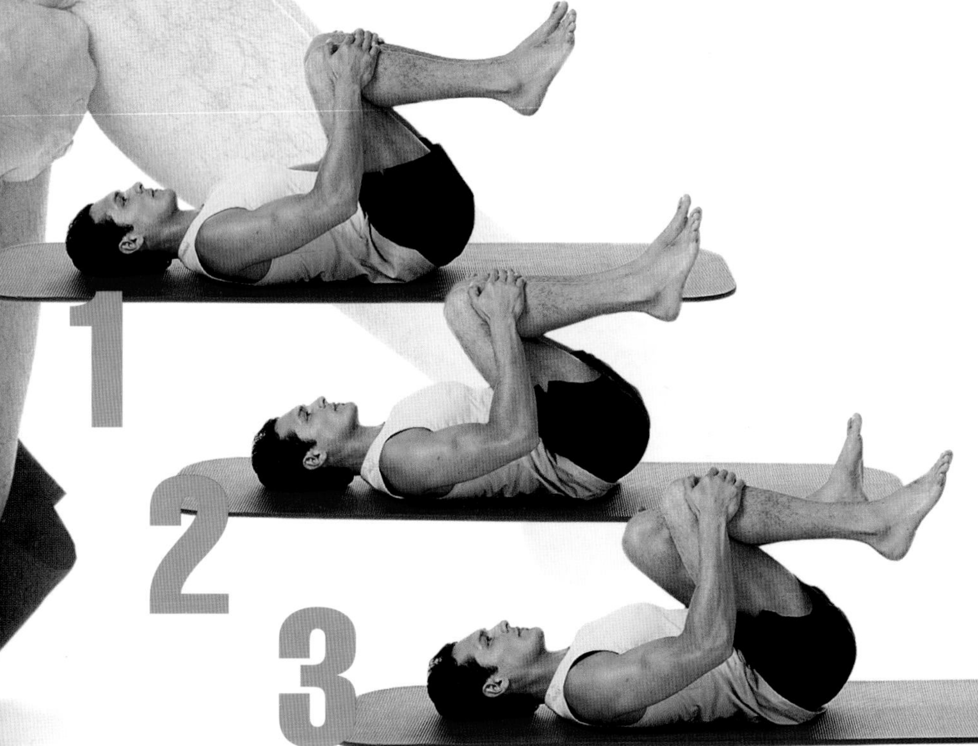

One to try ... releasing the back and neck

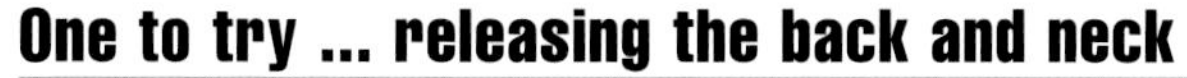

This exercise lengthens the muscles that run along the length of your spine, opening up your back. These muscles run right up to the base of your skull, so it also relieves tension and compression in your neck. Controlled breathing helps you to focus and relax.

1 Lie on your back and gently cradle your knees in your hands. Hold your knees slightly apart and in line with your hips and press your lower back flat against the floor. Pull your stomach in towards your spine and keep your abdominals tight.
2 Inhale. Then, as you exhale, gently draw your knees in towards your chest. Make sure your arms are not straining and your elbows are open and relaxed. Keep your spine flat against the floor. You should feel your chest and back begin to open out.
3 Inhale. As you exhale, slowly draw your right leg in towards your chest a little further. Inhale and release your leg, allowing it to return to the starting position. As you exhale again, slowly draw your left leg further in towards your chest. Repeat this sequence, coordinating it with your breathing for a total of 10 times.

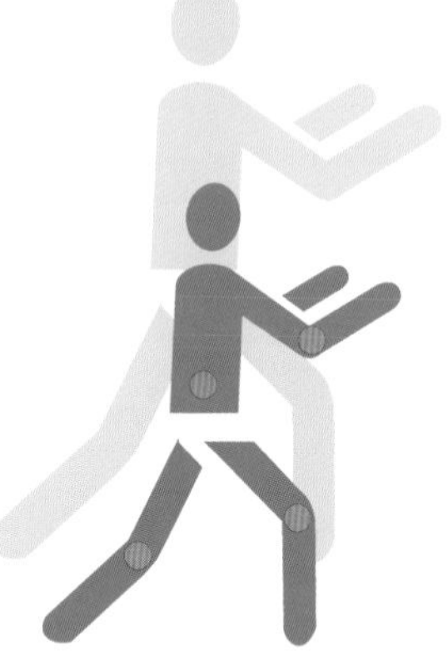

Tai chi

The ancient Chinese art of movement, tai chi, is sometimes described as 'meditation in motion'. As well as calming and focusing the mind, tai chi has many documented physical benefits, including increased flexibility, balance, muscle tone and good body awareness.

- Improves coordination and body control
- Aids balance and posture
- Tones muscles
- Increases range of motion
- Low impact
- Low risk of injury

SEE ALSO

>>58
>>164
>>191

Tai chi exercises use a continuous series of flowing movements, practised together in a sequence known as the Form. These motions are intended to help your 'qi' (internal energy) to move freely through your body, encouraging harmony between your mind and body. Whatever your faith in qi, there is no doubt that the controlled, flowing movements bring real physical benefits.

What will it do for me?

Practising tai chi keeps you aware of your body. The precise, repetitive movements, with their emphasis on the controlled use of gradual tension and relaxation, help you to achieve a heightened appreciation of the way your whole body moves. This in turn improves posture, coordination and balance, relaxing tense muscles and reducing many of the stresses on your bones and joints.

The slow, controlled motion of the exercises also helps to load your bones and works muscles in parts of your body that are often neglected by more conventional weight-training exercises. One study at the National Taiwan University Hospital found that 30 minutes of tai chi daily for six months increased leg muscle strength in the 50 to 60-year-old volunteers by up to 20 per cent.

One of the great advantages of tai chi is that anyone can practise it. It is low impact and carries little risk of injury, making it suitable for elderly people or those suffering from bone and joint problems. Because the exercises improve balance, it also reduces the risk of falls and fractures. Arthritis sufferers should find that the gentle movements lessen stiffness and improve flexibility.

Tai chi forms

Many different styles of tai chi have evolved over the centuries. The type most commonly practised in the West today, the Yang style, is characterized by mainly vertical postures and relaxed movements,

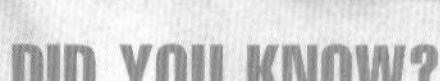

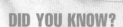

DID YOU KNOW?

A study at the Emory University School of Medicine, reported in the *Journal of the American Medical Association* in 1995, compared the effects of three types of exercise regime, including tai chi, on the likelihood of falls in older people.

- **The first exercise programme incorporated strength, balance and endurance exercises and reduced the risk of falls by 10 per cent.**
- **The second programme used balance training alone and reduced the risk of falls by 25 per cent.**
- **The third programme, consisting of tai chi exercises, reduced the risk of falls by a massive 47 per cent.**

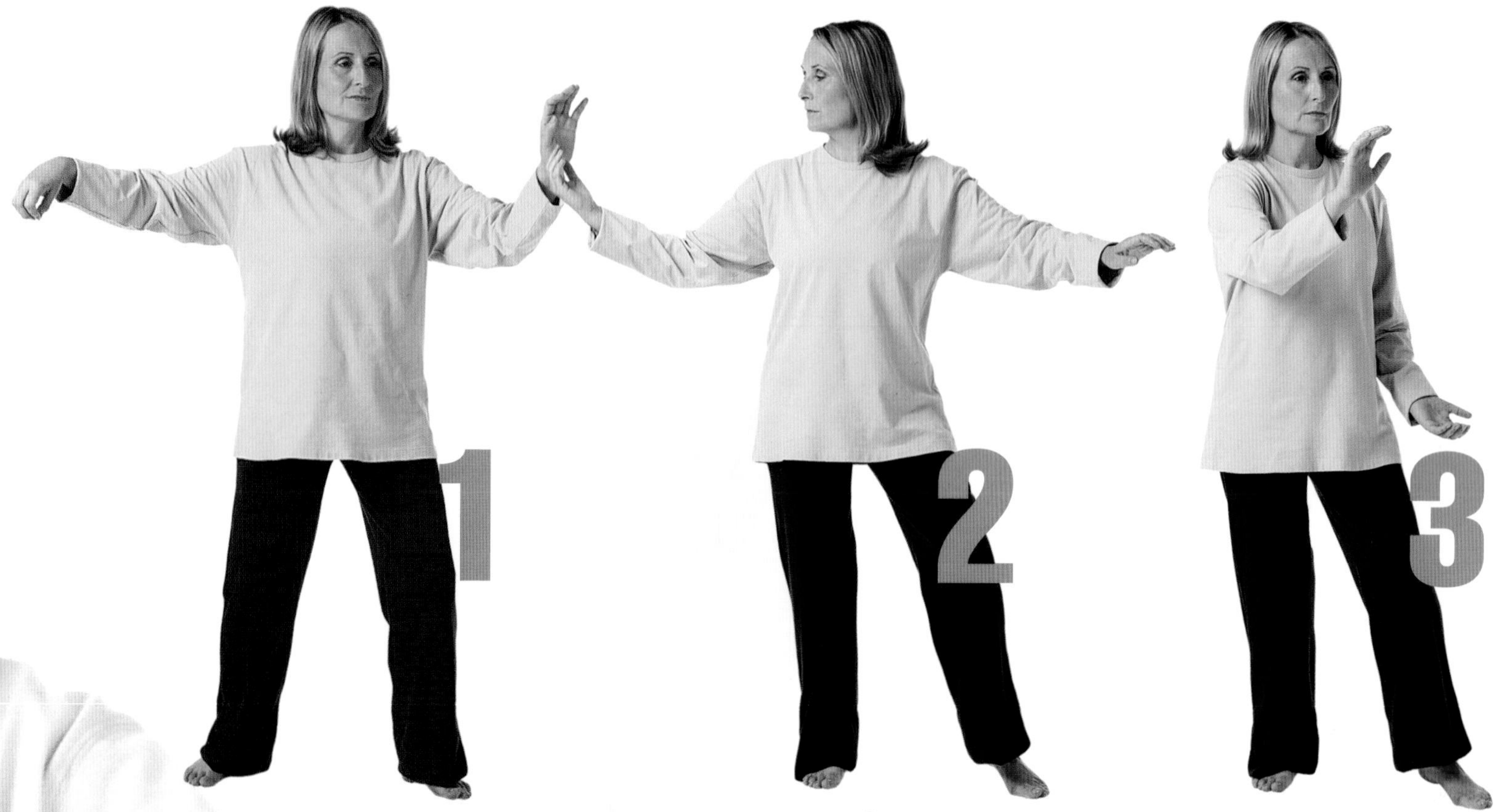

performed at a slow pace and complemented with calm, even breathing. There are several Forms in each style and the number of movements in a Form can vary from as few as 12 to as many as 108. It generally takes 5–15 minutes to complete a sequence of movements, depending on the Form.

Slowly but surely

When learning a tai chi Form, first try to familiarize yourself with one or two movements in the sequence and practise them regularly. Add more postures gradually, to give yourself time to learn each movement thoroughly. Although it might take only 10 minutes to perform a complete sequence, it can take several months to learn all of the movements that make up the Form.

Be patient – the more slowly you work through the exercises, the better you will understand and benefit from them. You may start to see any benefits to flexibility, balance and posture after only a few sessions but you may need to practise for much longer to see results.

One to try ... High Pat on Horse

1 Stand with your feet hip-width apart. Point your left foot directly ahead and keep your right foot a step back and pointing away at an angle – the classic 'Bow stance'. Form a 'beak' with your right hand and straighten your arm away from your body. Push directly ahead of you with your left hand, palm forward.
2 Begin to draw back your left foot, raising your heel. Move your right arm further to the right and open your hand up. Turn your left palm face down. Look over at your right hand.
3 Turn your head back to the left so that you are looking ahead of you. Move your right arm back across your body so that it is almost straight, palm facing down. Move your left hand down to your left hip, palm up.

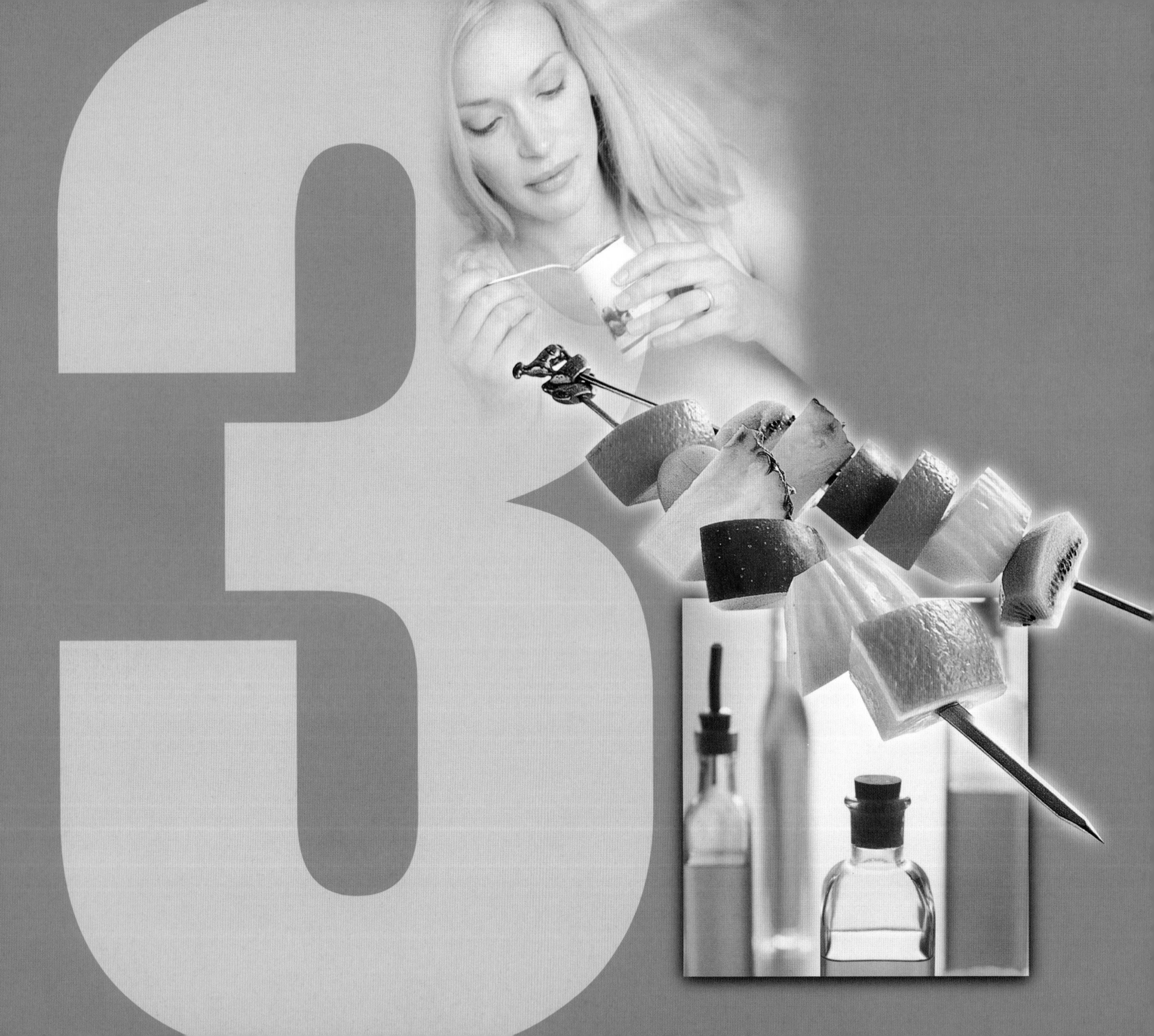

FOOD FACTS

Am I overweight? Should I eat dairy products? Do I need a supplement? The questions are endless and the answers often confusing and contradictory. In these pages you will find out which foods can positively affect your bones, muscles and joints (and which to avoid), as well as the supplements you might need at various stages of life for optimal musculoskeletal fitness.

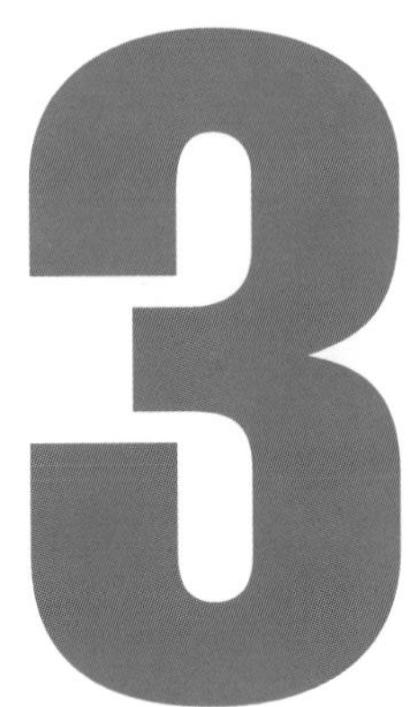

FOOD FACTS
Components of a healthy diet

Your muscles and the bones that make up your skeleton are active, living tissue; throughout your life this tissue is constantly renewed and repaired to keep you vigorous and strong. To do this well your body needs a healthy mix of vitamins, minerals and other nutrients.

It is easy to take your bones, muscles and joints for granted, but without proper nourishment, these vital tissues will soon start to deteriorate. Your diet provides the fuel your body needs to power your muscles and sustain tissue repair and growth. The protein in your diet is broken down into amino acids and used to build bones, cartilage and muscle. A range of other vitamins and minerals are essential to build healthy bones and muscles.

Diet is particularly important in bone health. A good calcium intake during childhood, adolescence and early adulthood, while your bones are still growing, will help to protect them throughout your life. As you get older, a calcium-rich diet is equally important to reduce loss of calcium from your bones.

DID YOU KNOW?

- **Your bones undergo a constant process of regeneration. It takes seven to ten years for an adult skeleton to be entirely broken down and rebuilt with new minerals.**
- **About 700mg of calcium enter your bones every day, deposited by the bone-building osteoblast cells.**
- **During rapid bone growth in childhood, your skeleton takes just two years to renew itself.**

126

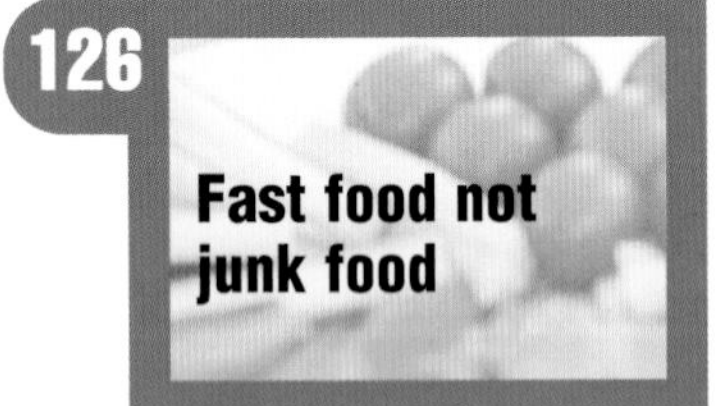

Fast food not junk food

200

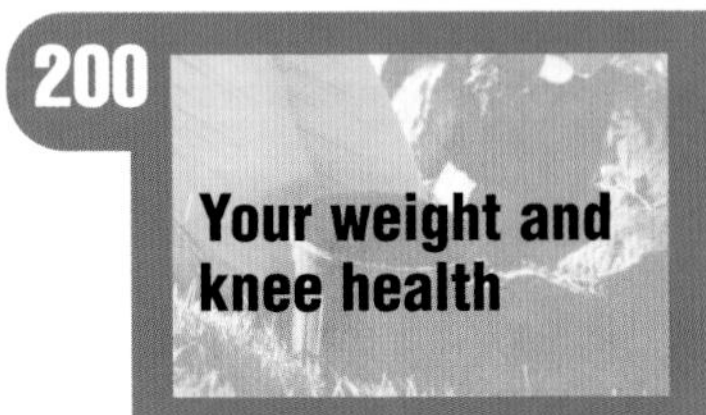

Your weight and knee health

268

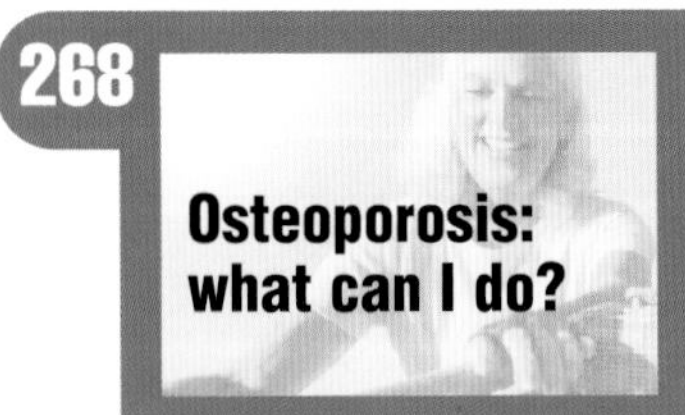

Osteoporosis: what can I do?

Getting the right balance

Sorting fact from fiction is not always easy when it comes to nutrition – hardly a week seems to pass without a new food scare hitting the headlines. The important thing to remember is that there is no such thing as a good or a bad food: the essential feature of a healthy diet is balance. To help you get a good balance, nutritionists divide foods into five main groups. You need to eat some foods from each group, each day.

- **Grains, cereals and potatoes** (such as bread, rice, pasta, noodles and breakfast cereals) provide fibre, protein, vitamins and minerals, but their main job is to supply the energy used to power your muscles. Foods from this group should provide the

DAIRY PRODUCTS

Aim to eat 3–4 servings a day. Choose reduced or low-fat alternatives such as skimmed and semi-skimmed milk where possible. You may find it difficult to get enough calcium if you don't eat dairy products – you could try calcium-fortified products or supplements instead.

What's a serving? 1 serving equals ⅓ pint milk, 1 small pot of yoghurt, or 30g (1oz) cheese.

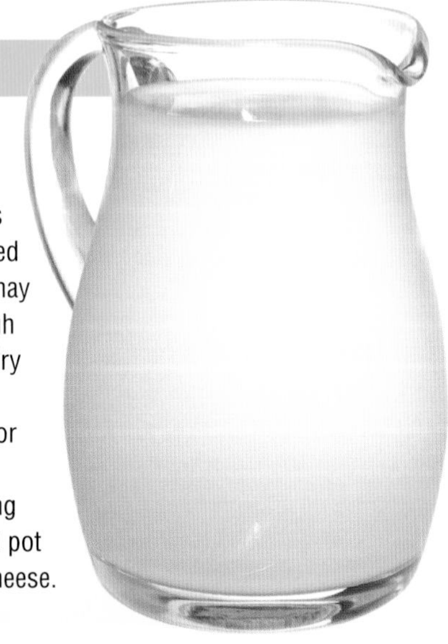

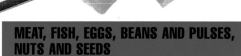

bulk of calories on your plate at each meal. Choose wholegrain varieties such as wholemeal bread, brown rice and high fibre cereals where possible.

■ **Fruit and vegetables** are a good source of many vitamins, minerals and phytochemicals. Eat a variety of different fruit and vegetables to gain the full range of different nutrients. Fresh, frozen, dried and canned fruit and vegetables, including tomato purée and baked beans, all count towards your total. Potatoes don't count, although other starchy vegetables such as parsnips and swede do. A small glass (150ml/5fl oz) of fruit or vegetable juice is one portion – but it counts as only one portion however much you drink, because it has very little fibre.

■ **Dairy products** (such as cheese, milk, yoghurt and fromage frais) are a vital source of calcium, essential for strong bones. They also provide protein, vitamin A, vitamin D vitamin B_2 and phosphorus. Dairy foods can be high in fat, particularly saturated fat, so choose low-fat options if possible.

■ **Meat and meat alternatives** (such as fish, eggs, beans, nuts and seeds) provide protein for growth and repair and for the production of vital enzymes, antibodies and hormones. Oily fish such as salmon, fresh tuna and mackerel are rich in omega-3 fats, which may help to ease arthritis symptoms and bring a range of other health benefits. Aim to eat oil-rich fish twice a week.

■ **Fats and sugars** Your body needs small amounts of fat to get essential fatty acids and absorb fat-soluble vitamins. But not all fats are equal: saturated fats (found in fatty meat, full-fat dairy products, butter and some margarines) can increase the risk of heart disease; fats in nuts and seeds, olive oil and oily fish are much better for your health.

Sugar provides 'empty' calories (calories that provide no protein, fibre, vitamins or minerals) so it makes sense to cut down on sugar where you can.

FATS AND SUGARS

Aim to eat 0–3 servings of fats and oils or 0–2 servings of high-fat or high-sugar foods per day. Reduce your saturated fats where possible.
What's a serving? 1 serving of fats equals 1 teaspoon of butter, oil or mayonnaise. 1 serving of high-fat, high-sugar food equals 1 packet of crisps; 3–5 boiled sweets; or 25g (1oz) chocolate

GRAINS, CEREALS AND POTATOES

Aim to eat 5–11 servings a day (depending on your appetite and calorie requirements).
What's a serving? 3 tablespoons breakfast cereal; 1 slice of bread; 2 heaped tablespoons boiled rice; 3 heaped tablespoons pasta; 2 egg-sized potatoes.

FRUIT AND VEGETABLES

Aim to eat at least 5 servings a day. This is the minimum requirement – the more fruit and vegetables you eat the better.
What's a serving? About 85g (3oz). This is equivalent to 1 apple, banana, or orange; 2 satsumas; 3 tablespoons of peas or carrots; 3 dried apricots; 1 tablespoon of raisins; 1 bowl of salad; ½ an avocado; 1 medium tomato; or 7 cherry tomatoes.

MEAT, FISH, EGGS, BEANS AND PULSES, NUTS AND SEEDS

Aim to eat 2–4 servings a day. Red meat is high in saturated fats, which raise cholesterol, so you should get most of your protein from fish, nuts, beans and pulses.
What's a serving? 90g (3¼oz) red meat; 125g (4.5 oz) chicken; 125–150g (4½–5½oz) fish; 5 tablespoons of baked beans; 2 tablespoons of nuts; or 2 eggs.

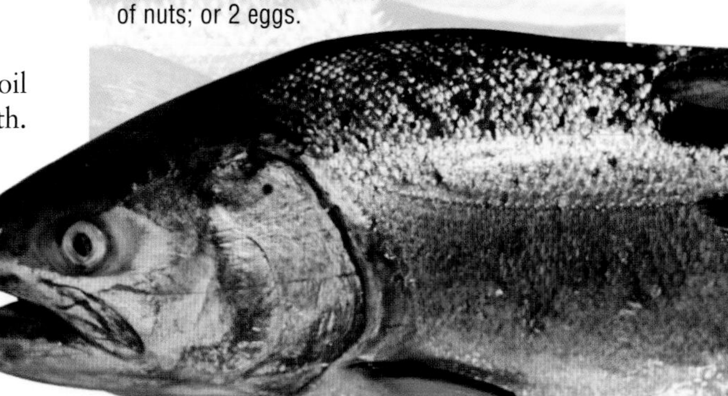

Nutrients for healthy bones, muscles and joints

A number of vitamins and minerals bring particular benefits for your bones, muscles and joints. These nutrients are all readily obtained from a varied, balanced diet (one that includes each of the food groups shown on pages 100–101). People who do not get enough of these nutrients in their regular diet may benefit from supplements.

Calcium

This is the single most important mineral for strong bones – your body contains around 1kg (over 2lb) of calcium, 99 per cent of which is contained in your skeleton. Calcium is also essential for blood clotting, muscle contraction and nerve function – if you do not have a high enough intake, your body takes calcium from your bones to supply your muscles, heart and nerves. This weakens your bones and puts you at risk of fractures and osteoporosis.

'According to the 2003 National Diet and Nutrition Survey, almost half of women in the UK do not get the recommended intake of calcium in their diet'

- In the average British diet, milk and other dairy products provide over 50 per cent of the calcium intake, but it is present in lots of other foods too.
- Non-dairy sources include beans and pulses, some green vegetables, nuts, fruit and canned fish that is eaten with the bones such as salmon and sardines.
- To find out how much calcium your body needs at different times of your life, from childhood to old age >>110–111. For a breakdown of the calcium content of some common foods >>268.

Vitamin D

This vitamin is essential for the efficient absorption of calcium from your gut to build strong bones. Lack of vitamin D also causes muscle weakness, aches and pains. In one Minnesota-based study of 150 patients with persistent musculoskeletal pain that had not been helped by ordinary treatment, all of the patients were found to have low levels of vitamin D.

Your body produces vitamin D when you expose your skin to sunlight – around 90 per cent of your intake comes from this source. Some groups, such as elderly, house-bound people, may not get enough sunlight to produce sufficient amounts of vitamin D. These people may benefit from a vitamin-D supplement (>>104–105). Most people, however, should be able to get enough from sunlight and from dietary sources.

- Around 15–30 minutes of sunlight on your face and arms each day during the summer months should be enough for your body to store most of the vitamin D it needs for the rest of the year.
- Vitamin-D rich foods such as oily fish, egg yolks, liver and margarine contribute the remaining 10 per cent.

Magnesium

This mineral plays an important role in both bone and muscle health. It promotes and regulates the parathyroid hormone, which stimulates calcium absorption in bones. Lack of magnesium affects the quality of bone calcification, weakening your bones.

Around half of the magnesium in your body is found in your bones, but most of the rest is found in the cells of your tissues and organs, where it is used to regulate a range of biochemical reactions. Some of these involve muscle and nerve function and, if your magnesium levels are low, your muscles may stiffen and cramp.

- Good sources of magnesium include Brazil nuts, sunflower and sesame seeds, bananas, pine nuts, cashew nuts and dark-green leafy vegetables such as spinach.

Omega-3 fatty acids

Unlike saturated fats, which have few health benefits, the essential fatty acids omega-3 and omega-6 play a key role in a range of vital body functions. Researchers are increasingly interested in the benefits of omega-3 oils in relieving stiff and swollen joints and reducing the general aches and pains often associated with ageing.

Omega-3s improve immune function, reducing symptoms of rheumatoid arthritis, and may help to relieve other inflammatory disorders such as osteoarthritis. Some studies have concluded that omega-3 fatty acids can also help to increase calcium levels, improving bone strength. Omega-3 fatty acids also bring considerable benefits for your heart and circulation.

- Omega-3 fatty acids are found in oily fish such as salmon, mackerel and sardines.
- Plant sources include linseed oil, rapeseed oil, pumpkin seeds and walnuts. A number of UK companies have recently introduced omega-3 fortified milks.

Other important nutrients

Other nutrients that play a key role in maintaining healthy bones, muscles and joints include:

- **Phosphorus** A good balance of calcium and phosphorus, combined in the form of calcium phosphate, is needed to build bone strength. Phosphorus is also essential for muscle contractions and helps to regulate other vitamins and minerals, including vitamin D, magnesium and zinc.

Phosphorus is found in many foods, notably dairy products, so deficiency is rare. Few people need to worry about getting more phosphorus in their diet – indeed, if levels are too high, your body may actually remove calcium from your bones to bind to the phosphorus and remove it from your bloodstream.

- **Vitamin K** Research suggests that this helps bones to lay down the minerals they need, like calcium. Friendly bacteria in your intestines produce about 80 per cent of the vitamin K that you need, the rest comes from foods such as spinach, broccoli, kale, sprouts and watercress.
- **Vitamin C** This helps the body produce collagen, a protein in bones, muscles and other tissues. It is an antioxidant and may boost your immune function. Vitamin C is found in most fruits and vegetables.
- **Potassium** Found in fruit, vegetables and pulses, especially green leafy vegetables, this regulates muscle and nerve function. Low levels can cause muscle weakness and cramps. It also balances sodium (salt) levels, helping regulate the water balance in your cells. Potassium has been shown to prevent calcium loss in postmenopausal women by offsetting the effects of a high-salt diet.
- **Other trace minerals** Your bones contain small quantities of minerals such as boron, zinc, manganese and copper. These trace minerals have a minor but important role in keeping bones and muscles healthy.

Zinc, which is found in food including red meat, seafood, eggs and dairy products, helps to regulate a number of enzymes involved in the bone building process. Boron (in fruits and nuts, vegetables and legumes) improves the strength and structure of your bone. Copper and manganese (found in shellfish, nuts and leafy vegetables) are also believed to play a role in bone formation.

CHECK THE LABELS

The pressures of modern life may mean that we don't always have the time to prepare fresh food. Fortunately, fast food doesn't have to be unhealthy. There is no reason why a meal from a packet or a jar needs to be any less nutritious than one that has taken hours to prepare.

When it comes to choosing convenience food, the secret is check the information on the label. Look at the amount of a particular nutrient and compare with the table below: where possible, choose foods that are high in fibre but low in fat, salt and sugar.

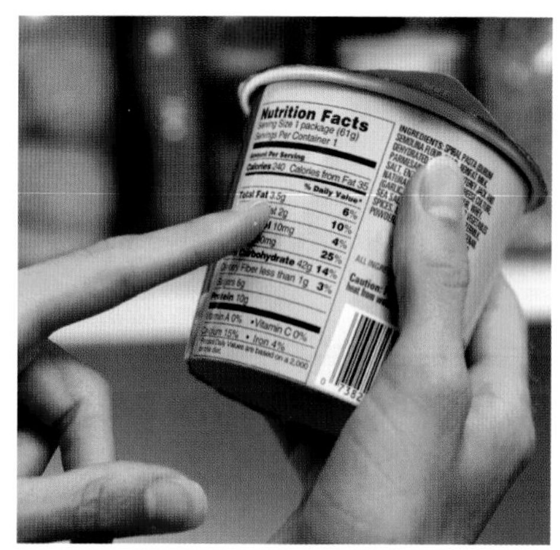

NUTRIENT	HIGH (per 100g)	LOW (per 100g)
Fat	more than 20g	less than 3g
Saturated fat	more than 5g	less than 1g
Sugar	more than 10g	less than 2g
Sodium (salt)	more than 0.5g (1.25g salt)	less than 0.1g (0.25g salt)
Fibre	more than 3g	less than 0.5g

How much should I take?

Although the government sets a Recommended Daily Allowance (RDA) for each of the essential vitamins and minerals we need in our diet, this only represents the minimum amount that you need to take in order to prevent a deficiency. In some cases, the amount you need to keep your bones, muscles and joints in peak condition may be higher.

A better indication of your optimal intake is the Recommended Nutrient Intake (RNI). This term describes the amount that is sufficient to meet the needs of most people in the population and takes age and sex into account. The RNI should be perfectly adequate for the vast majority of people – you should only take more than the RNI if you are advised to do so by your doctor or a qualified nutritionist.

It is important to bear in mind that both the RDA and RNI represent your overall intake of a certain nutrient – that is, your intake from diet and other sources and not just the amount you should take in a supplement. When calculating your intake, you should include all foods, including fortified foods as well as any supplements. If you get enough of a certain vitamin or nutrient in your diet, you will reach your recommended levels without needing to take any supplements at all.

CAUTION

It is possible to get too much of a certain vitamin or mineral, especially if you are taking high doses of supplements – a good reason to avoid taking a supplement unless you know that you really need it. The vitamins A, D, E and K are fat-soluble, which means they can be stored in the body; if large doses build up they can become toxic. Large doses of some water-soluble vitamins, like vitamin B_6, can also be harmful. High mineral intakes may inhibit the absorption of other key nutrients and can be toxic.

Do I need supplements?

Dietary supplements are no substitute for a healthy, balanced diet with plenty of fruit and vegetables and all of the food groups shown on pages 100–101. But for people who do not get an adequate supply of nutrients in their regular diet, supplements can be a useful way to 'fill the gap'. Reasons for taking supplements include:

- **A restricted diet** Our busy lifestyles mean that we often skip meals or eat too much fast food, which can limit the range of nutrients we obtain from our diet. Restricting your diet in other ways, by slimming or avoiding certain foods, may also lead to certain deficiencies.
- **Digestion problems** Bowel disorders such as coeliac disease and other problems can impair your absorption of nutrients.
- **Certain medical conditions** Some people may also benefit from taking supplements to help relieve the symptoms or slow the progression of a particular medical problem, such as osteoporosis.
- **Your age group** Nutritional needs vary at different periods of your life. Children need lots of vitamins and minerals to make strong bones and muscles, particularly during periods of rapid growth. Pregnant or breastfeeding women also need higher amounts of certain nutrients, including calcium, while elderly people may have trouble digesting some nutrients effectively.

NUTRIENTS	WHAT DOES IT DO?
Calcium	Vital for bone strength and formation; involved in muscle contraction
Vitamin D	Aids calcium absorption and helps to maintain muscle health
Magnesium	Aids calcium absorption; helps to maintain muscle and nerve function
Phosphorus	Builds bone strength and aids muscle contraction
Vitamin C	Antioxidant; aids wound healing and collagen production
Potassium	Regulates muscle and nerve function
Vitamin K	Aids bone formation
Omega-3	Improves immune function; may reduce inflammation in joints

Key nutrients for healthy bones, muscles and joints

RECOMMENDED DAILY ALLOWANCE (RDA)			DO I NEED A SUPPLEMENT?	CAUTION
Children	Adults	Elderly		
350–1000mg	700mg+	700mg+	700mg is the minimum. Breastfeeeding women, elderly people and people at particular risk of osteoporosis are likely to need more – around 1000mg – so may benefit from a supplement.	High levels can interfere with absorption of other minerals. Very high levels (over 2500mg a day) can be toxic. Has potential to react with some prescription drugs.
7mcg (1–3 years)	No RDI	10mcg (over 65s)	Most people get enough from sunlight. Older adults, people with limited sun exposure and people who are at risk of osteoporosis may benefit from a supplement.	High levels (over 50mcg a day) can be toxic.
85–280mg	270–300mg	270mg+	Supplements are usually only necessary on medical advice. Heavy drinkers or people at particular risk of osteoporosis may benefit.	People with kidney disease should talk to a doctor before taking supplements.
270-275mg	550mg+	550mg+	You should get plenty in your diet. Don't take supplements unless advised to do so by a doctor.	Too much phosphorus can affect your body's balance of other nutrients.
30-35mg	40mg	40mg	People who don't eat enough fruit and vegetables, heavy drinkers and elderly people may benefit from a supplement	Can interfere with some medicines. Women on the contraceptive mini-pill should not take high doses as same time as the pill.
800-3100mg	3500mg	3500mg	You should get enough in your diet. Don't take supplements unless advised to do so by a doctor.	High levels can be toxic. People with kidney problems should not take supplements.
No RDI: most vitamin K is produced by bacteria in the intestines.			Most people get enough due to action of gut bacteria – people with digestion problems may benefit from supplements.	Can interfere with blood-thinning drugs. Get medical advice before taking supplements if you are pregnant or breastfeeding.
No RDI. A typical dose for supplements is 2000mg, three times a day.			Supplements may be helpful if you don't eat a lot of oily fish, particularly if you suffer from rheumatoid or osteoarthritis.	Can affect blood clotting and regulation of blood sugar. Talk to a doctor before taking supplements if you are diabetic or take blood-thinning drugs.

Vitamin supplements

Vitamins are organic dietary compounds, essential in small amounts to help you grow, develop and function. A healthy, balanced diet should provide most of the vitamins you need, but certain groups (such as pregnant or breast-feeding women or people who don't get the full range of nutrients in their diet) may benefit from a suitable wide-spectrum multivitamin.

The National Osteoporosis Society recommends that older people with osteoporosis should take vitamin D and calcium supplements. Some studies have shown that vitamin D, used together with calcium supplements, may also be effective for reducing bone loss in postmenopausal women. For more details about supplements for osteoporosis >>268–269.

Mineral supplements

Mineral nutrients are the inorganic compounds (substances not made by plants or animals) you need to maintain healthy body function. There are a number of minerals involved in the formation of strong muscles and bones (>>102–103), but most of these are present in large enough amounts in a healthy diet. Calcium is the most common mineral supplement; there is usually no need to take other supplements unless advised to do so by your doctor or nutritionist.

> **'According to an article in the *British Medical Journal* in July 2005, almost half of UK teenagers do not get enough sunlight to make all the vitamin D they need for strong bones'**

Calcium compounds

Calcium is available in several forms, so check the amount of pure calcium before you buy. Calcium carbonate, the least expensive form, also provides the most elemental calcium (around 40 per cent).

Most compounds rely on acid in the stomach to break them down into a form that can be absorbed. The exception to this is calcium citrate. Older adults often lack sufficient stomach acid to absorb calcium carbonate; if you are over 65, try calcium citrate instead. Some people find that this compound is also less likely to cause flatulence, diarrhoea or constipation.

Other nutrient supplements

As well as vitamins and minerals, there are many other types of dietary supplement available, including amino acids, essential fatty acids (EFAs) and herbal supplements.

- **Fish oils,** available in capsules or as liquid, are rich in omega-3 essential fatty acids (>>102). Flaxseed oil is a vegetarian alternative. You should not take fish oil supplements if you are pregnant as they contain doses of vitamin A which can be dangerous to the developing foetus.
- **Glucosamine** is an amino sugar found in cartilage. There is some evidence to suggest that glucosamine supplements, extracted from crab or lobster shell, or animal cartilage, may help to reduce arthritic pain, but scientific opinion is still divided. Because glucosamine is not an essential nutrient there is no RDI: a typical dose is 1500mg glucosamine sulphate a day.
- **Chondroitin** is a protein molecule also found in cartilage. It is believed to help draw water into cartilage making it more spongy and relieving arthritic pain. Once again, more studies are needed before any definite conclusions can be drawn. A typical dose is 800–1200mg chondroitin sulphate daily.

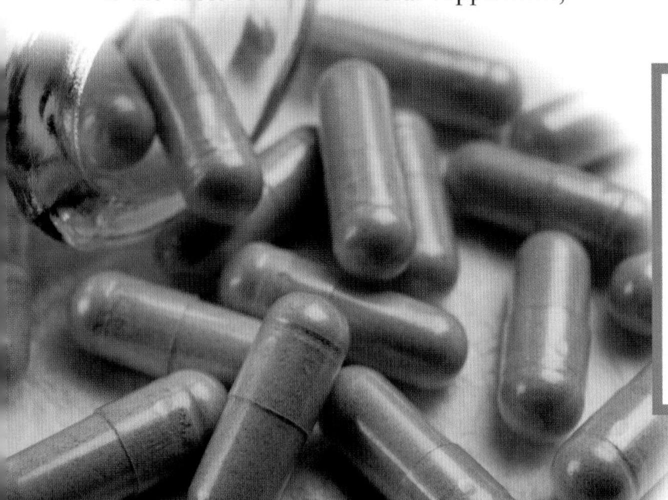

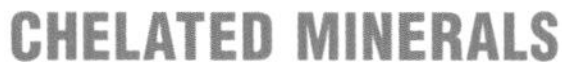

CHELATED MINERALS

The benefits of many minerals depend on how well your body absorbs the compound. A chelated mineral is one that has been bonded to an amino acid (or another organic molecule) so that it's more soluble and better absorbed by your body. It is hard to say exactly how effective chelated minerals are because very little impartial research has yet been published. While the chelating process probably does improve the solubility of some minerals, such as zinc, it is worth treating many of the bolder claims put forward by the health food industry with a degree of scepticism.

a visit to

THE NUTRITIONIST

A nutritionist can provide you with detailed, tailor-made advice on diet and nutrition. Approaches to treatment can vary, however, so make sure you find the right nutritionist for your needs.

Anybody can call themselves a nutritionist, so levels of qualifications and training vary widely. For professional, qualified advice in the UK, look for the letters RD (Registered Dietitian) after the nutritionist's name – this shows that the nutritionist is registered with the Health Professions Council. To make an appointment with a registered dietitian, ask your GP for a referral or contact the British Dietetic Association (www.bda.uk.com).

Another option is to visit a nutritional therapist. Nutritional therapy is a type of complementary therapy that places particular emphasis on the effects of toxins and waste products on the body. Although the principles of nutritional therapy are accepted by many orthodox medical professionals, nutritional therapists are not as well regulated as Registered Dietitians.

If you are in any doubt about your nutrient intake or diet, a qualified nutritionist can provide you with detailed, personalized advice and may have the experience to spot things that you or your GP have missed.

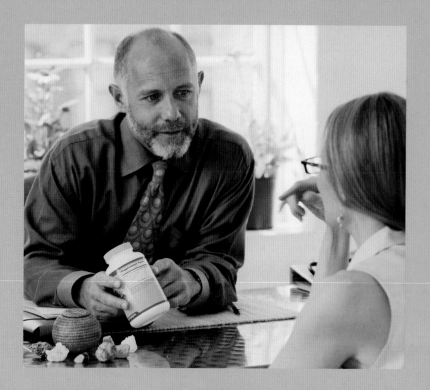

Assessment During your initial visit, the nutritionist may ask you questions about your medical and family history, your diet and digestion and your general lifestyle. Some nutritionists ask you to bring a food diary and a list of any herbs, supplements or medicines you take regularly. This will help the nutritionist to spot any potential problems.

Tests The nutritionist may organize laboratory tests (such as stool or urine analysis or blood tests) to find any deficiencies and test organ function. Some nutritionists also test for food allergies, which may play a role in certain musculoskeletal conditions. You should bear in mind that no reliable tests for food allergies are currently available and many of the tests on offer have little scientific basis.

Diet plan and advice Your nutritionist will be able to advise you on how to improve your general diet, avoid foods that may be making your problems worse or try foods or supplements that may improve your condition. The nutritionist may also compile an eating plan or nutritional guidelines specific to your condition or your particular nutritional requirements.

>> **Nutrients for healthy bones, muscles and joints:** page 102

Foods to avoid

Just as there are some foods that can help protect your bones and reduce the risk of osteoporosis there are others which when eaten in excess can increase the risk.

Salt (sodium)

Aim to keep your salt intake below 6g per day. A high salt diet increases the amount of calcium you expel in urine, weakening your bones. Food labels usually list the salt content as sodium: to convert sodium to salt, multiply by 2.5. Your sodium intake should stay below 2.4g per day.

Three-quarters of all the salt in our diet comes from processed foods. Ready meals, shop-bought sandwiches and canned soups are some of the worst offenders. Try to get into the habit of checking the labels of all processed foods As a general guide, a food with more than 0.5g of sodium per 100g is high in salt; 0.1g or less is low in salt.

Salt is an acquired taste – the more you use, the more you will want. If you cut down your sodium intake, you may find that your taste buds take a little time to get used to the change. Once they do, though, you won't miss the flavour.

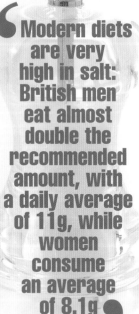

> 'Modern diets are very high in salt: British men eat almost double the recommended amount, with a daily average of 11g, while women consume an average of 8.1g'

Alcohol

Moderate drinking is not harmful – indeed a glass of wine each day may actually be beneficial to bone health. Experts believe that small amounts of alcohol may help to convert testosterone into oestradiol, a hormone that helps to prevent bone loss.

Excessive drinking is much more of a problem. Alcohol damages the cells that make new bone and can disrupt your digestive process, preventing your body absorbing nutrients properly. If you do drink, try to stay within the recommended limit of 2–3 units a day for women and 3–4 units a day for men. One unit is equal to one small glass of wine or half a pint of normal strength lager.

Caffeine and fizzy drinks

High intakes of caffeine can interfere with the absorption of calcium, although the detrimental effect of this on your bones is relatively small. One cup of coffee prevents the absorption of around 6mg of calcium – approximately the same amount as you would get from 1 teaspoon of milk, so drinking milky coffee helps to offset the problem.

Caffeine is most likely to be a problem if you drink a lot of cola or other caffeine-laden soft drinks. In addition, some experts believe that phosphoric acid, used as a preservative in many fizzy drinks, weakens bones: when phosphorus levels in your blood exceed calcium levels, your body takes calcium from your bones to compensate. Many soft drinks also contain lots of sugar, so it makes good sense to cut back.

> **CAUTION**
>
> Although protein is vital for healthy muscles and bones (it is broken down into the amino acids used to build body tissues), very high intakes can increase calcium excretion in your urine. Most people in the UK do not have a high enough intake to give cause for concern – but this could be a problem for anyone taking protein supplements or on a high-protein, low-carbohydrate diet.

Allergies and intolerances

The link between food allergy or intolerance and arthritis remains unproven. While it does seem likely that certain foods can aggravate the symptoms of rheumatoid or psoriatic arthritis in some people, this is not the case for all sufferers. Even if you suspect you have an allergy or intolerance, always talk to a doctor or a nutritionist before cutting any foods out of your diet.

Acidic foods

Some people believe arthritis can be made worse by eating foods such as oranges and tomatoes, but there is little firm evidence for this. Foods like tomatoes may taste acidic, but the acidity is low in comparison to the levels in your stomach. If you find that certain foods make your symptoms worse, it makes sense to avoid them – but make sure you get enough nutrients from alternative sources to compensate.

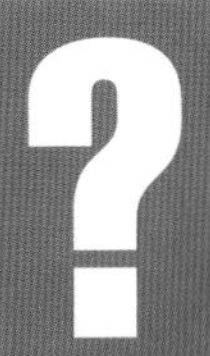

How healthy is my diet?

Answer the following questions as honestly as possible. Then check your score to see how healthy your diet is.

How many servings of fruit and vegetables do you eat a day?

- a) 0
- b) 3 or more
- c) 5 or more

How many servings of whole grain foods (such as wholemeal bread, brown rice or whole grain breakfast cereal) do you eat a day?

- a) 0
- b) 1
- c) 2 or more

What do you usually eat for breakfast?

- a) Nothing
- b) Cooked breakfast, muffin or pastry
- c) Wholegrain breakfast cereal or wholemeal toast

How many times each week do you eat fish?

- a) 0
- b) 1 or more
- c) 2 or more

How often do you eat ready-meals or takeaways?

- a) 3 or more times a week
- b) Once a week
- c) Occasionally

How often do you eat fried foods?

- a) Every meal
- b) Every day
- c) Rarely or never

When do you add salt to your food?

- a) In cooking and at the table
- b) Only in cooking
- c) Rarely or never

How much liquid do you drink each day?

- a) Less than 1 litre
- b) Between 1–1.5 litres
- c) Between 1.5–2 litres

How many servings of dairy products do you eat each day?

- a) None
- b) 1-2
- c) 3

HOW DID YOU DO?

For each (a) you have ticked, score 0 points, for each (b) score 1 point and for each (c) score 2 points. Add up the number of points and check your score below.

Less than 7 points: You need to take a careful look at your diet. Note the questions on which you dropped points to see how you can improve your dietary habits.

8–15 points: Your diet appears to be fairly healthy, but there is still room for improvement. Think about your shopping, cooking and eating habits to see where you can make changes.

16–18 points: Congratulations! Keep up the good work.

Your changing needs through life

From childhood, when you lay the first foundations of good bone and muscle health, through to old age, it is vital to keep your body healthy and nourished. But while the importance of a balanced diet stays constant, your specific needs do vary.

This is particularly true of your bones. Your muscle mass and composition is determined more by activity levels than diet; your bones, however, rely on a regular intake of vitamins and minerals such as calcium and phosphorus to stay healthy. For a breakdown of the calcium content of some common foods, >>268.

Strong bones through life

We tend to think of our skeleton simply as something to prop up our body, but bone is much more than that: your skeleton also provides an ever-changing pool of nutrients you can draw on throughout your life. It may be helpful to think of your bones as a sort of savings account. Imagine that you start off by depositing lots of money and withdrawing only a little; during later years, when you are no longer earning, your withdrawals increase and deposits decrease. This is exactly the same way that your bones work: during youth your bones accumulate lots of minerals and only lose a little; as you get older the reverse is true.

A good intake of calcium and other bone-building nutrients while you are still growing will increase bone density, making your skeleton stronger and preventing fractures later in life. The more bone you have 'in the bank' the more you can afford to lose before problems occur. But it's never too late to start looking after your bones – a good diet will help you to maintain bone strength, whatever your age.

CALCIUM INTAKE THROUGH LIFE

AGE	DAILY MINIMUM	NUMBER OF SERVINGS*
1–3 years	350mg	1–2
4–6 years	450mg	2
7–10 years	550mg	2–3
11–18 years, boys	1000mg	3–4
11–18 years, girls	800mg	3
Adult	700mg	3
Pregnant woman	700mg	3
Breastfeeding woman	700 + 550mg	4–5

*1 serving = 200ml milk, 1 piece of hard cheese the size of a matchbox, or 1 small pot (150ml) of yoghurt

DID YOU KNOW?

- As a general rule, the harder the cheese the more calcium it contains. Cottage cheese contains only low levels of the mineral while Parmesan is packed full of calcium.
- Low-fat dairy products contain as much calcium as full-fat versions. Indeed, pint-for-pint, skimmed milk contains slightly more calcium than full-fat milk. This is because calcium is contained in the non-creamy portion of milk.

Growing up strong

A calcium and nutrient-rich diet during childhood and adolescence, when your bones are still growing, will protect your skeleton throughout life. Even during periods of slow growth, children need two to four times more calcium per kilo of body weight than adults do. Water or milk are the best drinks for children and teens; too many fizzy drinks can leech calcium from bones.

Getting enough calcium and other nutrients is particularly vital for teenagers – according to a UK government survey in 2000, 25 per cent of teens have intakes below the recommended levels. Teenagers need to eat 3–4 servings of calcium-rich food a day (one serving is a 150ml pot of yoghurt or 200ml of milk) and take plenty of exercise to strengthen their bones.

You reach about 90 per cent of your peak bone mass by your early 20s, after which the process of bone building levels off. Calcium is still important to maintain bone density, however, and healthy adults should take in at least 700mg per day – equivalent to a 200ml glass of milk, a 150ml pot of yoghurt and a small piece of cheese.

Eating for two

If you are pregnant, you will need plenty of bone-forming nutrients in your diet to nourish your developing child. A good variety of fruit and vegetables, grains and protein will provide the growing foetus with all the nutrients required to lay down the foundations of a strong skeleton.

During pregnancy, a great deal of the your regular calcium intake is diverted to feed your developing baby and to produce breast milk. If there's not enough calcium in your diet, your baby will draw calcium from your bones, which may increase your risk of developing osteoporosis.

Despite all this, the government's recommended calcium intake is only 700mg per day – the same that is recommended for a healthy adult. This is because a pregnant woman absorbs calcium more efficiently and excretes less in her urine. Unless you are certain that you get at least this much calcium in your diet, however, it may be worth increasing your intake by around 30 per cent to protect your bones from osteoporosis. Teenage mothers, who may still be growing themselves, should pay close attention to the levels of calcium in their diet.

If you get enough calcium during pregnancy, childbirth may actually help to protect your bones. According to one study, giving birth significantly reduces your risk of hip fractures.

Breastfeeding

Breastfeeding women must be particularly diet-conscious. Calcium requirements and energy needs are much higher than during pregnancy – babies grow fast and rely on milk to supply all the nutrients they need to grow healthy bones and muscles. The National Osteoporosis Society recommends an extra 550mg per day – equivalent to about two glasses of milk. Eat plenty of fruit and vegetables, grains and protein. Drink lots of extra fluids, but avoid too much caffeine, soda and alcohol.

Managing the menopause

The decline in oestrogen levels that accompanies the menopause accelerates the loss of minerals from bone, which greatly increases the risk of osteoporosis >>148–149. Post-menopausal women need to ensure that their diet contains enough calcium and other essential nutrients such as vitamin D to reduce this risk.

CALCIUM IN WATER

Some brands of mineral water can contribute significant amounts of calcium. This may be useful for people who prefer not to eat dairy products. If you live in a hard water area, your tap water also contains calcium; your local water supplier should be able to give you an idea of exactly how much your water contains. In some hard water areas, tap water can contain as much as 250mg of calcium per litre.

CALCIUM LEVELS OF COMMON BRANDS

- San Pellarino: 208mg calcium/litre
- Badoit: 190mg calcium/litre
- Ashe Parke: 122mg calcium/litre
- Vittel: 91mg calcium/litre
- Evian: 78mg calcium/litre
- Volvic: 11.5mg calcium/litre

Growing old healthily

As you get older, your metabolic rate starts to slow and you need fewer calories but you still need all the same vitamins and minerals. Unfortunately your body becomes less efficient at absorbing nutrients and some prescription drugs, such as diuretics, interfere with your uptake, so make sure you get plenty of fruit and vegetables.

The older you are, the more likely you are to suffer from osteoarthritis and osteoporosis, so try to include plenty of oily fish and calcium in your diet. If you are unable to get out of the house very much you may also be missing out on vitamin D, so consider taking supplements.

TASTY TIPS AND INGREDIENTS

Even the most well-intentioned attempts to eat healthily won't get you very far if all you can find when you open the fridge are the remains of last night's takeaway, a three-week-old lettuce and half a jar of mayonnaise. The secret to eating well is to have plenty of healthy, appetizing food ready to hand, when you want it.

Having healthy ingredients and nutritious snacks there when you need them will help you to eat properly all of the time. Here is a selection of the many nutritious foods and ingredients that you can keep in your kitchen cupboard, fridge or freezer, ready for you to create a healthy snack or meal in a matter of minutes.

5 WAYS TO...

Boost your omega-3s

Oily fish such as mackerel are the best source of omega-3 fats but there are plenty of other ways to get omega-3s into your diet.

1 **Use omega-3 rich eggs** like Columbus eggs. Columbus hens are fed a special diet of cereal, pulses, seeds and green vegetables.

2 **Look for omega-3 fortified products**, such as fortified milk, bread and cereal bars.

3 **Use flaxseed oil** instead of olive oil to make salad dressings. Alternatively, mix the oil into yoghurts or add to smoothies.

4 **Add ground flaxseeds** to baked goods such as muffins or sprinkle over salads, soups or breakfast cereals. Stir a teaspoon of crushed seeds into yoghurt or add to smoothies

5 **Snack on nuts** such as walnuts, macademia nuts, brazil nuts and pine nuts that contain omega-3 fatty acids.

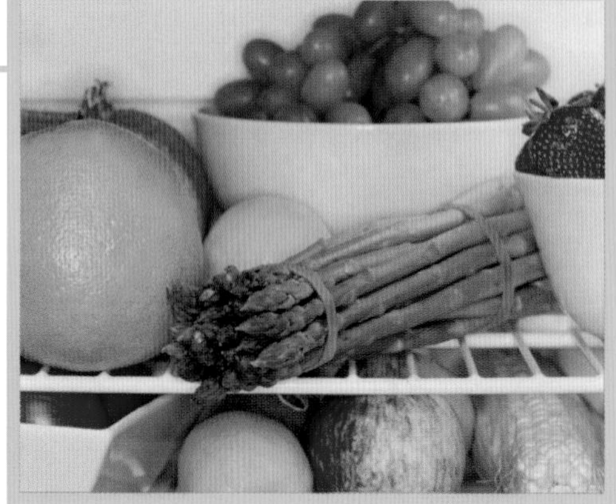

Foods to keep in the fridge

- **Fruit and vegetables** You are much more likely to reach your target of five a day if your fridge is full of tempting fruit and vegetables. Go for the ready-prepared options if you like – you'll pay a bit more for the convenience, but they'll still be cheaper and healthier than a takeaway. Make sure you keep plenty of green leafy vegetables like broccoli and spinach in stock – both are full of vitamin K and magnesium for your bones.
- **Ready-made fruit compote** Fruit compote is easy to stir into plain yoghurt for a quick dessert, blend with fruit juice to make a fruit smoothie or use as a sauce for frozen yoghurt or a tasty ice-cream treat.
- **Fresh soups** Serve with warm crusty bread for a quick lunch. Add a can of beans to increase the fibre content and sprinkle with some grated cheese to boost the calcium.
- **Ready roasted chicken** If you don't have the time to cook a chicken from scratch, go for the ready roasted option. To save time and space, strip off the meat (removing the fatty skin) and keep it in a plastic container. You can use it in sandwiches and salads or mix it with a bowl of pasta and a couple of spoons of pesto for a quick and easy meal.
- **Eggs** Scrambled or poached eggs on toast make a quick and easy lunch-time snack. If you don't eat oil-rich fish at least once a week choose omega-3 rich eggs such as Columbus.
- **Vacuum-packed smoked mackerel** Mackerel is rich in healthy omega-3 fats and goes very well in a salad. Alternatively, remove the skin and whiz the flesh in a blender with a little fromage frais for a quick healthy pâté to spread on toast.
- **Hummus** Spread over oatcakes or serve with vegetable crudités for a healthy snack. Buy ready made or make your own.
- **Salsa** Spread a couple of tablespoons over a piece of wholemeal pitta bread, top with grated cheese and grill for a quick and healthy pizza.

Foods to keep in the cupboard

■ **Canned beans and pulses** Rinse canned beans well to help wash away the sugars that cause flatulence. Add a can of beans to ready made soups to increase the fibre content.

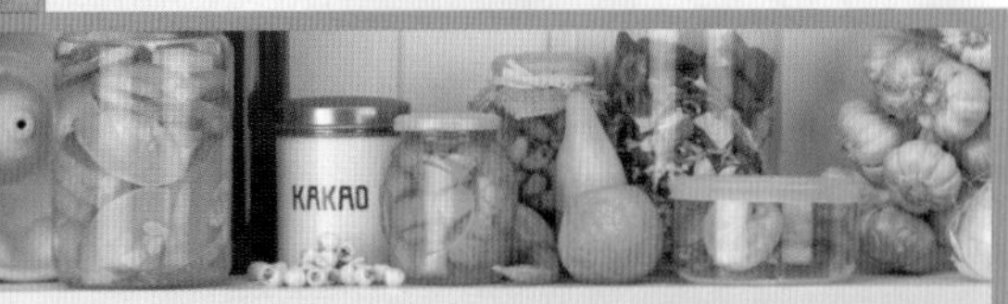

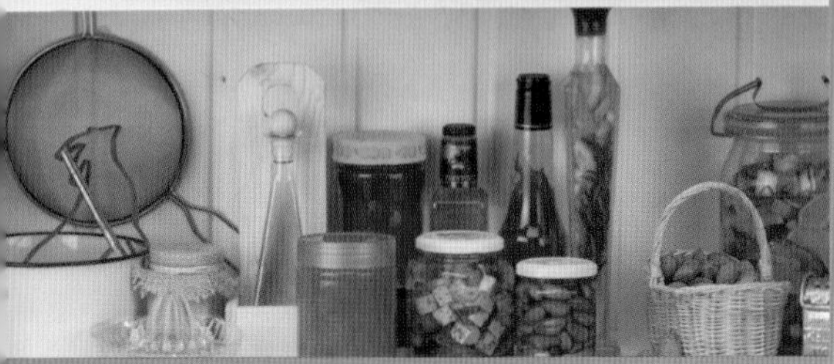

■ **Jars of pasta sauces** Vegetable-based sauces such as arrabbiata are healthier than creamy ones. Add a can of tuna or salmon to the pasta to boost your protein intake and a little grated cheese for calcium.

■ **Canned fish** Fish such as salmon, sardines and pilchards that can be eaten with their bones are an excellent source of calcium. Serve canned sardines on toast for a quick lunch or use canned salmon to make fishcakes.

■ **Couscous or bulgur (cracked) wheat** These grains require almost no cooking – pour over boiled water or stock, then simply stand for 15 minutes and serve.

■ **Ready-to-eat dried fruits** Dried fruits are a great way to satisfy your sweet tooth and get lots of vitamins, minerals and fibre at the same time. They make a great snack and good addition to rice, salad, stews or casseroles. Figs are a useful source of calcium.

3 WAYS TO...

Boost your calcium

If you don't eat any dairy products, there are plenty of other ways to boost your intake:

1 **Add almonds** to salads or stir-fries, sprinkle flaked almonds over cereals, or serve roasted almonds instead of peanuts with drinks.

2 **Mix sesame seeds** with breadcrumbs and use as a topping for bakes, add to stir-fries or baked goods or sprinkle over breakfast cereals.

3 **Choose calcium-fortified** products such as fortified soya milk or orange juice.

Foods to keep in the freezer

■ **Frozen vegetables** These make a great standby for occasions when you haven't got any fresh vegetables. Frozen spinach is a good source of calcium – use it to make soup or add a handful of spinach to dishes like spaghetti bolognese or curry.

■ **Grated cheddar cheese** Cheese freezes well and doesn't take long to defrost. For a quick snack or a light lunch, mix some grated cheese with a few tablespoons of milk and a little whole grain mustard, spread over a slice of wholemeal or granary toast, and grill.

■ **Frozen prawns** You can defrost frozen prawns in a matter of minutes by soaking them in cold water. Add them to stir-fries, salads or omelettes or fry them for a couple of minutes with a little fajita seasoning and stuff them into a pitta with some salad.

■ **Frozen ready meals** Ready meals are a good standby for days when you just don't have the time or the energy to cook. Many are very high in salt, though, so check the nutrition label on the back of the pack before you buy. Always serve ready meals with extra vegetables or salad to boost their nutritional value.

■ **Wholemeal pitta/tortilla wraps** These can be defrosted in a matter of minutes. Fill them with tuna or chicken and salad for a quick and tasty snack.

■ **Frozen summer berries** Whiz them up in a blender with milk and yoghurt to make a tasty smoothie or defrost and stir into yoghurt.

■ **Breadcrumbs** Instead of throwing away stale bread or the ends of the loaf, turn them into breadcrumbs and store in the freezer. Mix the breadcrumbs with grated cheese and use as a topping for vegetable bakes and cottage pie.

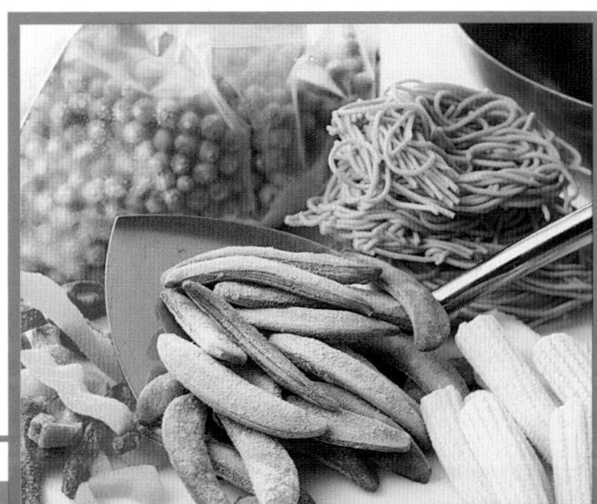

Your ideal weight

Keeping your weight within the ideal range for your height is one of the most important steps you can take to maintain healthy bones, muscle and joints. A good balance between energy intake and expenditure should ensure that you maintain a healthy body weight and get all of the nutrients your body needs to function effectively.

More than half the UK population is overweight and the proportion is increasing all the time. Excess weight puts an extra burden on your joints, increasing your risk from joint injuries, back pain and conditions such as osteoarthritis. But while it is healthy to keep your weight below a certain level, it is also important not to go too far the other way.

Losing too much weight too quickly may affect your body's ability to maintain and repair your bones and muscles and puts you at greater risk of conditions such as osteoporosis. Crash dieting, excluding food groups from your diet or losing too much, too quickly can starve your body of nutrients. A slimming diet still needs to provide all the nutrients your body requires.

Body mass index (BMI)

A good way to work out whether you need to lose or gain weight is to calculate your body mass index (BMI). To work this out using metric units, divide your weight in kilos by your height in metres squared. For example, someone who weighs 60kg (132lb) and is 1.65m (5ft 5in) tall will have a BMI of: 60 x (1.65 x 1. 65) = 22. Working out your BMI using imperial units is almost as straightforward: simply divide your weight in pounds by your height in inches squared and multiply by 703. Alternatively, look at the chart below.

A BMI between 18.5 and 25 is associated with the lowest health risks. Anything less than 18.5 and you might not be getting enough nutrients to maintain strong bones and keep your body healthy.

BODY MASS INDEX CHART

This chart represents the BMI scale visually – simply look at where your height and weight meet to find out where on the BMI range you fall. Your BMI provides a much better indicator of whether you are under or overweight than weight alone because it relates your body weight to your height.

- **If your BMI is 18.5 or below, you're underweight for your height and might not be getting sufficient nutrients in your diet**
- **If your BMI is between 18.5 and 25 you're a healthy weight for your height**
- **If your BMI is between 25 and 30, you're overweight, and should try to reduce your weight to below 25**
- **If your BMI is more than 30, you're obese: you may want the help of a doctor or nutritionist to lose weight**

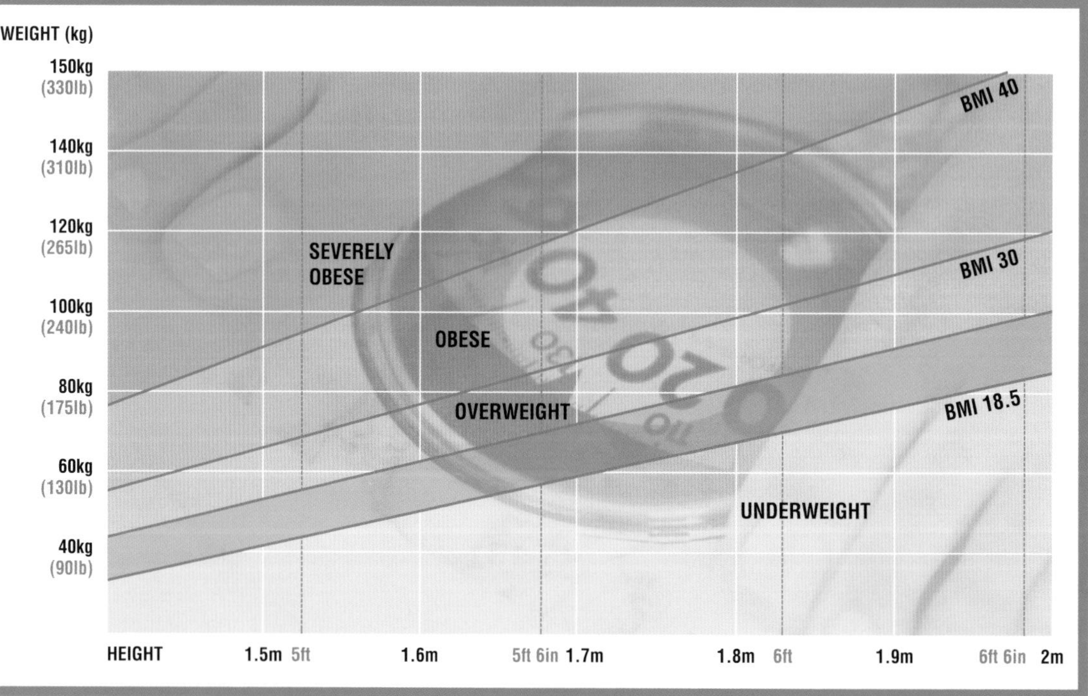

WHAT IS A CALORIE?

Strictly speaking, a calorie is a tiny amount – the amount of heat required to raise the temperature of 1g of water by 1°C. The more accurate term for the calories we eat or burn in exercise is kilocalories (kcal), the amount equal to 1,000 calories. This book follows common usage and refers to kilocalories simply as 'calories'.

The higher your BMI lies above 25, the more weight you need to lose: not only will this take stress off your joints, it will also lower your risk from problems including diabetes, heart disease and high blood pressure.

The energy balance equation

Your weight is a reflection of the balance between your energy intake and energy expenditure. If your intake is equal to your expenditure, your body weight will remain the same. If your intake exceeds expenditure, the excess energy is stored on your body as fat. To lose weight you simply need to tip the balance in the other direction, by increasing your expenditure, decreasing your intake, or a combination of both.

- **Energy intake** is determined by the amount and the type of food you eat.
- **Energy expenditure** is determined by your basal metabolic rate (BMR) and the number of calories you burn each day during daily activity and exercise.

Drugs such as steroids can increase appetite and cause weight gain, so if you are prescribed these drugs you need to be extra vigilant with your weight.

Choosing the right diet

Losing weight is not difficult – it is keeping it off that is the real challenge. Most people who lose weight later regain it because they choose the wrong sort of diet. There are no miracle cures: the only way to lose weight and keep it off is to make long-term changes to your eating habits and lifestyle.

The safest and most effective way to lose weight is slowly and steadily. Between 0.5–1 kg (1–2lb) a week is a good level of weight loss – if you lose too much too quickly you might lose lean muscle tissue as well as fat. Since the amount of lean muscle you have helps to determine your basal metabolic rate (the number of calories your body burns in order to function normally), it is a good idea to preserve it.

To lose half a kilo (1lb) of fat in a week you need to burn around 3,500 calories – about 500 calories a day. You can do this by restricting the calories you consume, but diet alone is rarely enough. To lose weight and keep it off you also need to increase the amount of calories you burn. The most effective way to lose weight is by combining a healthy diet with plenty of cardiovascular exercise (>>56–97).

When you need to gain weight

If you are underweight (with a BMI below 18.5), you might not be getting enough nutrients to keep your bones and muscles healthy. In particular, low weight is linked to a much greater risk of osteoporosis.

If you have a high metabolism or small appetite, gaining weight can be hard. The best way to increase your energy intake is to eat three healthy meals a day and plenty of nutritious snacks such as nuts and seeds, wholemeal toast or yoghurt. Avoid drinking with meals or for an hour before a meal as this can reduce your appetite.

7 WAYS TO...

A slimmer you

1 **Drink a glass of water** before each meal. Water will help to fill your stomach and prevent you from overeating.

2 **Eat breakfast**. Skipping breakfast will make you more likely to snack during the morning and overeat at lunch. If you can't face food first thing in the morning, pack a healthy snack to take with you.

3 **Trim the fat**. Weight-for-weight, fat contains twice as many calories as protein or carbohydrate. But don't fall into the trap of thinking low fat always means low calorie.

4 **Write a shopping list** and stick to it to avoid making impulse buys. Shop on a full stomach so that you're less vulnerable to temptation.

5 **Chew your food** thoroughly before taking a second mouthful and focus on what you're eating. When you eat slowly you're less likely to overeat.

6 **Take a break** before reaching for a second helping. Wait for 5–10 minutes and ask yourself if you really are still hungry before you help yourself to more.

7 **Don't eat on the go**. Make a rule that you can only eat when sitting down at the dining room or kitchen table.

WEIGHT-LOSS EATING PLAN

Does the very mention of the word 'diet' leave you depressed? Do you imagine tasteless meals of steamed vegetables and brown rice, a rumbling stomach and life without chocolate? The good news is that losing weight doesn't have to mean missing out on the foods you enjoy.

The key to losing weight is knowing which foods to eat and in what quantities. Some foods, particularly those that are high in fat, contain many calories – but this doesn't mean you need to avoid them completely, simply that you need to watch how much you eat. Other foods, such as fruit, vegetables, lean meat, fish and chicken are lower in calories and you can eat them in more generous quantities.

This weight-loss plan may look complex at first glance, but once you get the idea of the exchange system you will find it is very simple to follow.

STEP 1: Choose the right weight-loss plan

The number of calories you can expect to burn each day is related to physical activity as well as diet, so the first thing to do is work out whether you are inactive, moderately active or active. Then, decide how much weight you want to lose and use the table below to work out the most suitable weight-loss plan for you to follow.

LEVEL OF ACTIVITY	TARGET WEIGHT LOSS	WEIGHT-LOSS PLAN
Inactive (less than 5000 steps or under 30 minutes exercise a day)	Less than 1 stone (14lb) 1-3 stone (14–42lb) Over 3 stone (42lb)	1200cal plan 1500cal plan 1500cal plan
Moderately active (5000-10,000 steps or around 1 hour exercise a day)	Less than 1 stone (14lb)	1500cal plan
Active (more than 10,000 steps or over 2 hours exercise a day)	1-3 stone (14–42lb) Over 3 stone (42lb)	1800cal plan 1800cal plan

STARCHY FOODS

Type of food	One portion
Breakfast cereal	3 tbsp
Bread	1 medium slice
Bagel, croissant	½
Bread roll	½
Large pitta	½
Rye crispbread	3
Oatcakes, rice cakes	2
Pasta, noodles, couscous	3 rounded tbsp
Rice	2 rounded tbsp
Potatoes	2 egg-sized, 1 jacket
Oven chips	6
Malt loaf	1 slice

PROTEIN FOODS

Type of food	One portion
Chicken, turkey, lean ham	75g (3oz) cooked
Pork, lamb or beef	45g (1½oz)
Oil-rich fish	30g (1oz) cooked
White fish, prawns	60g (2oz)
Beans, lentils	2 rounded tbsp
Baked beans	2 rounded tbsp
Bacon	1 lean rasher
Fish fingers	2
Hummus, reduced fat	1 rounded tbsp
Eggs	1
Nuts	15g (½oz)

FRUIT

Type of food	One portion
Apple, orange, pear,	1 medium
Banana	1 small
Berries	1 cupful
Grapes	1 small bunch
Fruit juice	150ml
Dried apricots/prunes	3
Melon, pineapple	1 slice
Kiwi, satsuma	2
Passion fruit	2

STEP 2: How many portions?

Once you have worked out which weight-loss plan you want to follow, use the menu planner below to work out how many portions of each food group you can eat each day.

NUMBER OF PORTIONS PER DAY			
	1200cal plan	**1500cal plan**	**1800cal plan**
Starchy foods	5	5	5
Protein foods	4	6	7
Fruit	2	3	8
Vegetables	4	4	4
Dairy	2	3	3
Fats and oils	3	3	4
Snacks	2	3	4

SNACKS

6	ready-to-eat dried apricots
1	digestive biscuit
3	Jaffa cakes
1	crumpet, thinly spread with jam
1	mini chocolate bar
1	low-fat cereal bar
1	small bag of low-fat crisps
1	mug of hot chocolate with semi-skimmed milk

VEGETABLES

Type of food	One portion
Peas or carrots	3 tbsp
Salad	1 bowl
Avocado	½
Tomato	1 medium

Vegetables are allowed freely in this plan, so include as many as you want. Try to eat at least 2 servings of vegetable with each meal.

DAIRY

Type of food	One portion
Skimmed milk	300ml
Semi-skimmed milk	200ml
Yoghurt, low fat	1 small pot
Hard cheese	30g (1oz)
Brie/low-fat soft cheese	40g (1½oz)
Cottage cheese	2 heaped tbsp

FATS AND OILS

Type of food	One portion
Margarine, butter, oil	1 level tsp
Single cream	1 tbsp
Salad dressing	2 tsp
Low-fat salad dressing	1 tbsp
Oil-free salad dressing	2 tbsp
Reduced fat mayonnaise	2 tsp

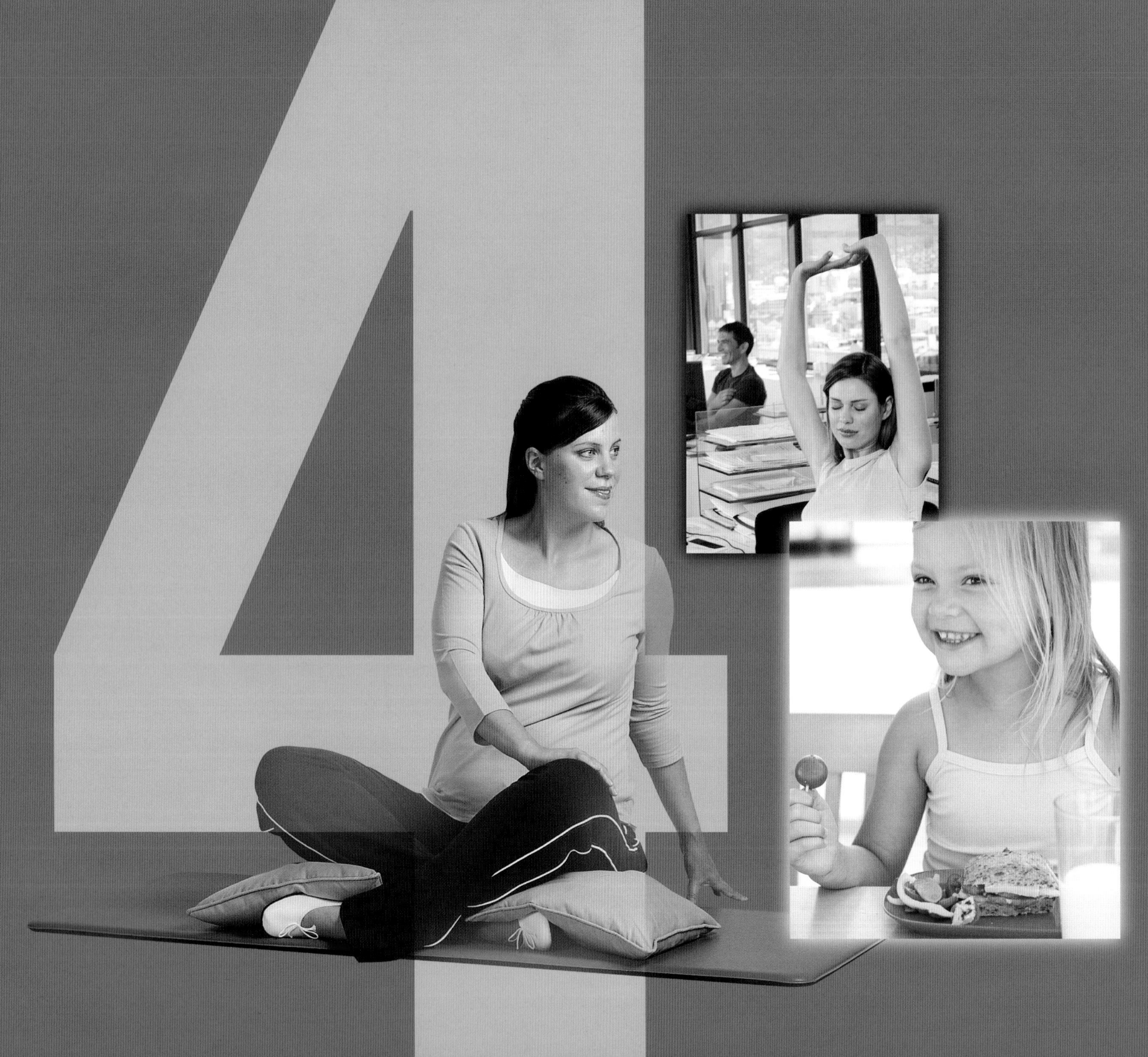

EARLY LIFE

Younger people are not immune to musculoskeletal problems and there are key times – such as in childhood or during pregnancy – when more care should be taken to ensure that poor posture or changes in body shape are not putting extra strain on the back or joints. These pages provide an assessment of the various stages at which problems can occur and outline specific and practical ways to prevent them – or limit any damage.

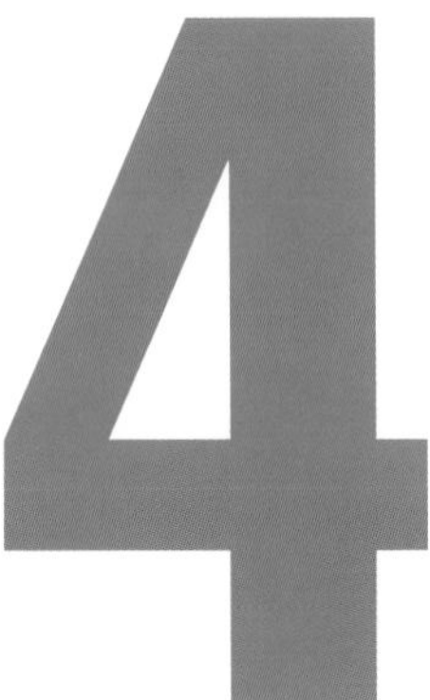

EARLY LIFE
Foetal growth and bone development

Two weeks after conception an unborn baby is no more than a bundle of cells. Already, however, these cells are starting to differentiate into the tissues that will soon form bone and muscle. Growth occurs at a rapid pace and the level of detail that can be seen in an nine-week-old foetus, still less than 6cm (2½in) long, is astounding.

Most skeletal development occurs during the first eight weeks of life, in the period between the appearance of the limbs as tiny bulges by the end of the fourth week and the formation of fingers, toes and joints by the end of the eighth. By the end of the embryonic period and the start of the foetal period in the ninth week of life, the entire skeleton is laid out. The process of ossification (hardening and calcification of the soft skeletal tissue) can begin.

Muscular development also occurs rapidly in the womb. By the time the embryo is four weeks old the heart muscle starts to beat and by the end of the sixth week it starts to move around inside the womb. As the nervous system matures and muscles begin to respond to stimulation from the brain, the foetus starts to practise movements and reflexes. By 16 weeks, entering the most active phase, the foetus can twist, turn, wriggle, punch and kick.

How bones are formed

Long bones (the tubular bones such as those found in the limbs), develop from rods of cartilage laid down as a 'model' which gradually harden (ossify) into bone. Sesamoid bones, such as the kneecap, develop in a similar way from tendon-like tissue. Most of the flat bones, such as the bones in your skull, develop slightly differently – instead of a cartilage model, the flat bones develop within a membranous cover.

The vertebral column develops from blocks of cells called somites that form along the back of the embryo. During the fourth week, the somites surround the tissue that will later go on to be the spinal cord and gradually develop into the vertebrae.

DID YOU KNOW?

- More than 300 separate bones are present at birth. As these harden some of the smaller bones, such as those in the base of your vertebrae, fuse and the number drops to 206.
- At birth there are two small gaps between the bones in the skull known as soft spots or fontanelles. These give the skull more flexibility during childbirth and let it mould to the shape of the birth canal.

110 Nutrition: your changing needs through life

176 Reducing the strain on your back

196 Common knee injuries

Ossification

The process of ossification (soft tissue becoming bone) begins around the eighth week of development as the cartilage gradually hardens. Cells called osteoblasts produce osteoid, a substance that, when calcified, becomes bone. For this reason, expectant mothers need to ensure they get enough calcium and phosphorus in their diet during pregnancy >>110–111. If the mother's intake of these minerals is too low, her body will remove calcium from her bones to compensate.

In long bones, the process of ossification begins in the centre of the shaft. Between this area and the bone ends (epiphyses) are the growth plates. As the centre of the shaft gradually ossifies into bone, cartilage cells in the growth plates multiply, lengthening the bone. By the time a baby is born, the shafts of the long bones have been largely ossified but the bone ends still consist mainly of cartilage. The growth and ossification process continues in the bone ends and growth plates through childhood and adolescence.

Muscle control

The baby's first movements – the twitching, rippling movements that occur from the sixth week – are produced by electrical activity in the muscles. As the brain and nervous system develops, however, the foetus takes more control of these motions.

By practising movements in this way, the baby's muscles get stronger, vital nerve connections are laid down and, eventually, the baby gains a sense of the various parts of its body and the ways in which they are connected. Each movement activates sensory pathways that the baby will need to control its muscles after birth.

FOETAL GROWTH

Measuring a foetus by ultrasound scanning can give a good idea of age and expected delivery date; it also provides a fascinating window into the private world of the womb. The speed of foetal development can be astounding: at eight weeks, when most of the major structural developments have taken place, the embryo is still only about 31–42mm (1¼–1⅔in) long. At 12 weeks the foetus only weighs about 50g (1⅘oz), yet by birth, a mere six months later, the baby is likely to weigh around 3.4kg (7½lb).

AGE (from conception)	APPROXIMATE LENGTH (crown to rump)
4 weeks	2–4mm (1⁄12–⅙in)
6 weeks	14–20mm (½–¾in)
8 weeks	31–42mm (1¼–1⅔in)
12 weeks	80–93mm (3¼–4in)
16 weeks	125–140mm (5–5½in)
20 weeks	190mm (7½in)
25 weeks	240mm (9½in)
30 weeks	270mm (10¾in)
Full term	300mm (12in)

Factors affecting development

The development of healthy bones and muscles in the womb relies on the foetus receiving an adequate supply of oxygen and nutrients, including glucose and amino acids (the building blocks to form proteins).

Various factors can affect the supply or delivery of nutrients and therefore growth. These include multiple pregnancies, poor maternal diet, excess alcohol and smoking. Anything that affects blood flow to the placenta, including some kidney diseases and maternal high blood pressure, can also affect foetal development.

In some cases a baby is small but growth through pregnancy is consistent – this may occur in first babies or if the mother's own weight is low. As long as growth is not restricted, a small baby is usually perfectly healthy.

The growing child

Your newborn's bones and muscles still have a great deal of developing to do. Throughout childhood and adolescence, your infant's bones and delicate muscles undergo a constant process of growth and remodelling. By the age of 17, when around 90 per cent of the final bone mass is present, bones are as strong as iron and around three times as light.

You child's bones are still rubbery at birth because the process of ossification, the hardening and calcification of soft tissue into bone, is not yet complete. Soft bones make it easier for your baby to squeeze through the birth canal and provide the potential for further growth, essential as the child grows bigger and taller.

By the time your baby is born, the shafts of the bones, the area where ossification takes place in the uterus, are close to their final structure. Although they will continue to grow thicker and harder for many years to come, the shafts now consist of hard compact bone on the outside and spongy cancellous bone and marrow in the centre.

HOW YOUR CHILD GROWS

The thick lines on this chart represent the average heights for girls and boys, but since 'normal' heights can vary considerably from the average, the thin lines show the range within which most children fall. Only 6 per cent of children fall outside this range.

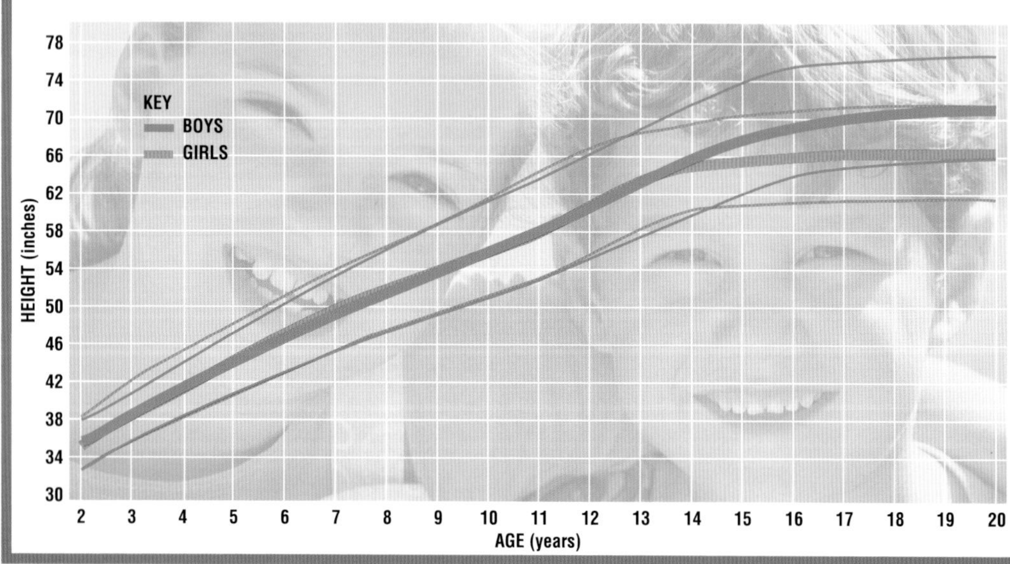

How bones develop

The process of ossification, which continues throughout childhood and adolescence, now shifts from the shafts to the ends of the bones. These remain soft to allow the bones to increase in length: between the shafts of the bone and the bone ends are growth plates that produce more cartilage, making the bones grow longer. Not until your early twenties do the ends of your bones finally harden, permanently fixing the length of the bone and therefore your height.

Bone density

This is not to say that bones no longer continue to develop after childhood – they grow thicker or thinner or change in density throughout life in response to the effects of diet and exercise. However, bone density during childhood goes a long way to determining peak density in later life: for every 5 per cent increase in bone density during childhood and adolescence, the risk of developing osteoporosis (>>264–275) or fracturing a bone in later life drops by as much as 40 per cent. For this reason it is vital to ensure that your child gets plenty of exercise and all the nutrients required to build strong bones.

Bone fractures in childhood

Children are very active – but not always well coordinated – and bumps and falls are a common feature of childhood. This puts your child more at risk of bone fractures: broken bones are the fourth most common injury in children under the age of six.

Luckily young bones are softer and more pliable than adult bones, and often bend rather than break. If they do break, partial (greenstick) fractures are more common than in older bones. A child's broken bones also tend to heal more quickly. They are surrounded by a thicker sheath of connective tissue than adult bones, which provides stability and ensures a good blood supply. And bones that are still growing tend to realign as they heal.

Despite this, childhood fractures do require immediate attention: although most heal well, breaks that occur near the bone ends can damage the growth plates, causing permanent growth problems. Your doctor will want to keep a close eye on the recovery process.

Puberty

The most dramatic increase in height and bone length occurs at puberty with a sudden growth spurt that lasts 2–3 years. Some children grow 10cm (4in) in a year during puberty. This growth spurt is related to the production of sex hormones such as testosterone, progesterone and oestrogens, which stimulate the growth of bone, muscle and other body tissues.

These hormones also play a role in the fusion of the growth plates that heralds the end of bone growth. Boys tend to have a growth spurt later than girls, around the age of 10–15 years compared to 8–13 years in girls. This gives boys time to grow taller and larger before the growth plates fuse.

> **'By the age of 17, about 24 per cent of a girl's total body mass consists of muscle – compared to 40 per cent of a boy's'**

How muscles develop

Your child's muscle fibres are virtually all present at birth but, like bones, these muscles are initially very small and weak. Newborns have a surprisingly strong grasp reflex, an evolutionary legacy that once allowed infants to grip tightly to their mother's fur. Other muscles, such as those in the legs or the neck, need time to develop their functional strength.

Like bones, your child's muscles will grow larger and thicker throughout childhood, with a growth spurt at adolescence. Both boys and girls follow this pattern, although hormonal differences mean that the increase after puberty is greater in boys than in girls. While bone growth – and therefore height increase – tends to peak around two years after the onset of puberty, muscle development peaks a little later. Indeed, muscles continue to grow even after teenagers reach their final height. Once again, the key to ensuring your child's healthy muscular development is to encourage plenty of activity and a nutritious diet.

Factors affecting good growth

A child's potential for growth is determined by genes inherited from both parents. But a number of other factors can influence whether this maximum potential is reached, including general health, nutrition and emotional well-being.

Sometimes growth is affected by a specific disease or disorder. Examples include hormonal disorders (such as a lack of growth hormone or an underactive thyroid), long-term illnesses such as chronic kidney failure and genetic disorders. These types of growth condition are rare, however. The most important way to help your child form healthy bones and muscles is to encourage a healthy diet and lifestyle.

HOW TALL WILL MY CHILD BE?

A child's adult height is determined by a number of factors, but gender and genetics are usually the most significant. The method of calculation given below provides a reasonably accurate prediction of a child's adult height, although the actual result can vary by as much as 12cm (5in) in either direction.

Father's height ....

Mother's height ....

Father's height plus mother's height ....

Divide result by 2 ....

For a boy: add 7cm (3in) ....

For a girl: subtract 7cm (3in) ....

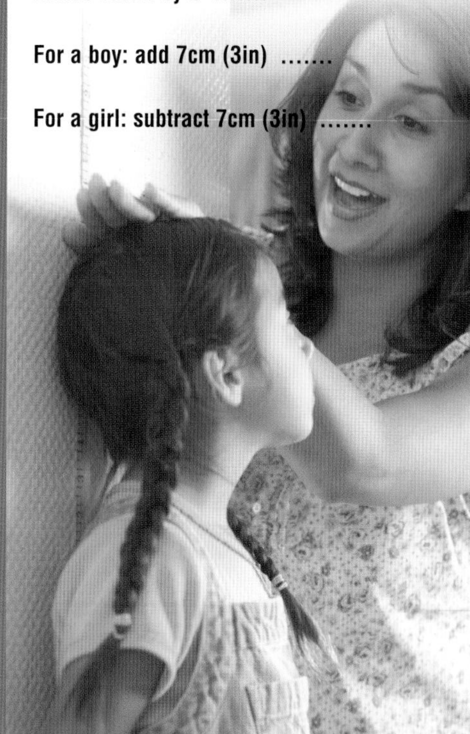

Exercise in childhood

Our increasingly sedentary lifestyles are a key factor in the rising levels of obesity in the UK, in children as well as adults. It is vital to establish healthy habits early in life as these tend to continue into adulthood.

Regular exercise in childhood not only reduces the risk of obesity, it also helps to prevent heart disease, strokes and diabetes. Exercise also strengthens bones and muscles at a time when your child is laying down the foundations for his or her future musculoskeletal health.

Very young children

From the moment babies first start to crawl they love being on the move and exploring their environment and are thrilled by the sensations of movement. As a parent, all you need to do is encourage this natural impulse and provide your child with a safe outlet for his or her energies.

At this age, your child needs simple activities that encourage physical development. You should gently guide him or her through the actions involved and, above all, make exercise fun.

CAUTION

During the first six months of life, babies are still developing the muscles they need to support their heads. Be very careful not to lift or hold your baby in such a way that the head flops too far forward or back.

- Give your baby the freedom to move in safety. For example, small babies like to lie on a mat and kick their legs.
- With older babies, try some simple exercises: hold the child in a standing position so that he or she can bounce up and down or walk along the ground.
- Make exercise times fun by singing songs or reciting rhymes.
- Encourage your baby but do not persist with something if the child is not interested.

Finding a safe balance

It is impossible to completely childproof your home or garden, so young children need to be kept under constant supervision as they experiment and find out what activities are safe. But don't err too far on the side of caution. Keeping a child penned in or discouraging natural exuberance will encourage unhealthy habits and may be counterproductive – children need the freedom to experiment, explore and even make mistakes if they are to learn how to calculate risks for themselves.

Age five and up

The Health Education Authority and the British Heart Foundation recommend that children aged 5–18 years get at least an hour of moderate-intensity exercise each day. Appropriate activities include brisk walking, swimming, cycling, dancing and active play outside. At least twice-weekly periods of an activity that promotes muscle strength, flexibility and healthy bones are also recommended. This may include skipping, climbing, jumping or gymnastics.

DID YOU KNOW?

- **Only a third of children in the UK spend two or more hours a week doing physical exercise, according to research in 2001. In some schools children have only an hour of scheduled physical education each week. In contrast, three quarters of children aged 11–16 watch more than two hours of television every day.**
- **The percentage of children who are obese has more than doubled over the past 30 years. Around 20 per cent of boys and almost 30 per cent of girls are now overweight.**

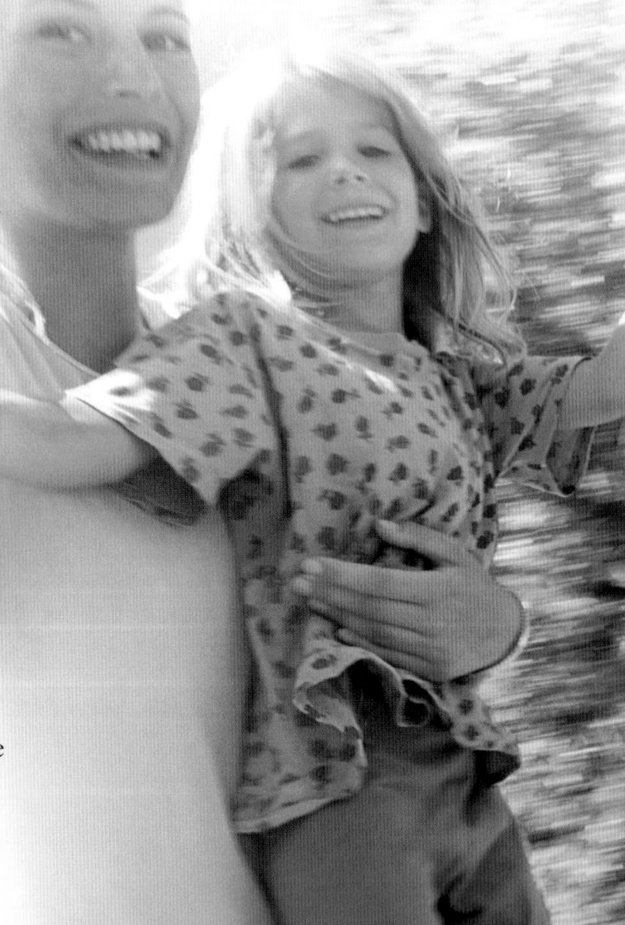

Once again, it is important to find a good balance between safeguarding your child and being overprotective. The number of children walking or cycling to school, for example, has fallen dramatically in the last 20 years. While parental concerns are understandable, over-reliance on cars can rob children of exercise.

Try to be a positive role model: walk your child to school, if possible, and take up a sport yourself to set a good example. Find an activity to enjoy as a family, such as walking, cycling and swimming, and encourage physical activity in preference to watching TV or playing video games. Take an interest in your child's sporting activities and, if your child finds a sport that he or she enjoys, offer plenty of encouragement.

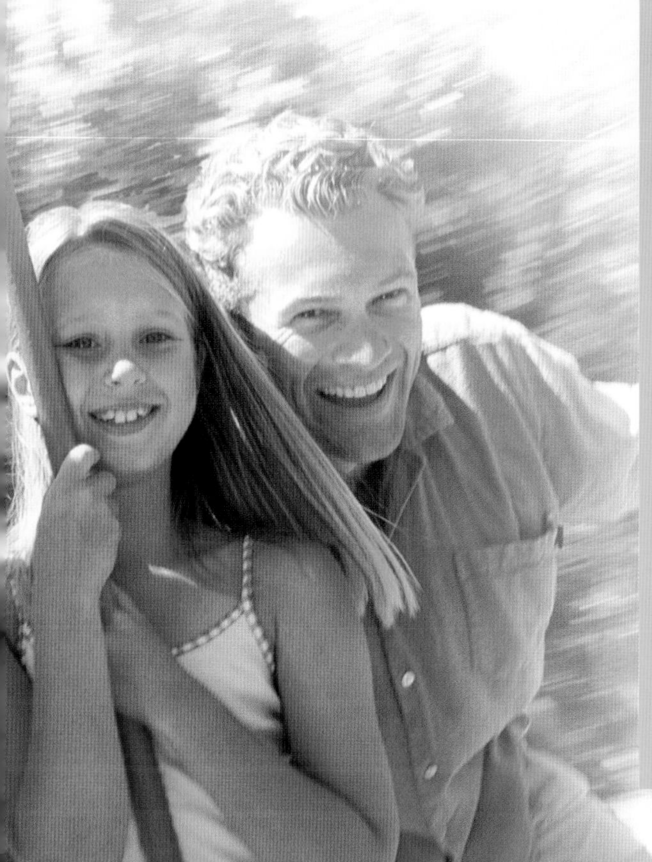

Does my child get enough exercise?

How much time does your child spend watching TV or playing video games?

- a) More than 3 hours each day
- b) 1–3 hours each day
- c) 1 hour or less each day

How often does your child walk or cycle to school?

- a) Rarely or never
- b) 2 or more times a week
- c) Most days

How often does your child get at least 60 minutes of moderate intensity physical activity?

- a) Less than once a week
- b) 1–2 times a week
- c) Most days

How often do you take part in physical activities with your child?

- a) Rarely or never
- b) Every week
- c) Most days

How often does your child play outdoors (excluding break-times)?

- a) Rarely or never
- b) 2 or more times a week
- c) Every day

How often does your child take part in extra-curricular sports or physical activities?

- a) Rarely or never
- b) Once a week
- c) Several times a week

HOW DID YOUR CHILD DO?

Mostly As: Your child is almost certainly not getting enough exercise. Think about where you could introduce some changes: you might need to reconsider your family exercise habits.

Mostly Bs: You child gets a reasonable amount of exercise but it is likely that he or she would benefit from getting more. Try to add a few more healthy activities into your weekly routine.

Mostly Cs: Great – your child gets plenty of exercise. Keep up the encouragement and build on this foundation so that your child maintains these healthy habits as a teenager and into adult life.

QUESTIONNAIRE

FAST FOOD – NOT JUNK FOOD

A nutritious, balanced diet is crucial for good bone and muscle health in childhood and in later life. It is important to encourage a healthy relationship with food and eating as early as possible.

Unfortunately, when it comes to persuading children to eat well parents have much to contend with: every day our children are exposed to a deluge of advertisements for fast food, fizzy drinks and processed snacks. Much as we all want to provide our children with the very best start in life, it can be difficult to find the time and energy to prepare good, fresh food when our children only seem interested in brightly-packaged junk.

But it doesn't have to be this way: with a little bit of imagination, fast, convenient and appealing meals can also be healthy. All of the nutritious snacks and meals shown here can be prepared in a matter of minutes.

Brisk breakfasts

Breakfast is the perfect time to boost your child's daily quota of fruit and ensure a good intake of bone-building calcium. Moreover, studies show that a wholesome breakfast improves children's concentration and helps stop mid-morning cravings.

- Fresh juice is a great way to boost your child's fruit intake. If you have a juicer, try making fresh apple, carrot or orange and mango juices – your child will have fun helping you feed the fruit into the juicer. If not, choose fresh (not from concentrate) fruit juice from a carton.
- A bowl of wholemeal cereal and milk is a good source of calcium, B vitamins and fibre (as long as you avoid over-processed children's cereals – these are usually laden with sugar and salt). Sprinkle some berries or a chopped banana on top.
- For a calcium and vitamin-rich smoothie that tastes like a treat, blend yoghurt and milk with berries and bananas.

Easy teas

The evening meal is a good time to make sure that your child gets some of her five daily portions of fruit and vegetables.

- Many children prefer cherry tomatoes or sticks of raw veg to cooked – a boon for busy parents. Simply chop up a variety of vegetables such as carrot, red pepper, baby corn or cucumber and add a ready-made but nutritious guacamole or hummus dip.
- If you don't have the time to make fresh soups, simply add some vegetables or canned beans to tinned or ready-made soups to boost their nutritional content.
- Instead of high-fat, poor-quality sausage rolls or hot dogs, use the best-quality sausages you can find inside a warm tortilla. This gives your child lots of protein for growth without all the unwanted additives.

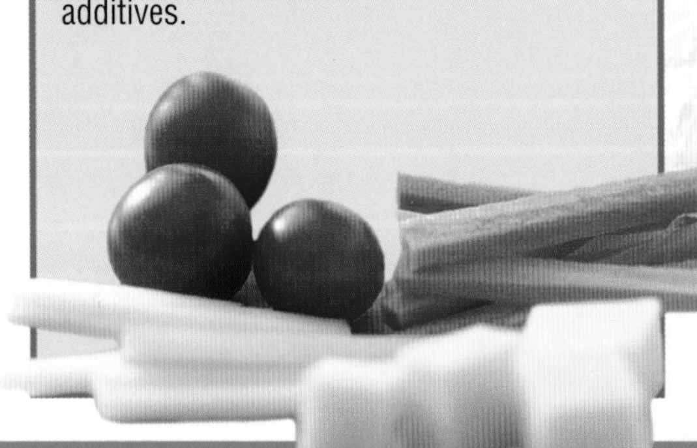

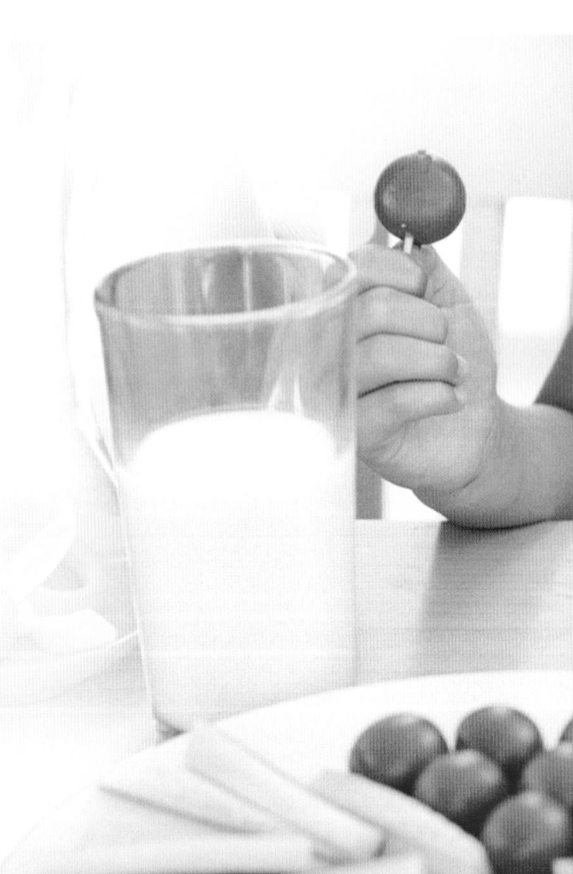

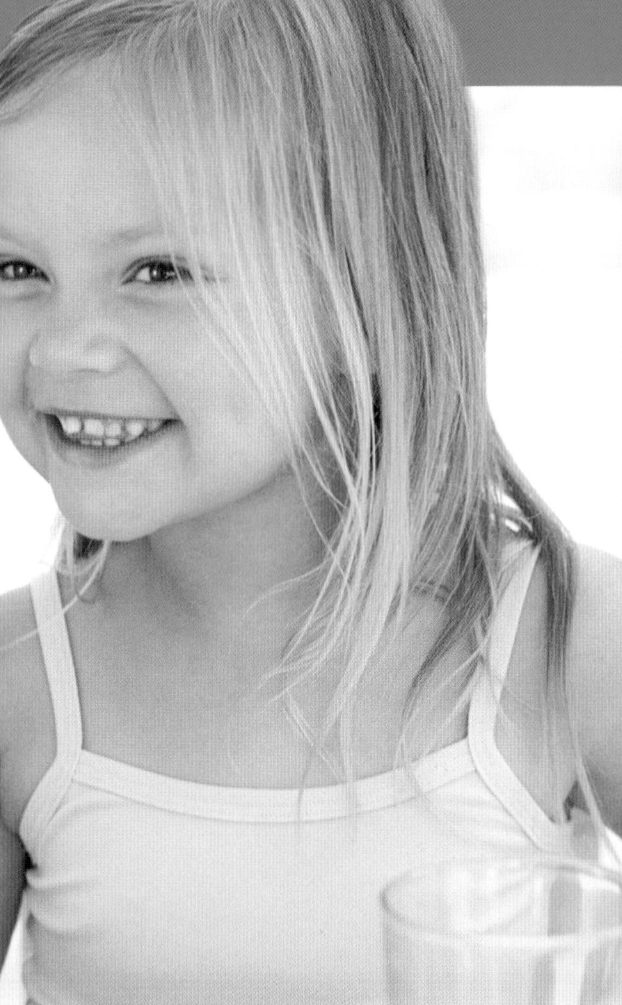

8 WAYS TO... Happy, healthy mealtimes

1 Eat a rainbow Offer a wide variety of fresh, colourful vegetables and try to present them in lots of different ways.

2 Go fruity Satisfy a child's sweet tooth naturally with ripe bananas, blueberries or pieces of dried fruit instead of processed snacks such as biscuits and cakes. Lay out a selection of fruit pieces on a plate for children to help themselves.

3 Check school meals Find out what type of food your child is eating at school and contact the school if you are concerned. If you provide a packed lunch, try to avoid processed foods and fizzy drinks and include some fruit.

4 Keep a healthy home Don't keep cakes, biscuits, or crisps in the house except for special occasions. Try not to offer sweet foods like biscuits as a reward for eating healthy foods.

5 Do it yourself Provide home-made food when possible – processed foods tend to be less nutritious and contain more salt and sugar.

6 Eat as a family Set a good example. A child who sees other family members eating and enjoying healthy foods is likely to do the same – you might not see the results immediately, but your child will be influenced in the long term.

7 Be positive Focus on being happy and healthy and making food interesting. Too much emphasis on weight sounds negative and could potentially encourage eating disorders.

8 Don't panic Many children go through a phase of fussy eating – sometimes just to get attention. If you ignore it and continue to provide a selection of delicious, healthy foods, your child will eventually adopt a more varied diet.

Speedy snacks

Children use up their stores of glucose more quickly than adults. Snacking between main meals used to be discouraged but most dietitians now recognize that children need to eat little and often. The key is to avoid over-processed, sugary snacks and drinks in favour of nutritious treats that release energy more evenly over the day.

- Chewy granola or fruit-and-nut bars make a great alternative to chocolate biscuits and processed snacks. Dried fruit, oats, nuts and seeds provide a nutritious combination of vitamins, minerals and essential fatty acids.
- Make fresh fruit lollies by pouring natural live yoghurt and puréed mangos, strawberries or peaches into moulds and freezing. For an even easier treat, freeze some fresh fruit juice, grapes or a banana wrapped in foil.
- A carbohydrate-based snack such as toast, a muffin or a crumpet an hour or so before bedtime can help your child to wind down before sleeping and will keep hunger pangs at bay during the night.

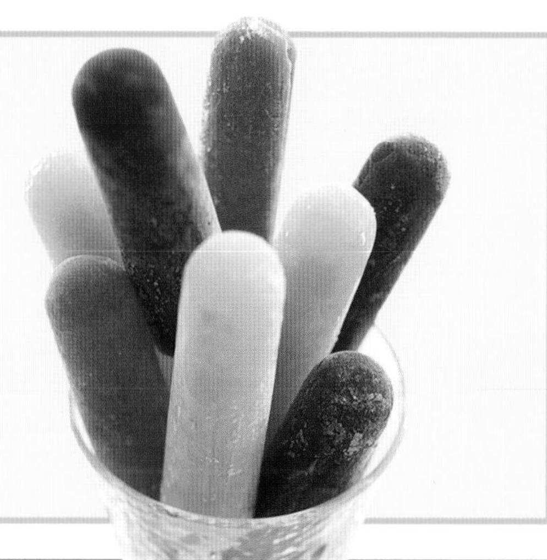

Posture problems in early life

Learning and establishing good posture in childhood is one of the best ways to protect bones, muscles and joints for life. The muscles and ligaments in your child's back are still developing and they may start to lengthen or shorten in response to poor postural habits. As a result, your child may become accustomed to these poor habits. Many posture-related complaints in adulthood can be traced back to poor habits learnt in childhood.

Poor posture contributes to a number of bone and muscle problems, most notably back pain. In one study, 44 per cent of 11–14-year-olds said that they had experienced low back pain in the previous month, with a slightly smaller proportion also reporting upper back or neck pain. In other studies, as many as 60 per cent of school children had experienced back pain by the age of 16. Poor postural habits can also lead to other aches and pains and can even contribute to the development of repetitive strain injury.

Problems at school

Very young children seldom spend long periods sitting still and significant postural problems are correspondingly rare. School-age children are much more vulnerable to problems: long lessons with little chance to move around, badly designed furniture and heavy school bags all place considerable strains on growing spines.

Education authorities are much more aware of these problems than in the past and have brought in a number of initiatives to promote better postural habits in schools. Nonetheless, it is worth talking to your child's school to find out whether any measures are being taken and to discuss any further initiatives that the school could take. Measures that may have a positive effect on posture at school include:

■ **Reviewing the timetable** The school may be able to schedule shorter lessons or provide short

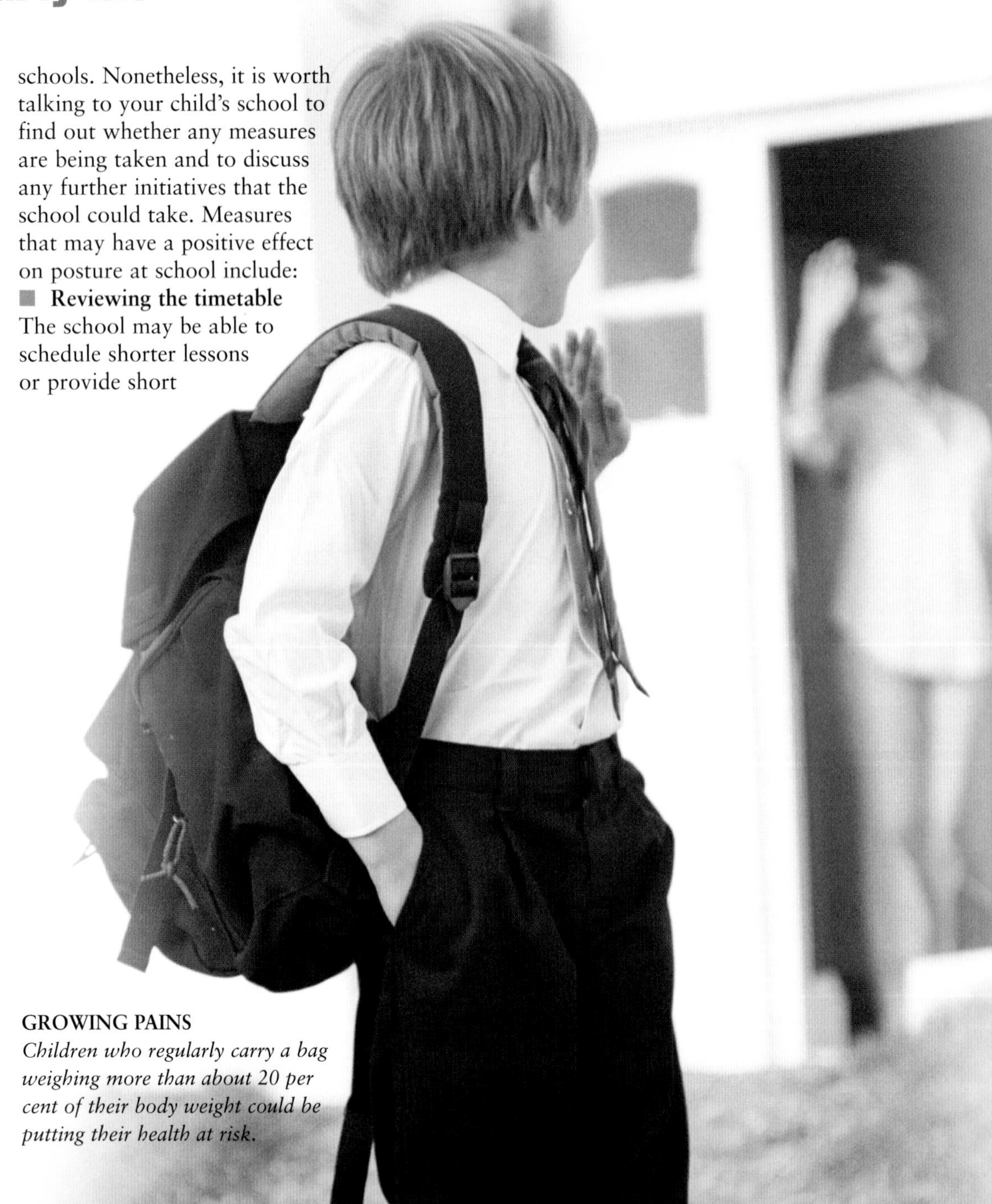

GROWING PAINS
Children who regularly carry a bag weighing more than about 20 per cent of their body weight could be putting their health at risk.

breaks during long lessons for the children to get up and move around. Children should have regular opportunities for physical activity, including a chance to get outside and run around during break times. Schools can also help by providing plenty of time for physical education and including activities such as gymnastics that promote muscle strength and flexibility.

- **Improving furniture** Many schools have standardized chairs and desks that make little allowance for size. British schools could benefit from the Scandinavian example, where most children have height-adjustable tables with tilting tops and adjustable chairs that take account of the natural S-shaped curvature of the spine. In the meantime, schools can take measures to improve existing furniture, such as providing seat wedges that give back support.

Safe back-packing

Children who carry heavy bags containing all the books and other equipment that they need for the day may be putting excessive strain on their spines. Not only can this result in short-term problems such as aches and pain, it may also have implications for back health later in life.

A recent study found that some children regularly carry as much as 60 per cent of their body weight on their backs. While this figure is clearly unacceptable there is no definitive answer as to how much is safe. As a guide, the American Academy of Pediatrics (APP) recommends that backpacks should weigh less than 15 per cent of a child's weight and never more than 20 per cent. Other measures to prevent excessive strain include:

- **Using both straps** Habitually carrying a bag over one shoulder places uneven weight on your child's spine and can cause your child to lean over to one side to compensate.
- **Finding the right bag** Look for a backpack with wide, padded straps that can be adjusted for comfort – the pack should hang just below the shoulders and rest against the base of the spine. Try to find one with padding against the lower back and separate compartments so that your child can distribute the contents more evenly around the bag.
- **Using lockers** Children are less likely to carry heavy bags around between lessons if the school provides lockers to store books and other equipment.

> **'Almost 70 per cent of children who watch more than two hours TV a day experience back pain, according to one study, compared to only 51 per cent of children overall'**

Home time

There is a limit to the control that you have over your child's posture during school hours, but there are many ways you can promote good habits in the home:

- **Encourage your child** to sit and stand without slouching or hunching over. Lead by example: rather than simply nagging your child, draw attention to your own good posture. For more tips on good posture at any age >>176–179.
- **Rearrange workstations** Most computer workstations are arranged for adult use – small children may have problems reaching the keyboard or placing their feet on the floor and may need to tilt their head back to read the screen. If your children have their own desks or computers, make sure they are suitable for their height. If you share a computer, show your children how to adjust the chair or the computer screen to suit their needs. For more information on good workstation posture >>177–178.
- **Limit time at the TV** A sedentary lifestyle does nothing to improve back health and the longer children spend hunched in front of a computer screen or slumped watching TV, the greater the strain on their backs. In one Scandinavian study, nearly 60 per cent of children who watched 1–2 hours of TV a day had experienced back pain. Among children who watched over 2 hours a day, the rate increased to almost 70 per cent.
- **Keep an eye on text-messaging** There are increasing reports of RSI in children and teenagers who send a lot of texts or spend long periods playing hand-held games consoles. Try to limit the time your children spend sending text messages to 5–10 minutes at a stretch and encourage them to use their fingers as well as their thumbs. For more information about avoiding RSI >>132–133.
- **Watch your child's weight** Ensure your child eats a healthy, balanced diet and does plenty of exercise. Being overweight increases the risk of back pain.

Starting work

A new job, particularly your first job, brings new stresses and responsibilities – some of which may have implications for your musculoskeletal health. It takes everyone a little time to adjust but you'll soon work out how to strike the right balance between work, health and relaxation.

One of the biggest changes that many people find when they first start work is that they have less time to devote to other aspects of life. You may find that you have less opportunity for sports or other pursuits and it can be tempting to abandon some of the activities you did at school or college. But regular exercise remains just as important during working life, especially if your job is stressful or does not involve much physical activity.

You will probably be spending a lot of time in a new environment but it is important not to let good habits, such as a healthy diet, start to lapse. There are other factors that you may need to think about: whether there is anything in your new job that could put your bones or muscles at risk, for example, and whether you feel confident that your employers are fulfilling all of their obligations to look after your health and safety.

Spotting potential problems

When starting a new job, it is important to consider whether there are any factors that could place your muscles, back or joints under particular stress. Jobs that involve long periods sitting in front of a computer are associated with an increased risk of back problems, for example. People in other occupations associated with a particularly high risk of back pain include:

- **Long-distance drivers** Workers who drive more than 25,000 miles a year take an average of 22 days or more off work with back problems, compared to only three days for low-mileage drivers.
- **Telephonists** Around half of office workers who use a telephone without a headset for at least two hours a day have neck pain and up to one-third also suffer from low back pain.
- **Supermarket cashiers** In one study, 57 per cent of people who had worked as a supermarket cashier for a year described themselves as suffering low back pain.
- **Nurses** Around 80,000 nurses injure their backs through bad lifting technique each year and many have to leave nursing.

Make sure that you do all you can to maintain good posture at work and minimize the risk of strain on your muscles and joints. If you spend long periods in front of a computer or drive long distances, or if your work involves a lot of lifting, try to follow all the guidelines for good posture while doing so >>176–179. It is also worth taking any occupational health advice offered by your employers.

Know your rights

All companies have a legal obligation to ensure the health and safety of their employees – and this includes taking steps to prevent work-related musculoskeletal disorders (WMSDs).

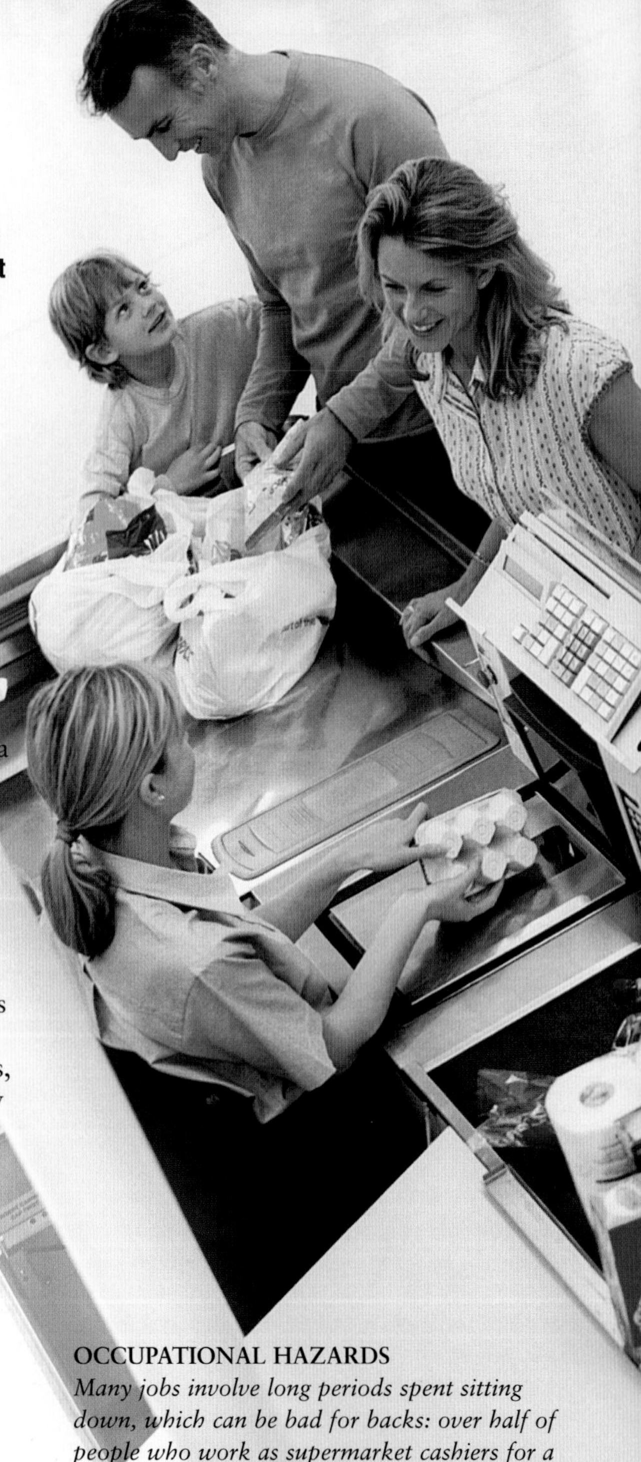

OCCUPATIONAL HAZARDS
Many jobs involve long periods spent sitting down, which can be bad for backs: over half of people who work as supermarket cashiers for a year or more suffer from low back pain.

If you regularly have to lift or carry heavy loads, for example, your employer must provide appropriate training or equipment. You should not be expected to work long periods without breaks or work in adverse conditions. Your employer should ensure you have a good working environment – which in an office may include considerations such as an adjustable chair and enough desk space to position your mouse and keyboard comfortably.

If you develop a work-related disorder such as back pain or repetitive strain injury (RSI), your employer should take steps to prevent the disorder from getting any worse – by modifying your workstation, for example, or investing in an ergonomic mouse or keyboard. If you have particular concerns or would like more information on your rights as an employee, contact the UK Health and Safety Executive >>336.

Maintaining activity levels

You may find it difficult to stay motivated or to find the time for exercise but regular activity remains vital for musculoskeletal health. If you establish a regular routine of exercise now, you will find it much easier to maintain these habits in the future.

- **Make the time** Aim to incorporate exercise into your everyday life so that it becomes a habit like brushing your teeth. The more convenient it is, the more likely you are to keep it up. Some people enjoy exercise early in the morning or find it convenient to jog or cycle into work; this helps to boost energy levels in preparation for the day ahead. Other people like to go for a run or visit the gym at lunch time. The hour or so after finishing work is also a good time to exercise – before you start winding down and lose motivation.
- **Make a start** Getting started is the most difficult part – once you're in a routine you'll find it much easier to continue. Start slowly and aim to build up to around 45 minutes 3–4 times a week. Don't overdo things: pain experienced when starting an exercise programme is likely to weaken your resolve to continue.
- **Stay motivated** Be patient and remember that it will take some time to build up fitness. To avoid exercise becoming a chore, make sure it is enjoyable and keep it fresh by changing your routine from time-to-time – you could start a new fitness class, for example. Many people find that exercising with others is the key to keeping up momentum.

> **'Around 1.2 million people in the UK suffer from musculoskeletal problems sustained during work – mostly back problems. Poor working posture and activities such as lifting are the major culprits'**

5 WAYS TO...

Stay healthy at work

It is all too easy to pile on the pounds when sitting at a desk all day or working late. With a little determination, however, it is easy to stay trim and keep your body healthy.

1 Get outdoors Take a walk at lunch time or stroll around the block during breaks. The change of scenery will do you good, help to keep you fit, and will boost your vitamin D levels from sunlight.

2 Snack sensibly Keep dried fruit and nuts and other healthy snacks on your desk. Healthy snacks will boost your nutrient intake and stop you craving fatty, salty junk foods.

3 Eat a good lunch If you use a work canteen, go for the healthy lunch options – salad, baked potato or fruit. Shop-bought sandwiches are often high in salt which is bad for your heart and bones, so you may want to prepare your own food the night before.

4 Drink enough Drinking plenty of water will contribute to your general health and can help you to stop snacking.

5 Stay active Walk to work, get off the bus a stop early or take the stairs instead of the lift. If you don't do other organized activities, try joining a gym near your work and going in early a few mornings every week.

AVOIDING RSI

Repetitive Strain Injury (RSI >>321) is a general term used to describe any soft tissue injury resulting from the repeated motion of a muscle or group of muscles. It therefore covers a range of more specific disorders, including tendinitis (>>330) and carpal tunnel syndrome (>>284). Other possible contributing factors include poor posture, lack of breaks and stress.

Because of the mechanism of injury – repetitive muscle use – RSI most commonly affects the muscles and tendons of the arms. Symptoms vary, but often include soreness, tingling, stiffness or numbness in the affected area as well as loss of function. In most cases symptoms ease and eventually disappear if the task or activity causing the problem is stopped.

Am I at risk?

Most risk factors for RSI relate to either muscles being placed under cumulative or repeated stress or to factors that make muscles more vulnerable to this stress.

Action and movements

- Do you regularly perform repetitive movements?
- Do you spend intense or extended periods performing repetitive movements?
- Do you find yourself holding static positions, including sitting positions, for long periods?
- Do you often make awkward stretching or twisting movements?
- Do you spend a lot of time pushing and pulling or handling heavy objects?
- Do you often make repeated or prolonged gripping actions?

Working environment

- Do you work in a cold environment or in poor light conditions?
- Do you find your workstation and your tools uncomfortable to use?
- Do you work for long periods without taking regular breaks?
- Do you use vibrating equipment such as drills?

Support and morale

- Do you feel your physical tasks lack variety?
- Do you feel under pressure to work quickly or reach deadlines?
- Do you feel you lack support from your manager or co-workers?
- Do you feel that you need more training to do your job?

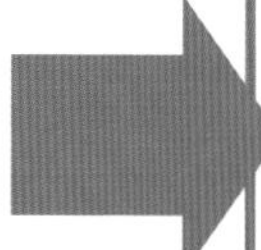

Will ergonomic products help?

Before buying any special devices, consider whether the product claims make sense to you and whether there is any research to back them up. The most important thing is that you personally find the item comfortable to use – even if other people find it helpful, it won't necessarily suit you. If possible, take it for a trial period.

- **Chairs** Look for a chair with a height-adjustable seat and an adjustable back rest that provides good support for your lower back. Ideally, arm rests should be height and width adjustable.
- **Keyboards** Some people find split keyboards more comfortable as they can reduce the need to twist wrists while typing. However, it is not certain that they reduce the up and down wrist movements that are often associated with RSI. A normal keyboard, correctly positioned, is probably adequate for most people.
- **Keyboard trays** These are usually height-adjustable with a negative slope (tilted away from the body) and can be

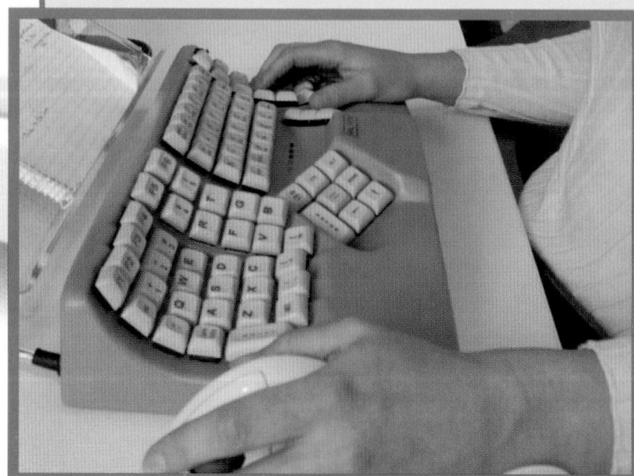

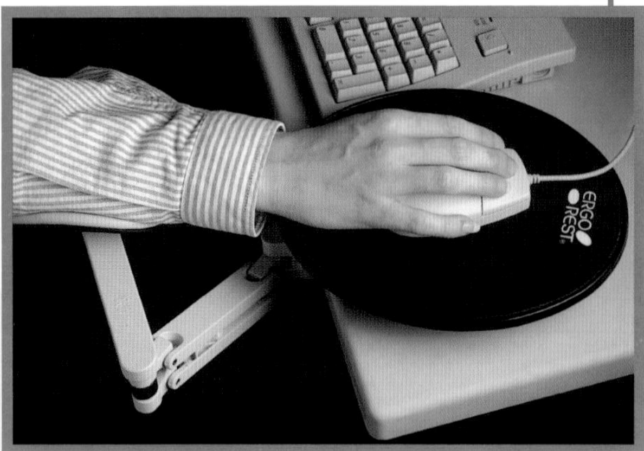

positioned at lap level so that you can hold your arms in a more natural position while you work. Research does suggest that this can improve wrist posture and comfort.

■ **Pointers** Various types of mouse and mouse-alternatives are available. Products requiring less wrist and forearm movement than a regular mouse include trackballs (which use a rolling a ball to move the cursor) and touch pads (which respond to the movement of a finger over a touch-sensitive pad). There is no research that singles out any one type of pointer as being the best ergonomically; it is a matter of personal preference. Size and positioning are often more important than design.

■ **Wrist rests** Research into the benefits of wrist rests is inconclusive and some people find they put more pressure on wrists. The rests should be about the same thickness as the base of the keyboard and not too soft: wrists can sink into soft rests, increasing twisting movements. You can also place rests between your wrists and elbows to support your forearms.

How can I avoid RSI?

RSI is usually work-related but leisure activities that involve repetitive actions, such as playing computer games, can also be a cause. Try the following to reduce your risk.

■ **Adjust your work area** If you work at a computer, make sure your chair, monitor and desk are at the correct height (make adjustments for different people if you share a workstation). Your eyes should be in line with the top of the screen. Organize your work area so that frequently used items are within comfortable reach, avoiding any unnecessary twisting and stretching. Ensure the light conditions and temperature are comfortable and the noise level not too high.

■ **Check your posture** particularly if you are working at a desk or a computer. Your wrists should be comfortable and the upper part of your arms should rest against your body rather than reaching forward to the keyboard. Your shoulders should be relaxed. For more information >>177–178.

■ **Move around** Avoid staying in the same position for extended periods of time. Most people type on keyboards in bursts, so try to shift position during these natural breaks. If your work involves repetitive actions, try to vary them as much as possible.

■ **Take regular breaks** Take a break every 30–60 minutes to give your mind and body a breather. If you are sitting down, get up and stretch your legs. Try to perform a few simple stretches every 1–2 hours: turn your head from side-to-side; raise and lower your hands at the wrists to relieve tension; make a fist and then spread your fingers out wide; bring your shoulder blades together to open up your chest; round your shoulders to stretch your upper back.

■ **Pace yourself** Try to plan your work so that you are not required to work too intensely for several days to meet a deadline. Talk to your employer about ways to avoid such situations occurring in the future. Avoid working through the comfort barrier: if you feel that you're placing your body under strain, stop and have a break.

■ **Use equipment properly** Avoid gripping pens too hard. If you use a computer mouse, try to use your forearm and not just your wrist. If you do a lot of text messaging, use both thumbs or use your thumbs and your fingers. Select tools and equipment that are appropriate for the job.

■ **Take regular exercise** Exercise relieves stress and keeps your muscles in good condition. Try to include aerobic and muscle strengthening elements as well as flexibility exercises such as stretching or yoga.

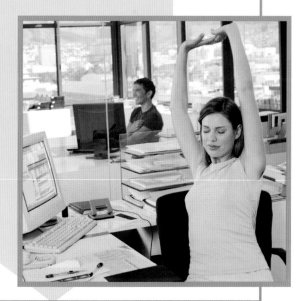

Avoiding sports and exercise injuries

Around one in ten musculoskeletal injuries in the UK are sports-related – and the majority occur in people under 30. Most of these sports or exercise injuries are muscle strains or sprains, although bone fractures and dislocations make up another 5–6 per cent. Exercise injuries can be defined either as acute or overuse injuries.

- **Acute injuries** occur as a result of a single, sudden trauma – a fracture caused by the impact between two footballers, for example, or a sudden pulled muscle.
- **Overuse injuries** develop gradually and occur when an area of the body is damaged as a result of the regular pressures of training over an extended period. Examples of common overuse injuries include stress fractures, shin splints and bursitis.

Although relatively few sports injuries are very serious, they can be painful and disruptive. Injuries cannot always be prevented but there are a number of ways that you can reduce your risk.

Avoiding excess stress

All physical activity places your body under stress. Usually this is desirable: your body responds to these demands by becoming physically more fit. Aerobic exercise, by making your heart and lungs work harder, improves the efficiency with which you take in oxygen and burn energy. Your bones and muscles respond to the strain of weight-bearing exercise by increasing in strength and mass. A degree of physical exertion is therefore vital if you want to get results – the key to avoiding injury is to keep these pressures at a level that your body can handle.

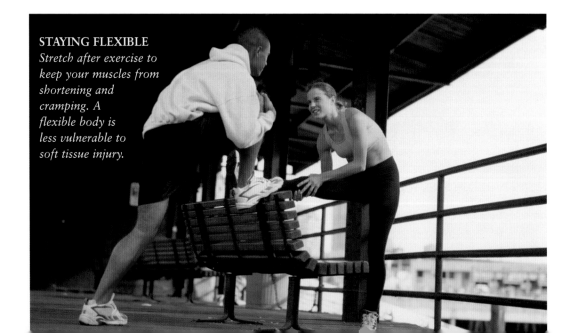

STAYING FLEXIBLE
Stretch after exercise to keep your muscles from shortening and cramping. A flexible body is less vulnerable to soft tissue injury.

DID YOU KNOW?

- **Approximately 40 per cent of sports injuries occur in people aged 10–19 years. Another 30 per cent occur in people aged 20–29. Only 25 per cent of sports injuries occur in people aged over 30.**
- **The type of injuries sustained also vary with age. Children are relatively more likely to sustain fractures and dislocations, while muscle strains and overuse injuries are more common in adults.**
- **Around 75 per cent of sports injuries involve the lower body, with the majority of these injuries involving the knees.**

Reducing the level of stress

You should not, of course, cut out strenuous activity altogether – this would lose you all the benefits of exercise. However, a selective approach can be useful if you know that a certain area of your body is vulnerable to injury. If you have problems with your knees, for example, the risk from a high-impact sport such as running may outweigh the advantages. You should also avoid sports such as basketball that involve demanding twisting and turning movements. There are other ways to reduce stress:

- **Warm up and cool down** Warming up before exercise prepares your body for exertion by warming muscles and increasing flexibility. It is particularly important to help prevent muscles and ligament strains and sprains >>64–67
- **Strengthen your body** Strong, balanced muscles will stabilize your joints. If you're unfit or out of shape you should therefore start slowly and build up intensity as your strength improves. Targeted resistance training can strengthen specific joints,

which will then protect the area during other activities. For some examples of knee strengthening exercises >>202–203.

- **Stretch** Lack of flexibility is a major cause of muscle strains, sprains and tendinitis, particularly in older people. For this reason, it is important to stretch after exercise >>66–67, 72–75.
- **Improve your technique** Lack of skill increases your risk of injury, making you more likely to misjudge movements. It is also important not to be too reckless.
- **Invest in good shoes** Very often, the most important piece of equipment is footwear. A good pair of trainers or boots is vital in many sports to provide support and absorb shock. Wear well-fitting, supportive shoes that are designed to be used for the sport you are doing >>48–49.
- **Check the surface** If you're a jogger, for example, running on soft grass or sand will place less strain on your hips and knees than hard roads. Uneven surfaces, tree roots and potholes can cause sprained ankles, while wet surfaces may be slippery.

Avoiding overtraining

Many sports injuries – and most overuse injuries – are a result of training for too long or training at too high an intensity. Your muscles need time to recover from exercise, so taking too few breaks or rest days can cause problems. Your body also needs time to adapt and build up endurance: too sharp an increase in the level of exercise is a common cause of overuse injuries such as runner's knee.

Whether or not someone is training too hard depends on an individual's own level of fitness, so it is hard to make specific recommendations. As a general rule, do not exercise strenuously every day and try to vary the type of exercise you do.

Avoiding re-injury

Past injury to an area of your body greatly increases your chance of injuring that area again. Only 50 per cent of sports-injuries are new injuries – the rest are recurrences of earlier problems. To reduce the risk:

- **Recognize why the injury occurred** in the first instance, so you can avoid making a similar mistake in the future. If your injury is connected to overtraining, for example, take things more slowly and include more rest days in the future.
- **Wait until you're fully recovered** before placing the injured area under stress. Many people resume exercise too early.
- **Strengthen the area involved** before resuming exercise. Even after the injury has healed, the area will be less flexible and the muscles around the injury weaker. You may need a programme of rehabilitation to rebuild strength. A physiotherapist can provide you with tailored advice on safe rehabilitation. For some examples of exercises to strengthen your knees >>202.

INJURY RATES FOR DIFFERENT SPORTS

Some sports are responsible for many more injuries than others. This chart shows the risk of injury per hour of activity, based on figures for various types of exercise published in *The American Journal of Sports Medicine*. Unsurprisingly, the sports which involve the greatest risk of injury are the full-contact sports such as rugby or high-impact sports such as basketball or soccer (not included in this survey). In other types of exercise, such as running, the main cause of injury is overuse rather than impact.

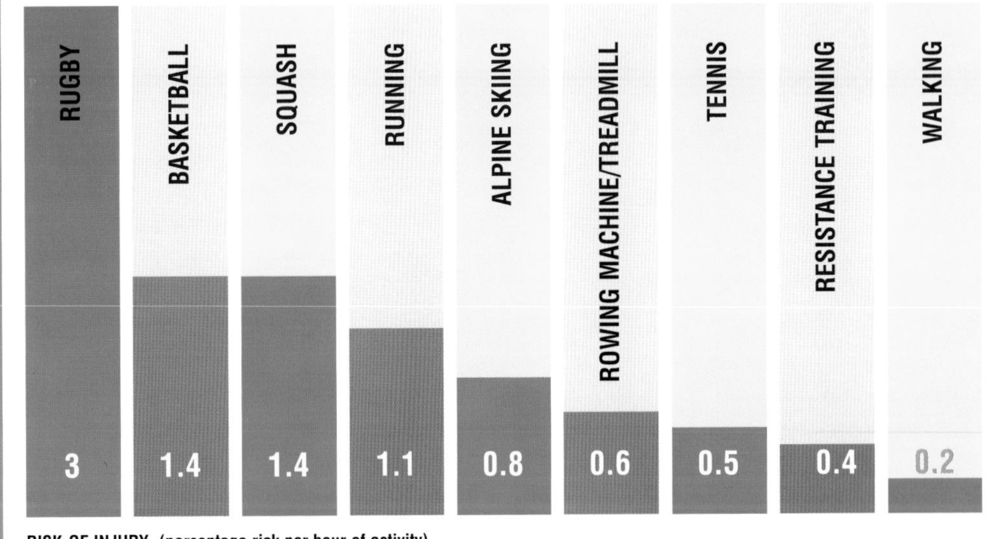

Your pregnant body

Pregnancy is a time of great change in most systems of the body and your musculoskeletal system is no exception. The major hormonal and physical developments that accompany pregnancy greatly increase the demands on your bones and muscles – but they also stimulate some incredible changes as your body prepares for birth.

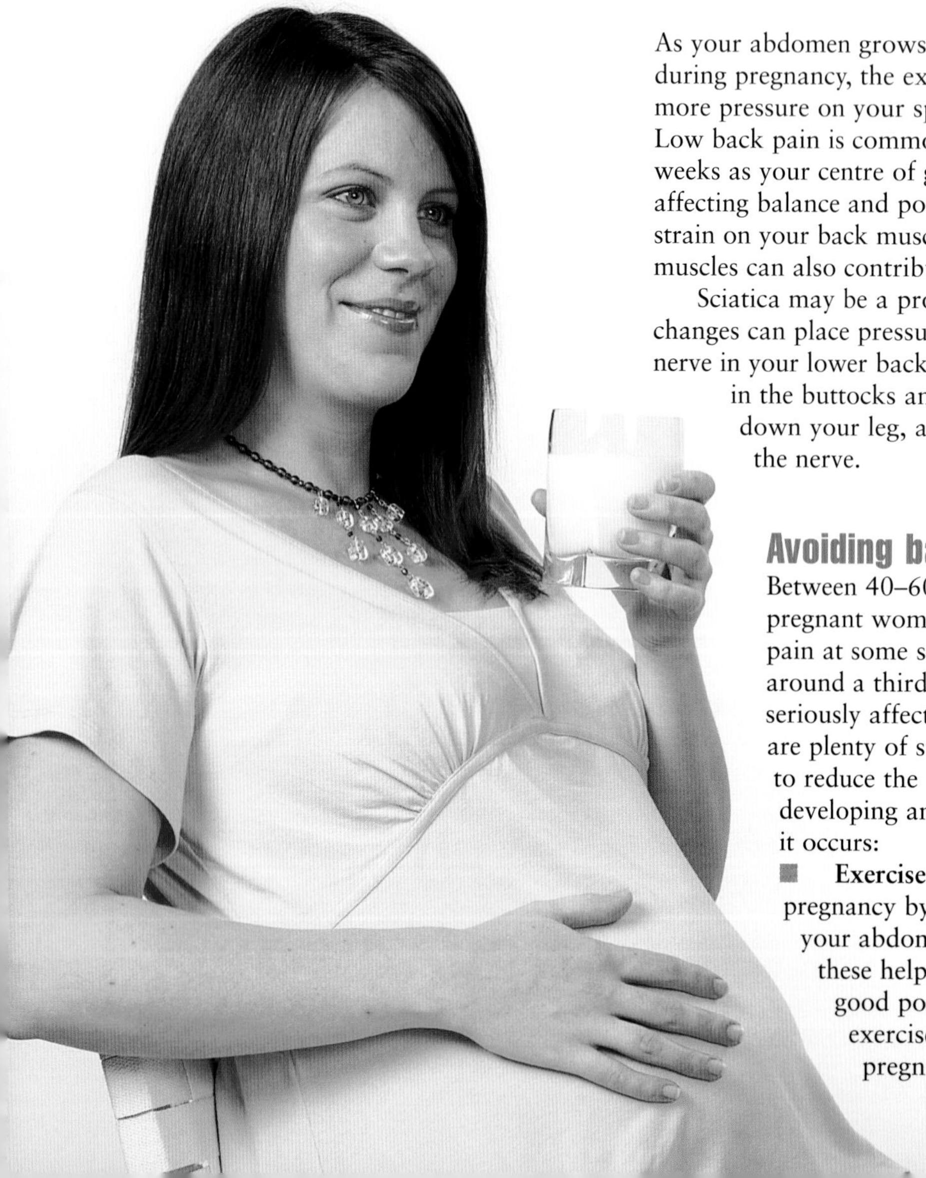

As your abdomen grows bigger and heavier during pregnancy, the extra weight places more pressure on your spine and vertebrae. Low back pain is common after about 12 weeks as your centre of gravity changes, affecting balance and posture and putting a strain on your back muscles. Weak stomach muscles can also contribute to back pain.

Sciatica may be a problem as postural changes can place pressure on the sciatic nerve in your lower back. Sciatic pain arises in the buttocks and may extend down your leg, along the course of the nerve.

Avoiding back pain

Between 40–60 per cent of pregnant women experience back pain at some stage – though only around a third of these will be seriously affected. Luckily there are plenty of steps you can take to reduce the likelihood of pain developing and to relieve pain if it occurs:

- **Exercise** Prepare for your pregnancy by strengthening your abdominal muscles – these help you to maintain good posture. Do back exercises throughout pregnancy to strengthen your back muscles and improve flexibility – exercise should also provide some pain relief. Swimming is an excellent exercise to help alleviate back pain because the water supports your weight. Breaststroke can make you arch your back, so stick to back stroke or crawl.
- **Posture** Avoid letting the weight of your bump pull your spine forwards when you are standing – stand tall and follow the same guildelines for good posture that you would normally >>176–177. When sitting, make sure your lower back is supported by the back of the chair or a cushion. Be particularly careful while lifting: keep your back straight, squat down, keep the object close to your body and use the muscles in your legs. Get help if you need to move a heavy object.
- **Support** Sleep on a firm, comfortable mattress – you may find it helps to use several pillows to tuck under your bump or under and between your legs. Consider wearing a pregnancy support girdle.
- **Relief** If your back is very painful, hold a heat pad or a wrapped hot-water bottle against it. Massage can also be an effective way to relieve pain.

Cramps and pains

Women often experience muscle cramps during pregnancy, and these cramps often occur more frequently or become more painful as pregnancy progresses. The cramps may be connected to circulation problems or to low levels of magnesium or calcium, minerals required for good muscle function. In addition, fluid retention during pregnancy can cause compression of the median nerve as it runs through your wrist (carpal tunnel syndrome >>284). This can cause pain or tingling in your hand.

Nutritional needs

A balanced diet plays a major role in promoting healthy pregnancy and a healthy baby. If you are already eating a nutritious diet, you will need to make only minor adjustments when you become pregnant. If you are not, now is the time to change!

Energy needs

Weight increases gradually through pregnancy with the greatest increase during the last three months. You should expect to put on around 11–16kg (25–35lb) over the course of the pregnancy, with 1–2kg (2–5lb) being put on in the first three months and then 1–2kg (2–5lb) every month for the next six months. You will need a small increase in calories in the first twelve weeks, then about 300 additional calories per day.

It may be difficult to maintain a balanced diet in the first 14 weeks or so of pregnancy due to the nausea that many women experience. Some women eat a great deal including large amounts of carbohydrates to stem the nausea and this can result in a major weight increase. Other women can lose weight if they have problems finding foods they can tolerate. If you suffer from nausea you may find that it helps to eat frequent, small meals.

Vitamins and minerals

Your pregnant body and your developing baby require a wide range of vitamins and minerals to stay strong and healthy. In theory, a balanced diet containing all of the main food groups and plenty of fruit and vegetables should include all the nutrients you need. The main exception to this is folic acid – studies have shown that the risk of a neural tube defect is dramatically reduced by taking a folic acid supplement during the first four months of pregnancy.

In the real world, of course, not everyone has a perfect diet and many women do need more vitamins or minerals during pregnancy. If you are worried about your diet, you should talk to your doctor about taking a daily antenatal supplement to boost your intake. But remember that a supplement is never a substitute for a healthy, balanced diet.

Calcium and iron

Certain nutrients are of key importance during pregnancy. In particular, it is vital to get enough calcium and iron in your diet – your baby needs calcium to lay down the foundation of strong bones in the womb and your body needs iron to form new red blood cells during pregnancy.

To some extent, your pregnant body does compensate for this by absorbing more calcium and iron from your food and excreting less in your urine. However, many women already have a lower intake of these minerals than recommended. According to the 2003 National Diet and Nutrition Survey, almost half of women in the UK do not get the recommended intake of calcium in their diet.

If your intake of these minerals is too low during pregnancy, you risk developing anaemia (deficiency of the oxygen-carrying haemoglobin in your blood) or losing bone minerals as your body redirects calcium from your bones to your baby. This can increase your risk of developing osteoporosis later in life.

For this reason, unless you are certain you already get enough of these nutrients, it is important to boost your levels. If you are under the age of 25, a good intake of calcium is particularly important as you might not yet have reached peak bone mass. Good sources of calcium include dairy products, dark green leafy vegetables and nuts. Good sources of iron include red meat and green leafy vegetables. For more information about good diet and nutrients for strong bones and muscles >>98–117.

PREPARING FOR BIRTH

In the course of your pregnancy, your body – including your bones and joints – will undergo some astonishing changes as it adapts to make room for your growing baby and to prepare itself for birth.

- ***18–24 weeks*** **The round ligaments along the sides of your uterus start to stretch to make room for your uterus to expand. This may cause pain in your abdomen, although symptoms usually disappear at around 24 weeks.**
- ***28 weeks*** **As your uterus starts to push up against your rib cage, your lower ribs begin to spread out to make more room for your baby. This may cause mild discomfort.**
- ***35 weeks*** **The pregnancy hormone relaxin starts to loosen your pelvic ligaments and the weight of your baby on your pelvic joints makes them expand in readiness for birth.**
- ***Birth*** **During labour your uterus, the largest muscle in your body, rhythmically contracts to squeeze your baby down the birth canal. Your cervix dilates to allow your baby to move under your pubic bone and through the opening in your pelvic floor muscles.**

Exercises to prevent backache in pregnancy

During the first few months of pregnancy, before your bump grows too big, you can perform the exercises for your back and shoulders shown in chapter 6 (>>180–183). These exercises will stretch and strengthen the muscles around your back and spine, helping to improve posture and prevent back pain later on in your pregnancy.

The exercises for your neck and upper back will continue to be useful throughout your pregnancy but, as your bump grows larger and heavier, the exercises for your lower back are no longer so suitable. You won't be able to lie on your front and you should avoid doing exercises on your back after the first trimester because this can place pressure on blood vessels and restrict blood flow to your heart and your baby.

To strengthen your lower back and reduce backache after the first trimester, try these exercises instead.

Sitting twist

The turning motion in this exercise helps to maintain the flexibility of your spine and release muscular tension in your upper back, neck and shoulders.

1 Sit on a cushion on the floor with your legs loosely crossed. If it feels more comfortable, place a cushion under each knee to support your legs. Keep your spine straight.

2 Keeping your spine held vertical, very slowly turn your upper body to the left. Place your right hand on your thigh above your left knee and your left hand on the floor just behind you. Hold and count to 5 before turning back to face the front. Repeat 5–10 times.

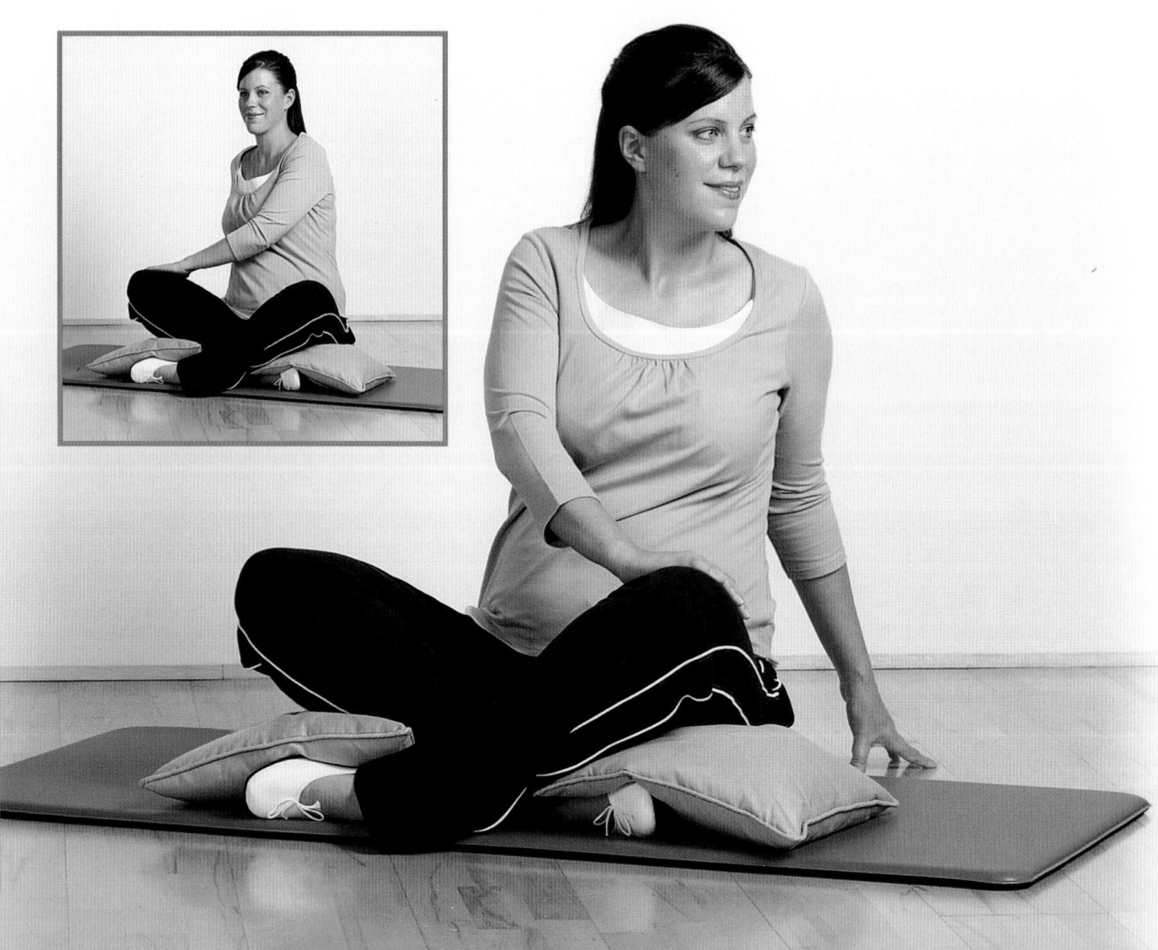

WATER EXERCISE

Your baby gets to float around all day in your womb, so why not get in on the fun with a visit to a pool? Swimming and aquaerobics are great ways to stay fit during pregnancy – the water supports the weight of your bump while you work out, taking the stress off your back and joints. The chlorine in the pool won't harm your baby – it simply keeps the pool free from bacteria.

Back curl

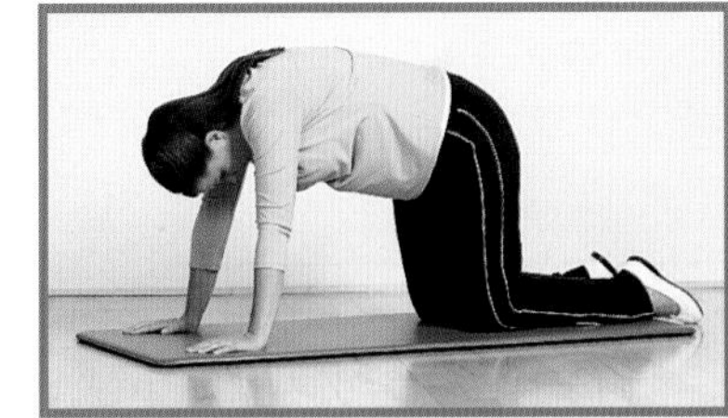

This aims to increase the suppleness in the lower back and can help to ease backache during late pregnancy. If you have carpal tunnel syndrome and the hand position causes discomfort, try using your knuckles instead of your palms.

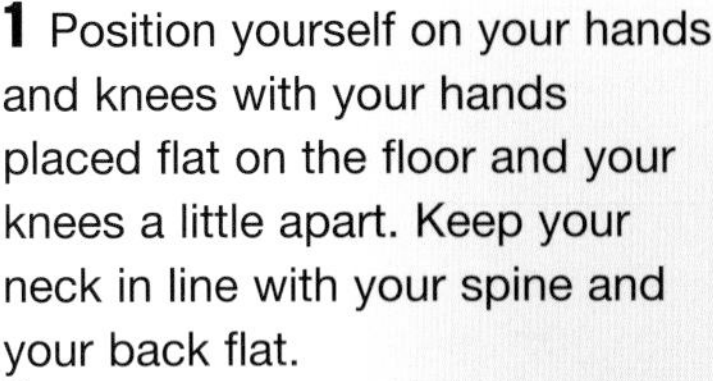

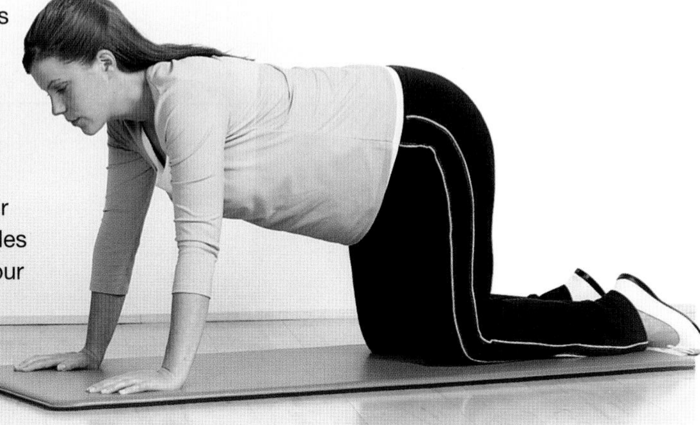

1 Position yourself on your hands and knees with your hands placed flat on the floor and your knees a little apart. Keep your neck in line with your spine and your back flat.

2 Tuck your head in towards your chest, clench your buttock muscles and tuck in your pelvis so that your back gently arches up into a hump. Hold and count to 5 before relaxing the back down. Repeat 5–10 times.

Back stretch

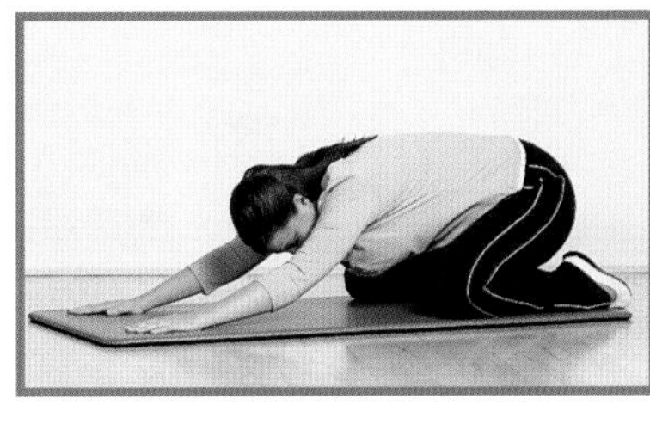

This exercise stretches your lower back and your buttocks. As your baby grows bigger you can move your knees wider apart to better accommodate your bump.

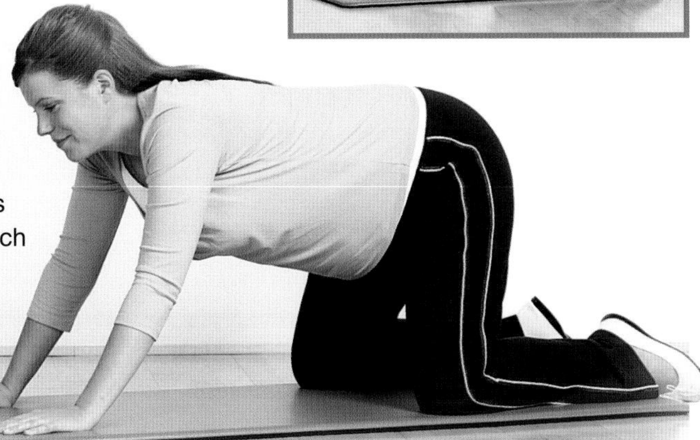

1 Position yourself on your hands and knees, with your hands placed flat on the floor and just in front of your head. Support your abdomen with a cushion if necessary.

2 Slowly rock back until your buttocks rest on your heels and your arms stretch forward. Walk your hands forward to increase the stretch slightly. Hold and count to 5 before moving back up. Repeat 5–10 times.

6 WAYS TO...

Exercise safely

It is important to bear the following points in mind when exercising during pregnancy:

1 Warm up and cool down before and after exercise. You may be more liable to injury when pregnant so it is important to prepare your body and give it a chance to wind down.

2 Drink plenty of fluids Pregnancy raises your body temperature so it is easy to become dehydrated. You should drink at least 2 litres (4 pints) a day and increase your intake when you exercise. Take a few sips every 15 minutes.

3 Don't lie on your back after about 12 weeks because this can interfere with your circulation as the heavy uterus presses against your blood vessels.

4 Avoid overstretching The hormone relaxin loosens your ligaments and softens your joints, making you more prone to injury. Take each stretch gently and avoid overextending.

5 Talk to your doctor or midwife who will give you personal advice about exercise and answer any particular questions you might have.

6 Know when to stop – you should stop immediately if you feel light-headed, dizzy or short of breath. If you have vaginal bleeding or if you feel any pains or contractions in your abdomen, stop and seek medical attention.

Regaining your pre-pregnancy shape

You'll have so much to think about after giving birth that it can be difficult to find the time to look after yourself. But a good diet, relaxation and gentle exercise will help your body to readjust to your post-pregnancy state and undo some of the unwanted effects of giving birth, such as loss of muscle tone and a weak pelvic floor.

When to start exercise

Almost as soon as the soreness begins to subside – as early as the day after the birth if the delivery was straightforward – you can start some gentle toning exercises to target the areas of your body that feel particularly weak. If you had a Caesarean section, you may need to wait a little longer – talk to your doctor about when to start.

First days

Start off with some gentle exercises to regain abdominal tone. To start, simply contract your stomach muscles: pull your stomach tight as you breathe out, hold a few seconds without moving your body, and relax. After this, progress to modified sit-ups: lie on your back on a firm surface and slowly raise then lower your head, keeping your shoulders on the floor. As your stomach muscles get stronger, you can start to curl your shoulders up, too.

You should also start exercising your pelvic-floor muscles as soon as possible. These muscles support your bladder, bowels and womb, helping to prevent urinary incontinence. The best way to strengthen them is to perform specially devised 'Kegel' exercises.

To do these exercises correctly, you need to get a feel for the muscles involved. Begin by trying to stop your flow mid-stream when you are urinating. Once you know what to contract, you can start by squeezing the muscles for a few seconds at a time and repeat 3–4 times. Try to do this several times a day and build up to holding the muscles for 10 seconds at a stretch and for 25 repetitions.

Establishing a routine

From a few weeks after birth, try to establish a daily exercising routine with a variety of gentle toning exercises such as abdominal curls or side bends. You can also do exercises with your child – lifting your infant is a great way to work your muscles and bond with your baby.

Walking is a good way to build up gently to a more strenuous aerobic-type exercise, as long as you avoid anything too demanding over the first few weeks. After a straightforward birth, you can usually start a more challenging aerobic exercise programme within 6–10 weeks. If you have had a Caesarean section, you may need to give your abdomen longer to recover – at least 10 weeks. Check with your doctor or health visitor to find out what type of exercises are appropriate.

Nutrition for new mums

Pregnancy and birth place high demands on your body, so you'll need to eat well to replenish your body's nutrients and get enough energy to care for your new baby. You're probably keen to get your old figure back after birth but you shouldn't be too hasty about dieting: even if you aren't breastfeeding, pregnancy will have depleted your stores of vitamins and minerals, so you should continue to eat well.

Breastfeeding

Good nutrition is particularly important if you are breastfeeding – your diet has to provide enough vitamins, minerals and energy to supply your needs and the needs of your growing baby. A vital part of breast milk is calcium for your baby's bones. The National Osteoporosis Society recommends that breastfeeding mothers get an extra 550mg of calcium per day – equivalent to about two glasses of milk. You should also eat lots of iron and vitamin-rich foods and get plenty of fluids.

You may need to increase your energy intake while breastfeeding – as a rough guide, you'll need an extra 500 calories on

DID YOU KNOW?

■ Women can lose 3–5 per cent of their bone mass during breastfeeding but this is rapidly recovered after weaning. Indeed childbirth may protect you against hip fractures: according to one study, being childless increases your risk of a hip fracture by around 44 per cent, while each additional birth reduces the risk by 9 per cent.

■ Breastfeeding may help to protect against rheumatoid arthritis (RA). Researchers have found that women who breastfed for 13–23 months had a 20 per cent reduction in the risk of RA compared with women who had never breastfed. Women who had breastfed for at least two years increased their risk reduction to 50 per cent.

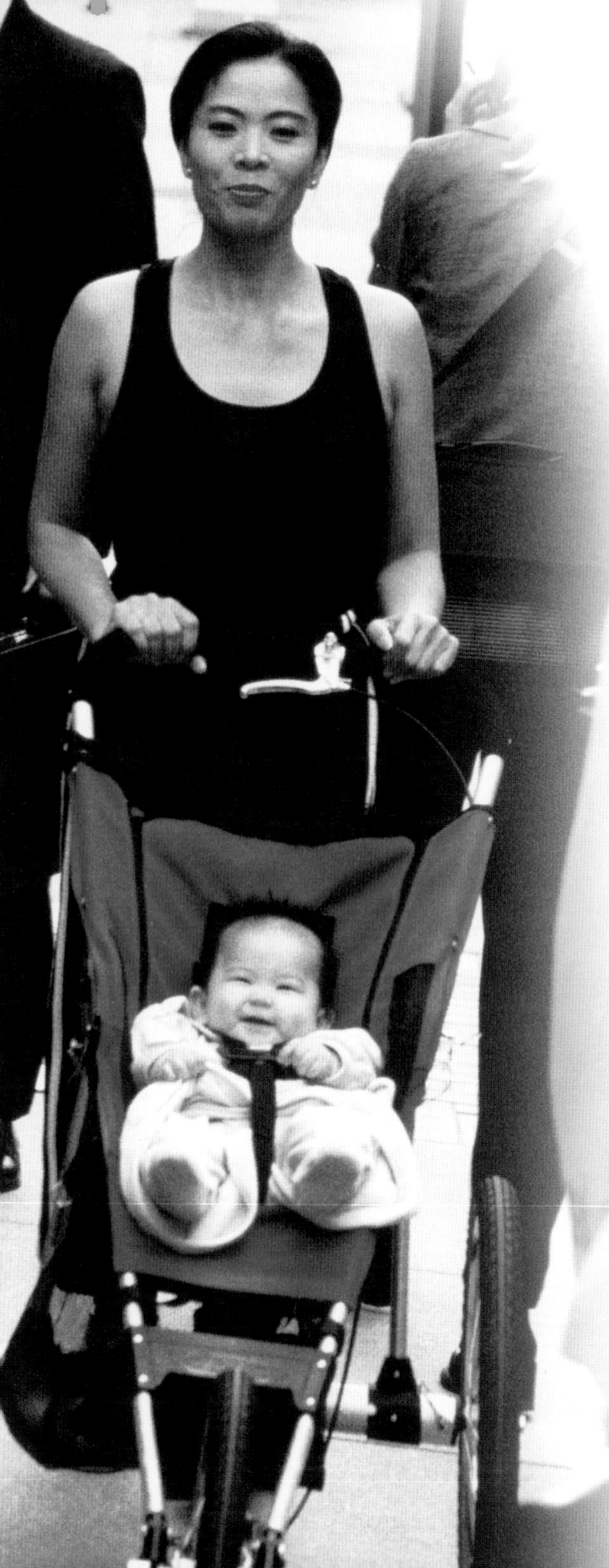

top of the 1950–2100 recommended for non-pregnant women. It you do wish to lose weight, wait until breastfeeding is well established before restricting your calorie intake in any way. Even then, take any weight loss slowly and gradually.

Lifting and holding your baby

Babies love to be hugged and held; it is one of the best ways to make your child feel loved and secure. Feeding, rocking, carrying and comforting helps you to bond with your baby – but must be done correctly as the extra weight can also place a lot of strain on your back and arms. By the time your baby is a year old, you may be regularly lifting and carrying a weight in the region of 8–12kg (18–26lb).

Carrying your baby

Newborns feel safe cradled in your arms while older babies may prefer a hip hold so they can watch the world. Unfortunately, cradling your baby with your shoulders or upper back rounded can cause muscle spasms. Regularly carrying your child on one side of the body, particularly with jutting hips, can cause muscular imbalance.

To avoid problems, make an effort to alternate and use both sides of your body. Try to keep your shoulders down and your stomach tight. Baby carriers and slings can exacerbate back problems; if you have backache, look for an ergonomic carrier with wide, padded, adjustable straps.

Holding for feeding

Over the first few months of life, you may need to feed your baby every 1–3 hours, so you should make sure that you use a chair with good back support. You may find it helps to use a footrest.

Many breastfeeding mothers hunch over to reach their babies, which can cause backache. Instead, buy a special nursing pillow to lift your baby up into a more comfortable position. If you have had a Caesarean section, try holding your baby at your side, feet tucked under your arm while breastfeeding: this type of 'football hold' can reduce pressure on your stomach.

SEPARATING STOMACH MUSCLES

Before starting any postnatal exercise programme, you should check that the vertical muscles in your abdominal wall have not separated during pregnancy: lie on your back with your knees bent, place two fingers horizontally below your belly button and gently push down – if you can feel a space between your stomach muscles more than about two fingers wide, your muscles may have separated, a condition known as *diastasis recti*. Talk to a doctor about modifying your exercise programme.

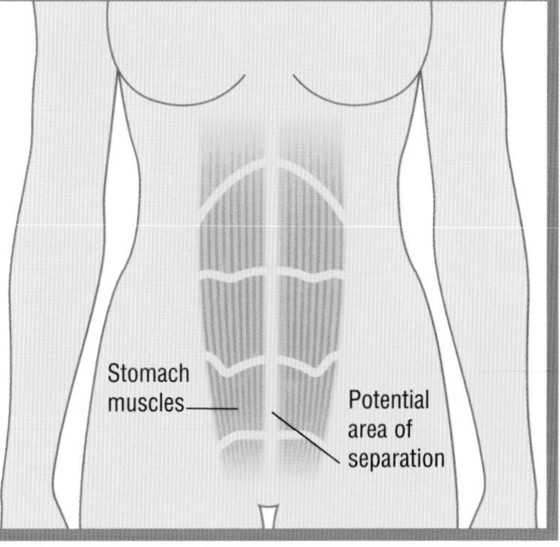

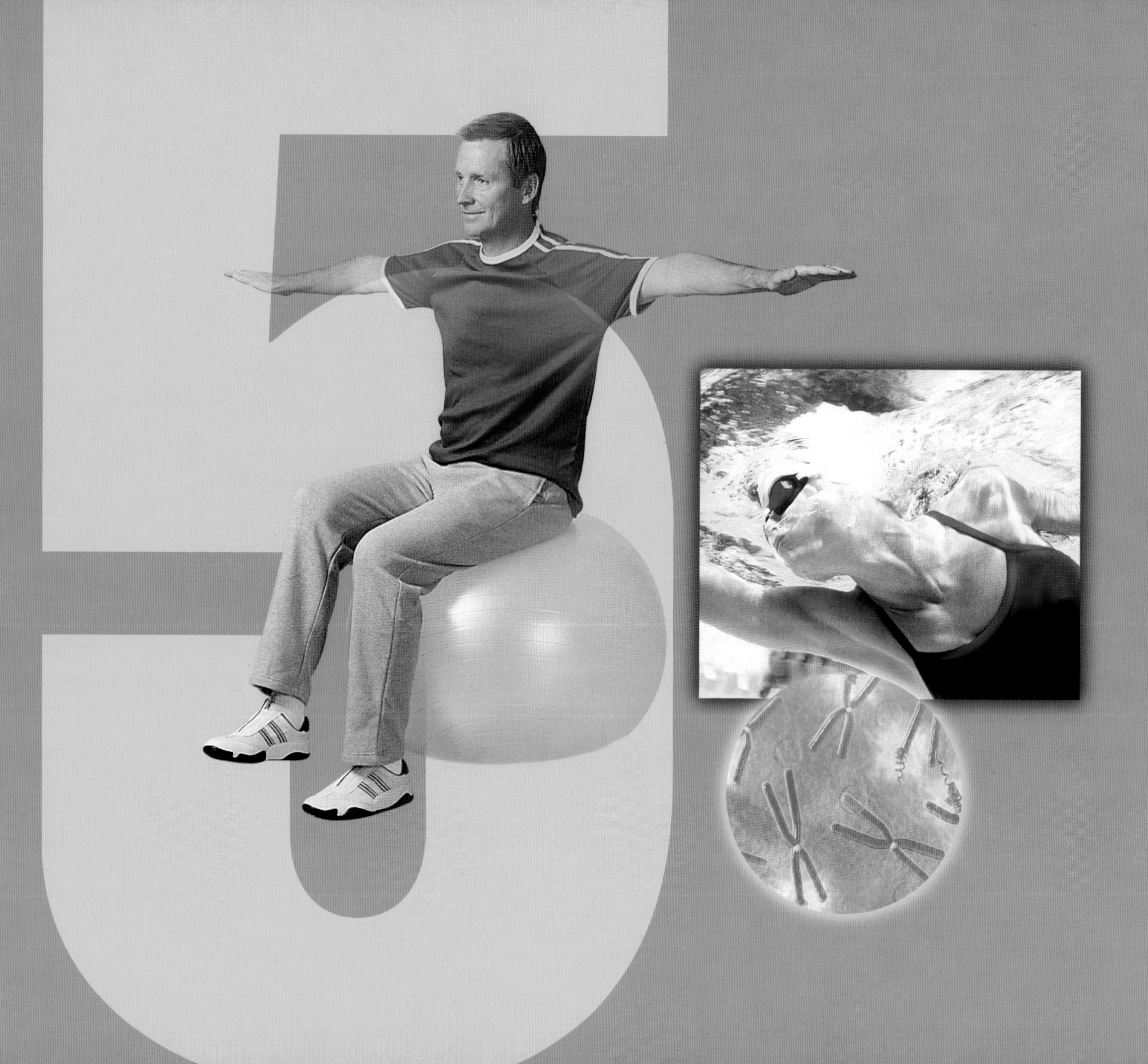

AGILE AGEING

There's no doubt that your body changes as you age but frailty and sickliness are *not* inevitable. The key to successful ageing is to take responsibility for your body and make sure it stays in good enough condition to withstand the many disorders associated with getting older. If this concept is new to you, it's time to make some small changes – be they in nutrition, exercise or lifestyle – that will lead to great benefits.

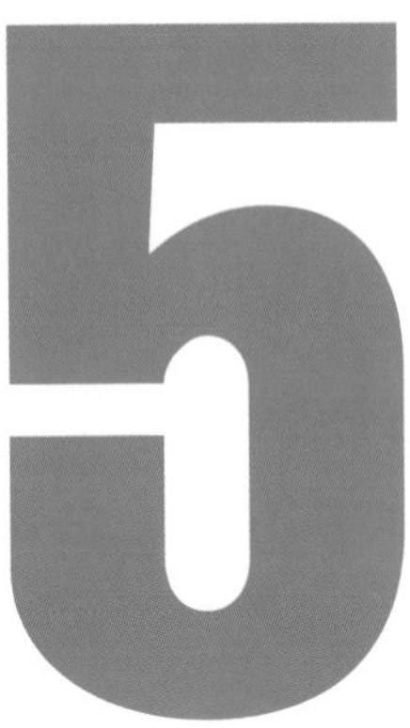

AGILE AGEING
Your changing body

Growing older is no longer something to be dreaded. Certain changes to your body are inevitable as you age but by staying active and eating well you can keep your bones, muscles and joints healthy and functioning well at any time of life.

Life expectancy in the Western world has risen steadily over the past half a century and, by the year 2025, more than a third of the UK population will be over 65 years of age. This increased longevity has brought many advantages, but with longer lifetimes has come an increase in the incidence of many age-related musculoskeletal problems, from minor arthritic aches and pains to fractures and osteoporosis.

218 Protecting your hips

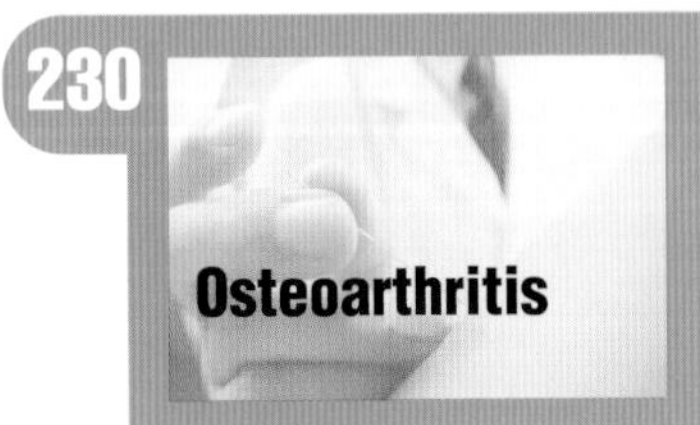
230 Osteoarthritis

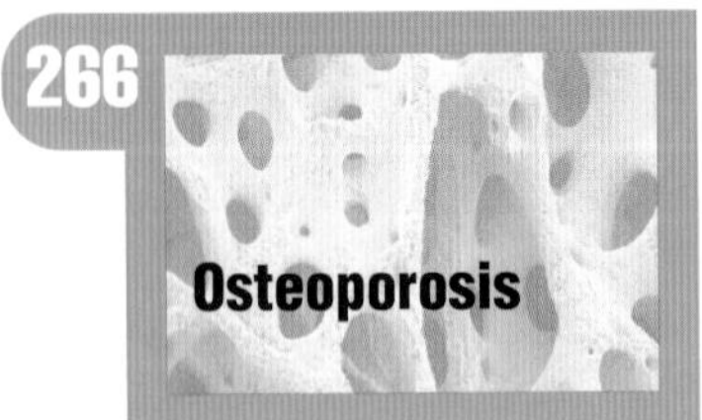
266 Osteoporosis

The ageing process

Bone and muscle mass tend to decline with age. Bone mass reaches its peak in your late 30s; after this time bone is gradually lost, a process that accelerates as you get older. Muscle mass undergoes a similar process: strength declines by about 15 per cent each decade after 50. At the same time, your connective tissues become stiffer, your joints less mobile and your metabolism starts to slow.

Many of these developments are connected to hormones. In women, the greatest hormonal change takes place with the menopause, usually between the ages of 45–55 (in the UK, the average age is 51). Low levels of oestrogen mean that women often experience an annual decrease in bone mass of 3–5 per cent in the years immediately following menopause. A similar, though more gradual, fall in the levels of some male hormones occurs in men.

At a cellular level, your body undergoes complex changes as you age. Within your musculoskeletal system, the cells that form new bone and cartilage (the osteoblasts and chondroblasts) become less effective. Degraded molecules start to accumulate and lower levels of hormones circulate to maintain tissues. At the same time tissue repair and wound healing are slower and fewer stem cells are present to develop into mature supporting tissue.

DID YOU KNOW?

- **Men lose bone mass by about 1 per cent each year after the age of 50, while women begin to lose bone in their early 30s, with a 2–3 per cent loss each year after the menopause.**
- **The risk of wrist fractures in women rises sharply after the menopause but stays the same or even declines after 65. In contrast, hip and spine fractures increase after 70 with a sharp rise after 80. This may be because older people have slower reactions and are less likely to use an arm to break a fall.**

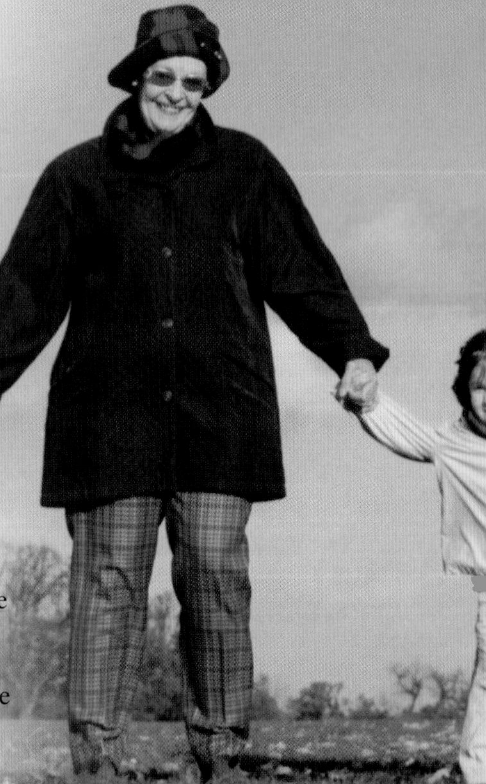

Trouble-free ageing

In time, these changes start to affect your posture and coordination. You may feel less stable and move more slowly. You may start to shrink with age, too: you can lose as much as an inch in height between the ages of 60 and 80 due to a combination of bone loss and reduced elasticity in your spine's intervertebral discs.

A number of musculoskeletal problems and conditions are also closely associated with the ageing process. As bone and muscle mass decreases and the cumulative wear on your joints builds up, both osteoarthritis and osteoporosis are much more likely to develop. Certain disorders, such as polymyalgia rheumatica and Paget's disease of bone, start to appear for the first time.

The combination of more brittle bones, weaker supporting muscles and reduced balance and mobility means that falls and fractures become more common. Reduced vision and hearing, which make falls and accidents more likely, can also contribute to the incidence of fractures. Around half of women and nearly a quarter of men over the age of 50 will suffer from an osteoporosis-related fracture at some time in their life.

Staying strong

Some of this ageing process is inevitable: the result of general wear and tear and the genetically determined 'biological clock'. Once our reproductive years are over, the theory goes, the body is genetically less disposed to continue to repair and maintain its systems into old age.

But there is increasing evidence that we can do much to offset the effects of age-related changes. You can avoid many age-related problems by taking care of your diet, getting plenty of moderate intensity exercise, avoiding tobacco and excess alcohol, and making judicious use of supplements such as vitamin D and calcium. Many of these same measures, allied with drugs and modern medical treatments where necessary, will help you to manage and in some cases even reverse problems when they do occur.

TELOMERES AND SMOKING

Your body's ability to regenerate as you age depends in part on strips of DNA called telomeres which cap the ends of your cell chromosomes to stop them unravelling. Each time a cell divides, its telomere gets shorter until eventually the chromosome starts to unravel. As a result, the cell can no longer divide, becomes older and eventually dies.

Studies suggest that smoking may actually accelerate this ageing process: telomeres in smokers are significantly shorter than in non-smokers. This may be one reason why regularly smoking 20 cigarettes a day doubles your risk of developing osteoporosis in later life.

Maintaining bone health

It is easy to take the good health of your bones for granted. Most people are only too aware of how their muscles and joints change with age, but brittle bones have few day-to-day symptoms.

Very often, the first time that someone is aware of a problem is when a fracture occurs. Even then, the root cause is not always addressed: doctors believe that many vertebral fractures go undiagnosed or are dismissed as generalized back pain.

Nonetheless, bone loss is one of the most common age-related conditions. Over half of people over the age of 50 have low bone mass, putting them at greater risk of fractures – and the consequences in elderly patients can be very serious. Half of hip fracture patients lose the ability to walk independently and up to 35 per cent are dependent on carers. As many as 1 in 5 patients over the age of 50 dies within six months of the fracture.

It is with some justification then, that osteoporosis has been called the 'silent epidemic'. Luckily, there is nothing inevitable about osteoporosis; there are plenty of measures you can take to keep your bones healthy, whatever your age.

> **'Only a quarter of women over the age of 50 have taken steps to have their bone health checked'**

What happens?

From middle age onwards, the amount of calcium in your bone gets less, a process that accelerates in women after menopause >>148–149. As mineral levels fall, your bone cortex – the hard outer layer that gives bone its great strength – starts to thin, notably at the femoral neck (the point at which your thigh bone meets your hip). Any type of stress on this weakened bone can lead to microfractures – tiny cracks in the bone that weaken it still further. The lower your bone mass, the greater the risk of breaking your bones; below a certain level you have osteoporosis >>264-275.

Why do you lose bone mass?

The pace at which bone is formed and broken down is controlled by cells called osteoblasts and osteoclasts. As you get older, the resorption of calcium from your bones by the osteoclasts starts to exceed the formation of new bone by the osteoblasts. This process is determined partly by changes to your hormones and your metabolism as you age, but the rate of change is also influenced by diet and lifestyle.

Exercise stimulates bone formation, but many people get less exercise as they get older. Any reduction in intake or our ability to absorb vitamins and minerals such as calcium and vitamin D may also play a role. The effects of other factors, such as too much alcohol or smoking can build up over time and suppress the function of the osteoblasts. So, while certain changes to your bone are inevitable as you grow older, you can considerably moderate the rate of the change by adopting a healthier lifestyle.

What can I do about it?

Because it is more difficult to reverse the process of bone loss than to maintain it, it is best to take preventative action before significant bone loss occurs. Your bones start to lose density from around the age of 35, so if you don't already watch your diet and get plenty of exercise, now is the time to start. Don't worry if you're older than

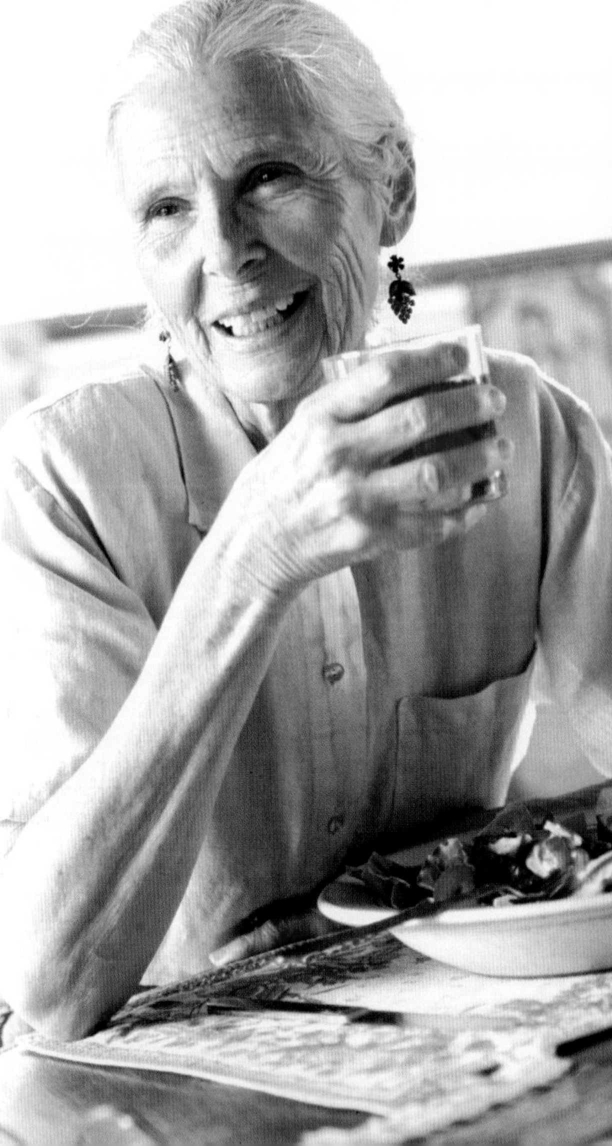

this, the right lifestyle decisions will help you to maintain the health of your bones, whatever your age.

■ **Diet and supplements** For strong bones, it is most important to get a balanced diet that supplies plenty of calcium and enough fluoride, phosphorus, vitamin D and protein. If you are worried about getting enough of these nutrients in your diet, consider taking a calcium and vitamin D supplement. For more information about good diet >>98–117.

■ **Exercise** Regular weight-bearing exercise such as walking or jogging will ensure that the protein and minerals you get in your diet are incorporated into your skeleton. Weight-bearing exercise loads your bones, stimulating the bone-building osteoblasts and improving the balance between bone loss and bone creation.

Modern life is full of labour-saving devices, so recreational exercise is more important than ever – in evolutionary terms we are designed for a mobile rather than sedentary lifestyle. The old adage 'use it or lose it' applies, but in moderation: too much stress can increase the risk of injury.

■ **Drug treatments** If you are diagnosed as osteoporotic, your doctor may prescribe drugs to slow the rate of bone loss. These include bisphosphonates (compounds that slow the action of osteoclasts), strontium ranelate (a compound of a mineral similar to calcium) or the calcium-regulating hormone calcitonin >>274.

■ **Hormone replacement therapy (HRT)** Treatment to replace lost oestrogen and progesterone in women may help to reverse some of the effects of menopause on bone, but has a number of potentially serious side effects. A safer alternative may be the family of drugs called selective oestrogen receptor modulators (SERMs) >>148-149.

? How healthy are my bones?

If you answer 'yes' to more than a few of the questions below, you may be at particular risk of fractures and osteoporosis. Talk to your doctor about getting a bone densitometry scan >>267.

YES	NO	
☐	☐	Are you over the age of 65?
☐	☐	Are you overweight?
☐	☐	Do you get limited exposure to sunshine?
☐	☐	If you are a woman, have you passed the menopause?
☐	☐	If you are a woman, did you have an early menopause?
☐	☐	Have you ever fractured a bone after an apparently minor bump or fall?
☐	☐	Do you eat few dairy foods, oily fish or leafy vegetables?
☐	☐	Do you get under 45 minutes moderately strenuous exercise a day?
☐	☐	Have you ever had to use steroids for a long period or suffered from an overactive thyroid or hypogonadism?
☐	☐	Have you ever had a long period of bed rest due to illness?
☐	☐	Do you smoke?

QUESTIONNAIRE

Managing your menopause

The menopause is a pivotal stage in a woman's life, the end of the reproductive cycle and the beginning of a new phase with its own conditions and considerations. Knowing what to expect and understanding all your options will help to ensure the continuing good health of your bones.

Throughout your reproductive years, your ovaries secrete oestrogen and progesterone on a cyclical basis. When ovulation finally ceases at the menopause your ovaries also stop making oestrogen: the abrupt fall in oestrogen is the immediate cause of most of the physical and emotional changes experienced during the menopause.

Every woman's experience of the menopause is different. Common symptoms include hot flushes, night sweats, mood swings, loss of libido and vaginal dryness. Some women find these changes upsetting or irritating; others are barely troubled by symptoms. Many women actually find it liberating to be freed from their hormonal cycle: even after the ovaries stop making oestrogen, the adrenal glands carry on for another 5–10 years and secrete hormones such as testosterone. Without the mitigating effect of oestrogen on these hormones, a woman can feel sexier, more energetic and more effective than ever before.

Bones, muscles and joints

Oestrogen stimulates the production of collagen, a structural protein found in muscles, bones, ligaments and tendons. Reduced cartilage production following the menopause can make your joints feel stiffer and your muscles weaker. As oestrogen also helps the absorption of calcium from your food, reduced levels of the hormone may affect the amount of calcium in your body. Calcium plays an important role in muscle function so low levels of calcium in your blood can cause cramps.

Menopause and your bones

Less immediately obvious, but of greater long-term significance, is the loss of bone mass after the menopause and the risk from brittle bones, fractures and osteoporosis – one reason why women make up around 80 per cent of osteoporosis sufferers.

Oestrogens help to prevent bone mineral loss. Without the powerful protective benefits of oestrogen, you can lose up to a fifth of your bone mass in the five to seven years following the menopause. This is why it is particularly important for menopausal and postmenopausal women to pay close attention to the health of their bones and be aware of the steps they can take to keep their bones healthy.

Hormone replacement therapy

Replacing lost oestrogen using hormone replacement therapy (HRT) can relieve many of the more unpleasant symptoms of menopause. Your doctor may prescribe oestrogen together with progestogen (a synthetic progesterone-like hormone) to reduce the risk of a thickened womb. Women who have had a hysterectomy can have oestrogen-only therapy.

DID YOU KNOW?

- **The health of your bones during and after the menopause provides a good indication of your risk of osteoporosis later in life; women who fracture a wrist within 10 years of entering the menopause have an eight times greater risk of hip fractures than the general population.**
- **Women are three times more likely than men to suffer from bone fractures. This may reflect the fact that men enjoy the protection of male hormones (androgens) for many years after women lose their oestrogens. Men do experience a gradual decline in the levels of sex hormones, sometimes called the andropause, often starting in their early 50s.**

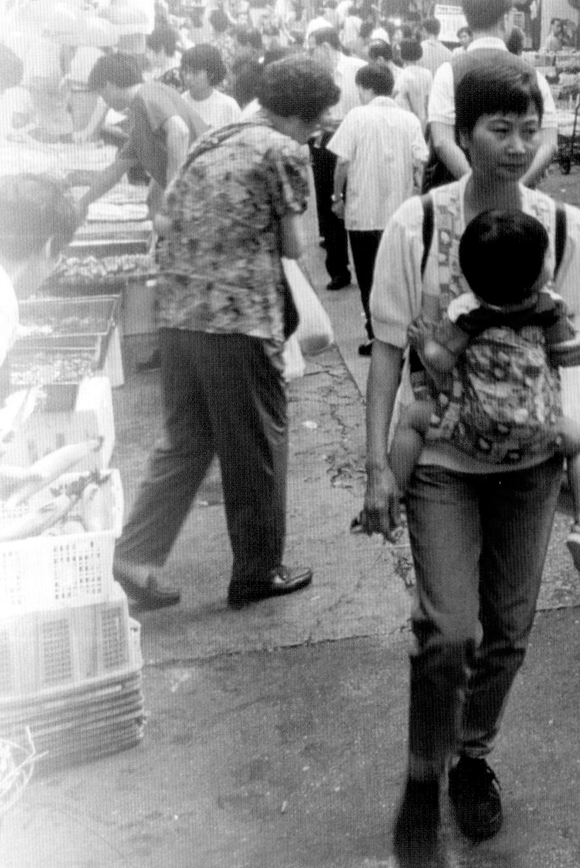

In the short-term, for the immediate symptoms of the menopause, this type of therapy is generally safe. Longer term use of HRT may increase your risk of breast and uterine cancer, blood clots and heart disease. The Medicines and Healthcare products Regulatory Agency (MHRA) recommends that the lowest effective dose be used for the shortest useful duration.

HRT and osteoporosis

It is these long-term risks that make the use of HRT to slow bone loss after the menopause so controversial. Hormone replacement can certainly help to maintain bone density but you'll need five or more years of oestrogen therapy for it to be effective – and you'll need to go on taking the hormone to maintain the benefits.

On balance, the risks of long-term HRT may well outweigh the benefits. For this reason, oestrogen therapy is not usually prescribed unless you are unable to take other osteoporosis treatments such as bisphosphonates >>274. In particular, women who have a family history of the breast or uterine cancers, blood clots or previous liver disease are not good candidates for HRT. As with any other type of preventative treatment for osteoporosis, you should never use HRT as a substitute for a good diet and plenty of exercise >>268–273.

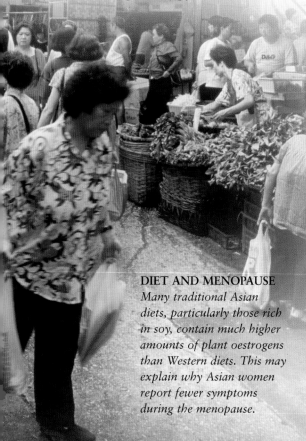

DIET AND MENOPAUSE *Many traditional Asian diets, particularly those rich in soy, contain much higher amounts of plant oestrogens than Western diets. This may explain why Asian women report fewer symptoms during the menopause.*

Alternatives to HRT

There are a number of alternatives to conventional hormone therapy, including drugs that mimic oestrogen's effects and other calcium-regulating hormones.

- **SERMs** (selective oestrogen receptor modulators) are a family of drugs that have oestrogen-like effects on some tissues but without many of the unwanted side effects. Raloxifene, for example, binds to oestrogen receptors in bone but not in the breasts or uterus, helping to prevent bone loss without increasing the risk from these cancers. A relatively new SERM, the synthetic steroid tibolone, has oestrogen, progesterone and androgen-like properties and has been shown to reduce the risk of osteoporosis without oestrogen's effects on breast tissue. SERMs may have various other side effects, including hot flushes, muscle soreness, weight gain and clot formation.
- **Estren** is a synthetic version of oestrogen that has proved as effective as HRT at preserving bone mass in initial tests in mice, without any apparent effect on breast cancer cells. This new class of drugs has been dubbed ANGELS (activators of non-genomic oestrogen-like signalling) and is also potentially suitable for treating men with osteoporosis.
- **Calcitonin** is a hormone that stimulates calcium absorption by your bones by inhibiting the action of the osteoclasts. It can help to counteract the effects of the fall in oestrogen after the menopause. Possible side effects include hot flushes, increased urination, nausea or rashes.
- **Teriparatide** is a new drug containing a fragment of parathyroid hormone, a hormone that regulates calcium levels. Parathyroid hormone stimulates both the bone-building osteoblasts and the bone-reducing osteoclasts. Continuous exposure to the hormone can reduce the amount of calcium in your bones, but intermittent exposure, such as a daily injection of teriparatide, stimulates the osteoblasts and encourages bone formation.

Phytoestrogens

Phytoestrogens are part of a large group of plant chemicals (phytochemicals) with medicinal properties. They include the isoflavonoids found in soya products and linseed and the lignins found in wholegrain cereals and pulses. Phytoestrogens have a similar structure to oestrogen and can mimic many of the hormone's effects – women who have a phytoestrogen-rich diet have a lower incidence of osteoporosis.

Unfortunately, there is some evidence that large amounts of phytoestrogens may increase the risk of certain cancers in much the same way as oestrogens. More research is required, but you should avoid non-dietary phytoestrogen supplements (pills or powders) which make it easier to ingest phytoestrogens in high doses.

A DAY IN THE LIFE OF YOUR BONES AND MUSCLES

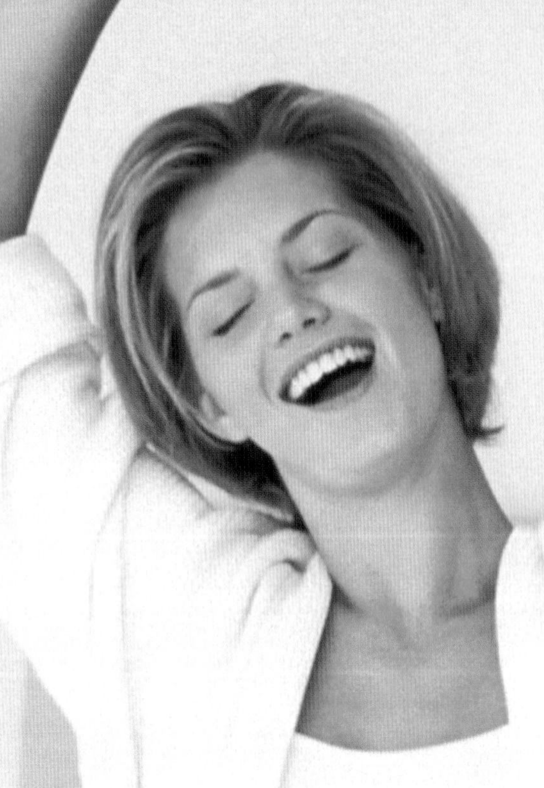

07:30

Rise and shine

During the night your bones and muscles have time to recover from the previous day's exertions. Without the effects of gravity on your spine overnight you may be up to half-an-inch taller in the morning than the previous evening. However, the lack of activity means your muscles may feel stiff in the morning.

■ **Limber up** Have a warm shower, relax your muscles and take 5 minutes to limber up and stretch. This will help to wake up your muscles and joints and prepare them for the day ahead.

■ **Wake up** A cup of tea or coffee first thing in the morning won't do you any harm, but too much caffeine can interfere with your uptake of bone and muscle-building nutrients such as calcium, iron and zinc. Try green tea instead: it contains less caffeine and has anti-inflammatory properties that may help to soothe rheumatic conditions.

■ **Refuel** A nutritious breakfast kick-starts your metabolism and makes you less likely to snack on unhealthy food later in the morning. A pot of yoghurt or a bowl of muesli or porridge with milk is a good way to get lots of calcium for your bones.

09:00

Out and about

Now you are ready for the day ahead. Your body needs to stay active to stay healthy – your muscles have evolved to work hard through the day, providing the mechanical power to move your bones. To keep your body in top condition, try to make as much use of your bones and muscles as possible.

■ **Get off early** Jump off the bus or the train a couple of stops early or park your car a little distance from your destination. You'll burn around 60 extra calories for every 10 minutes further that you walk.

■ **Stand up** Stay standing up when you use the bus or train. Hold onto the grab rail for support but use the muscles in your trunk and legs to roll with the motion – you'll improve your balance and work your core stabilizing muscles.

■ **Take the stairs** Walking up stairs rather than taking an escalator provides an aerobic workout similar to the step machine in the gym and strengthens the muscles in your legs and buttocks.

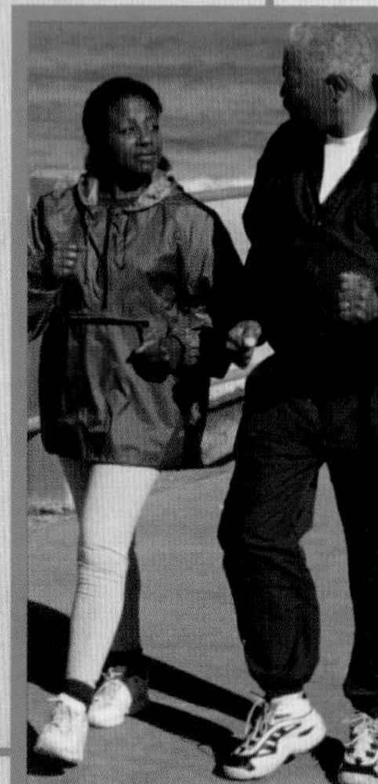

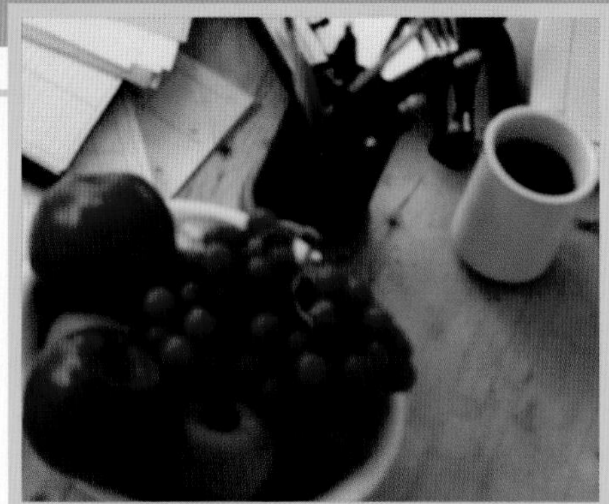

14:00

At your desk

Too much time spent sitting at a desk can store up problems for your back. Poor posture and lack of mobility places a lot of pressure on your muscles and joints, increasing your chance of back pain.

■ **Keep active** Try to get up and stretch your legs every 15 minutes or so to give your muscles and joints a chance to change position. Crumple up wastepaper before throwing it into the bin; clenching helps to ward off carpal tunnel syndrome.

■ **Fidget** Tap your toes or fingers, wriggle in your seat or tense your muscles while you're working. Research suggests that people who make lots of small fidgeting movements in everyday tasks burn a lot more calories – in one study the difference added up to as much as 350 calories a day.

■ **Snack healthily** Keep a bowl of fruit or some dried fruit and nuts on your desk. Fruit and nuts contain essential vitamins and minerals for bones and muscles and will help to keep your blood-sugar levels stable through the day, making you less likely to crave high-fat or salty snacks.

18:00

Keeping active

Regular activity – whether a trip to the gym or a brisk lunch-time walk – will keep your muscles and bones in peak condition and increase your chances of staying fit and active as you grow older. Doctors recommend at least 45 minutes of moderate-intensity exercise three times a week – and there are plenty of easy ways to stay active the rest of the time.

■ **Do the gardening** Even a couple of hours spent weeding or digging can burn around 1000 calories. Bend your knees, not your waist – this will tone your muscles and help prevent back strain.

■ **Be impatient** Pace up and down the platform when you're waiting for your train to arrive. If you're waiting for a bus, try walking to the next stop. If it means that you need to run for your bus, even better!

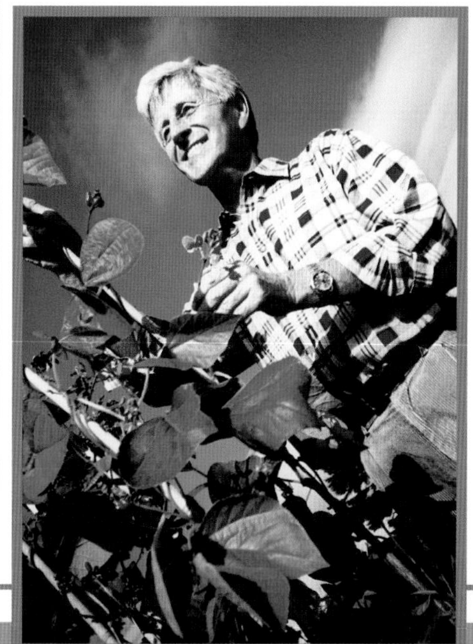

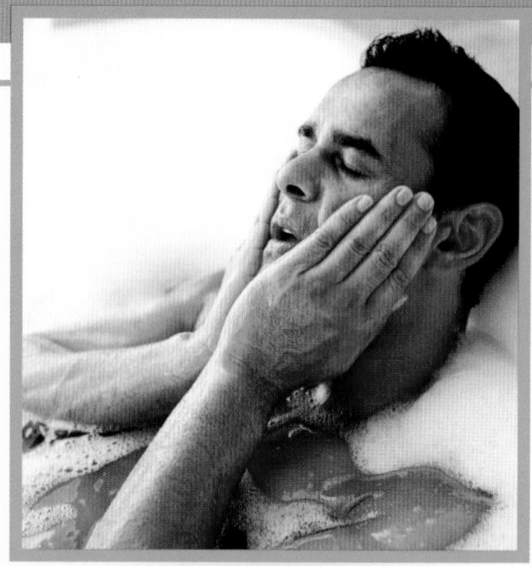

21:00

Winding down

Give your body a chance to relax before you go to bed – a warm bath will help to soothe your muscles and joints. Avoid simply collapsing in a sofa or armchair to watch television – lack of support and poor sitting posture can place stress on your back and spine.

■ **Sit and bounce** Instead of slumping in front of the TV, try sitting on an exercise ball – your posture will improve and you'll work your core stabilizing muscles.

■ **Hide the remote** Getting up to change the channel on your TV manually just 10 times an evening will burn around 3,500 calories over the course of the year – enough to lose about a half a kilo of body fat.

■ **Start laughing** Watch a good comedy or call a friend who knows how to make you laugh. Laughter releases tension, reduces stress and works your stomach muscles. Frequently laughing out loud over a 15-minute period can burn up to 40 calories.

Post menopause and beyond

Only a century ago, the average life expectancy in the UK was just 50 years. Today most people are expected to live well into their 70s or 80s and some women will live almost half of their lives after their menopause. This means it's more important than ever to look after your body.

Levels of physical activity tend to decline as people grow older. In the UK, according to government figures, only 17 per cent of men and 12 per cent of women aged 65–74 get the recommended levels of exercise (45 minutes of moderate-intensity exercise three times a week). This compares to 30 per cent of the general adult population.

Much of this decline results from changes to your body as you age, such as a slower metabolism and reduced muscle mass. Many people believe that a sedentary lifestyle is simply part and parcel of ageing.

But there is no inherent reason why activity levels should fall as you age – in some Asian countries where daily individual activities such as tai chi are a cultural norm, there is a levelling off or even an increase in activity from middle to old age. Your body does change as you grow older and your metabolism and musculoskeletal health may decline as a result – but you hold the keys to avert this decline.

The importance of activity

Throughout your life, your body relies on regular activity to maintain strong bones and muscles – lack of exercise causes a reduction in muscle bulk (sarcopenia) which contributes to the loss of physical endurance and mobility. The weaker you are, the less you can do and the more likely you are to avoid physical activity – a vicious cycle that condemns you to inactivity. Conversely, regular exercise will keep you fit and supple well into old age.

Maintaining your metabolism

Not only does inactivity increase your risk of age-related conditions ranging from general aches and pains to osteoporosis, it also lowers your body's metabolism. Most people's energy needs fall by around a third between the ages of 30–80 due to lower muscle mass and reduced energy expenditure. This can have a knock-on effect on your nutrient intake.

As your calorie requirements and therefore your appetite decline, it can be more difficult to get all of the nutrients that you need in your diet. Many of these nutrients, particularly calcium and vitamin D, are very important for your bones and muscles as you get older. Regular exercise not only keeps you fitter and stronger, it also boosts your metabolism and your appetite and helps you to remain active, whatever your age.

DID YOU KNOW?

- **A group of 50–73-year-old women who exercised for 1 hour a week for 8 months increased their bone mineral density by 3.5 per cent, according to a study in the journal *Clinical Science*. The sedentary control group lost density over the same period.**
- **Another study divided 40 postmenopausal women into two groups. The women in the first group, who did no extra exercise, lost both bone and muscle mass over the course of the study. The women in the second group increased their strength to the same level as women 15–20 years younger by the end of the study.**

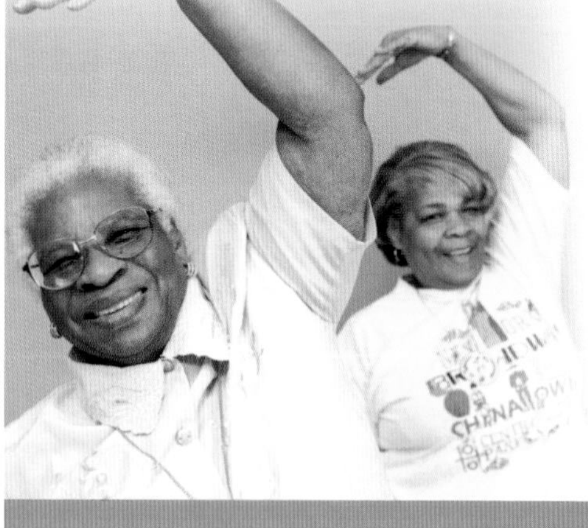

SLOWING METABOLISM

These pies represent the calories required per day to maintain the basal (resting) metabolic rate (BMR) of an average-size 30-year-old man – 1700 calories. The shaded slices show the reduction in the calories needed to maintain the BMR of the same man at 50 and 70 years of age.

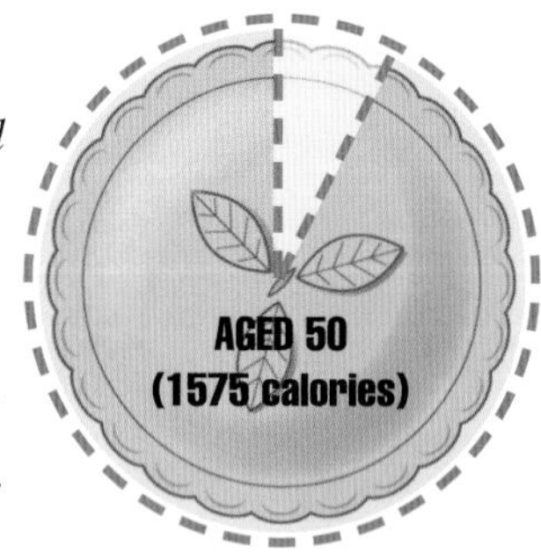

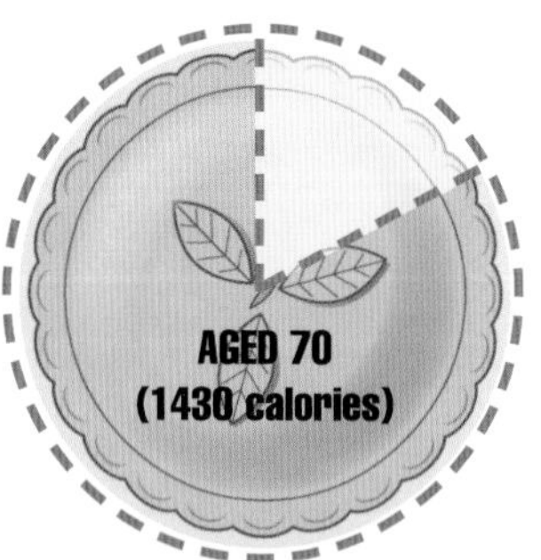

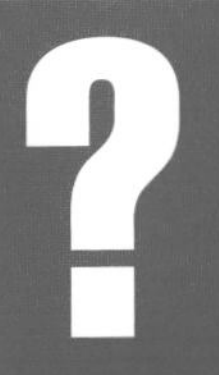

Am I at risk of musculoskeletal disease?

The following questions all relate to risk factors for the major age-related musculoskeletal diseases. Answer the questions as honestly as possible and check your score below to see how much you are at risk from muscle, bone or joint problems.

SCORE

How many of your close relatives have an arthritic condition?
Score 3 points for each relative affected.

How many of your close relatives have osteoporosis?
Score 3 points for each relative affected.

How many hours each day do you spend sitting down?
Score 1 point for each hour spent sitting down.

What is your girth at the waist?
Score 2 points for each inch that your waist is over 102cm/40in (men) or 97cm/38in (women).

Do you smoke?
Score 2 points for each year you have smoked over the last 5 years.

Have you ever had a bone fracture?
Score 2 points for each fracture.

How many units of alcohol do you drink, on average, each week?
Score 1 point for every 2 units that you drink over 21 units (men) or 14 units (women).

How many portions of fruit and vegetables do you eat each day?
Start with 10 points and subtract 2 for each portion.

How many hours of moderately intense activity do you get each week?
Start with 10 points and subtract 1 for each hour.

Are you male or female?
Score 5 points if you are female.

HOW DID YOU SCORE?

Under 30 points: Based on these questions your musculoskeletal health is good, but don't be lulled into a false sense of security: make sure you continue to eat well and get plenty of exercise.

30–50 points: You're at risk of developing musculoskeletal problems. Try to improve your score where possible by getting more exercise, eating more fruit and vegetables and drinking or smoking less. If you are over 50, talk to your doctor about getting a bone scan to check for osteoporosis.

Over 50 points: If you don't already suffer from bone or joint problems you are certainly at high risk of developing problems in the future. Talk to your doctor about getting a bone scan and make a firm effort to follow the advice in this book.

Common conditions that occur

Changes to cartilage, bone and soft tissues as people grow older mean that generalized musculoskeletal pain and stiffness are very common – nearly a quarter of people over the age of 55 describe themselves as having knee pain, while over the age of 70 nearly everyone has some stiffness and difficulty in initiating movement. A number of more specific musculoskeletal conditions also become more common with age – most notably arthritis and osteoporosis – some of which can cause considerable disability.

Rheumatic conditions

Rheumatism is a general term used to describe a variety of musculoskeletal aches and pains often accompanied by stiffness and inflammation. There are around 200 different rheumatic conditions, most of which can occur at any time of life but many of which are particularly common among older people. Rheumatic conditions such as arthritis are the leading cause of disability in people over the age of 65.

Arthritis

Inflammation of the joints, or arthritis, is the most common rheumatic problem – and one of the most common medical problems generally – among older adults. Arthritic conditions, notably osteoarthritis, rheumatoid arthritis and gout, affect around 50 per cent of people over 65.

■ **Osteoarthritis** is caused by the breakdown of the cartilage that cushions your joints and stops your bones rubbing together. Because it is a degenerative condition, the result of wear and tear or other types of trauma, the disease is uncommon before the age of 40. Although your likelihood of developing osteoarthritis does increase with age, the condition is certainly not an inevitable result of ageing. Many of the factors that affect your risk, such as your weight, the amount and type of exercise that you get and the amount of stress you put on your joints, are very much within your control. For more information about preventing and treating osteoarthritis >>228–247.

■ **Rheumatoid arthritis** is a painful condition caused when your immune system attacks the cells in your synovium, the layer of tissue that lines your joints. You can develop rheumatoid arthritis at any age, but around 80 per cent of people are first diagnosed between the ages of 35–50. The incidence tends to increase with age until around 75 when it starts to become less common again. The reasons why some people develop rheumatoid arthritis and others do not are not fully understood, although scientists believe that genetic factors and infections may play a role. For more information about diagnosing, managing and treating rheumatoid arthritis >>248–263.

- **Gout** is caused by the accumulation of crystals of urate in your joints. Gout accounts for around 5 per cent of arthritis cases and often first develops in men aged between the ages of 40–50. The condition can also occur in women, although rarely before menopause. Although genetic factors predispose sufferers to the condition, attacks are often triggered by certain foods, particularly rich foods, excess alcohol, dehydration or certain drugs. For more information >>294.

Polymyalgia rheumatica

This autoimmune disorder causes muscle pain and stiffness in your neck, hip and shoulders. It often strikes suddenly, sometimes after a flu-like illness. Around a quarter of people with polymyalgia rheumatica (PMR) also develop temporal arteritis, an inflammation of the arteries that supply blood to the head.

Doctors don't know exactly what causes the PMR, although genetic factors and infections may play a role. It is probably connected to the ageing process in some way since it very rarely appears in people under the age of 50. The average age of onset is 70 and many people who develop PMR are in their 80s or even older. Fortunately, symptoms respond well to corticosteroids and often disappear spontaneously within 18 months.

'Good attitude is just as important as good health: in one recent study, 50 per cent of over-70s described themselves as 'extremely' or 'very satisfied' with their health – compared to only 42 per cent of people aged in their 20s and 30s'

Soft tissue rheumatism

This is a general term used to describe inflammation of the ligaments and tendons of your joints rather than the bone or cartilage. Rotator cuff syndrome, for example, is characterized by inflammation of the tendons around your shoulder joint. A frozen shoulder occurs when the joint capsule in your shoulder becomes inflamed and stiff, possibly due to the formation of scar tissue in your joint, and tennis elbow (lateral epicondylitis) is caused by damage to the tendons around your elbow.

All of these soft tissue conditions are particularly common in people over the age of 40, probably as a consequence of the decline in collagen production and changes in tissue strength and structure as you age.

Osteoporosis and fractures

Low bone density is almost as common an age-related problem as rheumatism and often has even more serious consequences. Around 1 in 3 women and 1 in 12 men over the age of 50 suffer from osteoporosis, placing them at much higher risk of bone fractures: osteoporosis is implicated in around 70 per cent of fractures in people over the age of 45. Fractures are a major reason for loss of independence, hospitalization and even death in older people.

Osteoporosis is closely connected to ageing: you reach your peak bone mass in your early 30s, after which point bone is gradually lost. However, your rate of bone loss and your risk of developing osteoporosis are also determined by factors including the amount of weight-bearing exercise you get and the amount of bone-building nutrients such as calcium and vitamin D in your diet. For more information about preventing and treating osteoporosis >>264–275.

Paget's disease

This disease accelerates the rate at which bone is formed and broken down, increasing it by up to 40 times. Doctors don't know exactly why the condition develops, although it seems to be at least partly genetic and may be connected to a childhood virus. Despite this, it usually affects people over 40 and becomes more common with age. Around 5 per cent of people over 50 have Paget's disease.

In some cases the growing bone can squeeze nearby nerves or cause joint problems, leading to pain and deformities. Although the bone usually expands it also grows softer and more porous than normal bone, making it more likely to bend or fracture. In most cases, however, the disease causes few obvious symptoms.

Avoiding falls and other problems

The key to taking care of your bones, muscles and joints into old age is to stay active and eat well. Although your genes play a role in your susceptibility to certain conditions, a healthy lifestyle will both reduce your likelihood of problems and ensure you avoid the worst effects of any problems that do occur.

Keep active

Physical exercise is crucial to your independence in later life: an active lifestyle will help you to perform everyday exercises safely and effectively, whatever your age.

You don't have to set aside time for a specific exercise programme – you can gain a great deal simply by having active hobbies such as gardening, golf, rambling or dancing. Even a regular brisk walk to the shops will help to keep you mobile. The recommended level of exercise is 45 minutes of moderately stressful exercise three times a week. But if you can do more, you're likely to experience greater physical and psychological benefits and stay independent for longer. Where possible, try to incorporate the following elements into your activities:

- **Cardiovascular exercise** helps you to maintain a good body weight, a healthy appetite and a strong heart. Any exercise that gets your heart beating faster, such as a brisk walk or dancing, will burn calories and keep your heart and lungs in condition.
- **Weight bearing exercise** keeps bones and muscles strong. The most effective way to build bone and muscle mass is to use weights such as dumb-bells (or your own bodyweight) to target specific areas of your body. However, almost any physical activity, from walking to tai chi, will provide some benefits. For examples of some gentle weight-bearing exercises >>168–171.

> **'The number of damaging falls suffered by one group of 70–92 year olds halved after six months of weekly tai chi classes, according to a study in 2005'**

- **Balance and flexibility training** keeps you mobile and helps you to avoid falls. Yoga, Pilates and tai chi are all excellent ways to improve your balance and flexibility, but most physical activities will improve your general mobility to some degree. For good exercises to keep you supple and steady on your feet >>160–167.

FALL ALARMS

If you feel unsteady on your feet or live on your own, you might want to think about getting an emergency fall alarm. If you suffer a fall and can't reach a telephone, this will allow you to contact a 24-hour response centre simply by pressing a button on a pendant or a wristband that you wear all the time. Staff at the centre will then call out a relative, a neighbour or the emergency services to help you. Most local authorities run community alarm schemes and the charity Help the Aged (www.helptheaged.org.uk) also runs a telephone response service.

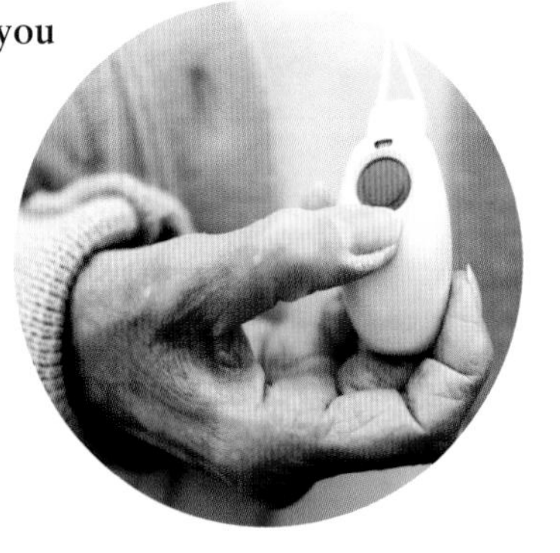

Eat well

Most people find their energy requirements decrease with age, which can make it more difficult to maintain a good intake of bone and muscle-building nutrients. In addition, the amount of acid in your stomach decreases as you get older making it harder to absorb some nutrients, including zinc, calcium and iron. Some prescription medicines can interfere with your uptake of certain vitamins and minerals.

It is therefore more important than ever to eat plenty of fruit and vegetables and get enough protein-rich foods in your diet. If you find meat too tough, cook it longer in stews or casseroles or eat protein-rich alternatives such as beans, nuts, pulses or fish. Oily fish also contains omega-3 fatty acids which are very good for your joints. If you are taking diuretics, make sure you get enough potassium and magnesium-containing foods in your diet:

bananas, meat, potatoes, oranges and dried fruit are all good sources. For more information on healthy eating >>98–117.

Supplements

Because it may be difficult to get enough vitamins and minerals in your regular diet, you may also benefit from taking a broad-spectrum multivitamin. This should provide most of your vitamin and mineral needs, although older people may also benefit from taking extra vitamin D and calcium for strong bones.

Most of your vitamin D intake should come from the action of sunlight on your skin (although 10 per cent comes from your diet). Elderly people with mobility problems may find it difficult to enjoy enough direct sunlight, making supplements particularly important. Vitamin D promotes muscle as well as bone strength so may also help you to avoid falls.

A typical supplement for older adults or people with osteoporosis is 500–1000mg calcium and 10–20mcg vitamin D. Bear in mind that any multivitamins you are already taking may contribute towards this intake. For more information on supplements >>104–106.

Spot potential problems

A number of health checks are available on the NHS, so it makes sense to make the most of what is on offer. Early diagnosis of weak or brittle bones is essential so that you can prevent fractures and take steps to improve your bone health. If you haven't already had one, talk to your doctor about getting a bone densitometry scan – this X-ray scan takes around 20 minutes and gives a good indication of your risk of fractures. For more details >>267.

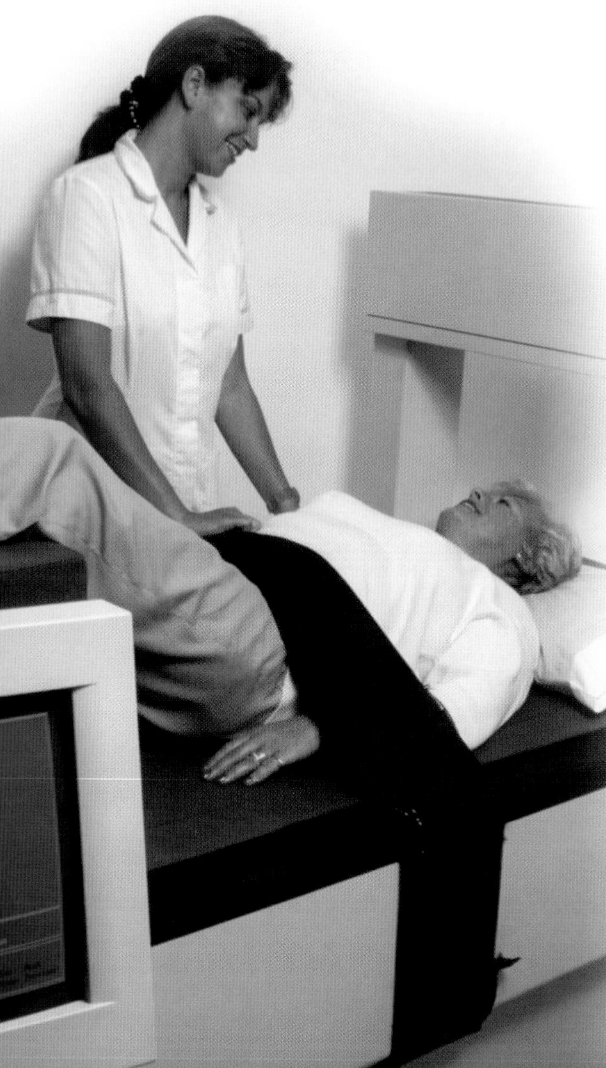

BONE DENSITOMETRY SCAN

The machine shown here uses X-rays to measure the calcium content of bones, usually in the lower back and hips, and check for brittle bones. Portable scanners, which measure mineral density in the heel are also now available.

4 WAYS TO...

Avoid falls

1 Replace those slippers. Worn-out or ill-fitting slippers are a significant cause of accidents – 9 per cent of casualty patients who've had falls blame their slippers. In a recent slipper exchange scheme in Tyne and Wear, elderly people were given "safety slippers" with special fastenings and non-slip soles. Falls were cut by 60 per cent and the scheme is to be extended across the UK.

2 Check your eyesight. Vision plays an important role in your sense of balance, so it is a good idea to have your eyesight checked regularly, even if you don't feel you need glasses. Eye tests are free if you are over the age of 60.

3 Fall-proof your home. Around 60 per cent of falls occur in the home. Make sure you have good lighting, especially on stairs, and arrange your furniture so that you don't bump into things. Keep floors free of trailing flexes, loose carpets and clutter, and close cabinet drawers and doors so that you don't stumble into them. Fix handrails, grab bars and other safety devices where necessary.

4 Check your medicines. Some prescription and over-the-counter medicines can make you feel faint or unsteady: let your doctor know if any of your medicines have this effect. Illnesses such as flu can also make you unsteady on your feet, so ask for the flu jab each winter.

EXERCISING WITH BONE AND MUSCLE PROBLEMS

Bone, muscle and joint problems are no reason to curtail your exercise routine. Many people assume that rest rather than activity is the best way to deal with injuries but while this may be true initially, it is also important to maintain a good level of fitness, whatever your condition.

Muscle power diminishes rapidly when muscles are not used; the proteins in surrounding muscles start to break down within 24 hours if a joint is completely immobilized. If you allow the muscles and ligaments that support and control your joints to deteriorate, you make yourself vulnerable to further injury – setting up a vicious circle of injury–rest–re-injury.

It is also vital to stay fit if you suffer from a long-term condition such as arthritis or osteoporosis. It can be tempting to avoid physical activity, particularly if your joints are sore or you are worried about falls, but this will only increase your problems in the long-term. Exercise can relieve pain, strengthen bones and muscles, improve flexibility and help you to avoid falls and fractures.

RECONDITIONING AFTER INJURY

Even after a soft tissue injury such as muscle strain or a ligament sprain appears to have healed, you may still find it difficult to exercise the area without aggravating the injury. This may be because the tissues involved and the muscles, tendons and ligaments around the area are still weak. You need to build up strength slowly – a process known as reconditioning.

- **Start with exercises that involve static, pain-free stretching to increase flexibility around the injured area.**
- **Next, move on to resistance exercises to increase muscle strength around the site of the injury. Aim to increase the intensity of the exercises gradually: if you feel more than a slight sensation of pain during exercise, move back to a lower intensity. If you feel significant residual pain an hour or so after exercise, you may have gone too far and should rest for a few days before starting the process again.**
- **When your muscles are stronger and you no longer feel any sensation of pain during exercise, you can move on to exercises that involve a wider range of movements. Build up slowly until you are back to your full range of movement.**

TAKE IT SLOWLY

Warm up before activity to prepare your body (>>64–67) and always exercise at a comfortable, steady pace. During balance and flexibility training it is always better to perform each exercise slowly and completely rather than attempting to do lots of repetitions at a fast pace. During strength training, make sure that you give your muscles adequate time to relax between each set.

PROBLEM	WHAT TYPE OF EXERCISE SHOULD I TRY?	WHAT TYPE OF EXERCISE SHOULD I AVOID?
Mild osteoporosis **>>264**	Weight-bearing exercise such as walking, stair climbing or resistance exercises can help to maintain bone mass. Balance exercises can reduce your risk of falls and fractures.	Avoid contact sports or sports with a high risk of falling such as skiing. Water-based activities, such as swimming or aquaerobics, do not significantly increase bone density.
Severe osteoporosis **>>264**	Almost any level of stress on your bones risks fractures. Water aerobics and swimming are useful because the water supports your body weight while you exercise. Posture, balance and coordination exercises will help you to avoid falls.	Avoid contact, high-impact or jarring sports or any activity where there is a significant risk of falling over. Avoid any excessive twisting, flexing or bending movements.
Osteoarthritis **>>228**	Weight-bearing exercise will keep your joints strong and stable. Aerobic exercise will help you to maintain a healthy weight, taking pressure off joints. Swimming or aquareobics will support your weight and reduce impact during exercise.	Avoid high-impact exercises that place stress on your joints.
Rheumatoid arthritis **>>248**	Aerobic exercise will help you to maintain a healthy weight, taking pressure off joints. In the short term it may reduce pain by releasing of endorphins. Swimming or aquaerobics will support your weight and reduce impact during exercise.	During flare-ups you may need to rest your joints completely. Avoid high-impact exercises that may aggravate your joints further.
Muscle and ligament injuries **>>299, 328**	You will need to rest the injured tissues for at least 2–3 days to let inflammation subside; If the injury requires longer to heal, do aerobic exercises that don't use the site of injury. Work back to former fitness levels slowly and pay attention to muscle strength and balance around the injured area.	Avoid contact or high impact sports. Avoid activities that require twisting or pivoting motions of the joints involved (throwing a Frisbee, playing squash). Avoid any activity that causes pain in the injured area.

LISTEN TO YOUR BODY

If something causes pain, stop: pain is your body's early warning system. You don't need to stop what you are doing altogether – just decrease the intensity or change the focus of the exercise to see if the pain improves. Where possible, avoid taking painkillers before exercise: these mask the sensation of pain and make it much harder to recognize when you are doing something wrong.

KNOW YOUR AIMS

It is always good to include elements of strengthening, aerobic and flexibility training, but particular conditions may benefit from a specific emphasis. If you have osteoporosis, for example, you may want to concentrate on bone-strengthening and balance activities. If you have damaged the ligaments in your knee, you may need to strengthen the muscles around the joint. See table for more guidance.

KNOW WHAT TO AVOID

Different medical conditions require different precautions. If you have osteoporosis, for example, the main risk is fracturing a bone: avoid leaning or bending your upper body too far forward since this can cause spinal fractures. Stooping or rotating the shoulders is also a risk. With sports injuries the main risk is aggravating the injury further, so avoid movements such as twisting or pivoting that put damaged tissues under stress.

Improving your balance

It is easy to take your sense of balance for granted – at least until you start to lose it – but good balance is one of the most essential components of physical fitness. Without good balance even the most simple physical tasks, from walking up a flight of stairs to picking up an object from the ground, become difficult or hazardous. Balance is vital in old age to prevent falls.

Understanding balance

Your sense of balance relies on the sensory input from your eyes, your inner ear (your vestibular system) and the special receptor cells in your muscles, joints and tendons (your proprioceptive system). You respond to these sensory cues by tensing your stabilizing muscles, in particular the 'core muscles' in your abdomen, buttocks and lower back, to correct your position and keep you stable.

TAKE CARE

If you experience any of the following symptoms, you may have a balance disorder of some sort. Talk to your doctor to determine the cause of the problem before attempting any balance exercises.

- **A sensation of dizziness or vertigo**
- **Frequent falls**
- **A sensation of falling**
- **Light-headedness**
- **Visual blurring**

As you grow older these stabilizing muscles grow weaker and your reflexes become slower. Your proprioceptive and vestibular senses become less sensitive and your eyesight may be less sharp. Poor balance can also be a side effect of certain medications or medical disorders.

As a result of these changes, falls are responsible for more serious injuries among people over the age of 65 than any other type of accident. Almost 90 per cent of serious bone fractures in older people are the result of falls and around half of those who break their hips never walk again. But because balance and coordination are at least partly dependent on good physical condition and on skills that can be learned and practised, a great many of these falls could have been avoided. One study in New Zealand showed a 40 per cent reduction in falls in women over 80 years of age who participated in simple strength and balance training.

Improving your balance

Almost any type of physical activity improves your ability to balance simply because most exercise requires good balance. Indeed, one of the main reasons that falls tend to increase with age is that people become more scared of falling as they get older and take less exercise.

Any type of activity that improves balance tends to improve one or more of the three basic elements of good balance: your sense of equilibrium, the strength of your stabilizing muscles and your general coordination. Particularly good activities for older exercisers include dancing, which requires good body-awareness and coordination, and low-impact activities such as yoga, Pilates and tai chi. In particular, a number of studies have suggested that tai chi, with its emphasis on controlled, choreographed movements, is very effective at cutting falls.

DID YOU KNOW?

- **Could vibrating shoes provide the solution to balance problems? Scientists have developed special gel-filled insoles that vibrate just below the level which a human can feel but at the right level to stimulate the nerve cells in the soles of your feet. You rely on these nerve endings to sense pressure changes as you walk or stand but as you grow older these nerve endings can lose sensitivity.**
- **According to research published in *The Lancet* in 2003, the volunteers who tested the vibrating insoles showed marked improvements in their sense of balance and less side-to-side swaying.**

Balance and osteoporosis

Falls and tumbles can be particularly dangerous if you suffer from brittle bones. This means that it is even more important to develop and maintain good balance – but also that you need to be careful how you approach exercise. Take each exercise slowly and make sure you have a stable object to hold on to in case you lose your balance. If you have severe osteoporosis, however, you should talk to a doctor or physiotherapist before trying any of these exercises. You may be better performing balance exercises in a pool where there is less risk of hurting yourself if you fall.

Balance routine

The exercises shown here should only take 10 minutes to perform. If you train regularly – around three times a week – your balance will greatly improve within two or three months.

Follow the instructions for each exercise precisely. Some of the exercises have variations. These should only be attempted once you are comfortable with the standard exercise and are best avoided if you have a history of falls or balance problems (see box, left).

Side to side

1 Stand with your feet shoulder-width apart and your knees slightly bent and place your hands on the front of your thighs.

2 Slowly lean your body over to your right, bending your right knee a little more as you do so. Next, lean your body over to your left, bending your left knee a little as you do so. Move from side to side 10 times in a smooth, fluid manner.

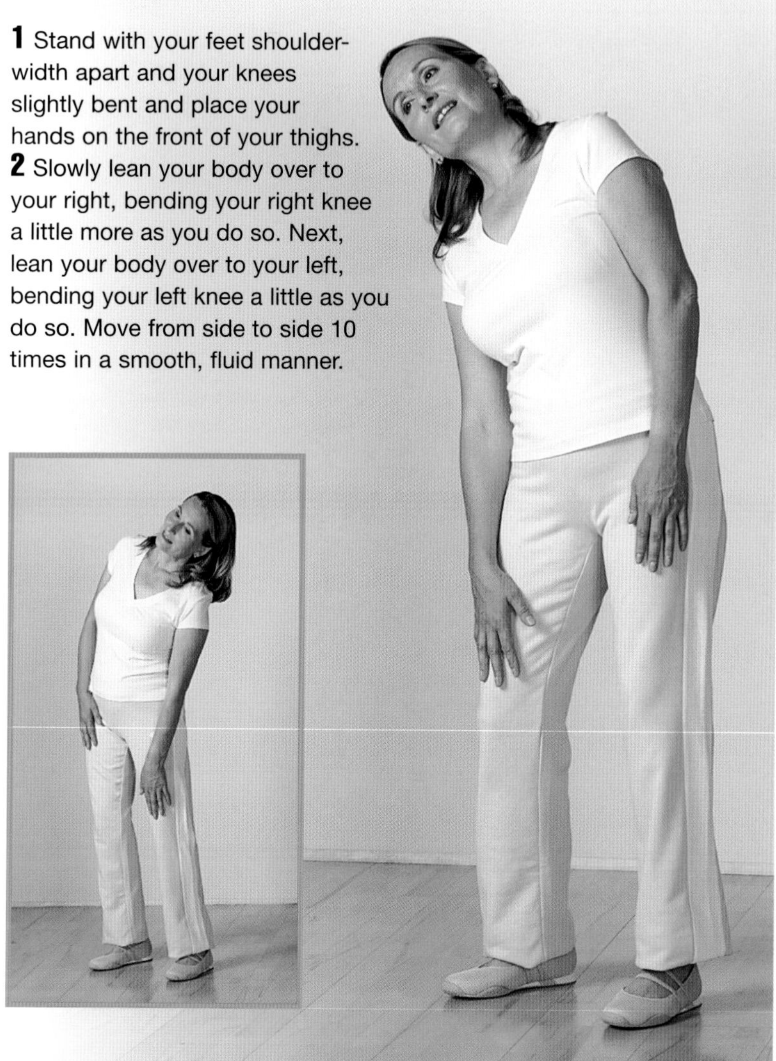

Leg circles

1 Stand next to a stable chair. Rest one hand lightly on the chair back but don't use it for support unless you feel you are about to lose your balance. Keeping your leg straight, raise your right foot a few centimetres off the ground.

2 Slowly circle your leg 10 times in a clockwise direction. Rest your foot back on the ground for a moment then lift it again and repeat the circling motion 10 times in an anticlockwise direction. Switch legs and repeat the exercise using your left leg.

- Once you can perform 25 circles in each direction, try bending your supporting leg a little. This makes it more difficult to balance and works the muscles around your hips, knees and ankles.

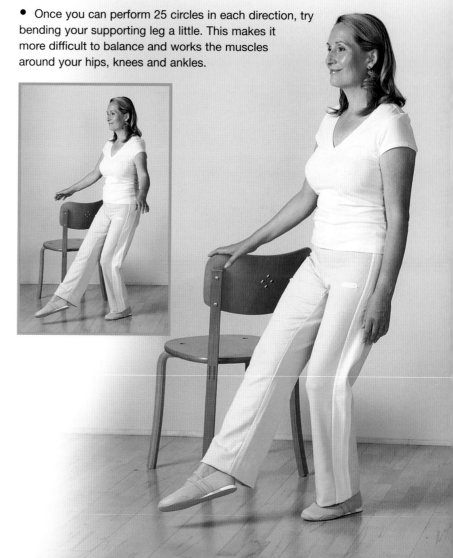

Stand on one leg

1 Stand next to a wall or the back of a stable chair. Rest your hands lightly against the wall or the chair back but don't use it for support unless you feel you are about to lose your balance.
2 Lift your right foot off the floor so that you are standing on one leg. If you can, lift your knee as high as your hip. Try to stand like this for 8 seconds. If you begin to lose your balance, simply use the wall or the chair to steady yourself. Repeat the exercise using your left leg.

- Once you can stand on one leg for 8 seconds without needing to steady yourself, try to increase the time to 10 or 12 seconds or even longer. This is a great way to monitor your progress.

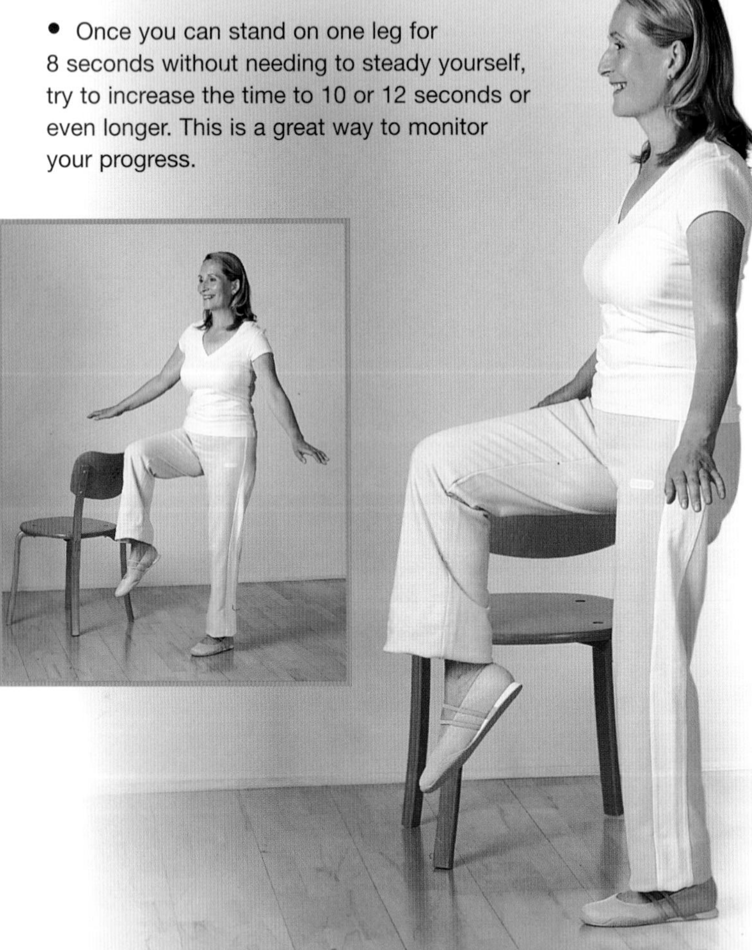

Tandem walk

1 Stand sideways on to a wall and place one hand on the wall for support. Keep your other arm relaxed by your side. Place the foot nearest the wall directly in front of the other so that your feet form a straight line.
2 Move your weight onto your front foot. Bring your back foot forward and place it directly in front of your other foot. Take 10 steps forward in this manner, turn slowly and take 10 steps back.

- If you feel confident moving along in this manner, try moving away from the wall and stretching your arms out to the side as you move forward.

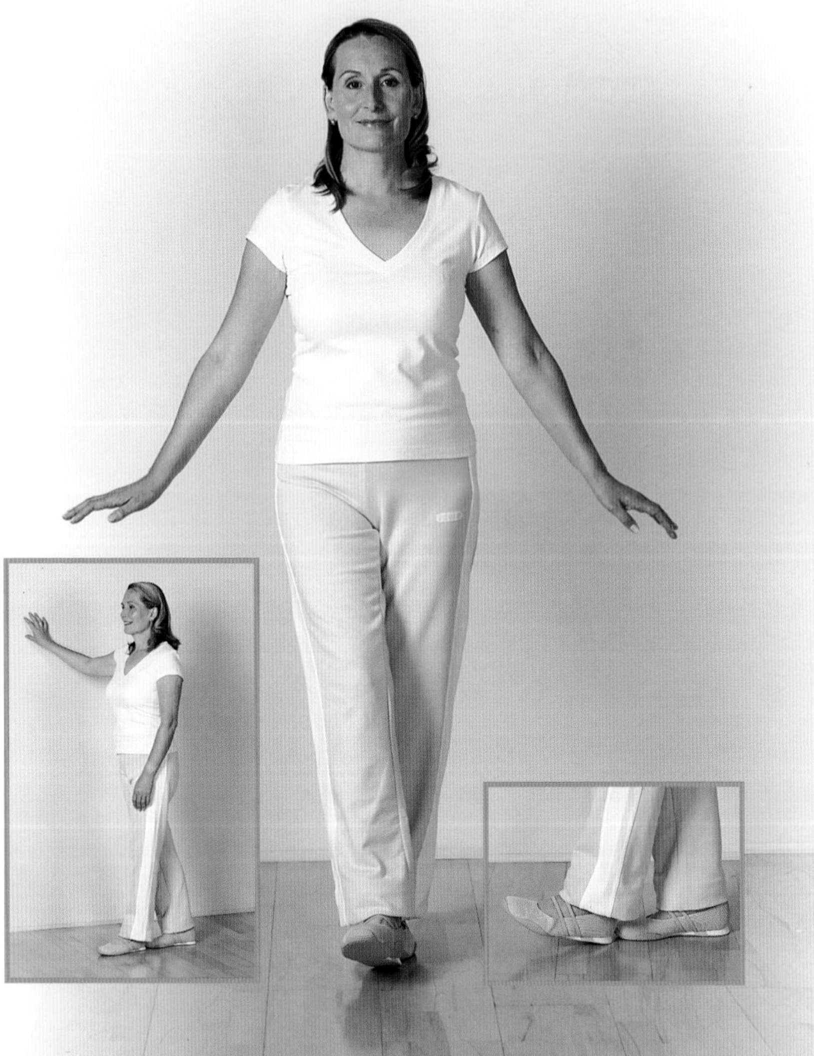

Toe walk

1 Stand sideways on to a wall and rest one hand on the wall for support. Keep your other arm relaxed by your side. Lift your heels and place your body weight on the balls of your feet.
2 Using the wall for support, walk 10 steps forward on your toes. Make sure your weight is over your big and second toes: do not let your feet roll outward on to your little toes. Move back onto your flat feet, turn slowly, and take 10 steps back on your toes.

- If you feel confident moving along in this manner, try moving away from the wall and lift your arms above your head as you move forward.

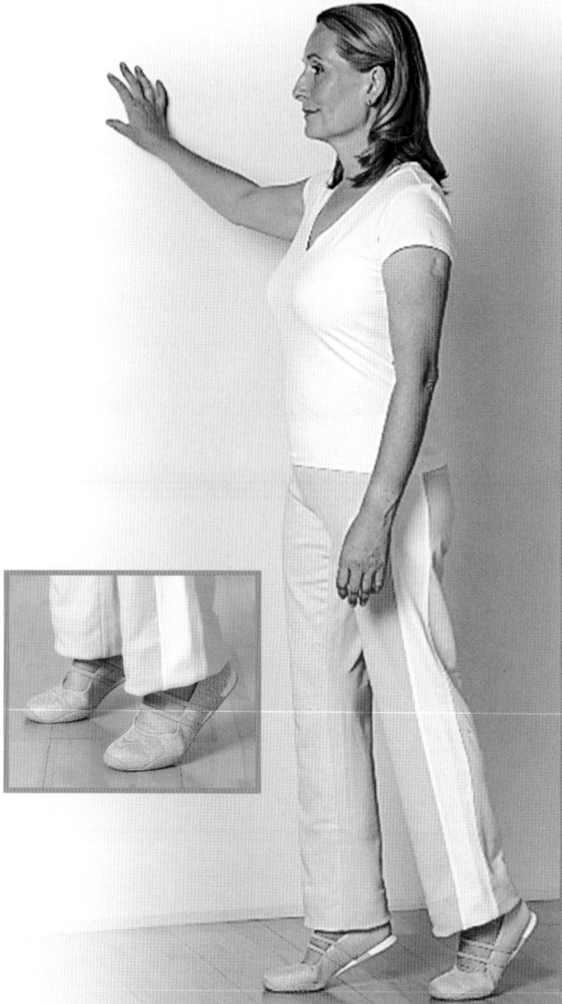

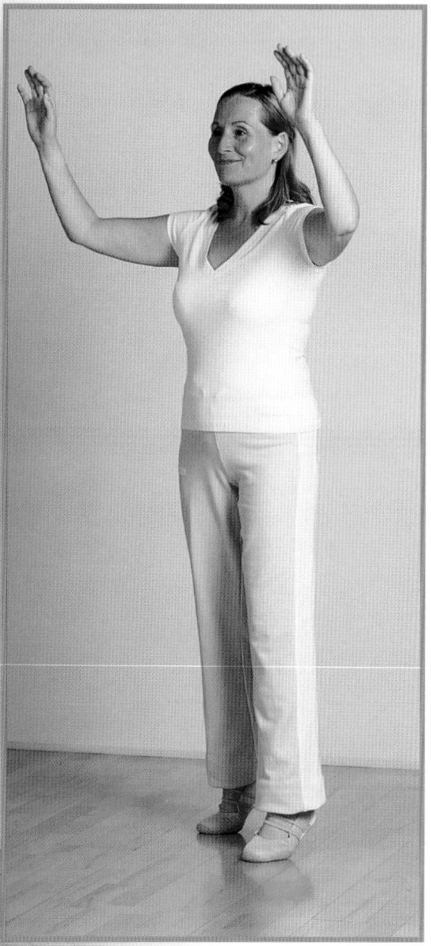

Exercise ball

The exercise ball (Swiss ball) is very useful for developing balance. Because it is an unstable base from which to work, almost any exercise involving a ball uses a wide range of supporting muscles. Simply sitting on the ball, for example, places your body in an unstable position, making your leg and abdominal muscles contract to maintain your balance. If you are concerned about falling and injuring yourself, it's also possible to buy balls and half-balls with flat bases or supports.

Try sitting on a ball with your legs bent and your feet flat on the floor. Lift your arms out to your sides to help with your balance. If you feel stable in this position, lift one leg slightly off the ground. If you still feel confident, try bouncing a little.

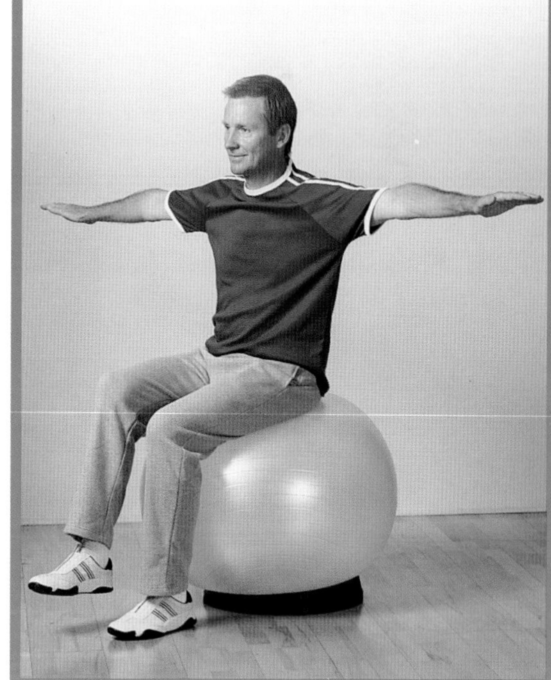

Keeping flexible

It is always important to maintain your body's flexibility, but as you get older and can no longer rely on youthful resilience to keep you supple, the benefits of flexibility training become ever more pronounced.

Most people's bodies acquire a measure of tension and stiffness over time – even sportsmen and keep-fit enthusiasts rarely make use of their full range of motion. As the years go by, habitual muscular tensions may start to pull your posture out of alignment and you may lose much of your youthful flexibility. Regular training is a useful way to counteract this process, particularly if you suffer from joint and muscle pain. By keeping limber, you'll move more freely, feel more energetic and perform life's daily chores more easily.

Stretch and relax

The key to maintaining your body's natural flexibility and being able to move freely and easily lies with stretching. Controlled, sensible stretching releases tightness in your muscles, improves the range of movement in your joints, prevents stiffness and cramps and can help you to maintain good body alignment and mobility. Even if your joints are inflamed and arthritic, a programme of gentle, regular stretching can help to ease the pain and discomfort and reduce inflammation.

Yoga and tai chi

Many people still regard stretching in purely functional terms: as a necessary but unexciting follow-up to the main workout. In the East, however, flexibility is almost a religion: mind-body therapies such as yoga and tai chi place the emphasis squarely on stretching, relaxation and good posture. Both tai chi and yoga offer an excellent way for older people to stay flexible, relaxed and tension free.

Relaxation

Your emotional state can have an effect on your flexibility. If you feel stressed, for example, the muscles at the top of your shoulders and neck contract and tighten. This can lead to headaches, sore neck and even joint compression. Flexibility training counteracts these problems by releasing the tension in your muscles, making you feel more relaxed. You may find that listening to music and focusing on your breathing can also aid relaxation as you stretch.

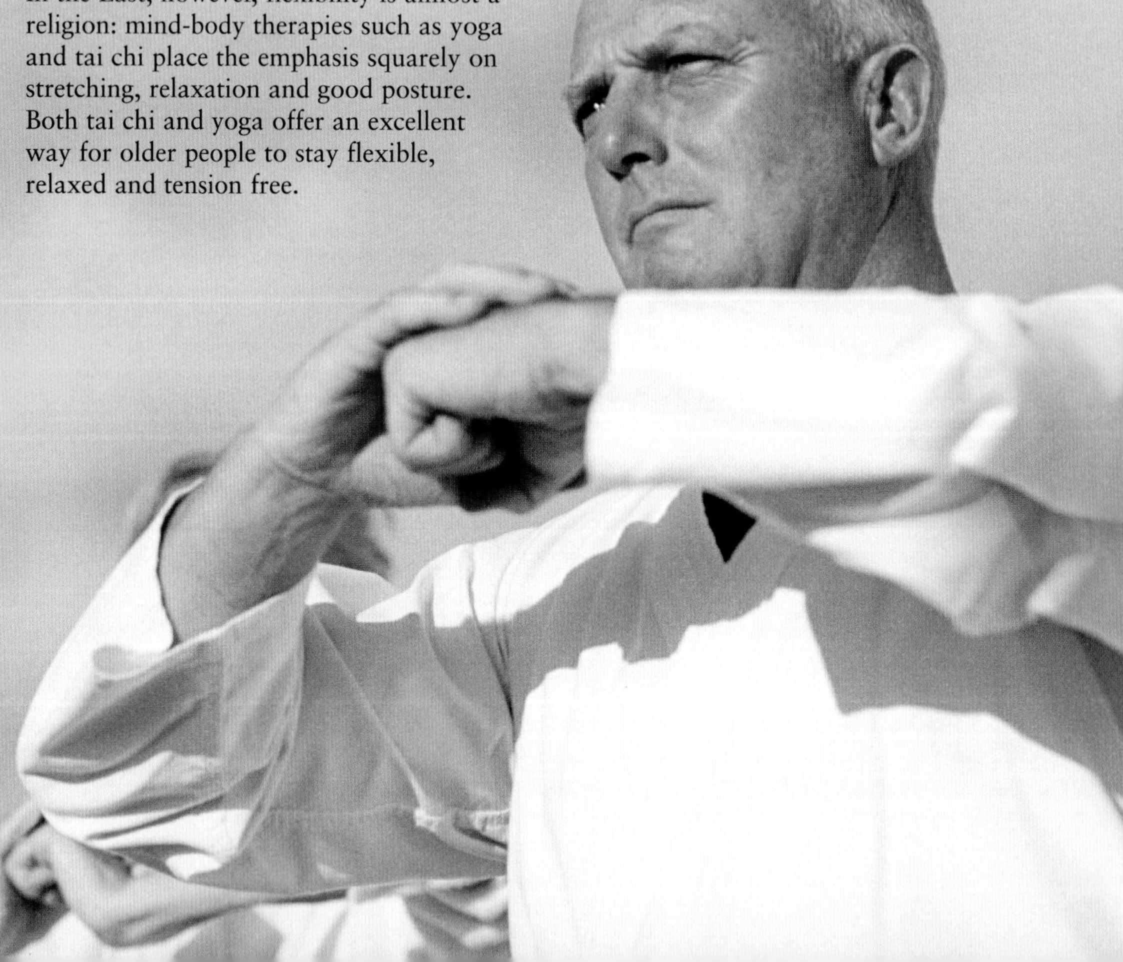

‘Tight muscles are a common cause of back pain: tight hamstrings in particular may play a role in as many as 80 per cent of cases of low back pain.’

Flexibility routine

To get the most benefit from this routine, try to perform the following exercises at least 2–3 times per week. Avoid stretching first thing in the morning when your muscles are still stiff and always warm up thoroughly before you begin >>64–67. Repeat each stretch 3 times.

Never take a stretch to the point of pain. Stretch until you feel a slight tug or a sensation of mild discomfort but don't try to push beyond that point.

The key to success is consistency: the real benefits come with continued stretching over months, not days. When you first start stretching it is quite normal to feel stiff. Your chest, shoulders and the backs of your legs are often particularly tight. The more you perform these exercises, the looser you will become.

Chest

1 Sit on a chair with your back straight. Hold your arms straight out in front of you and raise your forearms so that they are at right angles to your upper arms. Place your forearms and palms together.

2 Open your arms out wide, keeping your elbows at shoulder height and pushing your shoulder blades together. Hold for 15–30 seconds then move your arms back together.

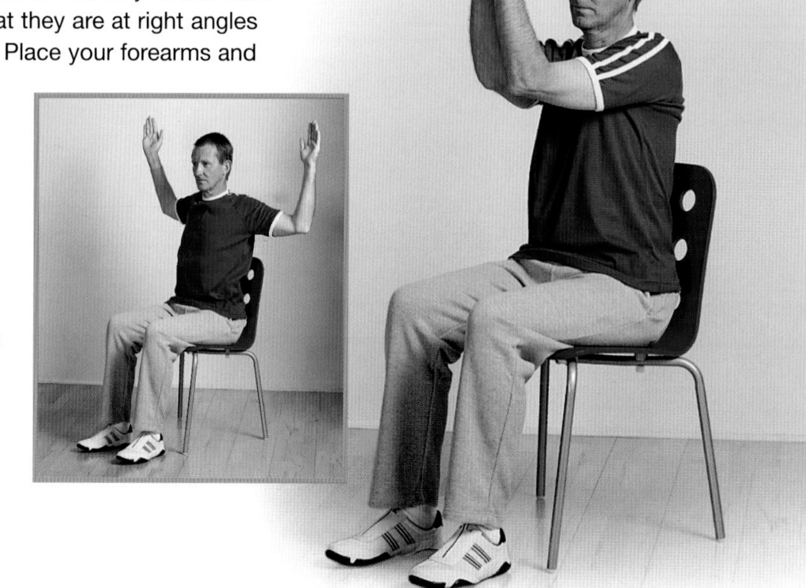

Shoulders

If you are unable to get down to the floor safely, you can perform this exercise on a bed.

1 Lie on your back and point your toes. Interlock your fingers and extend your arms straight above your head with your palms pointing towards the ceiling.

2 Keeping your arms straight, slowly move your hands back behind you until you feel a stretch in your shoulders. Hold for 15–30 seconds then return your arms to an upright position.

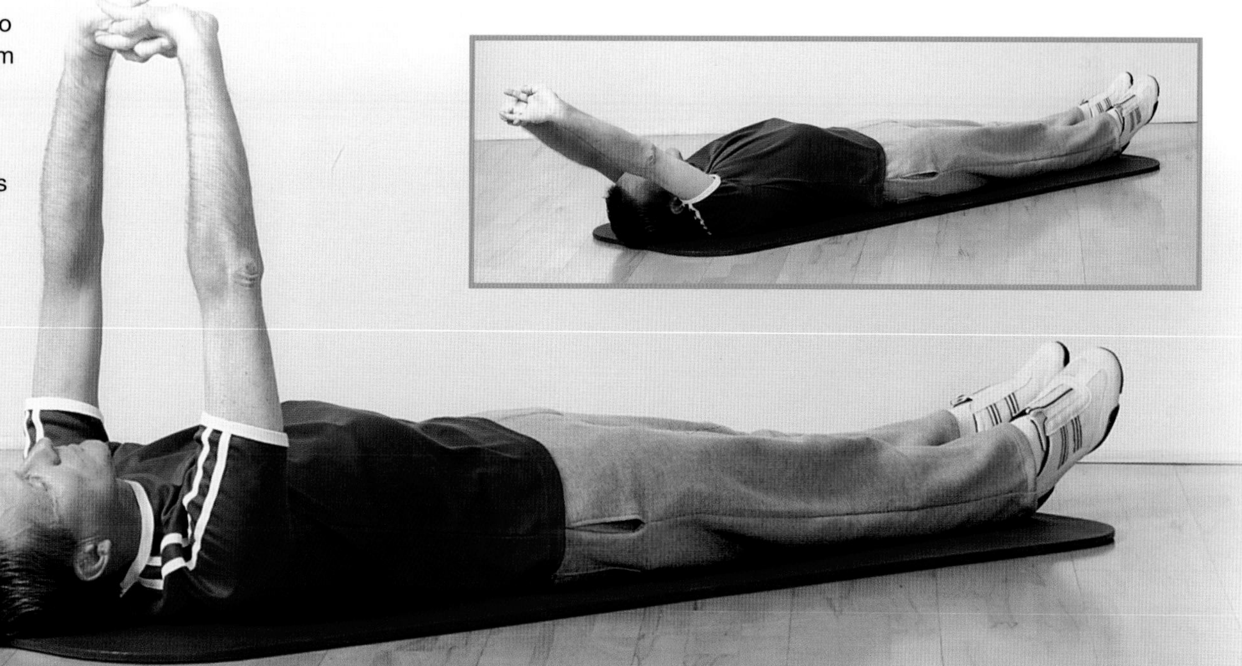

Flexibility routine (continued)

Back

1 Sit on a chair with your back straight. Interlock your fingers and extend your arms straight out in front of you with your palms away from you.
2 Round your back and push your arms away from your body until you feel a stretch along your upper back. Hold this stretch for 15–30 seconds and then relax.

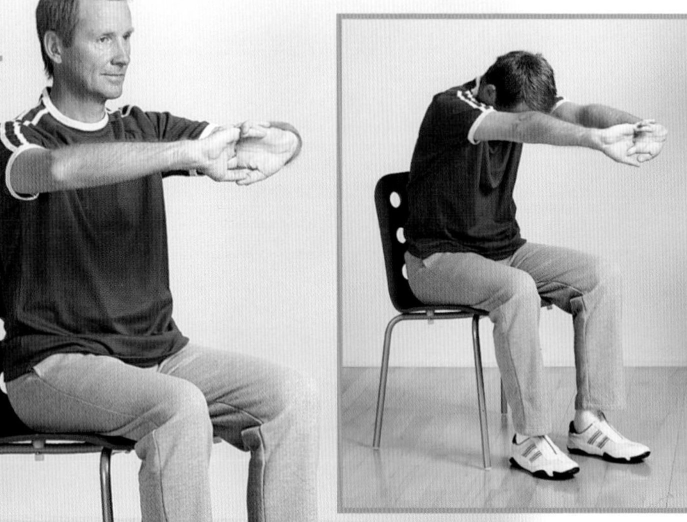

Torso

1 Stand with your feet shoulder-width apart and your arms by your sides.
2 Exhale as you gently lean over to your left side until you feel a stretch on your right side. Hold this stretch for 15–30 seconds, then repeat on the other side.

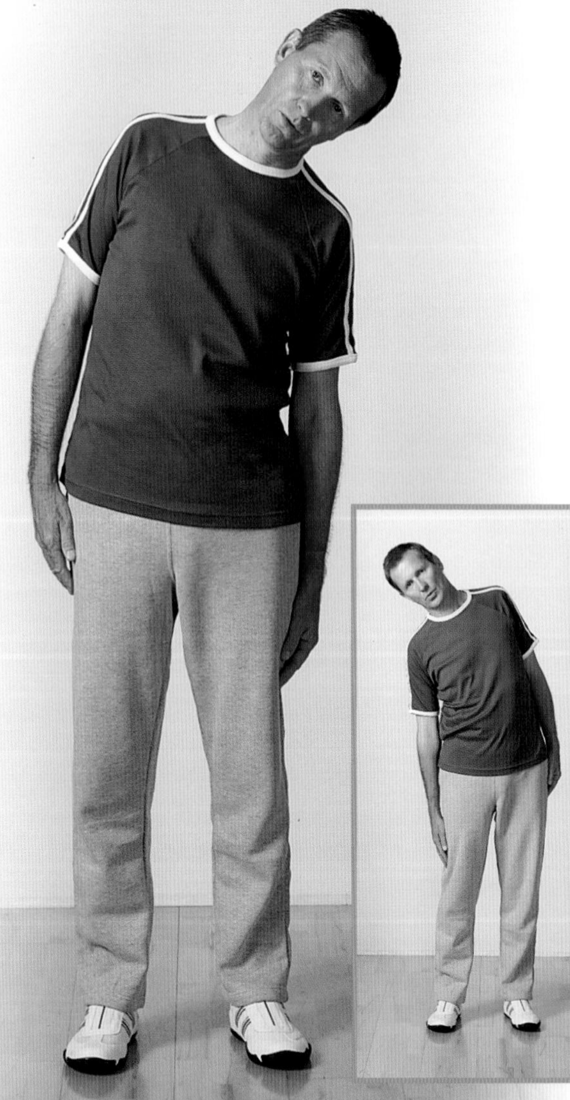

Hands

This exercise is very good for people suffering from arthritis in the hands.

Extend your arms out in front of you at chest height and spread your fingers as far as possible. Do not stretch your fingers to the point of pain. Hold this position for 5 seconds before relaxing and bringing your arms comfortably down to your sides. Rest for a moment and repeat.

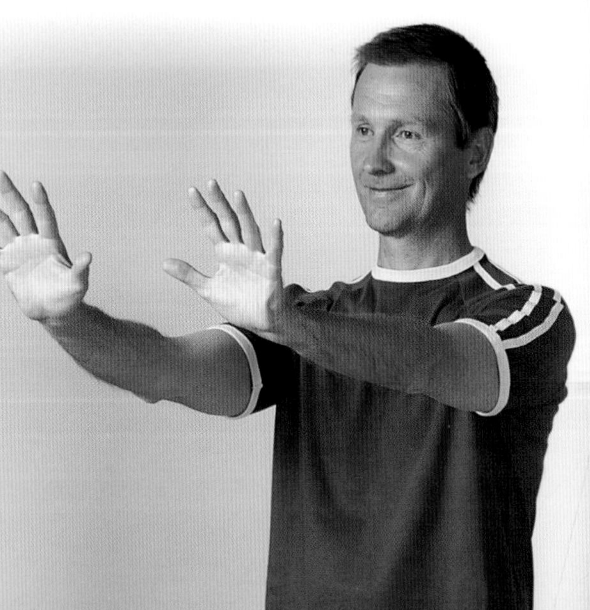

Front of leg

If you are unable to get down to the floor safely, you can perform this exercise on a bed.

1 Lie on your right side with your knees bent and your head supported by a cushion or pillow. Take hold of your left foot with your left hand. If you have trouble reaching, use a towel wrapped around your foot.
2 Gently pull your heel towards your buttocks until you feel a slight stretch along the front of your thigh. Hold the stretch for 15–30 seconds, then repeat the exercise lying on your left side.

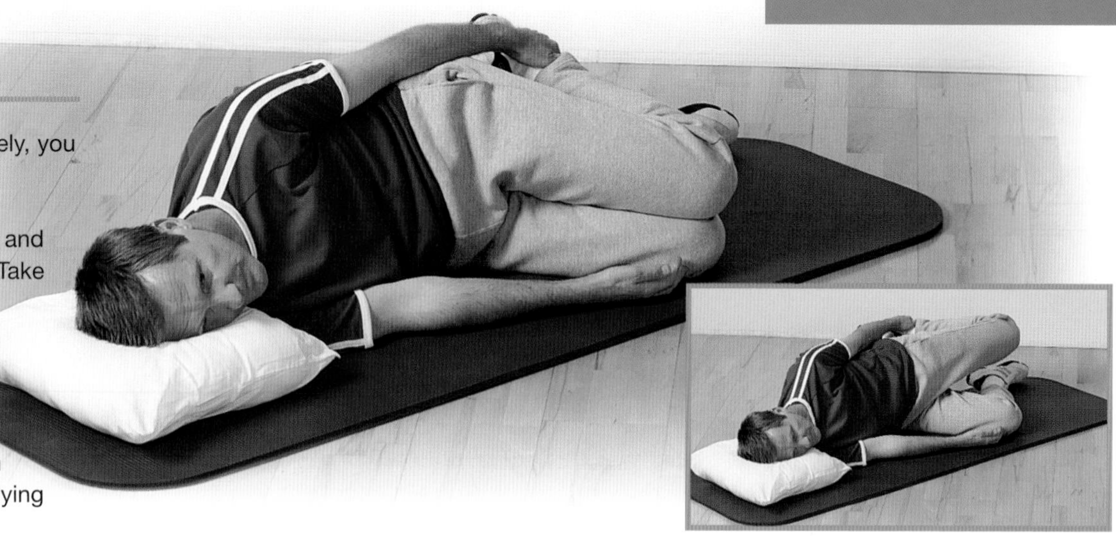

Rear of leg

If you have had a hip replacement, check with your doctor before doing this stretch.

1 Sit on a chair with another chair in front of you. Place one leg straight out in front of you on top of the chair. Keep your other foot flat on the floor.
2 Keeping your back straight, slowly lean forward until you feel a slight stretch along the back of your leg. Hold this stretch for 15–30 seconds, then repeat using your other leg.

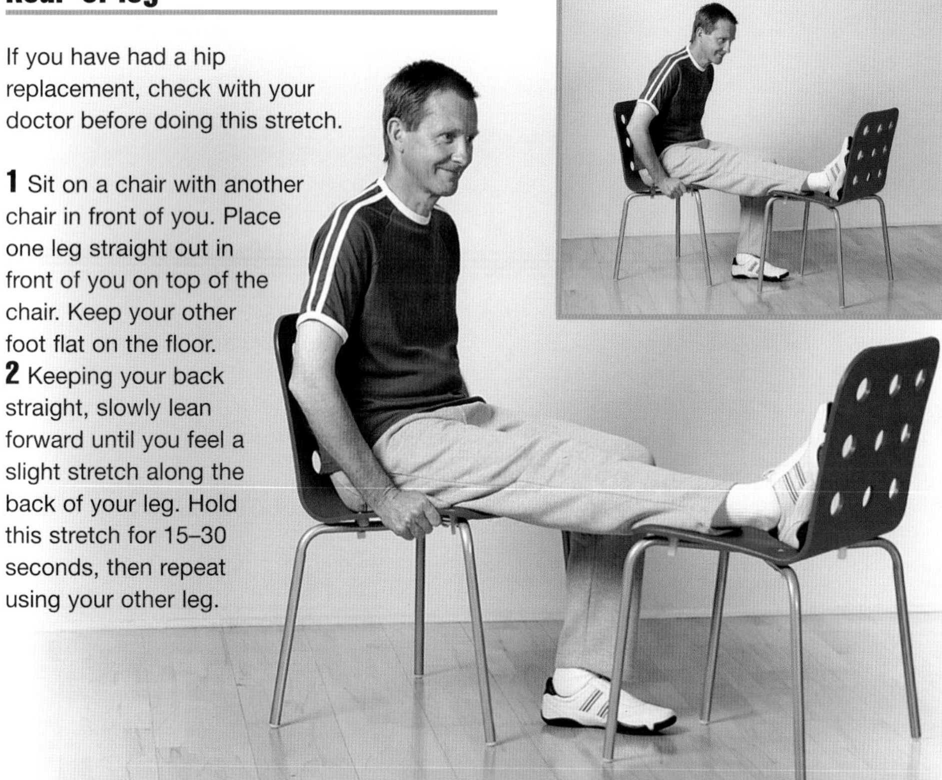

Calf

1 Stand with your feet hip-width apart. Step your left leg as far forward as you can without lifting your right heel off the ground.
2 Keeping your right foot flat on the floor, bend your left leg and lean forward until you feel a slight stretch along your right calf. Hold this stretch for 15–30 seconds, then swap legs and repeat.

Maintaining muscle strength

Muscular strength usually starts to decline after the age of 40 with an acceleration in the decline after 60. By 75, around a quarter of men and two thirds of women have difficulty lifting objects weighing more than 4.5kg (10lb). This kind of decline can significantly interfere with your independence and everyday quality of life.

Luckily, it doesn't have to be this way. Most muscle loss is a result of not using muscles enough – according to a report by the US Centers for Disease Control and Prevention, only 11 per cent of over-65s do enough load-bearing exercise to maintain muscle strength. Strength training will prevent and recover much of this loss in muscle size and strength. Strong muscles also help to protect against joint injury and can help you to avoid falls and fractures by keeping you balanced and mobile.

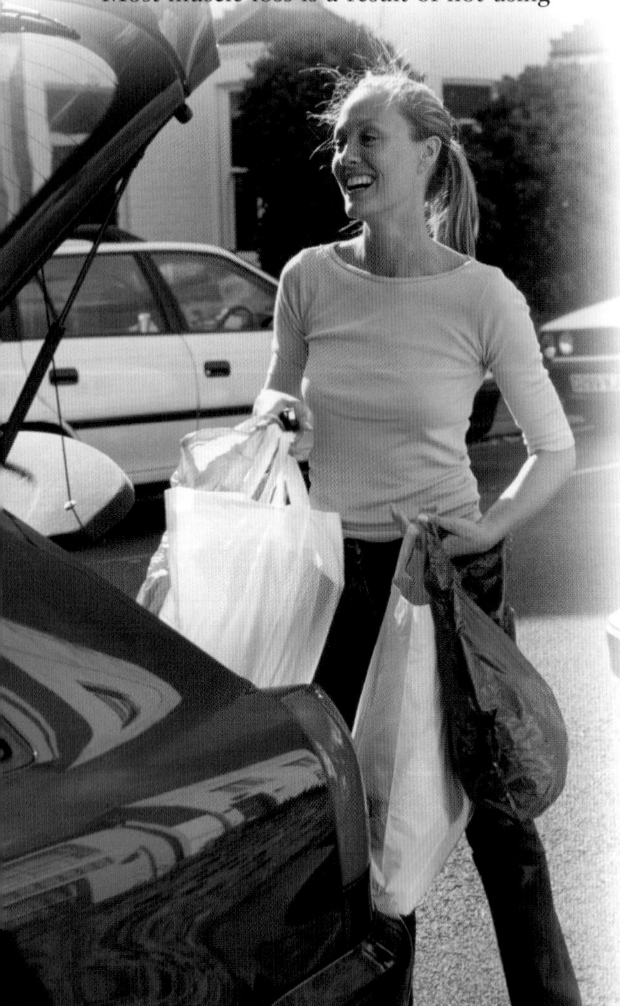

Strength-training also keeps your bones in good condition. Healthy bones are important at any age, but the older you get the more likely you are to experience significant problems. Bone mass decreases by approximately 10–20 per cent after the age of 65 and 20–30 per cent after the age of 80. This makes you much more susceptible to osteoporosis and fractures as you grow older – particularly if your supporting muscles are also weak.

Exercising safely

Before you begin each workout, it is vital to warm up properly >>64–67. This will ready your muscles and joints and reduce the chance of injury. At the end of each workout, make sure you also cool down.

When performing the exercises, try to use the full range of movement set out in the individual instructions. Over time not only will your strength improve but you may find that your range of movement improves without even trying. For some people, especially those with existing joint problems, these ranges may be limited. The key is to listen to your body. Never force any movements.

DID YOU KNOW?

- **There is no upper age limit for strength training; indeed, the weaker your muscles the greater the potential gains. In one study at Tufts University, a group of 87–101-year-old men and women increased knee extensor strength on average by almost 175 per cent. The oldest participant, a 101-year-old retired dentist, managed 200 per cent!**
- **Strength training does much more than just give you stronger muscles. Another study at Tufts University took a group of postmenopausal women: after only two days a week strength training over the course of a year they showed on average a 75 per cent increase in strength, a 13 per cent increase in dynamic balance and a 1 per cent increase in hip and spine density.**

Strength-training routine

Ideally you should try to do the strength-training exercises shown here 2–3 times a week. Perform each exercise for one set of 8–12 repetitions, rest for a minute, and perform a second set of 8–12 repetitions.

Choose a weight that will allow you to perform each exercise for 8 repetitions. If you don't have any dumb-bells, you can use any object of a suitable weight: bottles of water, shopping bags holding tins of food or even a pot of paint.

Over the weeks you will notice that you are able to lift the weight for more repetitions. When you can perform the exercise comfortably for 12 repetitions, increase the weight. This way your muscles will continually adapt and grow stronger. For exercises that don't use extra weights, you can increase the number of repetitions.

Chair-assisted squats

This exercise works the quadriceps muscles in your thighs and your buttock muscles and improves bone density in your hips and legs.

1 Stand behind a chair with your legs shoulder-width apart. Rest your hands on the back of the chair for support.
2 Inhale and slowly bend your legs to lower yourself down towards the floor. Keep your back upright and do not bend your legs past a 90-degree angle. Hold for a moment, then exhale as you push yourself back up to a standing position.

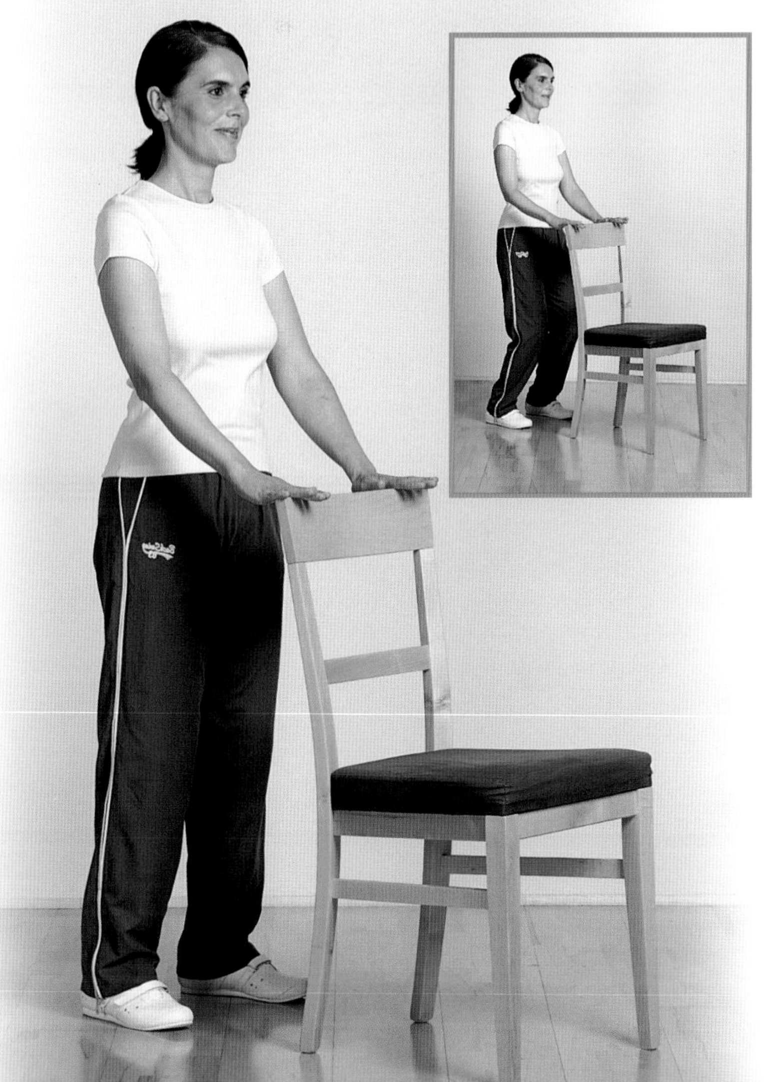

Leg curl

This exercise concentrates on your hamstrings, the muscles along the back of your thighs, and improves bone density in your hips and legs.

1 Stand facing a wall, about an arm's length away, with your feet hip-width apart and your right foot placed about a step back. Place your palms flat on the wall at shoulder height and lean in towards the wall.
2 Exhale as you bend your right leg to curl your right foot up behind your buttocks. Do not bend your leg any further than feels comfortable. Hold for a moment, then inhale as you lower your foot back down to the ground. Repeat with your other leg.

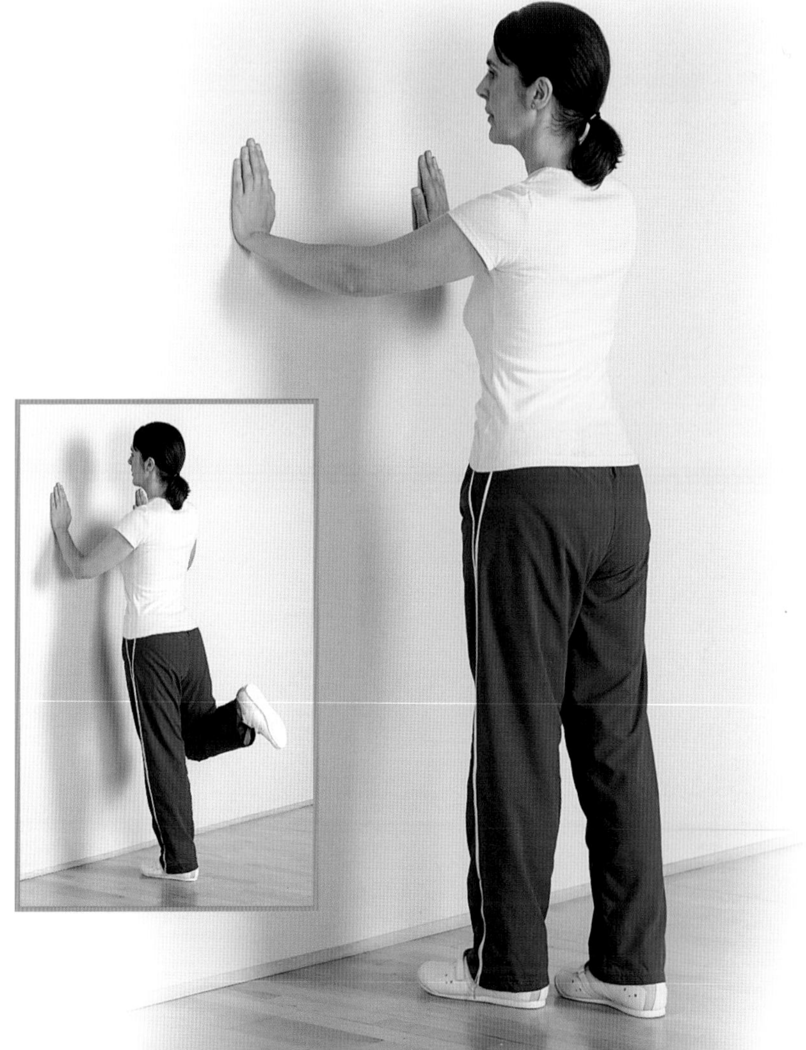

Standing chest press

This exercise works your chest and shoulder muscles and triceps and improves bone density in your arms and shoulders.

1 Stand facing a wall, about an arm's length away, with your feet shoulder-width apart. Put your palms flat on the wall at shoulder height and slightly wider than shoulder-width apart.

2 Inhale and slowly bend your arms, leaning your body in towards the wall. Keep your stomach tight and your back straight. Exhale as you push yourself back up to the starting position.

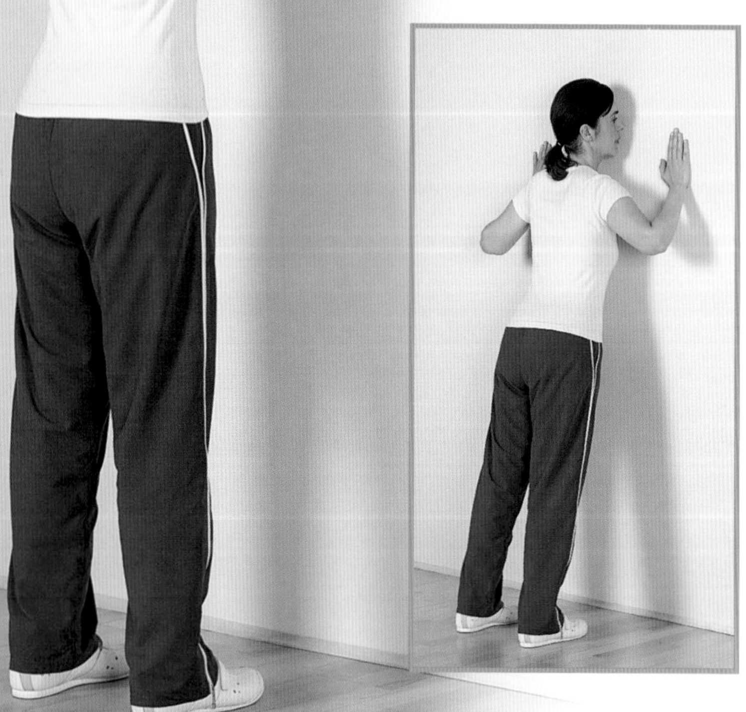

Bending lift

This exercise uses your shoulder muscles and the muscles in your back and improves bone density in your arms and shoulders.

1 Stand close to a chair with your legs shoulder-width apart, holding the weight in your left hand with your left arm extended downwards. Inhale and lean over from the waist, placing your right hand and right knee on the chair seat.

2 Exhale as you bend your arm and pull the bag upwards until your hand is level with your chest. Keep your back straight, hold for a moment, then inhale as you slowly lower your arm. Move to the other side of the chair and repeat with your other arm.

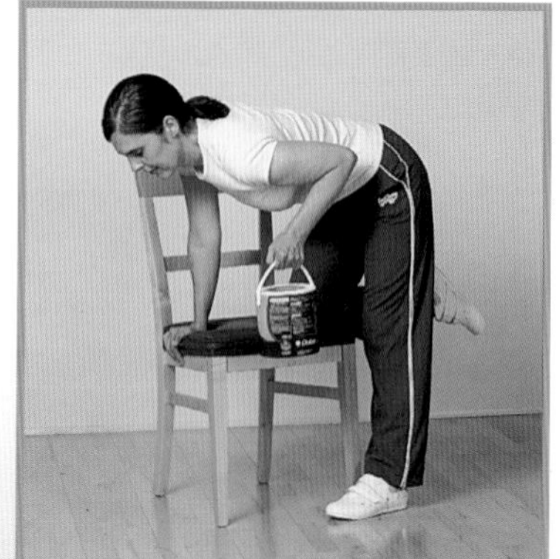

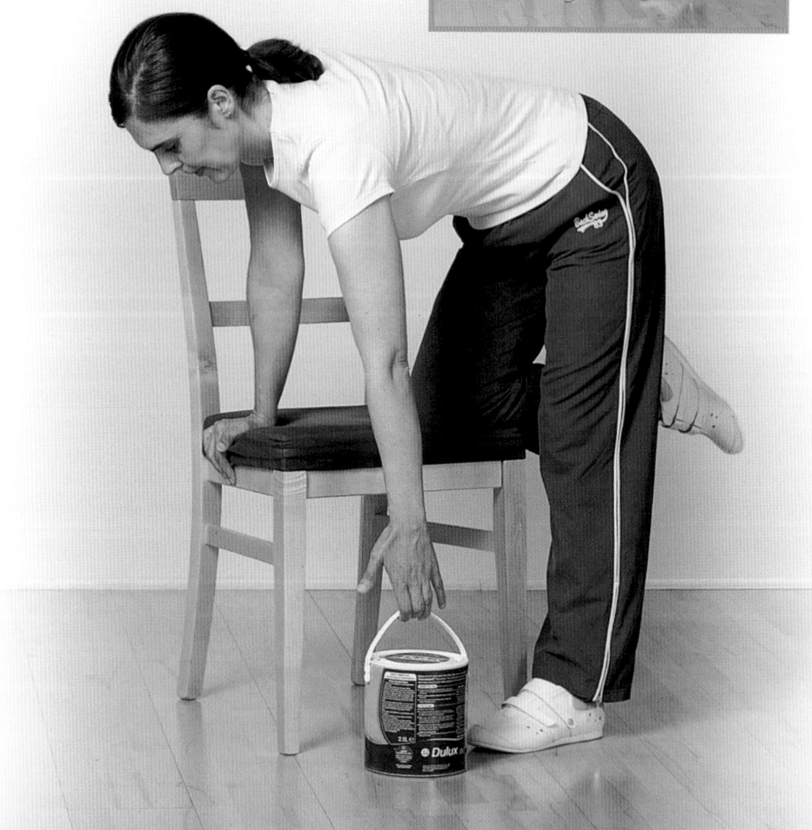

Arm raise

This exercise works the muscles in your shoulders that you use to lift your arms to the sides and increases bone density in your arms.

1 Stand with your feet shoulder-width apart and your arms down by your sides and relaxed. Hold a weight in each hand.
2 Exhale as you raise your arms up and out to your sides until they are horizontal to the floor. Hold for a moment, then inhale as you slowly lower the weights back down.

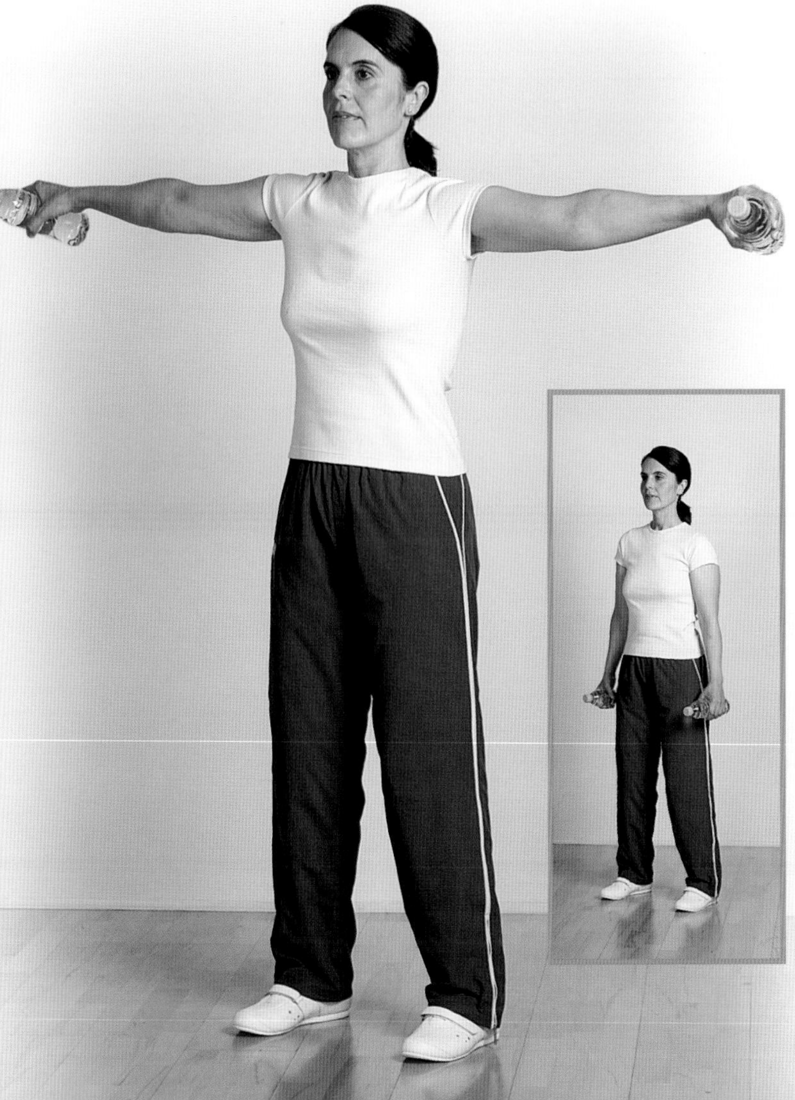

Static wrist curl

This exercise strengthens the muscles in your shoulders and forearms and increases the bone density in your wrists.

1 Grip a pole or a broom handle with one hand in an underhand grip and one hand in an overhand grip. Keep your arms about shoulder-width apart. Rest one end of the pole or broom handle on the back of a chair for support.
2 Try to rotate the pole in one direction with one hand and in the opposite direction with the other hand. Because you are turning in opposite directions, the pole should not move at all. Breathe evenly as you count to 5. Change over hand positions and repeat.

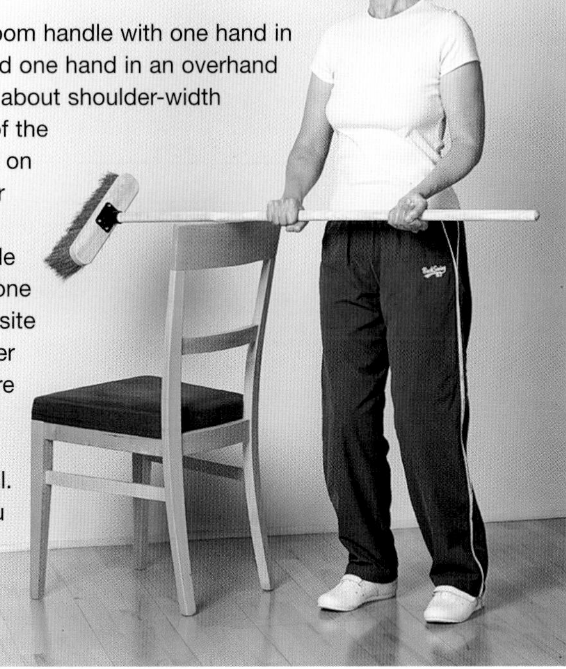

BALL GRIP

Grip strength is often ignored during strength training but a good grip is vital to help you pick things up, unscrew stiff jar lids and perform a host of other everyday tasks.

To improve your grip, grasp a soft foam ball or tennis ball in one hand. Slowly squeeze it as hard as you can and hold the squeeze for 3–5 seconds before releasing.

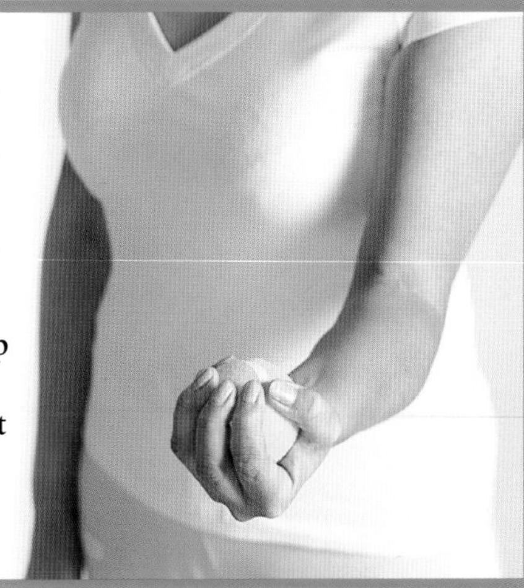

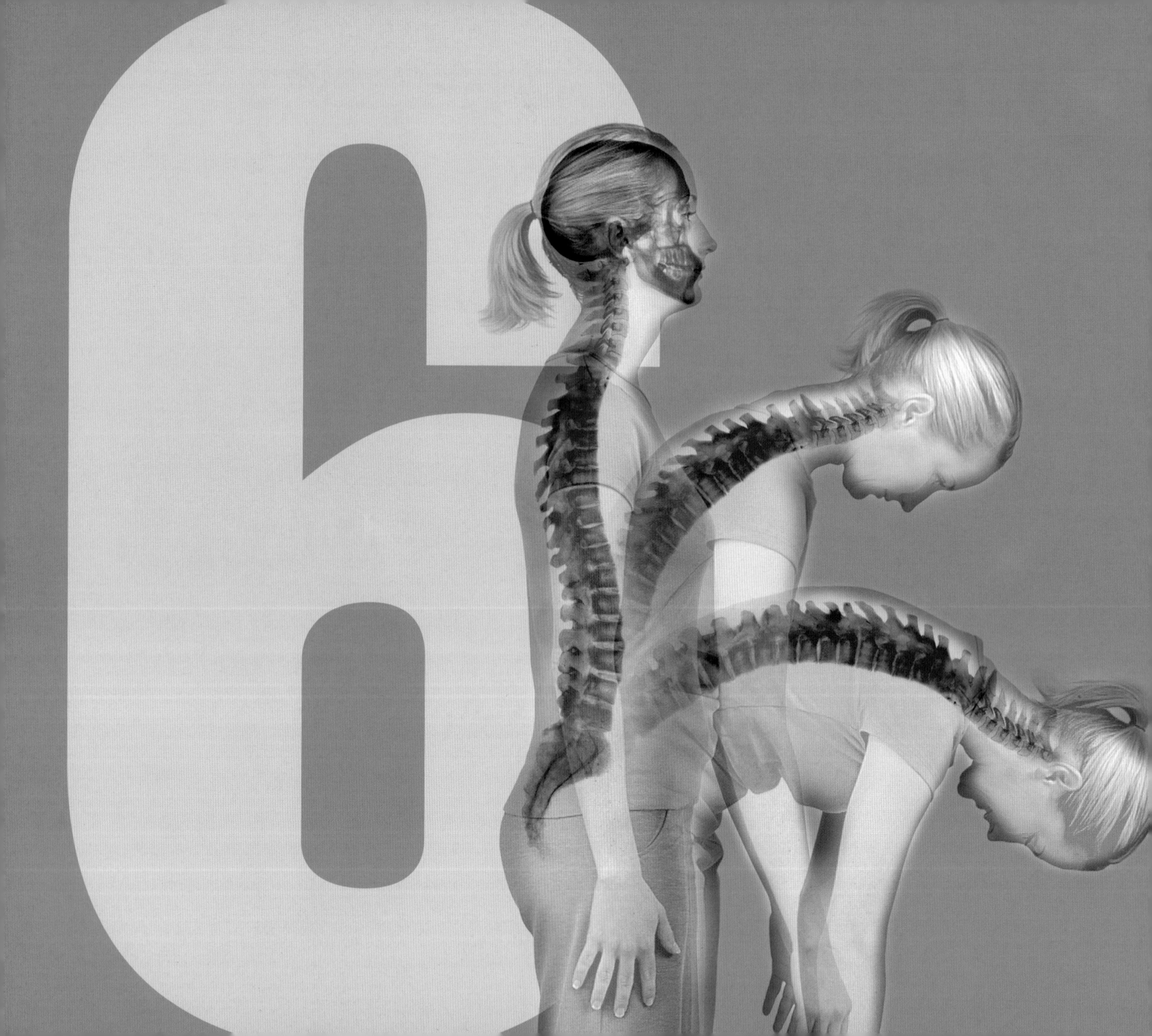

A HEALTHY BACK AND SPINE

With the spine's complex structure of bone, discs, nerves, ligaments and muscles, it's no wonder that back pain is so common. And it is not confined to the older population: over half of the nation's children are affected. In these pages you'll find out how your back works, which activities cause it the most stress, how to minimize the symptoms and the therapies that can help.

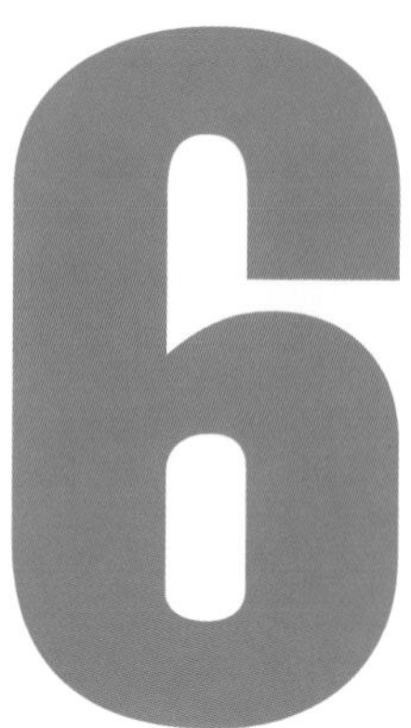

A HEALTHY BACK AND SPINE
How your back works

Each year more than 9 million people across the UK visit their GP or consult a specialist because of back pain. Your back is an amazing piece of engineering, but this very complexity makes it vulnerable to all the stresses and strains of daily life.

Your spine

Your spine is a column of 33 bony segments called vertebrae that run from the base of your skull down to your pelvis. This column provides the central scaffolding for your body, supports your head and torso, protects your spinal cord and provides anchorage points for your ribs, muscles and ligaments.

The vertebrae at the base of your spine fuse by adulthood, leaving 26 separate bones in all. It is the movement between these bones that gives your back its flexibility, letting you bend forwards, backwards and to the side or twist your torso. Movement between individual vertebrae is relatively restricted – the flexibility of your back depends on the combined movement of groups of vertebrae.

The joints in your spine

Each vertebra in your spine is connected to its neighbour at three points: through an intervertebral joint at the front and two small facet joints at the rear. Although these joints are very small in comparison to a joint such the knee, they are every bit as complex.

- **Facet joints** These hinge-like joints link your vertebrae together. Each facet joint is surrounded by a capsule of connective tissue and bathed in synovial fluid. Facet joints are in almost constant motion with the spine and the cartilage covering the bone can become inflamed or worn out over time, causing arthritis.
- **Intervertebral joints** Within these joints the vertebrae are separated by a fluid-filled pad of cartilage, the intervertebral disc, which acts as a shock-absorber. As your muscles pull on your spine these discs compress at the points where they're placed under pressure, letting your spine move, lengthen and shorten. Standing, sitting and bending can place a lot of pressure on these discs and as you get older the amount of fluid decreases, reducing flexibility. The discs can sometimes bulge out to the side, pressing on nerves.

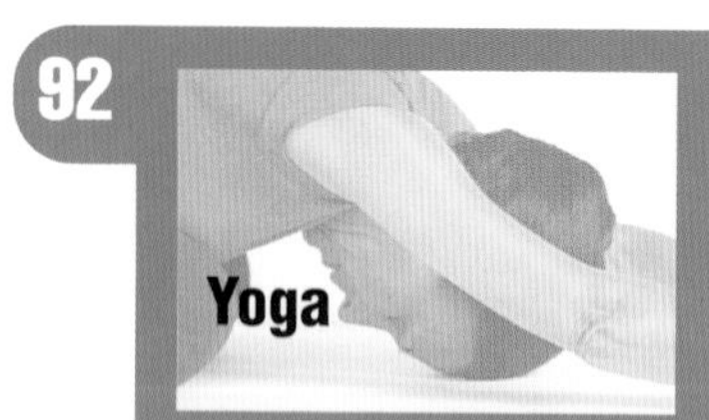

92 Yoga

128 Posture problems in early life

138 Exercises to prevent backache in pregnancy

CERVICAL CURVATURE
This section supports your head and extends down your neck. The cervix contains seven vertebrae.

THORACIC CURVATURE
This region of the back contains twelve vertebrae and forms the attachment point for your ribs.

LUMBAR CURVATURE
This is the main weight-bearing portion of the spine and the area where the most movement occurs. It contains five, sometimes six, large vertebrae.

SACRAL CURVATURE
The is where your spine meets your pelvis. It contains four fused sacral vertebrae and five fused coccygeal vertebrae in your tailbone.

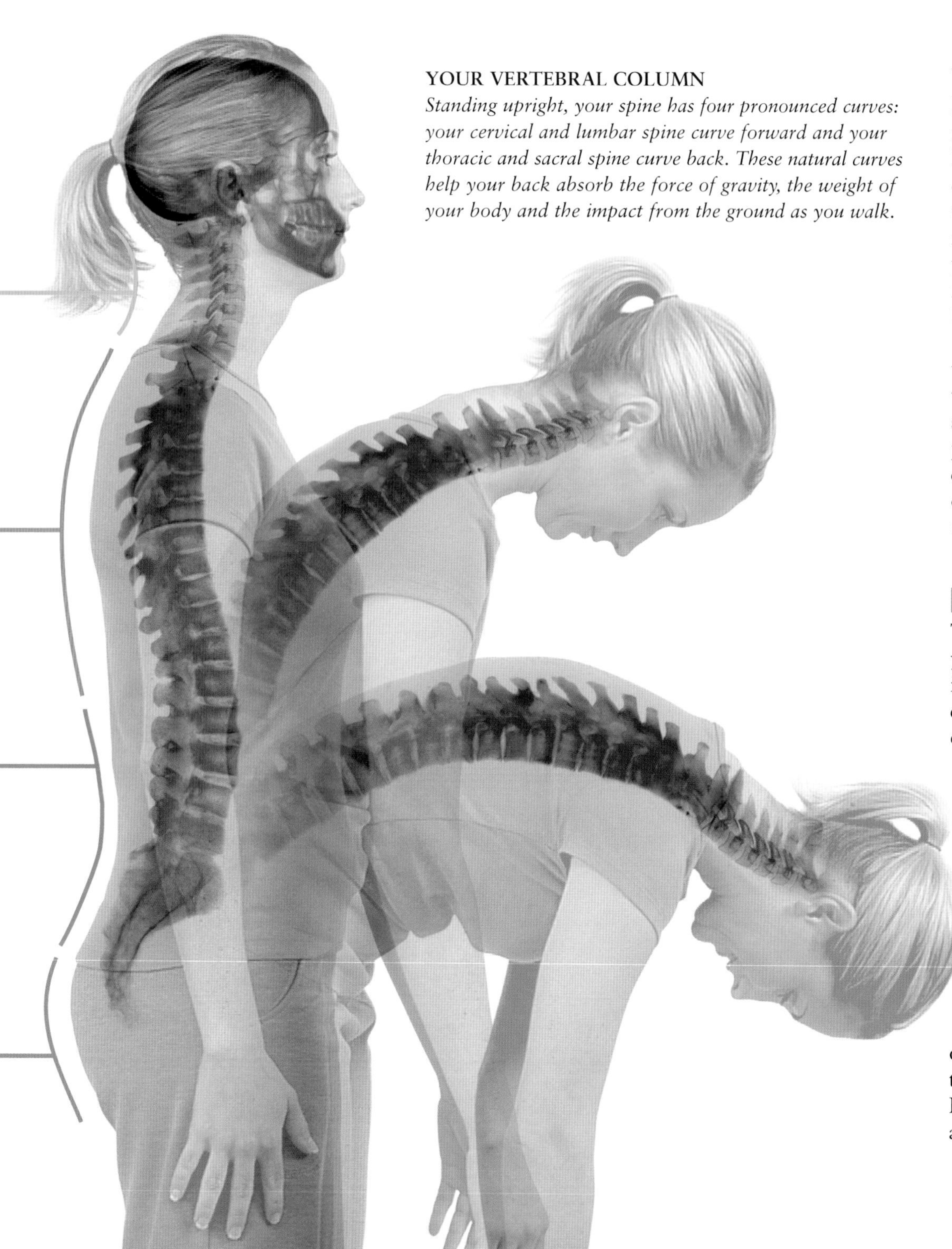

YOUR VERTEBRAL COLUMN
Standing upright, your spine has four pronounced curves: your cervical and lumbar spine curve forward and your thoracic and sacral spine curve back. These natural curves help your back absorb the force of gravity, the weight of your body and the impact from the ground as you walk.

The spinal cord

Each vertebrae has a hole through the middle; when they stack up together these holes form a hollow tube called the neural canal. This tube protects your spinal cord, the bundle of nerve tissue that carries messages from your brain to the rest of your body. Pairs of nerve roots branch off from your spinal cord and out of gaps between each vertebra.

The fact that almost all of the body's vital nerves begin in the spine is one reason why back pain is so common and can feel so agonizing. This also explains why the pain from a trapped nerve in your back can sometimes seem to radiate down to other parts of your body such as your arms (brachalgia) or your legs (sciatica).

Muscles and ligaments

There are three main layers of muscles in your back: the small inner layer connects individual vertebrae; the next layer connects groups of vertebrae; the large outer layer of muscles, your erector spinae, connects your spine from top to bottom. Your erector spinae works together with your abdominals to maintain your spine's curves. A number of other muscles, such as your shoulder muscles and buttocks, are also involved in back movements.

Because of the number of muscles involved in moving your back and maintaining its curves, it is easy for muscle imbalances to pull your back out of alignment or for muscles and ligaments to suffer from painful strains and sprains. Ligaments also have a poor blood supply and do not heal easily when damaged.

Reducing the strain on your back

Back pain is usually the result of lifestyle, ageing or accident. Of these three factors, lifestyle plays a central role in how well you age and in your chances of accidental injury. Good lifestyle habits – correct posture, good lifting techniques and plenty of exercise for a strong, flexible back – will keep your risk of back pain to a minimum.

The single most important way to look after your back is to respect the natural curves of your spine. Any habitual pose that changes your back's regular curves – from an awkward sleeping position to a poor driving posture – can increase the pressure on your spine.

Good posture means holding your body in its correct alignment. While it is important not to slouch, you should also be careful not to overcompensate. Holding your back too straight puts your spine under almost as much pressure as when it is too arched. Poor posture can quickly become a habit: over time, the muscles and ligaments in your back begin to lengthen or shorten, making your posture feel natural.

> 'Picking up a mug of coffee from the opposite side of a table can produce as much force against your vertebral discs as lifting a 10kg (22lb) weight next to your body'

Good posture in your car

People who drive more than 25,000 miles a year take an average of 22 days a year off work with a bad back, according to the National Back Association, compared with just over three days for low mileage drivers. Part of the problem is the posture that drivers adopt: the RAC Foundation, among others, has noted that motorists often adopt a 'banana' posture while driving, leaning into the wheel and stretching their legs to reach the pedals.

Driving also gives you little opportunity to adjust your posture or to stand up and move around. Vibrations from the road exacerbate the problem, increasing muscle fatigue and compression of the intervertebral discs.

There is no way to remove this stress entirely – even the best driving position puts a greater strain on your back than standing. There are, however, ways for you to protect against long-term damage to your back.

■ **Choose the right car** If you have an existing back problem, consider getting an automatic car to avoid frequent gear changes that put stress on the spine. A car with power steering reduces the awkward shoulder and trunk movements you need to park the car. Choose a car with cloth seats

6 WAYS TO...

A strong back

The key to maintaining a healthy back is to be aware not only of your posture, but also of the everyday movements that place your spine and back muscles under unnecessary pressure.

1 **Assess your posture** regularly, both sitting and standing – it's easy to pick up bad habits without noticing. Take a good look at yourself whenever you pass a mirror.

2 **Change your position** regularly. If you have to stay in one position for an extended period of time, in a car or at a desk, for example, try to take a break every 20 minutes or so to move around and stretch.

3 **Avoid wearing high heels** for long periods. High heels accentuate the normal curve of your back and tip your pelvis, which can contribute to knee and back problems.

4 **Use both shoulders** when you are wearing a backpack. If you carry a heavy bag, a briefcase or a suitcase, try to alternate the arm that you use to carry it.

5 **Watch your wallet** when you are sitting down. A bulging wallet in your back pocket can place pressure on the sciatic nerve.

6 **Don't snooze in front of the TV** as an armchair or sofa won't take pressure off your lower spine. Snoozing prevents you shifting when your back starts to feel uncomfortable.

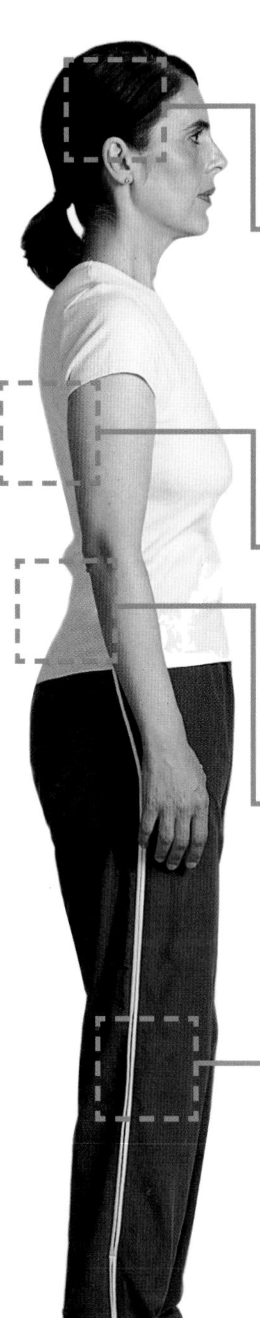

PERFECT POSTURE

HEAD AND NECK

The crown of your head, not your forehead, should be the highest point of your body. Keep your head and chin neutral: neither jutting out nor tucked too far in.

UPPER BACK

Lift your chest and keep your shoulders down and back, but not so far that your pose feels forced or unnatural.

LOWER BACK

Pull your stomach and your buttock muscles tight. Try not to over-arch or round your lower back.

LEGS

Keep your knees slightly bent and your toes pointing forwards. If you need to stand for long periods, rest one foot on a step to relieve pressure on your lower back and change feet every 5–15 minutes.

rather than leather or vinyl, as cloth provides friction and grip and stops you sliding into a slouching position.

- **Get in carefully** Try not to twist your body when you get in or out of your car. If this is a problem, get into the car by sitting sideways on a seat then turning your whole body around; when getting out turn your body towards the door, then put your feet on the floor and stand up. A swivel cushion may help.
- **Adjust your seat** Set the seat back in an upright or slightly reclining position as this stops you slouching and reduces the effects of vibration on your spine. Position the seat so that you can easily reach the pedals and make sure that your hips are higher than your knees. If you share a car, always readjust the seat before you drive.
- **Adjust the headrest** To prevent whiplash injuries, ensure that the top of the head restraint is level with the top of your head and certainly no lower than eye level.
- **Hold the wheel correctly** Don't grip too hard and make sure you hold the wheel in the correct '10 minutes to 2' position. If your car has an adjustable wheel, set it at a comfortable angle.
- **Take regular breaks** However good your posture, you'll need to change your position regularly. The Highway Code recommends a 15-minute break at least once every 2 hours. During your break, take a short walk or do a few simple neck and back exercises >>180–183.

Sleeping soundly

Although the weight of your upper body on your spine is considerably reduced when you're lying down, it is easy to adopt an awkward position without realizing it when you're asleep. In particular, try to avoid lying on your front with your neck twisted to one side and try not to stay in one position for too long.

Most people spend 6 to 8 hours a day in bed, so it is well worthwhile making sure that your mattress and pillow give you the best possible support:

- **Bigger is better** A spacious bed will stop you adopting a cramped position. Try out a range of beds. Lie on a bed for several minutes and turn over a few times before you make a decision.
- **Choose a good mattress** Look for a moderately firm mattress: not too hard, not too soft. Choose one that yields enough to adapt to your contours, but is not so soft that you sink into it: your spine should maintain its natural curves. Remember to turn your mattress regularly.
- **Choose a good pillow** Your pillow should support your neck in alignment with the rest of your spine. An overstuffed pillow or too many pillows may push your head too far forward; a pillow that's too limp or flimsy may tip your head back.

Good posture at your desk

Poor sitting posture is a major cause of lower back problems. Sitting places much greater pressure on your spine than standing or walking – even when you sit upright, the weight of your upper body exerts around 50 per cent more pressure on your lower spine than when standing. If you sit slouched over, the pressure on your spine is up to 150 per cent greater than when standing.

Good sitting posture is particularly important if you have to spend long periods at a desk or in front of a computer. Try to get up and walk around every 20 minutes or so. Do some neck stretches,

SITTING AT YOUR DESK

■ *Eyes* Make sure that the screen is at the right height so that your eyes are level with the top of the screen – place some large books under the monitor if necessary.

■ *Body* Do not slouch. Keep your pelvis tucked in and make sure that your lower back is fully supported by your chair. Position the monitor and keyboard so that you don't need to twist your hips or neck to use them.

■ *Arms and wrists* Your work surface should be just lower than your bent elbows. Your wrists should be level with your hands while typing – use a wrist pad if necessary.

■ *Legs and feet* Set the seat height so that your legs are bent at right angles and your feet are flat on the floor or on a foot rest. Your legs should fit underneath the work surface so you don't lean forward.

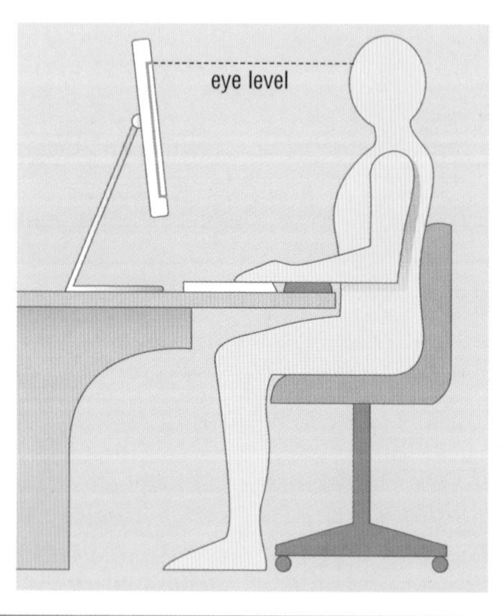

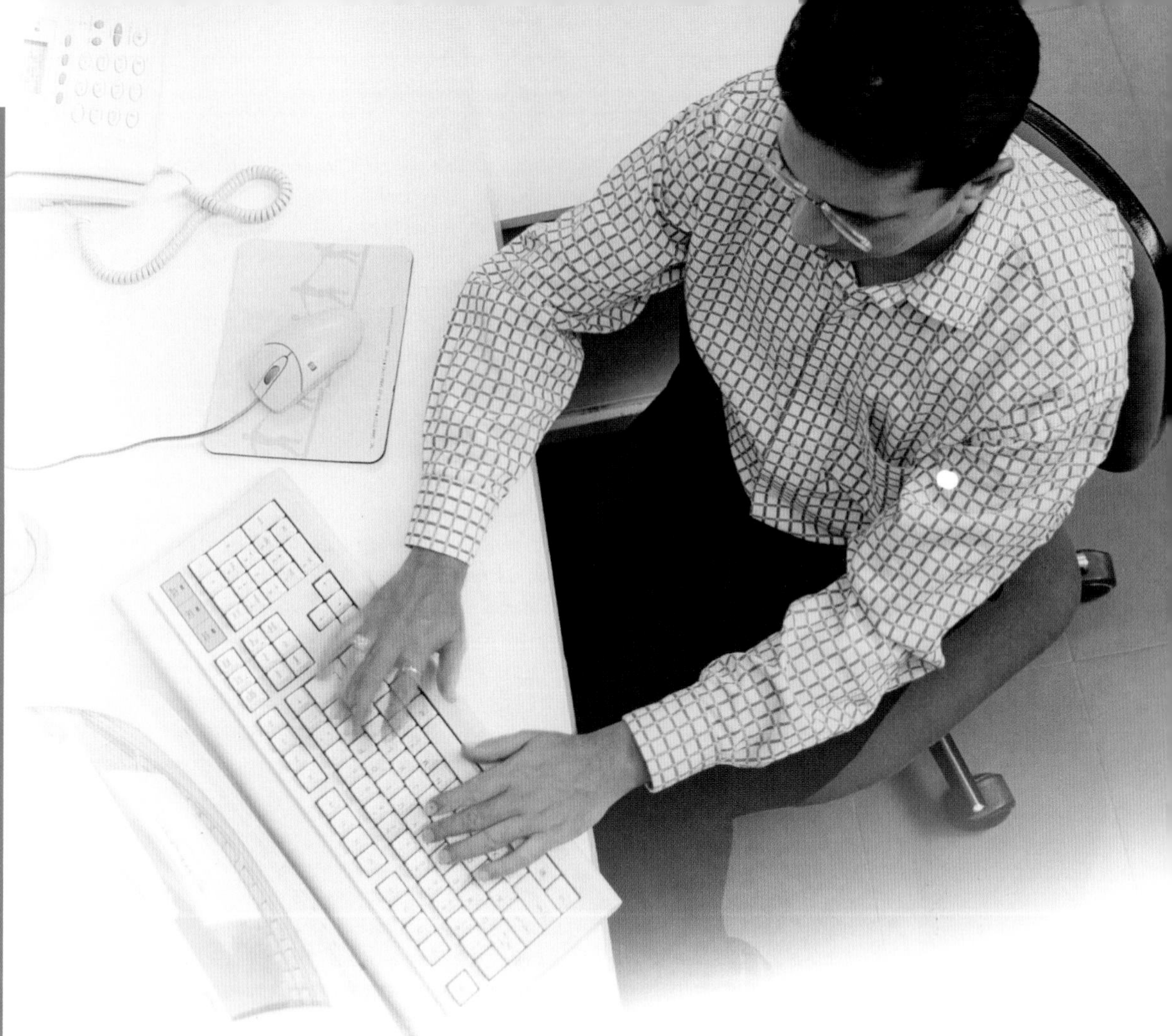

shoulder rolls, shrugs, arms stretches, neck rolls and back stretches to loosen up your spine >>180–183. It is fine to assume other sitting positions for short periods, but try to spend most of your time sitting in the optimal position (>>box, left).

Exercise and your back

Doctors no longer recommend bed rest for back pain: the muscles, ligaments and joints in your back, like any other area of your body, need regular exercise to stay healthy. Without movement the intervertebral discs start to dry up and shrink, your ligaments begin to lose their elasticity and the muscles around your spine grow weaker. Exercise also helps you to maintain a healthy body weight, reducing extra strain on your spine.

You need strong muscles around your back to protect your spine. Weak muscles do not contain enough tension to brace your spine and absorb the stress of movement. It is also important to keep muscles on opposing sides of your body balanced: in particular, weak abdominals and strong lower back muscles are a common cause of lower back pain.

This is not to say that physical activity does not hold any risks, simply that the benefits far outweigh the dangers. To avoid potential problems such as strained or torn ligaments it is vital to warm up thoroughly before exercise >>64–65. Always exercise within your limits, avoid sudden twisting movements in your trunk and stop immediately if anything hurts. For a programme of simple exercises to increase the strength and flexibility in your neck, back and shoulders >>180–183.

Lifting and pushing

Poor lifting technique is the single most common cause of acute back pain and, because it exacerbates any existing

> **‘Pushing and pulling heavy objects can also contribute to back sprains and strains. Given the choice, always push a heavy object rather than pulling it’**

weakness, can also cause longer-term back problems. Manual workers and people whose job involves a lot of lifting are most at risk: around 80,000 NHS nurses injure their backs each year, often as a result of lifting patients. You can reduce your risk of injury by using the correct lifting techniques (>>box, below).

Even the best technique won't remove the risk altogether, though, so check the weight of the object before you pick it up: if you find that you're straining you may need to get someone to give you a hand. If you have to lift an object that's higher than your shoulder level, use a stable step-stool or ladder to avoid over-reaching.

Pushing and pulling heavy objects can also contribute to back problems, sprains and strains. Given the choice, always push a heavy object rather than pulling it – this puts less pressure on your lower back. Bend your knees and use your legs rather than your back for power and watch out for sudden changes in resistance.

LIFTING OBJECTS SAFELY

You can reduce your risk of injury by making sure you use the correct technique: check the weight of the object before you lift and follow the guidelines shown below:

1 Stand with your feet hip-width apart and as close to the object as possible. Place one foot slightly in front of the other. Bend your knees and squat down, keeping a straight back and tight stomach.

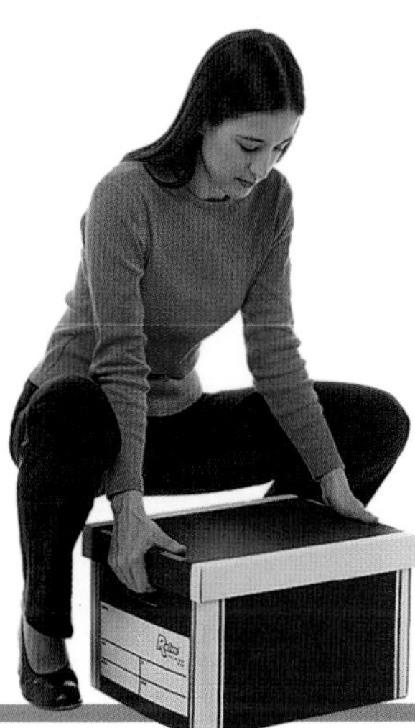

2 Hold the object close to your body as you stand up. Keep your back straight and use your legs and not your back to provide the power.

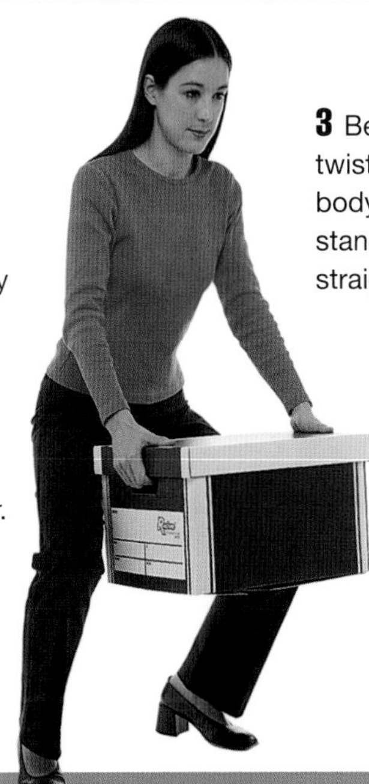

3 Be careful not to twist or turn your body until you are standing up straight.

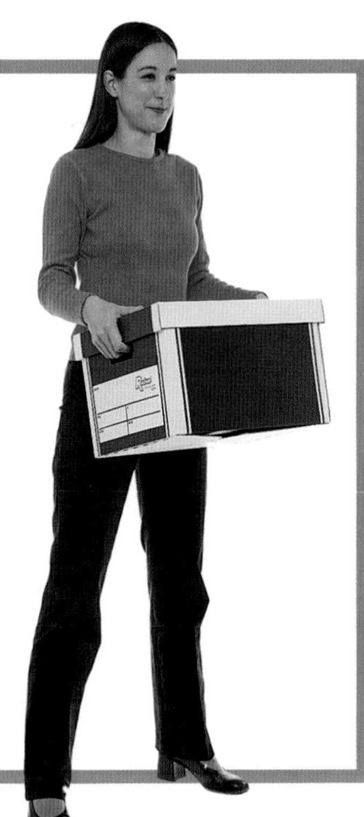

Exercises for your neck

Your cervical spine (the portion of your spine in your neck) supports the weight of your head and protects the nerves that travel from your head to the rest of your body. The average human head weighs 4–6kg (10–12lb) – about the same weight as a small bowling ball – so the vertebrae in your neck are under considerable pressure, even when you're standing still. Your head is also positioned slightly forward over your spine rather than directly above, which means that your neck muscles have to work continuously to balance the weight of your head.

The muscles and joints in your neck control the nodding and rotation movements of your head and let you bend and twist your neck. Holding your head in an awkward position for any length of time can cause muscle tension and compress your neck vertebrae, which may have a knock-on effect throughout your back and spine, causing pain and discomfort.

With regular practice, the simple exercises shown here will help you to maintain neck strength and mobility. If you have any existing problems, the exercises may also help you to regain loss of motion in the neck region and control pain.

- Perform each movement slowly for five repetitions, resting a short time in between each set of movements.
- If any of these exercises makes you feel uncomfortable or dizzy, slow down, reduce the extent of the stretch or skip the stretch altogether.

Head rotation

Rotate your head to one side until you can't turn it any further. Bring your head back to the centre point, rest a moment, then turn your head to the opposite side.

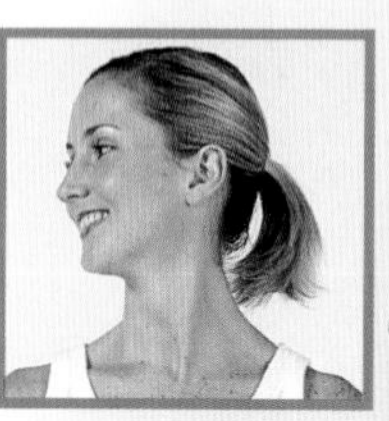

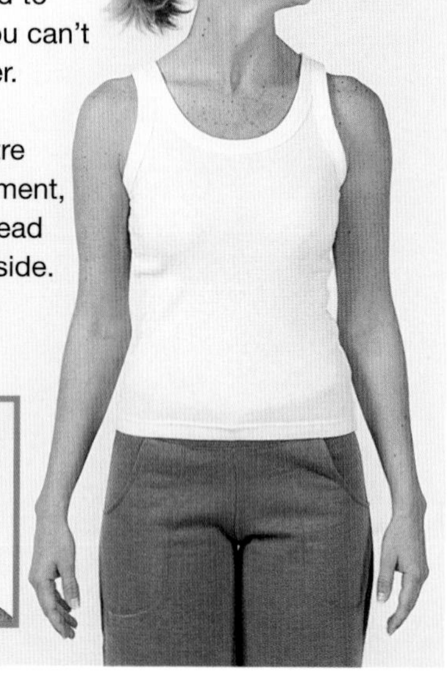

Neck flexion/extension

Bend your head forward until your chin touches your chest and your eyes look straight down at the floor. Bring your head back up, rest a moment, then bend it back until your eyes look directly at the ceiling.

Neck retraction

Draw your head back and bring your chin down slightly. This exercise counteracts the natural tendency to poke your head too far forward.

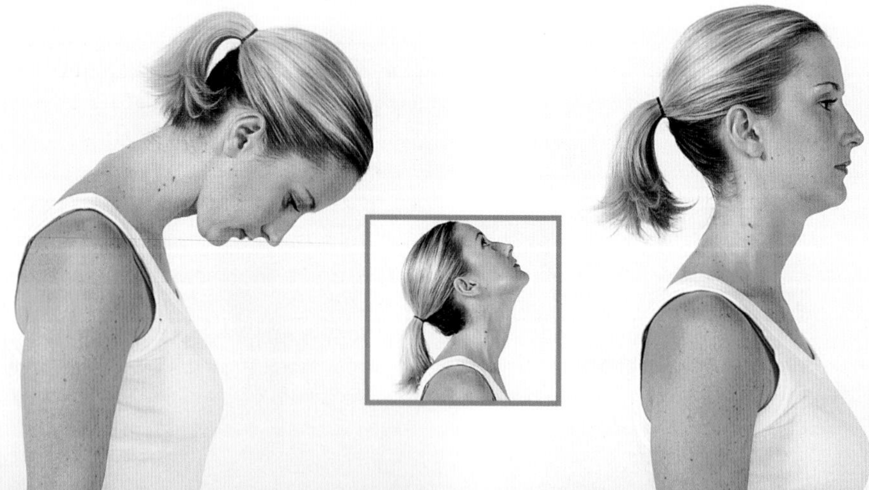

Side flexion/extension

Keep your head facing forward and move your ear down towards your shoulder until you feel a stretch along the opposite side of your neck. Bring your head back to the centre, rest a moment, then move your head over to the opposite side.

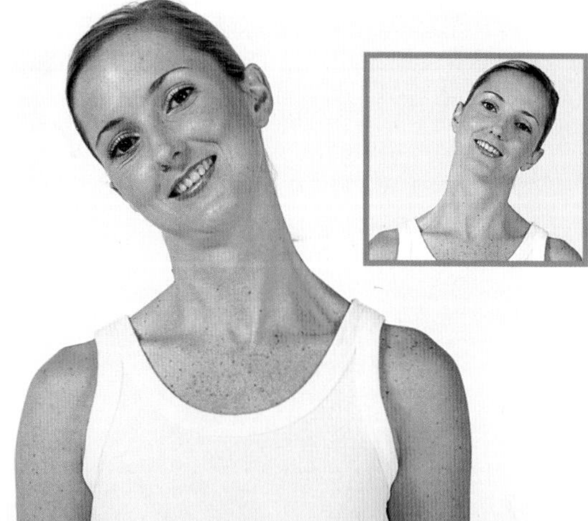

Exercises for your upper back and shoulders

Your thoracic spine, in your upper back, does not have such a wide range of motion as your neck or lower back, so injuries are relatively rare. However, irritation or excess tension in your back and shoulder muscles can be very painful. In particular, poor posture and hunched shoulders – common among people who sit at a desk all day – can tighten your chest muscles and overstretch the muscles in your upper back. This may compress the vertebrae in your spine and lead to areas of painful, knotted muscles and tension headaches.

The exercises shown here are intended to strengthen the muscles around your upper back and shoulders, open your chest and reduce tension in the muscles and ligaments. Try each movement slowly for five repetitions, resting a short time in between each set of movements.

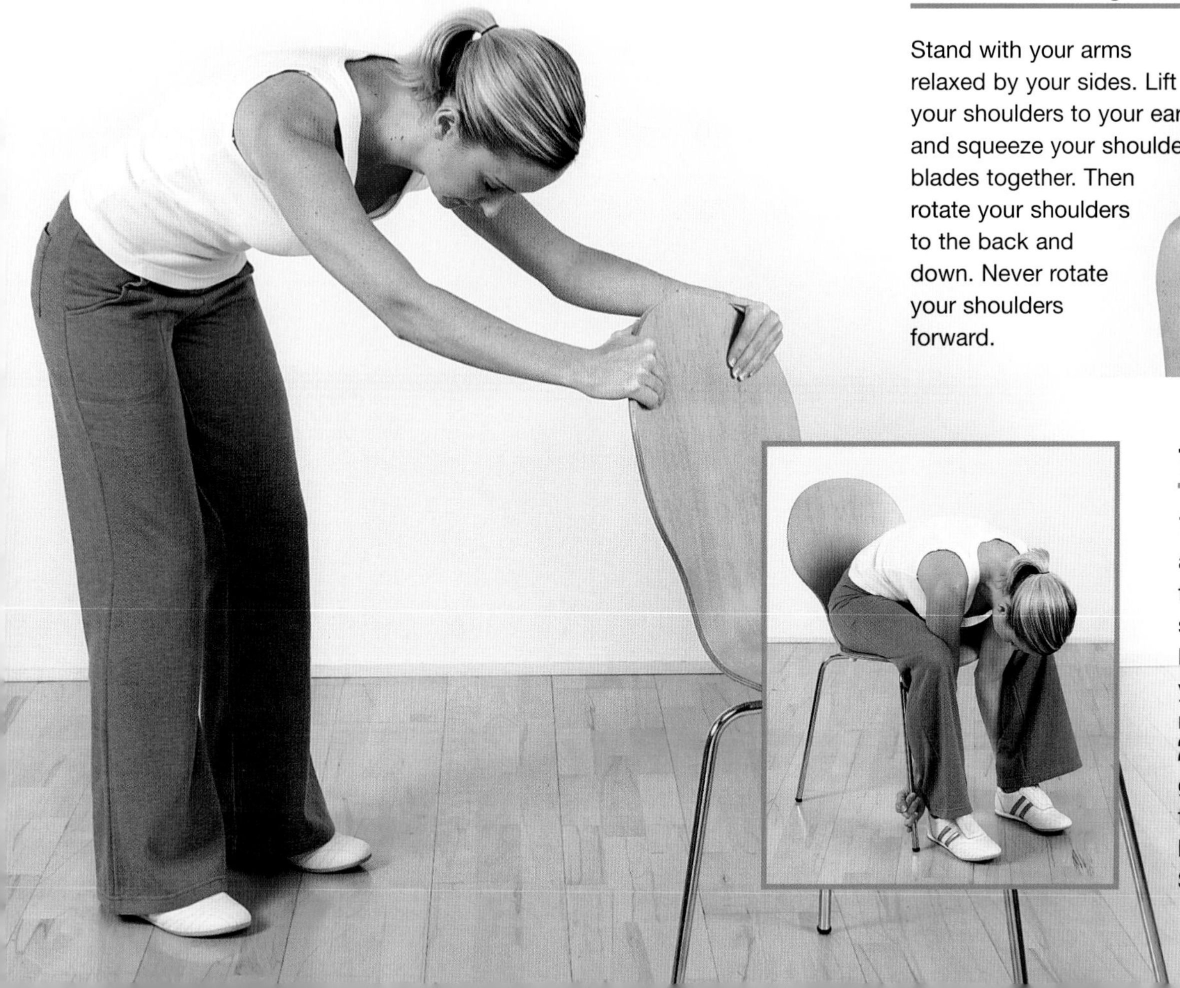

Shoulder brace

Stand with your arms relaxed by your sides. Bring your shoulders as far forward as possible and then bring them right back, pulling your shoulder blades together.

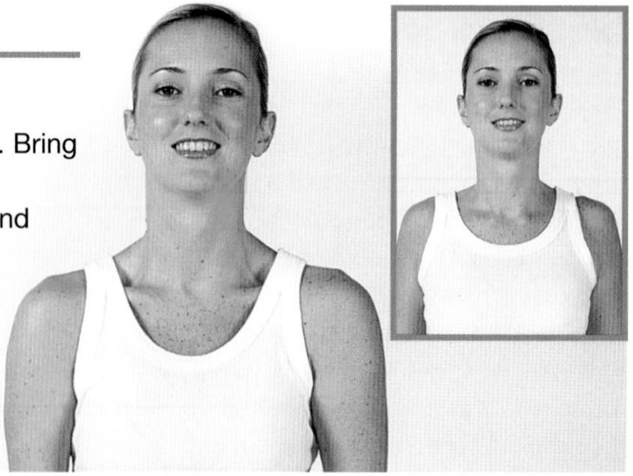

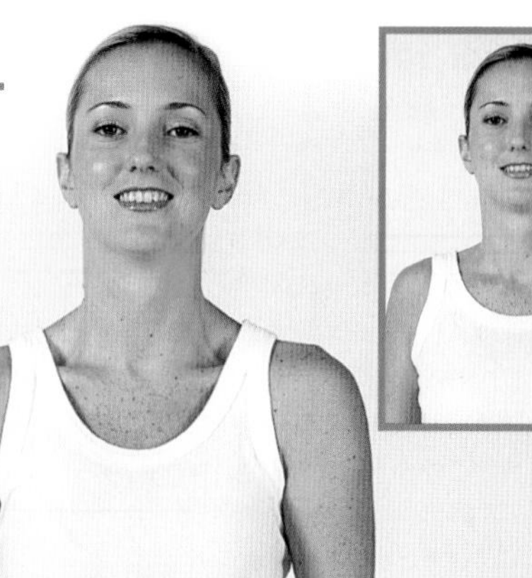

Shoulder shrug

Stand with your arms relaxed by your sides. Lift your shoulders to your ears and squeeze your shoulder blades together. Then rotate your shoulders to the back and down. Never rotate your shoulders forward.

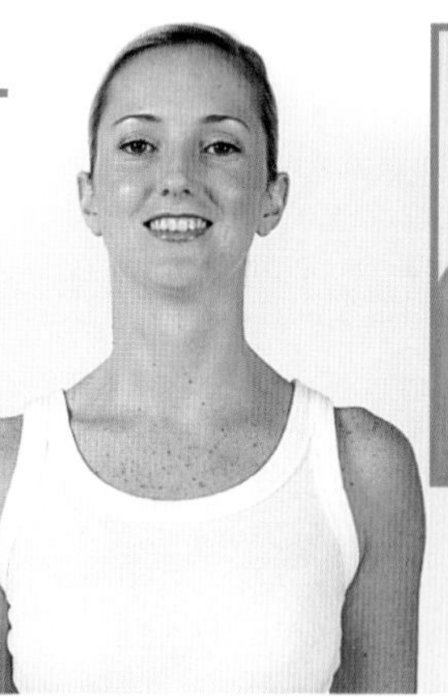

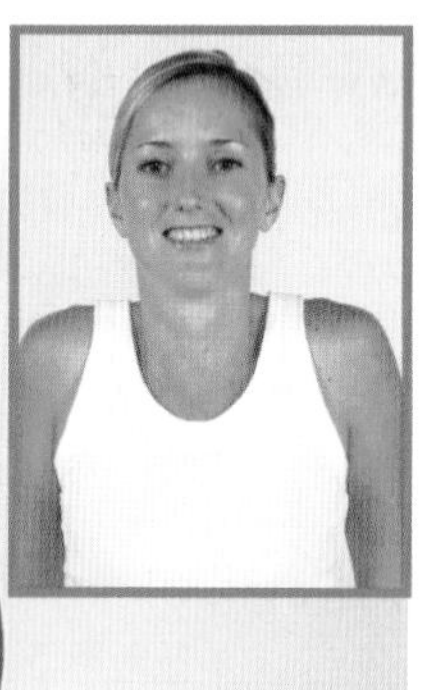

Thoracic stretch

1 Stand with your feet about shoulder-width apart and your knees slightly bent. Bend over from the waist and hold onto a stable support such a chair back. Push your bottom backwards until you can feel a stretch along your upper back. Hold for a count of 15 before moving back up.

2 Sit on a chair with your feet flat on the ground. Gradually roll your upper body forward from the waist. Reach your hands between your legs to grip the legs of the chair. Slowly curl back up.

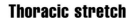

Exercises for your lower back

The lumbar region in your lower back is the most frequently injured area of the spine. This is mainly because your lower back carries the full weight of your torso and allows for a much greater range of movements than your upper back. The majority of episodes of lower back pain (lumbago) are caused by muscle strain: back muscles – like other muscles – need exercise to maintain strength and tone.

Exercises to prevent and treat low back pain usually focus on strengthening the spine flexors (your erector spinae and gluteal muscles), spine extensors (your abdominals) and the muscles along the sides of your torso (your oblique abdominals). Another important group of muscles are your hamstrings, the large muscles in the back of your thighs. Tight hamstrings limit the motion in your pelvis, which can cause lower back pain.

With regular practice, the exercises shown here will help you to maintain the strength and flexibility of the muscles in your lower back. Do not strain or force the movements, and stop if you feel any discomfort. Try each movement slowly for five repetitions, resting a short time in between each set of movements.

Knee roll

Lie on your back with your knees bent and your feet flat on the ground. Keep your knees together. Roll your knees steadily from side to side.

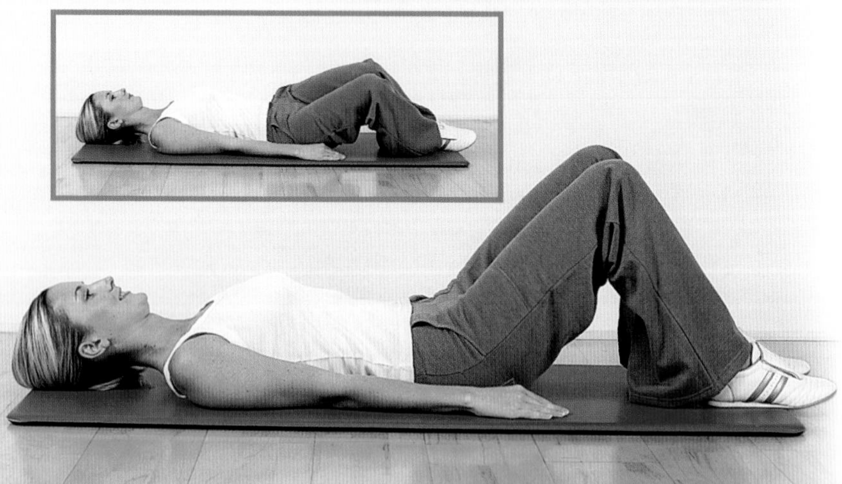

Forward bend

Stand with your feet hip-width apart. Without bouncing, slowly reach one hand down towards the opposite foot. Let your other arm swing up behind your body. Return to a standing position. Don't worry if you can't reach your toes – your flexibility should improve with practice.

Pelvic tilt

Lie on your back with your knees bent and hip-width apart and your feet flat on the ground. Press your lower back down to the floor, then arch your lower back up off the floor. Let your tail bone tip down to the mat and do not lift your buttocks.

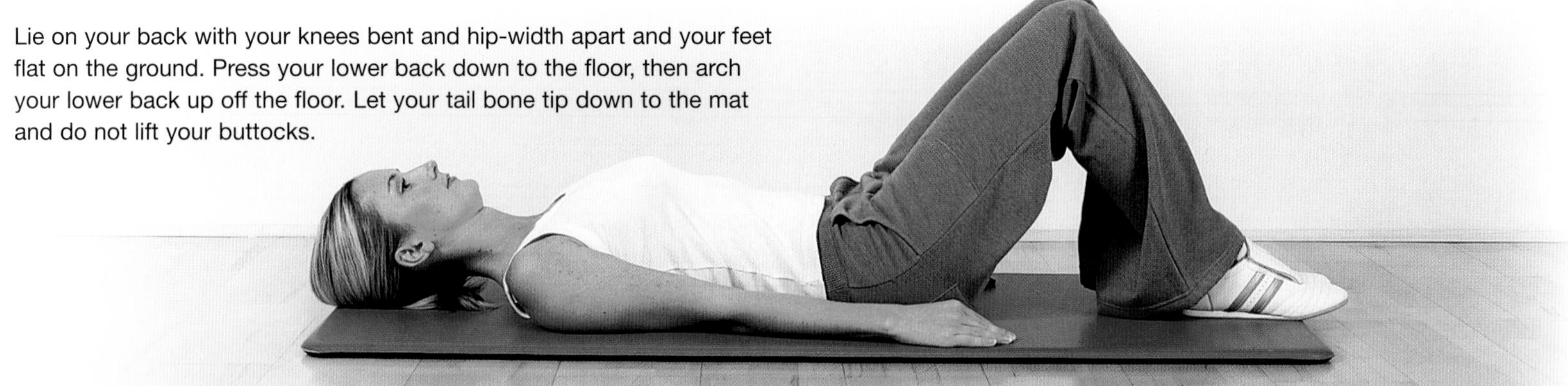

Abdominal curl

Lie on your back with your knees bent and your feet flat on the floor. Cross your hands over your chest and pull in your stomach muscles. Slowly curl your shoulders and upper back up off the floor. Try to keep your lower back in contact with the floor.

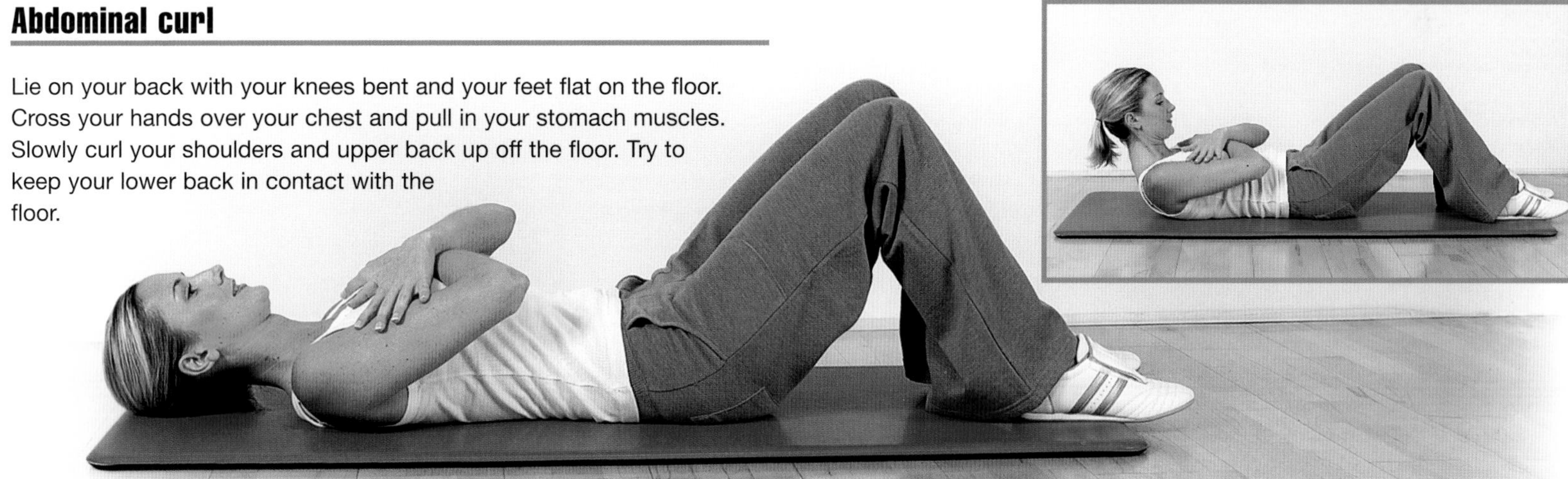

Back extender

Lie on your stomach with your hands laced underneath your forehead. Use your lower back muscles to slowly lift your head and shoulders about 20cm (8in) off the floor. Be careful not to strain your neck.

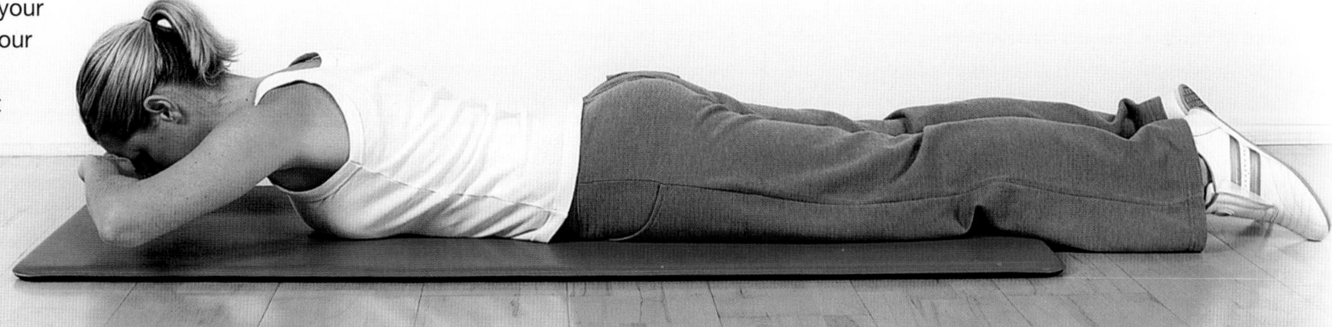

COMPLEMENTARY THERAPIES FOR YOUR BACK

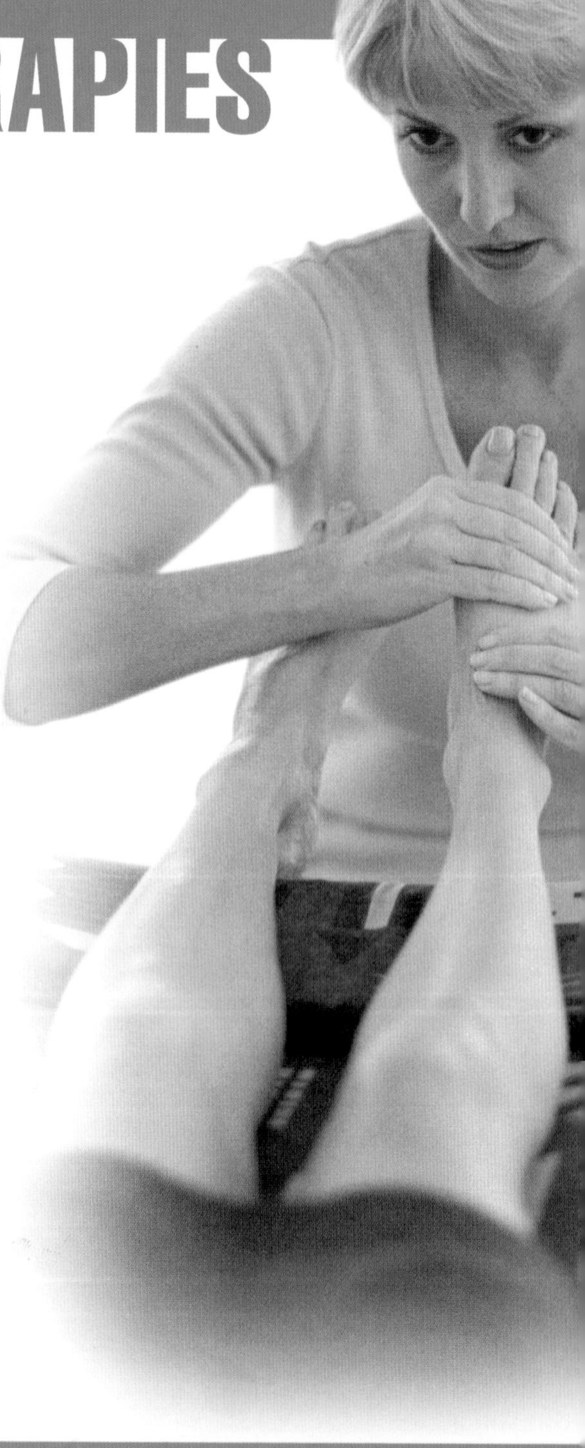

Around a third of people in the UK use some form of complementary therapy and many treatments are now recognized by the medical establishment as a useful addition to orthodox medicine. Approaches and training vary considerably: some therapies, such as osteopathy, are very widely accepted; other therapies are less well regulated.

Because complementary therapies often take a holistic approach, addressing problems on a mental, emotional and physical level, they may be useful for persistent musculoskeletal problems such as back pain. Here are some of the potentially useful therapies available.

Acupuncture

This traditional Chinese therapy uses fine needles inserted into specific 'acupoints' around the body in order to promote the flow of energy or 'qi'. Proponents believe that acupuncture can treat a range of conditions, including back pain, and a number of studies suggest that it does have genuine pain-relieving properties: brain scans on patients show that the treatment activates regions of the brain known to be involved in pain modulation.

This effect is relatively short lived, lasting for hours or days after a session. Nevertheless this may provide a window in which to introduce other treatments such as physiotherapy. Acupuncture may also stimulate the nervous system and improve circulation. The therapy is now available in many NHS pain clinics. Alternatively, your GP can put you in touch with a qualified practitioner in your area.

Shiatsu

A Japanese massage therapy intended to stimulate energy flow through the body. The word shiatsu means 'finger pressure' although practitioners also use palms, thumbs, feet and sometimes knees to apply rhythmic pressure to points around the body that correspond to the 'acupoints' used in acupuncture. The therapy also incorporates assisted-stretching techniques. Treatment can be fairly physical but you should feel relaxed or invigorated afterwards.

Shiatsu is deeply rooted in the language and philosophy of Traditional Chinese Medicine (TCM) which makes it difficult to evaluate all of the claims made for this therapy scientifically. Studies do suggest shiatsu has some genuine relaxing and pain-relieving effects and it may be a useful way to relieve muscle tension in problem backs and necks.

What to ask your therapist

Before making an appointment to see a complementary therapist, your should ask the therapist the following questions:

- Are you registered as a trained practitioner with the appropriate professional body?
- Are you experienced in treating conditions similar to mine?
- Are there any risks involved in the treatments?
- Are there any medications or other treatments that might interfere with the therapy?
- How long does the treatment last and how many sessions are required?
- How much do you charge?
- Do you have professional indemnity and public liability insurance?

Reflexology

An ancient system of foot massage based on the principle that there are reflex points in your hands and feet that correspond to particular body systems and organs. Reflexologists believe that pressure on these points can reduce tension, improve circulation and remove energy blockages along the nerve pathways to particular areas of the body such as the spine or sciatic nerve.

Many people find this type of foot massage relaxing and this may help to relieve muscle tension and therefore pain in your back. There is little research to support the more theoretical claims on which reflexology is based and most doctors remain largely sceptical about the therapy's wider benefits.

Chiropractic and osteopathy

These manipulative therapies have a common origin in the traditions of bonesetting and continue to share many techniques and approaches today. Osteopathy uses manipulation, massage and stretching to improve the alignment and function of bones, joints and muscles all over the body. Chiropractic therapy tends to focus more closely on the spine and is based on the principle that vertebral misalignments underpin most musculoskeletal disorders.

Most doctors consider the therapies to be a potentially valuable way to treat many musculoskeletal disorders. For more information >>189.

The Alexander technique

A system of practical postural exercises developed at the turn of the century by an actor named Frederick Matthias Alexander, who discovered that he was able to enhance his voice and reduce tension in his neck by improving his posture. He created a programme of exercises to encourage beneficial ways of standing, sitting and moving.

The technique uses the repetition and practice of specific movements and postures. Teachers instruct students orally and may also use touch and hand pressure to train students how to hold their bodies according to their natural strengths. The Alexander technique is a useful way to deal with back pain caused by poor posture and is especially useful as a preventative measure. In some areas the therapy is available in the NHS.

Pilates

Developed in the early 20th century by an athlete named Joseph Pilates, this physical therapy uses resistance and control exercises to stretch and strengthen muscles and joints. The exercises are designed to work with natural body mechanics to improve posture, breathing and release tension. Some instructors use special Pilates apparatus to create a variable resistance to work your muscles against. For more information >>94–95.

Common back problems

One third of adults suffer from back pain at any one time, according to the British Chiropractic Association, but in the majority of cases the exact cause of the problem is never identified. Doctors have a good understanding of the mechanisms that cause back problems, but it is often difficult to identify the exact source of the pain.

Many episodes of back pain are trivial, if unpleasant, and tend to resolve without treatment or the need for further investigation. In most cases symptoms are probably due to poor muscle tone, muscle tension or spasm, or back sprains and strains. Nonetheless, back pain may at times be a sign of something more serious and it is important to be aware of how the different conditions can affect your back.

Sprains and strains

The most frequent cause of back pain is a small injury to the soft tissues in your back, such as a muscle or tendon strain or a ligament sprain. Most strains and sprains occur during day-to-day activities such as lifting or twisting: any excessive physical demand on your back can over-stretch your tissues. Even snoozing in an armchair can place your muscles and ligaments under uneven pressure and may result in minor damage. Your lower back, in particular, is susceptible to muscular strains because it forms the pivot around which you move your upper body.

When you stretch or tear the muscles or ligaments in your back, the tissues swell up, causing pain, tenderness or stiffness. You may feel pain immediately or it may develop over the course of several days. An injured muscle may also 'knot up' and start to spasm. This type of spasm is a common response to injury, designed to immobilize the painful area and prevent further damage, but can cause excruciating pain. Because the tension affects neighbouring muscles a localized spasm may cause pain and tension over a wide area of your back.

Most strains and sprains resolve within a few weeks, but you may find painkillers or heat treatments such as warming packs and baths help to relieve discomfort.

CAUTION

Back pain with any of the following symptoms may indicate a serious problem such as a dislocated or fractured vertebra or a spinal tumour. You should contact your doctor immediately.

- Unexplained fever with back pain
- Loss of bowel or bladder control
- Back pain after a severe blow or fall
- Redness or swelling on your back or spine
- Pain travelling down your legs or weakness or numbness in your buttocks, pelvis or legs
- A burning sensation when you urinate or blood in your urine
- Pain that keeps you awake at night or worsens when you lie down
- Very sharp pain

Joint problems

The complexity of your spine makes it particularly vulnerable to structural problems. Each of the 26 bones that make up your spine (the remainder of your vertebrae are fused) is connected to its neighbour by three separate joints. This means there are multiple points of wear and friction within your back.

Osteoarthritis

The degenerative joint disease osteoarthritis – sometimes called spondylosis when it occurs in the spine – is marked by the slow deterioration and thinning of the cartilage that cushions the joints. This can occur at any point in your spine, but the lumbar and cervical vertebrae in your lower back and neck are most vulnerable because they are the areas of your back under the most pressure during day-to-day life.

The loss of cartilage results in narrowed joint spaces and grinding between vertebrae, causing inflammation, pain, swelling and stiffness. Sometimes the body attempts to compensate for cartilage loss by growing bony spurs around the joints, which may compress nerve routes and cause sciatica (>>188). For more information on preventing and managing osteoarthritis >>228–247.

Ankylosing spondylitis

This is a type of arthritis that mainly affects the joints of the spine, particularly the joints that connect the spine to your hips. Unlike osteoarthritis, which is primarily due to wear and tear, the causes of ankylosing spondylitis are not fully understood, although genes probably play a part. The condition affects around 1 in every 200 people.

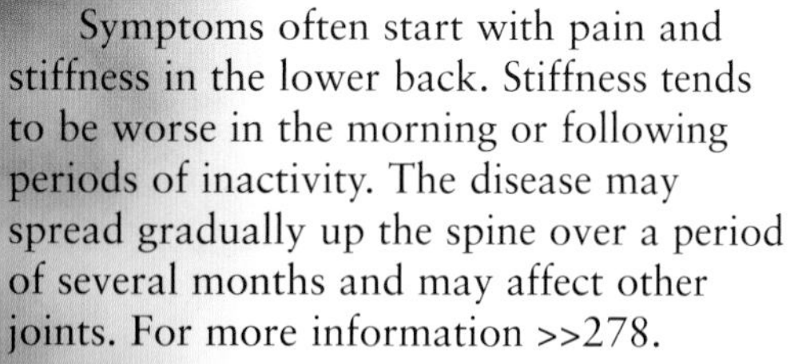

Symptoms often start with pain and stiffness in the lower back. Stiffness tends to be worse in the morning or following periods of inactivity. The disease may spread gradually up the spine over a period of several months and may affect other joints. For more information >>278.

Prolapsed (slipped) disc

The discs between the vertebrae in your spine absorb a great deal of the stress during everyday movements. Each disc has two parts: a soft, jelly-like centre called the nucleus pulposus and a strong outer ring of ligament fibres called the annulus. A prolapsed or herniated disc occurs when the jelly-like nucleus pulposus bulges through a tear in the outer ring.

Prolapsed discs are commonly called slipped discs, although the disc itself does not slip out of position.

As the discs themselves have almost no nerve supply, a prolapsed disc doesn't tend to cause pain unless it pinches a nerve root, in which case you may feel radiating pain down your arms or legs. If you avoid placing further stress on the disc, the herniated bulge may dry out, taking pressure off the nerve, and scar tissue should start to form over the tear in the annulus. Painkillers or manipulation by an osteopath may help to relieve symptoms.

GET IN THE SWING

Swinging a golf club requires a sharp twist of the spine that places a lot of stress on muscles, ligaments and vertebrae. To minimize problems, always warm up thoroughly and, after every few holes, take a couple of swings in the opposite direction to even up the stress on your spine.

Prolapsed discs are responsible for around 1 in 20 cases of acute back pain. More than 80 per cent of prolapsed discs occur in the lower back and are most common in people between the ages of 30 and 50: between these ages the annulus weakens. After the age of 50 the nucleus pulposus starts to harden, making problems less likely. Slipped discs in the neck are most common among 40 to 60-year-olds.

Spinal fractures

As you get older and the amount of calcium in your bones decreases, you become increasingly vulnerable to the brittle-bone disease osteoporosis. This condition affects all the bones in your body but certain areas of your skeleton, including the vertebrae in your spine, are at particular risk of fractures.

> **'An estimated 8 out of 10 people will experience an episode of lower back pain lasting more than a day at some point in their lives'**

Spinal fractures tend to be compression fractures: tiny breaks that cause the vertebrae to collapse vertically. These often develop from the stress of everyday activities and may cause gradual loss of height, back pains and aches. As vertebrae start to crumble, you may develop a range of other back problems such as trapped nerves, muscles spasms and arthritis.

The sometimes gradual onset means that many people are never properly diagnosed but doctors believe that

ABNORMAL SPINAL CURVES

Seen from the side, the curves of your back should resemble a very soft 's' shape. These curves help your spine to absorb pressure and impact – if you hold your back too straight or too arched, your spine tends to absorb a lot more pressure and the muscles and nerves in your back are placed under much more stress. If you have postural problems or other back disorders, the natural curves of your back may look irregular or exaggerated. Types of abnormal spinal curve include:

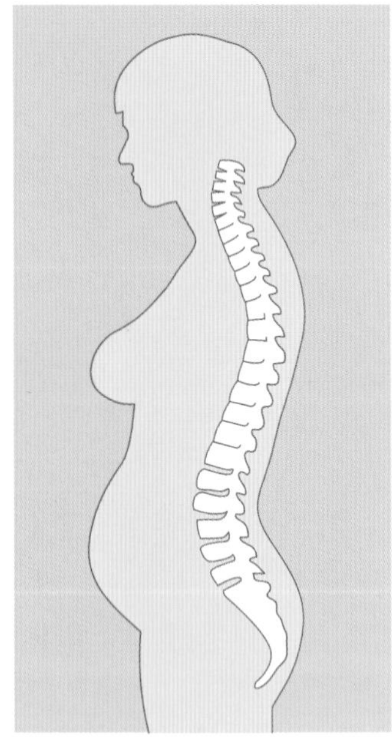

Lordosis (swayback). This is an exaggerated inward curve of the lumbar spine (lower back), or very occasionally the cervical spine (neck). It may be due to poor posture, a congenital deformity of the spine, neuromuscular problems, back surgery or a hip problem. It is fairly common in young children and pregnant women.

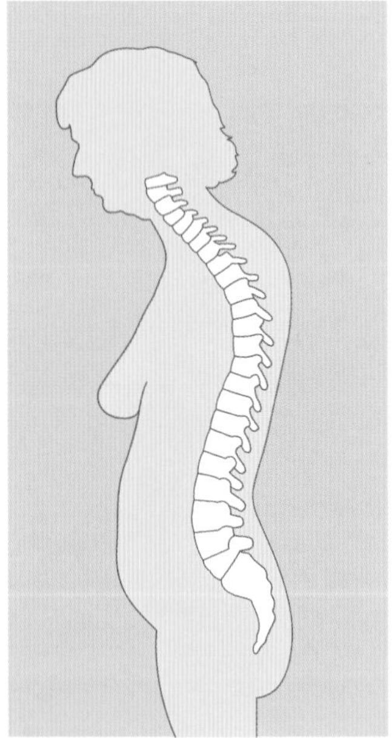

Kyphosis (dowager's hump). This an exaggerated curve of the thoracic spine giving the back a hunchback appearance. It is often caused by collapsed vertebrae and cartilage degeneration and most commonly occurs in people who suffer from osteoporosis or osteoarthritis of the spine. Adolescent kyphosis is known as Scheuermann's disease.

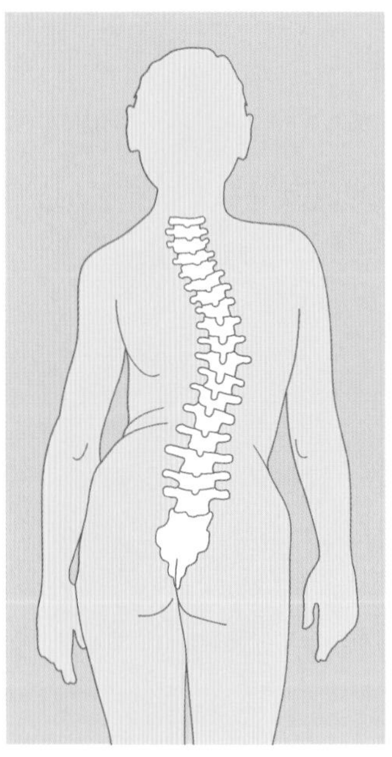

Scoliosis This is a sideways bend in the spine, so that it forms a 'c' or 's' shape when seen from behind. This can be due to habitual poor posture or unbalanced muscles but sometimes develops for no obvious reason, often during the adolescent growth spurt. It affects around 2 per cent of the population. For further information >>323.

osteoporosis is a very common cause of chronic back pain among older people. If you are over 50 and suffer from long-term back pain, talk to your doctor about getting a bone density scan >>268. For more information about preventing and managing osteoporosis >>264–275.

Neural problems

Because your nerves travel through your spine on their way to your brain, pain that originates in another part of your body can sometimes feel as though it comes from your back. This is known as referred pain. Conditions that can produce referred back pain include ulcers, kidney disease, ovarian cysts and pancreatitis.

This can also work the other way. Damage to the nerves in or around your spine may cause pain that seems to radiate down to other areas. Conditions that cause or result from nerve damage include:

- **Central canal stenosis** Any narrowing of the spinal canal puts pressure on your spinal cord, which may cause pain and numbness, pins and needles, muscle weakness or bowel and bladder problems. You may feel pain in areas such as the buttock, thigh or leg. Possible causes of central canal stenosis include physical abnormalities that are present at birth, prolapsed discs or osteoarthritic bone spurs that protrude into the spinal canal.
- **Sciatica** The sciatic nerve is the largest nerve in your body and the main nerve travelling down your leg. A pinched sciatic nerve in your lower back, which may be caused by a prolapsed disc or a bony spur pressing against the nerve, is one of the most common causes of referred pain. Sciatic pain radiates all the way down from your lower back to your toes.

a visit to

THE OSTEOPATH OR CHIROPRACTOR

Osteopaths and chiropractors physically manipulate joints and tissues to relieve a wide range of musculoskeletal conditions. The two therapies take a very similar approach, although chiropractors tend to focus more closely on the spine.

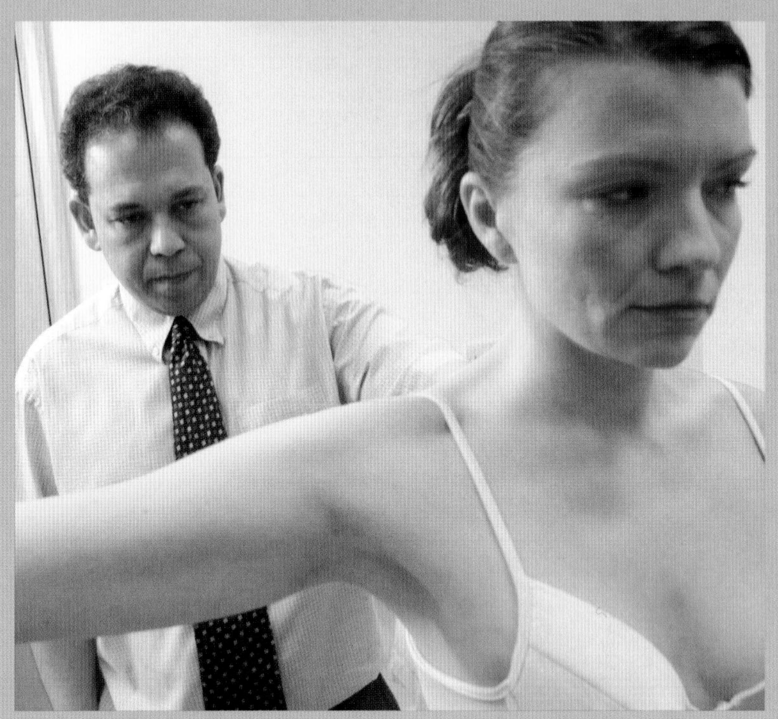

Although osteopathy and chiropractic are complementary therapies, most conventional medical professionals recognize them as an effective way to treat many back problems. The UK Clinical Standards Advisory Group recommends both therapies in its advice to GPs. Therapists should not treat certain conditions, such as severe osteoporosis.

If you feel you could benefit from visiting an osteopath or a chiropractor, your GP may be willing to refer you to a suitable practitioner. Alternatively, contact the General Chiropractic Council (GCC) or the General Osteopathic Council (GOsC) for details of registered therapists in your area – all osteopaths and chiropractors have to be registered with these professional bodies by law.

A session normally lasts around 20–30 minutes. The number of sessions that you will need varies considerably depending on your problem, but two to ten sessions is normal, initially every week or so. Most practitioners charge £20–£30 for a consultation.

Initial consultation At your first consultation the osteopath or chiropractor will examine you to diagnose any problems and may use X-rays or other tests. An osteopath may also use touch (palpation) to identify points of weakness and problem areas and will check overall postural balance. The osteopath may ask you to remove some clothes and perform a series of movements.

Manipulation Osteopaths and chiropractors use many of the same techniques. A chiropractor will tend to focus on your back and place more emphasis on freeing up and mobilizing the spinal column. An osteopath will tend to manipulate limbs, joints and soft tissues all over your body. Neither treatment should be painful, although some people experience minor side effects such as muscle soreness.

Aftercare After manipulating or massaging your back, the osteopath or chiropractor may show you how to achieve better posture and give you advice on changing any aspects of your life that are making your problem worse. The therapist may also teach you some simple exercises that you can do at home to relieve pain and stop problems recurring.

>> **Complementary therapies for your back:** page 184 >> **A visit to the physiotherapist:** page 243

Minimizing the symptoms of back problems

Most episodes of back pain resolve in time without the need to visit your GP. In the longer term, however, problems often recur. This may be because the immediate cause of the pain – a muscle spasm, sprain or strain, for example – is merely a symptom of a wider problem such as muscle weakness or postural misalignment.

For this reason it is important not to ignore the long-term treatment of back pain. Simple first-aid measures such as rest, heat treatment or over-the-counter analgesics can help relieve immediate symptoms. Persistent back pain may need professional treatment from a specialist such as a physiotherapist or an osteopath. For further information about low back pain >>301

First-aid treatment

Cold treatments such as ice packs may help to reduce swelling and inflammation from back strains and sprains during the first 72 hours or so after injury. Wrap the ice pack in a towel rather than placing it directly on your skin and apply for no more than 20–30 minutes every couple of hours. Once the initial swelling subsides, heat treatments such as warming packs, hot water bottles or hot baths may help to ease muscle spasm and block the sensation of pain.

Painkillers

Non-prescription painkillers such as paracetamol are often useful in the short term to relieve back pain. Certain painkillers, known as non-steroidal anti-inflammatories (NSAIDs) also reduce the inflammation that often accompanies back injuries, strains and arthritic conditions. Unfortunately some NSAIDs, including ibuprofen, have been linked to an increase in the risk of heart attacks. For more information, see box >>280.

Avoid taking painkillers for long periods. Long-term use of painkillers to control chronic back pain may indicate that you need higher doses to achieve the same effect. If you need to use painkillers for more than a few days you should see a doctor to determine the underlying problem.

Rest and activity

Doctors used to recommend bed rest for almost any back problem and there is no doubt that rest is important. Lying down reduces pressure on your spine and prevents friction between inflamed bones and discs. However, doctors now understand that extended periods of bed rest can actually slow recovery and increase the risk of problems recurring. Complete rest may be recommended during the acute phase (the first day or so after an injury) or during painful flare-ups of chronic conditions. But as a general rule, it is vital to get mobile again as quickly as possible.

Light activity encourages circulation (which aids healing), improves flexibility and maintains strong muscles around your spine. A number of studies have found that people with back pain who get back to normal activities quickly feel healthier, take fewer painkillers and are less distressed than those who limit their activities.

Back supports

You should never wear back or neck braces for extended periods unless specifically advised to do so by your GP or specialist. Long-term use of such supports stops you using your muscles and they will quickly start to atrophy, placing you at much greater risk of further injury.

Sports and activities

Although exercise is a great way to relieve painful backs, certain activities do have potential risks. Sports that involve constant impact, such as jogging, can aggravate low back pain and contact sports such as football can be dangerous if you have neck problems. Cycling can easily jar your back, particularly when riding over rough terrain or if your seat is set at the wrong angle or your bike is the wrong size. On the other hand, certain activities bring real benefits. Good sports for bad backs include:

- **Swimming** and other water-based activities such as aquaerobics are useful because water counteracts some of the effects of gravity, reducing compression in your lower spine. Swimming is very low

DID YOU KNOW?

- **The longer you are off work with back pain, the lower your chances of returning to work at all – only half of those who take six months off return to work; once you've been off for a year your chances of getting back to work are only 5 per cent.**
- **An eight-week study at Queensland University found that important postural muscles become switched off during bed rest. In all 19 previously healthy volunteers, the lumbar multifidus muscles (the muscles that keep the vertebrae in position in the lower back) grew wasted and inactive.**

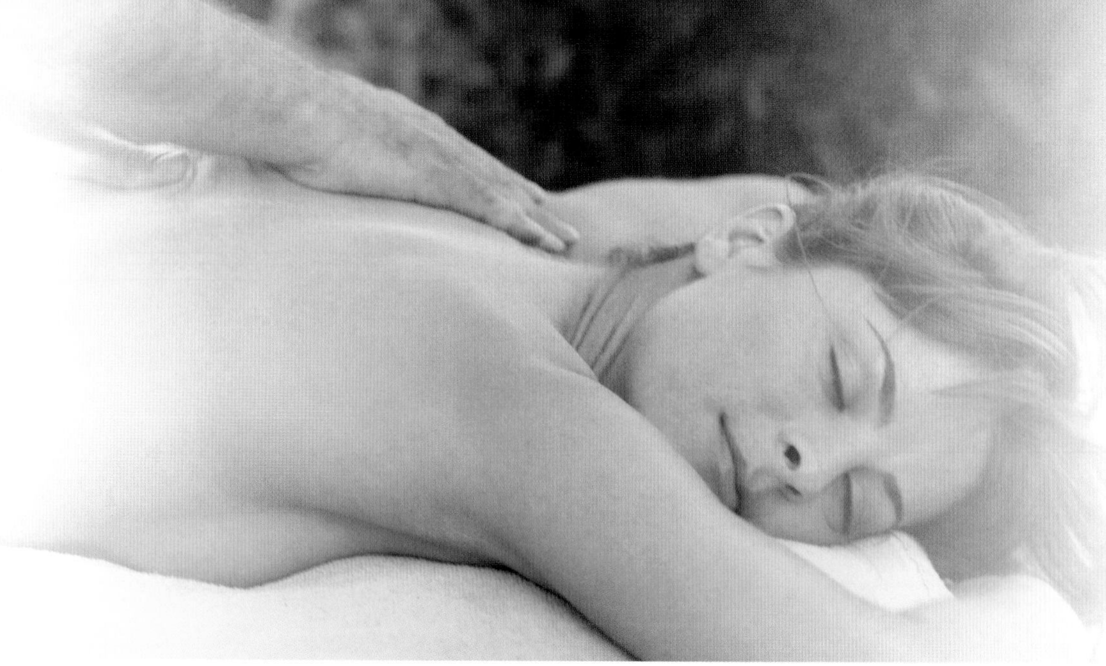

impact and warm water can help to ease muscle spasm. Backstroke is particularly beneficial as it opens up the chest and shoulders. For more information >>86–87.

- **Walking** is low-impact and helps to strengthen your back and stomach muscles without placing them under too much strain. Try to walk with your body held tall and always wear supportive, well-cushioned boots or shoes. For more information >>90–91.
- **Exercise balls** can help you to target your core muscles. The ball places you in an unstable position, so you automatically engage the muscles in your abdomen, back and pelvic-girdle region. These are the core muscles that support your lower back and spine, help you to maintain posture and control your twisting, reaching and bending movements.
- **Tai chi and yoga** are both enjoyable ways to improve mobility, flexibility and muscle tone. The deliberate, flowing movements of tai chi and the controlled stretching required by the yoga poses encourage good postural awareness without straining or jarring your back. For more information, >>92–93 and 96–97.

Physical therapy

Many of the most common causes of back pain, such as muscle spasm and muscular tension, misaligned vertebrae and some postural problems, respond well to physical manipulation. Common types of physical therapy for problem backs include:

- **Massage** to improve circulation, aiding muscle recovery, and reduce tension. There is much to be said for a relaxing rub down from a friend or loved one but there are also a number of professional massage techniques which may particularly help your back. These include neuromuscular therapy, a technique which focuses on areas of muscle spasm (trigger points). If you opt for a professional massage, make sure you choose a fully qualified masseur.
- **Physiotherapy**, which involves a range of physical and manipulative techniques that improve movement, strength and flexibility. Treatment should also address underlying factors that contribute to the physical problems; to get the full benefit it is vital to follow the therapist's advice outside the sessions and to practise any recommended exercises. For more information >>243.
- **Osteopathy and chiropractic**, which are specialized manipulative therapies that focus on combating structural misalignments in the musculoskeletal system. For more information >>189.

Back surgery

Surgery remains a treatment of last resort for back problems. It is unlikely to be used unless other treatments have failed and, even then, the majority of back conditions are not suitable for surgery. Conditions that may benefit from surgery include pinched or compressed nerves and vertebral deformities or fractures.

- **Tissue removal** During a laminectomy, the surgeon removes a small portion of vertebra or a bony spur to stop it pressing against your spinal cord or the nerves leaving your spine. In a discetomy, the surgeon removes a portion of an intervertebral disc such as a prolapsed disc (>>187) that is pushing against a nerve.
- **Spinal fusion** The surgeon may wish to fix two or more verterbrae together using bone grafts and metal plates, screws or rods. This may be to prevent instability from a fractured vertebrae or to correct a spinal deformity. The fused section of the spine is more stable and can bear weight better, but you lose flexibility and mobility.

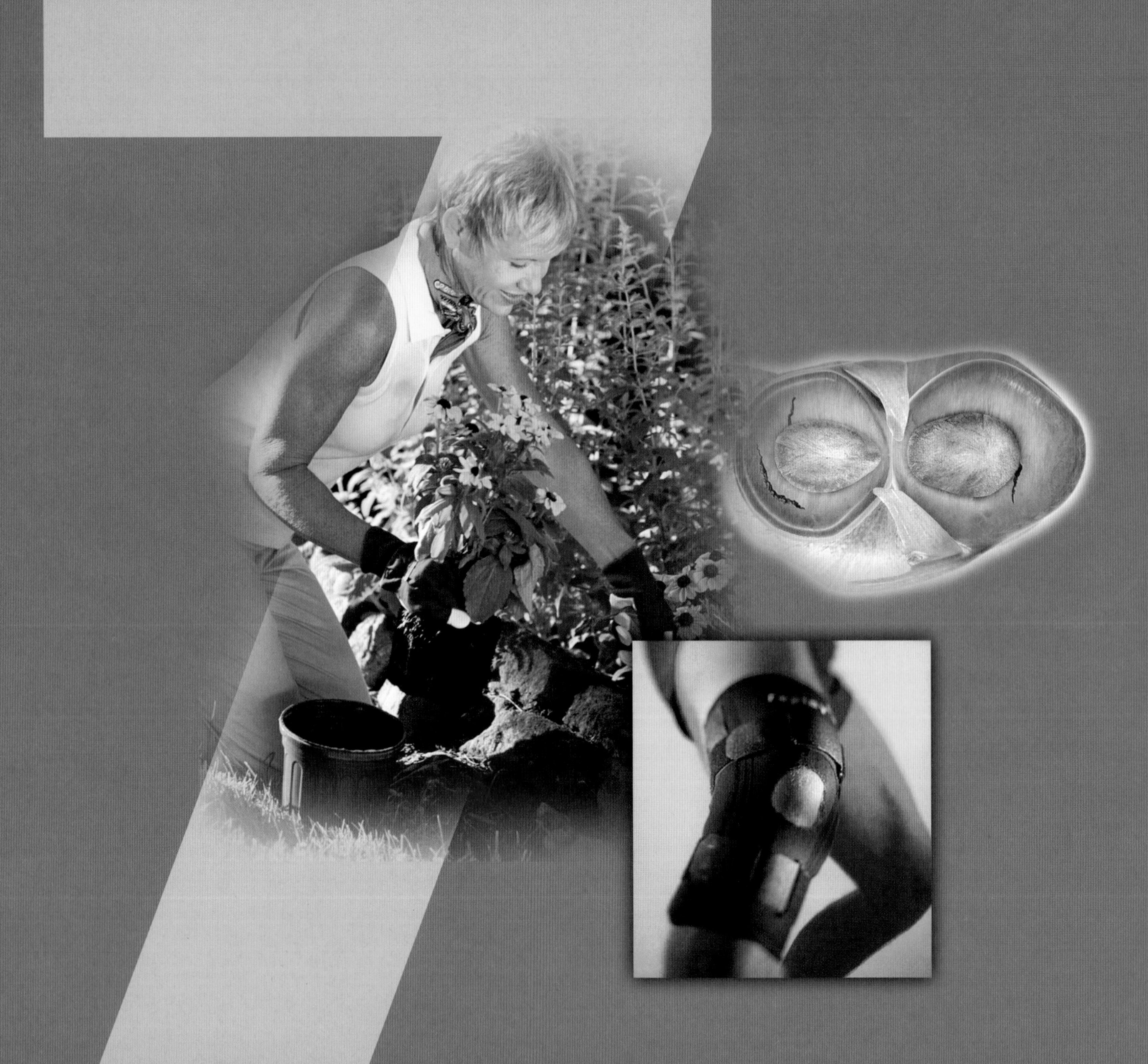

SAFEGUARDING YOUR KNEES

We subject our knees to tremendous stresses throughout life, from acute injuries suffered on the sports field to the longer-term burden of chronic conditions such as obesity. In these pages you will find out how you can maintain optimum knee flexibility for life, how to tackle any problems that might occur and the latest knee replacement techniques.

SAFEGUARDING YOUR KNEES
How your knees work

Formed by the intersection of three bones – your calf bone (tibia), thigh bone (femur) and kneecap (patella) – the knee is the largest and most complex of all the joints of your body. The knee bends with an essentially hinge-like motion; when your leg is fully extended, however, a small rotary movement locks the joint to help you balance.

From the outside, your knee looks a simple enough joint – the only visible motion as you flex and extend your leg is a straightforward back-and-forth motion, similar to the way a door opens on a hinge. Under the skin, though, the mechanism is rather more complex.

In the first place, your knee actually consists of two separate joints: one between your thigh and calf bones (around which most of your leg movement occurs) and another between your thigh bone and kneecap. In addition, the superficially simple hinge-like motion of the knee also involves a certain amount of gliding and rotation.

Controlling the movement of these joints is an elaborate arrangement of muscles, ligaments and tendons, which must all interact precisely to keep your bones in place as you move your leg. The complexity of this joint is one of the reasons why so many people suffer from persistent or unexplained knee problems.

Your bones and muscles in movement

The end of your shin bone, or tibia, has two elliptical indentations, similar in shape to the curved bottom of a wine glass. The rounded ends of your thigh bone fit into these shallow cavities, forming a joint known as a condyloid joint. It is this joint that controls the flexion and extension of your leg.

It also allows for a controlled screw-like movement. Small amounts of rotation occur with each step, locking your joint straight so that your muscles require less effort to maintain balance.

The kneecap

Your kneecap, or patella, is a disc-like (sesamoid) bone embedded into the tendons around your knee. This bone defends the knee joint against front-on injury and spreads the force of any impact.

Arteries and nerves

Several important blood vessels and nerves travel through the knee joint, including the popliteal artery, the main blood supply to your calf and kneecap. An injury such as a dislocated knee may cause damage to the popliteal artery, which can seriously impede the blood supply to your lower leg.

CARTILAGE

Two C-shaped flaps of tough, rubbery cartilage, the menisci, absorb impact and increase stability (for a plan view of the menisci >>197). The ends of your bones are covered by articular cartilage. This tissue absorbs shock and forms a low-friction surface so your bones glide smoothly over one another. The consistency is similar to the tissue in your ear lobes or on the tip of your nose.

54 Fit for life

228 Osteoarthritis

248 Rheumatoid arthritis

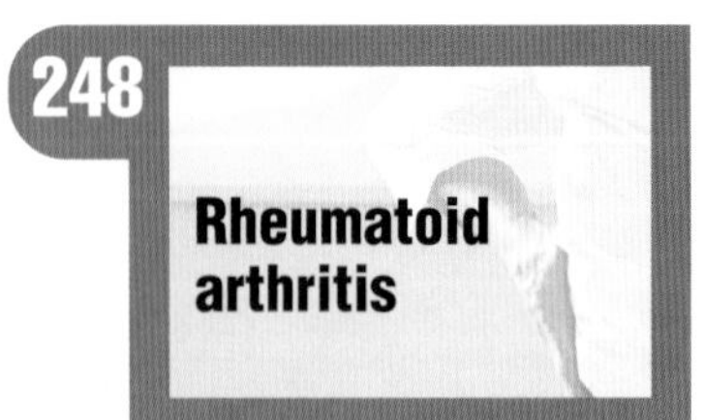

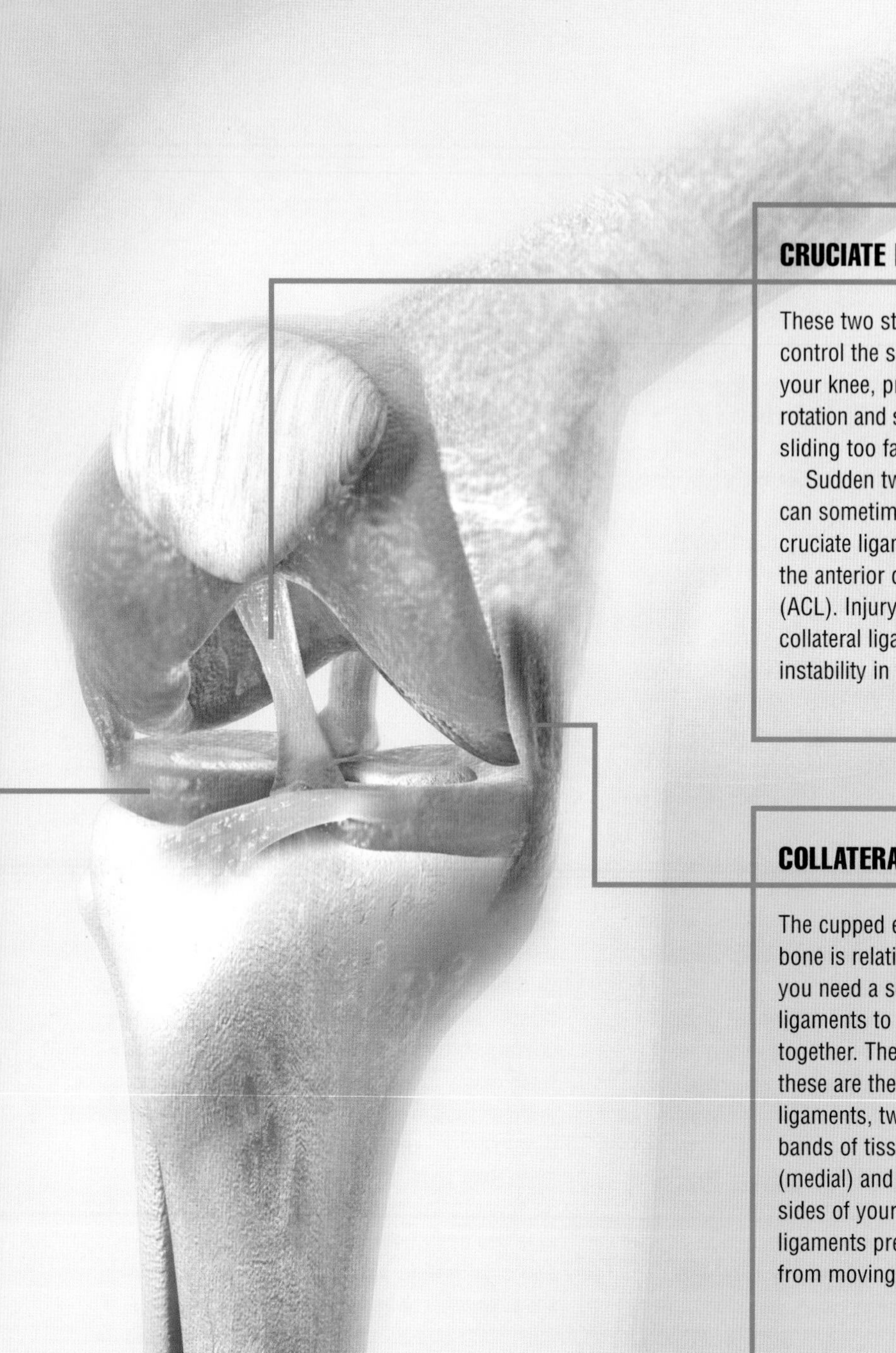

CRUCIATE LIGAMENTS

These two strong ligaments control the screw-like motion of your knee, preventing excessive rotation and stopping your bones sliding too far forward or back.

Sudden twisting movements can sometimes tear your cruciate ligaments, particularly the anterior cruciate ligament (ACL). Injury to cruciate or collateral ligaments may cause instability in your knee.

COLLATERAL LIGAMENTS

The cupped end of your shin bone is relatively shallow, so you need a series of strong ligaments to hold the knee together. The most important of these are the collateral ligaments, two very strong bands of tissue on the internal (medial) and external (lateral) sides of your joint. These ligaments prevent your knee from moving sideways.

The joint between your kneecap and your thigh bone is known as a gliding joint because the flat surfaces of the joint allow only sliding or back-and-forth motion.

When you straighten your leg, your kneecap presses back into a special groove in your thigh bone. This stops the tendons that attach the muscle to the bone from dislocating sideways, helping to make your joint more stable.

Muscles

The muscles in your thighs power movement around your knee joint. Strong muscles also maintain knee stability – one reason why most sport injuries occur when athletes are tired.

- **Quadriceps** This is the largest of the muscle groups around the knee. It consists of four main muscles that stretch along the front and sides of your thigh and connect to the kneecap via the patellar tendon. Your quadriceps muscles work together to straighten your leg at the knee.
- **Hamstrings** Your hamstrings run directly behind your thigh bone and connect the thigh bone to the bones in your calf. They bend and rotate your leg, control the deceleration of your knee and help your foot to land smoothly.

Your joint capsule

The knee joint is surrounded by a capsule, which consists of a tough fibrous membrane on the outside and a thin synovial membrane, similar to the lining on the inside of your mouth, on the inside. Within this capsule, the joint is lubricated with clear, viscous synovial fluid, similar to saliva. Diseases such as rheumatoid arthritis and gout cause inflammation in the synovial cavity.

Common knee injuries

Knee injuries vary greatly with age and activity. Problems are relatively rare during childhood, although still-growing bone tissue can cause problems. The most frequent knee injuries in young adults are sports related, such as tears of the menisci or ligament injuries. Fractures around the joint are more common in older patients with weak bones.

The structure of the knee and the demands placed on the joint during strenuous activities make it one of the most frequently injured joints in adolescents and young adults. Sports-related injuries include sprains (a stretched or torn ligament) and strains (torn muscles or tendons). Most mild sprains and strains heal well with rest; more serious injuries may need to be immobilized using a cast or, more rarely, operated on. Tears to the menisci, the flaps of cartilage that cushion your joint surfaces, are also common.

As you grow older, the bones around your knee may become weak due to osteoporosis, making them more likely to fracture and causing serious joint problems. As the cartilage covering and cushioning your joint surfaces wears down over time, you are also more likely to develop osteoarthritis – around 40 per cent of people over the age of 75 suffer from some degree of knee osteoarthritis. For more information about these conditions >>228–247 and 264–275.

Meniscal injuries

The menisci, the tough C-shaped layers of cartilage between your thigh and shin bones, are among the most frequently injured tissues in the knee. The menisci help to cushion and stabilize your knee joint and take much of the force of impact on your knee; sudden twisting or pivoting motions in your leg can tear the tissue.

Meniscal tears often cause pain and swelling in the front of the knee, although there are not always any symptoms. In some cases, a flap or a ring of cartilage may float loose inside your joint, locking your knee completely. As your menisci age they become weaker and less elastic and degenerative tears can occur with little or no trauma. Around 60 per cent of people over the age of 65 have some type of degenerate meniscal tear.

Treating meniscal problems

Minor tears on the outer edges of the menisci, where the blood supply is good, usually heal in a couple of weeks with no treatment other than resting the affected joint. Surgical removal of the damaged tissue used to be routine for more serious injuries, but this is now avoided where possible. Although patients often recover knee function well after surgery, the lack of cushioning increases wear on the cartilage covering the bone ends, meaning they have a much higher risk of osteoarthritis.

Several less drastic techniques of repair and transplant have been developed, with varying degrees of success. These include meniscal repair, where the surgeon attaches sutures to hold the edges together.

DID YOU KNOW?

- **Women are much more likely than men to suffer from ligament injuries, particularly tears to the anterior cruciate ligament or ACL (>>right).**
- **Statistics gathered by the National Collegiate Athletics Association show that female football players suffer over twice as many ACL tears as male players, and female basketball players suffer almost four times as many tears. Secondary school girls require knee surgery around five times more often than boys.**
- **This may be because women tend to have larger pelvises and therefore a larger angle between shin and thigh bones, placing greater stress on the knee. Another suggestion is that women have a narrower femoral notch (the space at the bottom of the femur through which the ACL runs).**

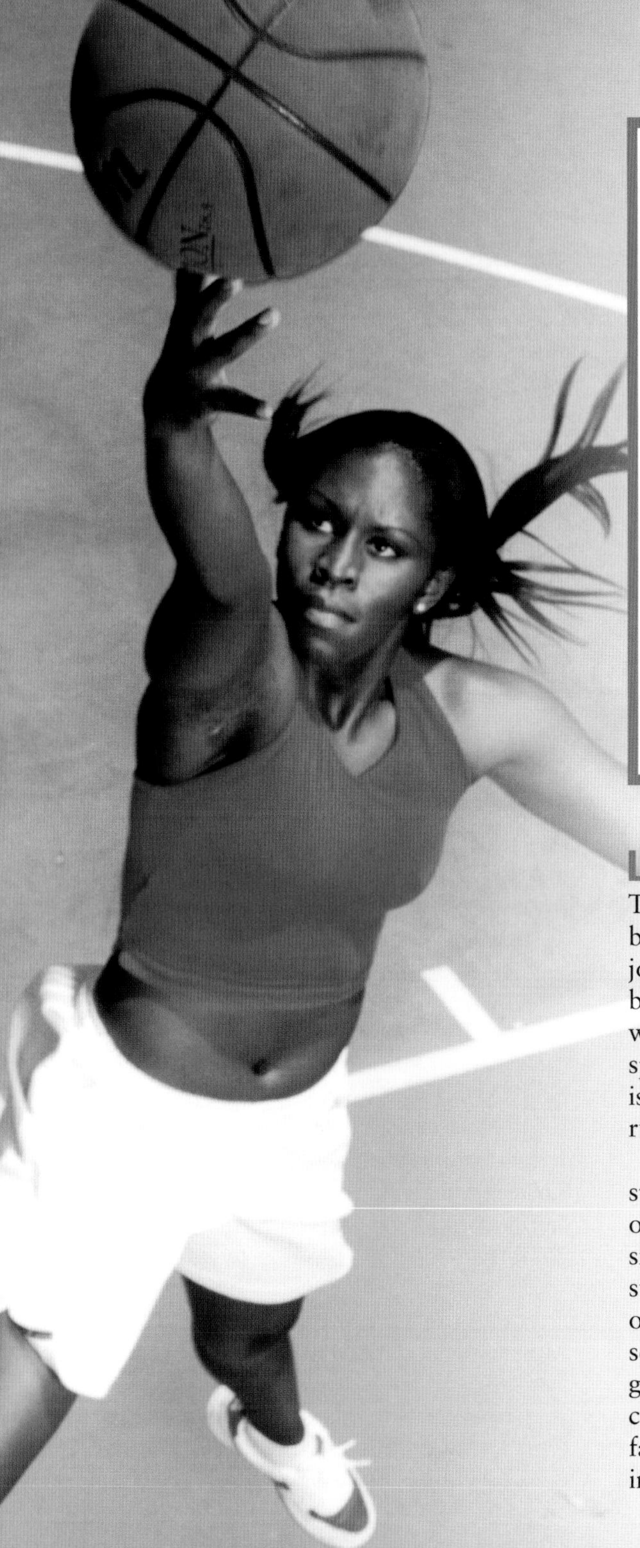

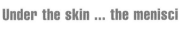

Under the skin ... the menisci

Tears in the meniscal cartilage (seen here from above) are common but can be very difficult to repair. The most important factor is the location of the tear: the outer edge of the meniscus has a good blood supply, meaning that tears heal relatively easily. The blood supply towards the centre of the tissue, however, is very poor and injuries along the inner edge heal very slowly, if at all.

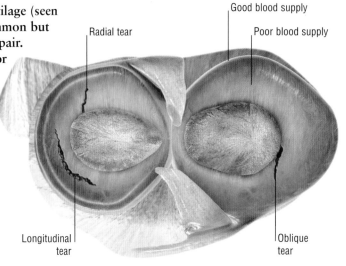

Ligament injuries

These strong bands of tissue fasten the bones in your knee together and keep your joint stable. A healthy ligament can stretch by around 5 per cent of its regular length without damage – any further and it may sprain or rupture. In a sprain the ligament is stretched or partially torn; in a complete rupture the ligament may be severed.

Torn ligaments often occur during strenuous activities, such as contact sports or exercises involving twisting or side-to-side movements. Particularly risky are sudden, forced, twisting motions, which often occur in sports such as basketball or squash, where one foot is planted on the ground and the rest of your body rotates clockwise and back. A sudden knock or a fall can also cause an injury. For more information about ligament tears >>299.

Anterior cruciate ligament (ACL)

This is one of the most serious types of ligament injury, because it restricts mobility and can be very slow to heal. Your ACL limits the twisting and forward motion of your knee. If you tear this ligament you may feel a ripping sensation or hear a pop in your knee. It will probably be painful and may quickly swell. Your knee may give way and feel unstable, particularly if you attempt to stand or put weight on it. In most cases, you will have to stop any physical activity.

Because your ACL keeps your knee stable, a damaged ACL makes your knee more vulnerable to other injuries. Around 50 per cent of ACL tears are accompanied by cartilage tears and 20–30 per cent involve damage to other ligaments.

Do I have a ligament sprain?

If you answer 'yes' to any of the following questions, you may have sprained a ligament in your knee. Seek advice from your doctor.

YES	NO	
☐	☐	Did you feel a popping or snapping sound in your knee at the time of injury?
☐	☐	Does the pain seem to come from inside your joint, rather than from the surface of your knee?
☐	☐	Does your knee feel loose or unstable, as though it might give way if you put your full weight on it?
☐	☐	Does swelling or bruising persist for more than a few hours after the time of injury?
☐	☐	Can you feel any fluid behind your kneecap?

QUESTIONNAIRE

Treating ligament problems

Mild ligament sprains usually heal well after a period of rest. Follow the RICE procedure (>>204) to reduce pain, bruising and swelling. Pain usually lasts around five to seven days and should ease a little each day. If you have a more serious sprain, your doctor may prescribe painkillers, anti-inflammatories or a programme of exercises to strengthen the joint – strong quadriceps muscles will help to prevent your knee from sliding forward.

Serious ligament injuries, including most types of anterior cruciate ligament tear, are unlikely to heal by themselves. If you wish to continue high-level athletic activities you may opt for surgical reconstruction, but many patients prefer simply to give up sports that place stress on the knee. If you choose surgery you'll need to commit to a programme of rehabilitation and accept the small but real risk of complications such as infection, stiffness and scarring >>208–209.

Other common knee problems

A number of other conditions can cause nagging aches and pains in your knee – certain knee problems are particularly common among specific age groups and genders or among people who practise certain hobbies or activities.

> 'Around 75 per cent of all sports-related injuries involve the legs – and one third of these are injuries to the knees'

- **Tendinitis** Irritation of the tendons – the stiff cords that attach your muscles to bone – can cause pain or swelling in the front of your knee or just below your kneecap, particularly during running, jumping or climbing activities. Athletes such as runners and cyclists are especially prone to inflammation of the patellar tendon, the tendon that connects your quadriceps to your shin bone. For more information about tendinitis >>330.
- **Bursitis** Inflammation of the bursae – the small sacs of fluid that help your tendons and ligaments glide smoothly over the joint – causes pain and tenderness on the inside of your knee, usually around 5cm (2in) below the joint. Bursitis often results from prolonged periods of kneeling, and the condition is more common in carpet fitters, plumbers and gardeners. It can occur in athletes such as runners (the condition is sometimes called runner's knee) and may be caused by overstraining. Bursitis is also associated with osteoarthritis of the knee in older patients. For more information >>283.
- **Dislocated kneecap** This occurs when your kneecap slips slightly out of position – the kneecap is then pushed sideways each

time you contract your quadriceps, compressing it against your thigh bone. You may be able to see or feel the dislocation and you will probably feel pain or swelling and have difficulty straightening your knee. Strengthening the muscles around your knees, specifically your vastus medialis (the quadriceps muscle along your inner thigh) should improve the balance and function of your kneecap. For more information about dislocated joints >>288

- **Osgood-Schlatter disease** Children and teenagers, particularly boys, sometimes suffer from a type of growing pain in the knee. Osgood-Schlatter disease causes pain and swelling in a bony prominence called the tibial tuberosity, which is located just under the knee in the centre of the shin bone. Symptoms usually improve with rest and should disappear completely once bones stop growing. For more information about Osgood-Schlatter disease >>308.
- **Chondromalacia patellae** Stress on the joint between your kneecap (patella) and thigh bone can soften and deform the cartilage between the bones. This causes pain and stiffness and sometimes a clicking sensation when your knee is bent. This condition is most common in very active teenagers. Mild cases should resolve with rest but severe cases may require surgery. For more information >>286.

Chronic knee conditions

Pain or stiffness that is present for several weeks and does not appear to be caused by an accident or injury may be due to chronic inflammation of the joint. For more details, see the pages on osteoarthritis (>>228–247), rheumatoid arthritis (>>248–263) and gout (>>294).

? Do I need medical attention?

Most minor strains and sprains heal without any formal treatment after a period of rest. If you tick 'yes' to any of the following questions, however, you should get your knee checked by a doctor.

YES	NO	
☐	☐	Does your knee fail to respond to RICE treatment (rest, ice, compression, elevation)?
☐	☐	Has your knee been painful for more than two weeks?
☐	☐	Can you feel any sharp, shooting pains in your leg while you are resting?
☐	☐	Do you limp when you walk?
☐	☐	Can you see or feel any sort of deformity in your knee?
☐	☐	Can you feel any numbness or tingling in your knee, lower leg or foot?
☐	☐	Do your lower leg, foot or toes feel cold or have they turned blue?
☐	☐	Do your lower leg, foot or toes feel hot and red?
☐	☐	Is the knee pain accompanied by any feelings of weakness, sickness or fever?
☐	☐	Do you suffer from recurrent knee pain?

QUESTIONNAIRE

Your weight and knee health

The anatomical structure of your knee joints means that even relatively small increases in body weight can greatly increase the stress placed on your knees. Being overweight significantly increases your risk of joint injury and exacerbates the effects of general wear and tear on your knees. It may also aggravate any existing joint conditions.

Your knees and hips are the main weight-bearing joints in your body. Of these two joints, your knees are particularly vulnerable to injury because the weight of your upper body is conducted and amplified by the bones in your thighs. Your centre of gravity is located roughly around the level of your navel and the distance between this point and your knees acts as a kind of lever, magnifying the effects of gravity on your knees as you walk.

This means that the forces applied to your knees during normal walking may reach four or five times your actual body weight. During more strenuous sporting activities – when you place your joints at unusual angles or land hard on the ground – the forces on your knees may be up to 12 times your normal body weight. These everyday stresses on your joints mean that even small increases in your body weight can have a significant impact on your likelihood of damaging your knees.

DID YOU KNOW?

- **Excess weight accounts for around half of all operations to repair the cartilage in the knee.**
- **According to a study at the University of Utah in 2005, men with a body mass index of 27.5 and women with a BMI of 25 (just over the healthy range) are three times more likely to suffer from meniscal tears than those with a BMI under 25.**
- **Being just 1kg (2.2lb) overweight can increase your chance of developing osteoarthritis by as much as 10–15 per cent.**

What can go wrong?

Evolution has developed some ingenious mechanisms to protect your joints from wear and tear. The layers of cartilage covering your joint surfaces and the pads of cartilage (menisci) between your bones help to distribute your body weight evenly around the joint. The synovial fluid in your knee capsule has an important lubricating effect – when you stand upright, the fluid forms a thin film between your joint surfaces, reducing friction almost to nothing, spreading the weight and preventing direct contact between your bones. The circulation of fluid is also important to keep the cartilage cells lining your joint healthy, since the cartilage tissue contains no blood vessels.

If these mechanisms work properly, your knees should stay largely problem free. Unfortunately, over-use of your joints, joint injuries, and inflammatory or infectious diseases can damage or wear down the cartilage covering your knees.

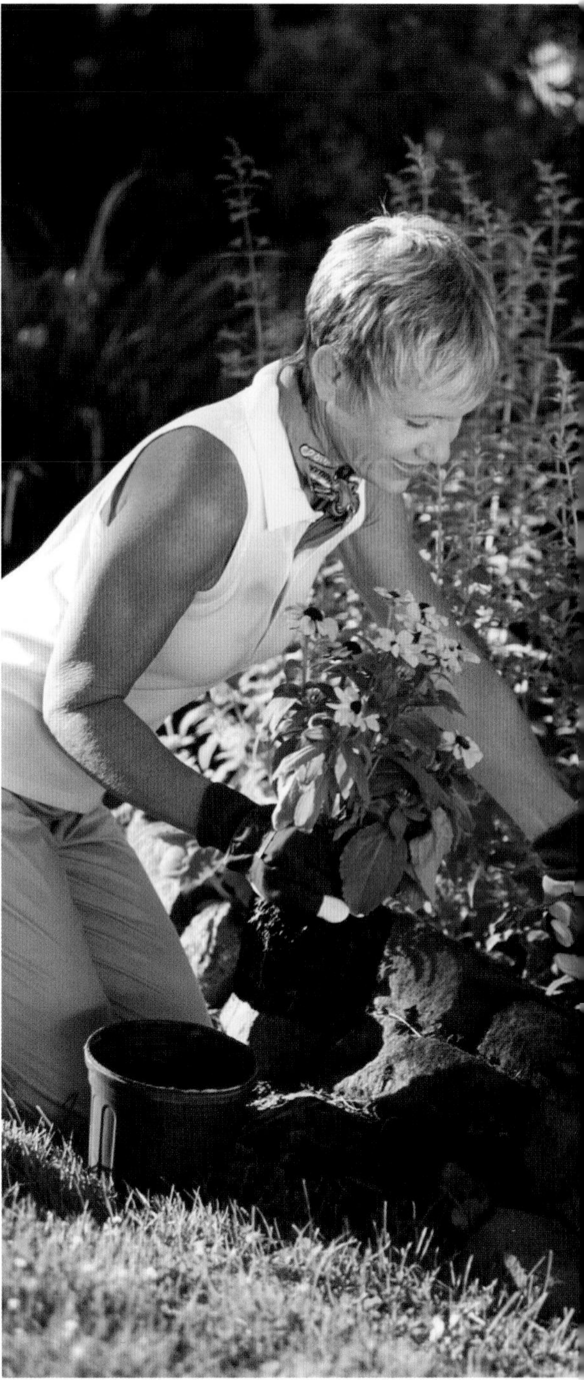

Am I at risk from knee injuries?

Q I'm a keen gardener. Am I at risk?

A Long periods spent kneeling can cause bursitis (inflammation of the lubricating fluid sacs in your knee) or push your kneecap out of alignment. People with professions that involve a lot of kneeling, such as plumbers and carpet fitters, often have problems.

Q Does my weight increase my risk?

A Excess weight places more pressure on the muscles, ligaments and tendons that support and protect your knee, making injuries such as sprains and strains more likely. It also increases wear on the cartilage in your knee, making you more likely to develop osteoarthritis as you grow older.

Q Is my child likely to have problems?

A Growing bones below the knee can cause pain and swelling – a condition known as Osgood-Schlatter disease. This condition is particularly common among active 10–15-year-old boys. Chondromalacia patellae, swelling of the cartilage under the kneecap, is also more common in active teenagers.

Q I do a lot of running. Are there any problems I should watch out for?

A High-impact sports such as running and basketball are associated with a range of knee problems including bursitis (or runner's knee), shin splints and Achilles tendinitis.

Q What about other sports?

A Sports that involve twisting and pivoting motions, such as squash or basketball, put a lot of strain on the tissues that stop your knee slipping sideways, making you more likely to suffer ligament or meniscus tears. Female athletes are at particular risk.

Q I'm slightly bow-legged and I've heard this can increase my risk of some knee conditions. Is this true?

A Rolling your feet too much as you walk (over-pronation >>50–51) and other structural misalignments of your legs can affect the distribution of weight around your joint. This will increase your risk of short-term injuries such as strains and long-term conditions such as osteoarthritis.

This can lead to meniscal tears and long-term degenerative conditions such as osteoarthritis (>>228–247). Excess body weight has a double impact on this process: it both increases the likelihood of injuries occurring in the first place and – once damage has occurred – speeds the process of degeneration.

Excess weight increases pressure and wear on your knee cartilage, intensifies the load on your supporting muscles and ligaments during activity, and amplifies the effects of any existing misalignment of your joints. Knee alignment also plays an important role in weight distribution. According to researchers at the University of Boston, in osteoarthritis sufferers who are moderately bow-legged or knock-kneed the condition is 8 per cent more likely to get worse for every two point increase in their body mass index. Patients with well-aligned knees do not face the same risk.

How much weight is too much?

Body mass index (BMI) is a good way to pinpoint the most appropriate weight range for your height. Generally speaking, a BMI of between 18.5 and 25 is associated with the lowest health risks – although very muscular people may have higher BMIs without an increased risk of medical problems. For further details >>114–115.

If your BMI is more than 25, your knees are more vulnerable to problems. Aim for a combination of a healthy, balanced diet and plenty of cardiovascular exercise – swimming, walking and cycling are good aerobic exercises that will not place too much stress on your joints.

Maintaining knee strength through exercise

Prevention is better than a cure. People tend to ignore their knees until something goes wrong, but strong, well-prepared muscles will protect your knee ligaments and menisci from excess strain and help you to avoid injuries before they occur. A good exercise programme can also alleviate pain and rehabilitate injured joints.

To ensure that your knees stay supple and injury free it is vital to keep your joints strong and flexible. Weak muscles are a leading cause of knee injuries, so it helps to strengthen your quadriceps and hamstrings, the muscles that support your knees. But it is not just the size of your muscles that is important – balance and stability training will train the muscles around your knees to work together more effectively.

Simply building up stronger muscles can actually be counterproductive, making your muscles tight and inflexible. To keep muscles supple and prevent sprains, always warm up before any strenuous physical activity. Stretch at the end of each session to stop your muscles tightening.

Muscle balance

Keeping muscles in balance is important to long-term knee function. Unbalanced muscle groups – weak hamstrings and strong quadriceps, for example – can pull your joint out of alignment.

Individual muscles within groups can also cause problems. A strong outer thigh muscle (vastus lateralis) can overpower your inner thigh muscle (vastus medialis), pulling your kneecap out of place. This creates friction and wear on your cartilage, causing knee pain and eventually even osteoarthritis. This may be a particular problem in women, because wider hips cause a greater angle of pull to the side. The straight leg raise exercise is a good way to work your vastus medialis.

Exercising with injured knees

Injuring your knee doesn't mean you have to stop being active, but it may mean that you may need to change the way you exercise. Where possible, avoid high-impact activities that jar your joints, such as running and football, or sports that involve sudden twisting or pivoting motions. Activities such as swimming and aquaerobics are a great way to maintain aerobic fitness without putting excess strain on the knees.

Who, when and where?

The exercises shown here are designed to strengthen your muscles and protect your knee joints from future injury. You could try incorporating the exercises into your regular stretch routine after exercise.

Everyone will benefit from strong joints, but people who need to pay particular attention to their knees include athletes (especially female athletes) and people who are at greater risk of injury, such as the elderly or overweight. The exercises may also be useful as part of the rehabilitation programme after injury or an operation, but you should always get proper medical advice first if you have existing injuries.

Knee extension

In this exercise you strengthen your quadriceps by straightening your leg against resistance. This uses a good range of knee motion, although you should stop before your leg reaches its full extension. Adjust the weight used to suit your strength and fitness levels – if your muscles are weak or injured, perform the exercise without any extra weight. If you have access to weights machines, a leg extension machine is a good way to perform the exercise in a safe, controlled manner.

1 Sit on a chair with your body straight and your back pressed against the back rest. Hold onto the sides of the chair seat for stability.

2 Inhale as you slowly straighten one leg until it is almost parallel to the floor. Do not lock your knees or completely straighten your leg. Hold the position for a second.

3 Slowly lower your leg back down and repeat on the other side. Perform three sets of 10 reps.

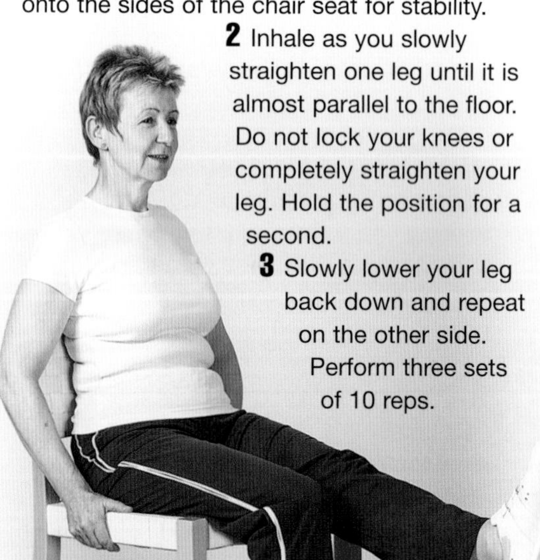

Hamstrings curl

It is important to maintain a balance between opposing muscle groups. If the muscles that straighten your leg (your quadriceps) are stronger than the muscles that bend your legs (your hamstrings), you risk straining your hamstrings. Strong hamstrings also help prevent your tibia (calf bone) sliding too far forward during knocks and falls.

Use ankle weights to perform the following exercise.

1 Lie face down on a mat with your legs straight, but not locked.

2 Inhale as you slowly bend one leg at the knee, lifting your lower leg off the mat. Continue to bend your knee until your lower leg points upwards at 90 degrees to the floor and hold your leg there for a second.

3 Slowly lower your leg back onto the mat. Perform three sets of 10 reps.

Straight leg raise

This exercise works all of the four quadriceps muscles around your knee, particularly your vastus medialis. You keep your leg straight throughout the exercise, so that your quads contract isometrically (without movement) – isometric muscle contractions help to stabilize your joints. Because your leg is straight as you lift, you can perform this exercise with a bandaged or immobilized knee.

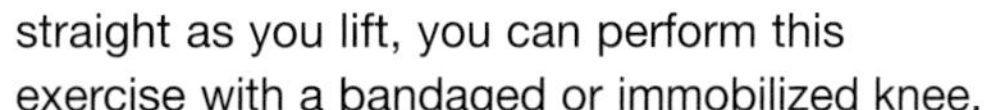

1 Lie on your back on a mat. Bend one knee and place your foot flat on the floor to stabilize your pelvis. Keep your other leg straight, without locking your knees.

2 Inhale as you slowly raise your leg about 25cm (10in) off the mat and hold your leg there for a count of three.

3 Slowly lower your leg back onto the mat. Perform three sets of 10 reps.

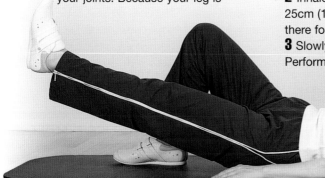

STANDING AND LATERAL JUMP

Sudden twisting and pivoting movements are a common cause of ligament and meniscus sprains. These jumping exercises use the muscles around your knee dynamically, as you would use them during sports and other strenuous activities but in a more controlled manner. They should teach the muscles around your knee to work together more effectively, reducing your risk of landing badly and twisting your knee.

- Stand with your fingers interlocked behind your head, squat down slightly and jump as high as possible. Bend your knees slightly as you land and come back down into the squatting position. Increase the number of repetitions as you get more proficient.

- Imagine a straight line on the ground heading away from you. Stand on one side of the line, about 30cm (12in) away. Jump to the side, over the line, and land with your knees slightly bent on the other side. Jump back to your original position.

Minimizing symptoms if problems occur

Although they are often painful, most minor knee injuries heal well by themselves and are easy to treat at home using basic first aid, over-the-counter medicines and measures to prevent the symptoms worsening. Even more serious knee problems will usually respond well to these measures, although you should get you knee checked by a doctor too.

There are a number of simple, self-help measures you can take, both at the time of the injury and in the days or weeks following, to reduce symptoms and minimize pain in your knees. These steps are not a substitute for proper medical treatment or advice, but they are sufficient to treat most minor injuries and are unlikely to cause further problems if your injuries do turn out to be more serious.

If you have any persistent or long-term problems with your knees, you should always seek professional help before starting any programme of home treatment or exercise. If there is any suggestion that you may have a fractured bone in your knee, you should get it checked out at a hospital. For more detailed advice about treating the symptoms of chronic knee conditions such as osteoarthritis and rheumatoid arthritis >>228–263.

Remember RICE

Almost all acute (rapid onset) knee injuries, such as sprains, strains and painful knocks, will cause much less pain and swelling if they are treated immediately using RICE treatment. The acronym RICE stands for rest, ice, compression and elevation.

- **Rest** will give injured tissues time to recover; using a joint too soon after injury can increase any tissue damage. Try to keep your joint rested for 2–3 days after an injury and avoid repeating the activity that caused the problem until your knee seems to be completely healed.
- **Ice** causes blood vessels in your knee tissues to constrict, reducing swelling, bruising and inflammation in the joint. It also numbs your tissues, reducing pain. Apply ice to the joint immediately after injury and for up to 72 hours later. Wrap the ice pack in a towel rather than placing it directly against your skin and apply for a maximum of 20–30 minutes every couple of hours. A bag of frozen peas works well. Once swelling has subsided (probably no more than 72 hours later) you can change to heat treatment, such as warming packs and hot towels, to increase blood flow and reduce stiffness.
- **Compression** of your joint directly after injury also reduces swelling and bleeding and helps to limit movement. Firmly wrap a bandage around the joint but not so tight that you restrict blood supply. If you feel a strong throbbing when wrapping the joint, re-bandage it more loosely. Keep the bandage on your joint for the rest of the day following the injury but remove it at night. You can apply the wrap over or underneath an ice pack.
- **Elevation** of the joint above your heart level stops blood pooling in the affected joint, reducing swelling and bruising. Keep the joint elevated during the night following injury by sleeping with a cushion or pillow underneath your knee.

Reduce stress on your knees

Any damage to your knee, whether the result of an isolated injury or a combination of minor injuries that are starting to affect joint function, will reduce your knee's ability to deal with high-impact, joint stressing activities. Brisk twists and turns and sudden starts and stops place high demands on your knees and activities that involve these sorts of movements, especially contact sports, are best avoided.

Maintain your fitness

Although you may need to curtail some of your activities, this should not stop you from keeping fit. Activities that will help you maintain cardiovascular fitness without compromising the stability of your knees include walking, swimming, aquaerobics and cycling. Several types of gym machine are suitable for weak knees, including the elliptical trainer, rowing machine and cross-country ski machine.

Whatever type of exercise you choose, always wear good, well-fitting trainers to reduce jarring. Your knee may also benefit from some type of brace during exercise. See box, right, for more details.

It is also important to keep the muscles around your knee in good condition. After only a week of bed rest, your muscles can lose around 10 per cent of their strength. Weak muscles will make your joint susceptible to further injury. Try some of the gentle, knee-strengthening exercises shown on pages 202-203.

Consider drug treatment

A number of drugs are available over the counter or on prescription to relieve the pain and inflammation caused by a knee injury. Because these drugs only treat the symptoms of injury, it is very important that you do not neglect the underlying cause of the injury.

- **Analgesics** such as paracetamol or co-dydramol are readily available and often useful in the short term to relieve pain.
- **Non-steroidal anti-inflammatory drugs** (NSAIDs) such as aspirin, ibuprofen, naproxen and diclofenac may be used on a temporary basis to suppress inflammation and reduce pain, swelling and stiffness. Although many of these drugs are available over the counter, prolonged use can cause side effects including intestinal bleeding. A new generation of NSAIDs, the Cox-2 inhibitors, are much less likely to cause gastrointestinal problems and until recently were believed to be largely risk-free. Unfortunately, a number of studies have recently linked both Cox-2 inhibitors and some older NSAIDs (including ibuprofen) with an increased risk of heart attack. Advice on these drugs may change so you should talk to your doctor about the latest guidelines. If you are at risk of heart attacks you should avoid taking NSAIDs unless advised otherwise by your doctor.
- **Corticosteroids** similar to the hormones produced by your adrenal glands, are the most powerful anti-inflammatory drugs available. They are injected directly into your joints for short-term pain relief, but should not be used over long periods because of the risk of high blood pressure, lowered resistance to infection and weakened mucles and bone. However, one or two injections in a painful joint should not generally have any major side effects.

CAUTION

Modern painkillers suppress the pain from injured knees very effectively – but your pain is there for a reason. Pain provides a major incentive to keep your joint still – without these signals you are more likely to move or damage your joint further. You are also less likely to seek medical help. Never use pain-relieving drugs for more than two weeks without getting your doctor's advice.

ORTHOPAEDIC BRACES

Knee braces made from neoprene or other types of elasticated material are widely available in high-street sports shops and health stores. These braces stabilize your knee by supporting the natural action of your ligaments and provide warmth and compression to ease soreness and prevent swelling. Many braces have an opening around the kneecap to keep the bone in position. Special rehabilitative braces, designed to limit certain types of movement while your knee is healing, are also available, often featuring hinged plastic or metal supports.

For support braces to work well, you should wear them during any activity that puts you at risk of injuring your knee. Make sure the hinges are at the places where your knee bends and check the placement of the support regularly to make sure it hasn't moved. Don't let the braces lull you into a false sense of security – even the most advanced knee support won't protect you if you try to push your body too hard.

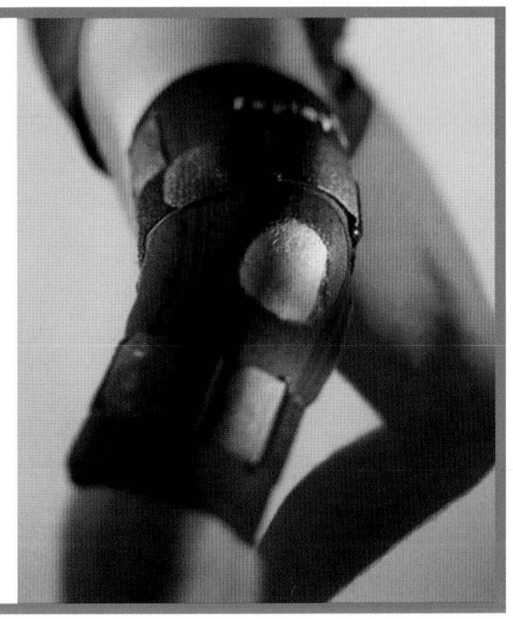

Medical advances

Surgeons are now able to reconstruct damaged joints and joint tissues more successfully than ever before. Patients experience less trauma and recover more quickly and most can expect a level of joint function that would only rarely have been achieved in the past.

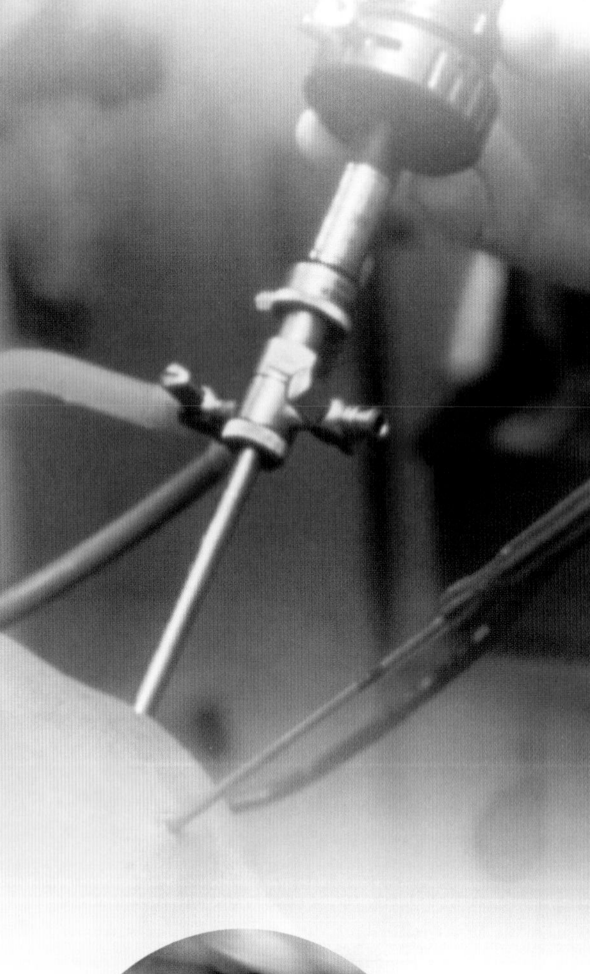

Recent developments range from new anti-inflammatory drugs and better surgical techniques to general improvements in our understanding of the body's processes. In the field of surgery, the greatest advances have been in joint replacement, keyhole surgery and the use of biomaterials such as artificial ligaments.

Arthroscopic surgery

The less injury that a surgeon causes to the tissues around the knee, the more effective the rehabilitation of the joint after surgery. As early as the 1930s, surgeons made attempts to perform surgery with minimal skin incision, but these operations were hampered by the lack of adequate equipment, both to produce images and to perform the operations necessary.

The key to the success of this type of keyhole surgery was the development of an instrument called the arthroscope in the 1960s. It has taken time and technological refinements for arthroscopy to become a truly effective surgical technique, but today it is one of the least invasive ways to diagnose and operate on knee problems.

What happens during the operation?

The arthroscope is a narrow fibre-optic tube that can be inserted into a small incision in your knee. The fibre-optic cables transport light into the joint and convey images back to a video screen by the operating table. Since arthroscopy requires only tiny incisions, many procedures are performed on an outpatient basis with only local anaesthetic.

During an arthroscopic operation, your joint is injected with a saline solution to open up space inside the joint for the instruments and protect your joint tissues from irritation. The arthroscope is then inserted into the joint, allowing the surgeon to see the interior of your knee on a monitor. The surgeon operates on your knee using instruments inserted into the joint through another small incision or, occasionally, by using precision tools mounted at the end of the scope. The surgeon can then trim, stitch or even replace damaged tissue, as appropriate.

Total knee replacement

Total knee replacement is not new – the operation has been performed worldwide for over 30 years. During this time, however, the procedure has been refined and improved. Better surgical techniques,

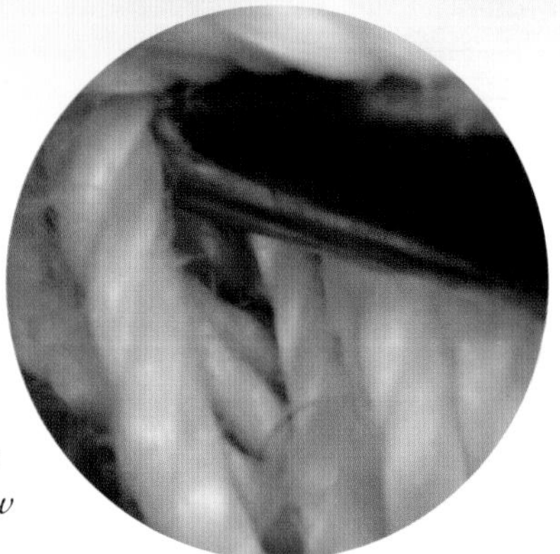

KNEE ARTHROSCOPY

A surgeon uses an arthroscope and probe to examine the inside of a knee with minimal trauma to the patient. The view through the arthroscope (shown below right) is of artificial ligament fibres, which allow doctors to reconstruct damaged ligaments.

prosthetic designs, bearing surfaces and methods of fixing the implants mean that the operation is safer, recovery is quicker, and implants last longer than ever before.

One of the most interesting recent advances in knee replacement is the development of computer assisted (CA) surgery. The components of an artificial joint must meet at precise angles to prevent premature wear, but until now surgeons have had to rely on manual measurements and their own experience to set the joint straight. Computer assisted surgery makes use of infrared cameras, digitized bone images and tracking devices to calculate exactly where the surgeon should cut with far less margin for error. For a more detailed look at the knee replacement operation >>208–209.

ACL reconstruction

There are also a number of new techniques to reconstruct damaged anterior cruciate ligaments (ACLs) under development. These include the use of artificial ligaments and the use of grafts from other tissues such as the patellar tendon and tendons of the hamstrings. The advantage of using artificial ligaments is that you don't need to lose any healthy tissue from elsewhere in your body. To date, however, no artificial materials can withstand the loads that your ACL has to bear for very long. Even the toughest artificial materials will last no more than five to seven years, depending on your level of activity.

There are several alternatives under investigation. One reason that living cartilage stays strong for so long is that your body's repair systems constantly repair minor damage. Researchers are looking into materials that will allow your body cells to grow into and fuse with the artificial tissue, forming a repairable structure. Scientists have developed several absorbable materials, designed to be slowly substituted by your body cells, although none are yet strong enough to substitute a ligament such as the AC entirely.

Most ACL reconstructions are performed under arthroscopic guidance, meaning there is minimal damage to the joint and surrounding soft tissues. You should be able to start a rehabilitation programme on the day of the operation, although it may be several months before the repairs reach full strength.

MAGNETIC RESONANCE IMAGING

Doctors have used MRI scans since the 1980s to diagnose soft-tissue damage in the knee, such as tears to ligaments and cartilage. MRI scanners use the energy from a powerful magnet to create cross-sectional images of an area of the knee – and unlike CAT scans, they can show the joint from almost any angle and produce no ionising radiation.

Recent advances in MRI technology means that it may soon be possible to assess cartilage quality and volume as well as looking for actual tears. This means MRI scans could be used to assess the likelihood of future cartilage problems, such as osteoarthritis, in the same way that bone density testing is currently used to check for future bone weakness before fractures occur.

Meniscal reconstruction

Until relatively recently, the complete removal of damaged menisci was routine. Although removal of the meniscus did alleviate the symptoms in the majority of the patients, it also deprived the knee of the cartilage's cushioning properties – as a result, many patients later developed osteoarthritis of the knee. Today, doctors avoid total meniscectomy where possible.

One of the problems with surgical treatment of your menisci is that the central portions of the tissue lack blood vessels. Rips along the periphery, where the blood supply is relatively good, can usually be rejoined and stitched using arthroscopy. Along the inner edge, where blood supply is poor, the tears tend not to heal.

Several alternative techniques have recently been developed or are undergoing research including meniscal transplant, where the surgeon replaces a damaged meniscus with a normal one from a donor. This operation relieves activity-related pain and swelling in 80–90 per cent of cases. Doctors do not yet know whether meniscal transplant will actually help to slow the development of osteoarthritis and other degenerative changes in the knee.

Cell therapy

Autologous chondrocyte implantation (ACI) is a process whereby healthy cartilage cells are harvested from a patient and then injected back into the joint to replace damaged articular cartilage (the cartilage covering the bone ends in your knee). Unfortunately ACI therapy is not suitable for treating meniscus injuries, although it may offer some relief from the chronic pain of osteoarthritis. For more information about advances in treating osteoarthritis >>246–247.

KNEE REPLACEMENT SURGERY

Knee replacement surgery (knee arthroplasty) is one of the most common surgical procedures in the UK: around 40,000 operations are performed each year. It is usually very successful in relieving knee pain – around 90 per cent of patients are left pain free or with minor, residual pain. It is, nonetheless, a major procedure. Your doctor is unlikely to recommend it unless you have long-term arthritic knee pain that does not respond to other treatments. Knee replacement surgery is not suitable for treating problems such as torn ligaments or menisci which can, in any case, often be repaired using much less invasive arthroscopic surgery >>206.

The principle of the knee replacement operation is to remove the injured cartilage and some of the bone underneath it and apply an artificial cover over the remaining bone. Depending on the condition of your knee, the surgeon may perform a total knee replacement (semi-constrained arthroplasty) or a half knee replacement (uni-compartmental arthroplasty). Half-knee replacement is used if only one side of your knee is damaged and is usually a simpler operation with a quicker recovery time.

Unfortunately, all artificial joints have a limited lifespan. Most artificial knees will last 10 years or more, even in young, active patients, but every joint will need to be replaced eventually. Subsequent operations are often less successful than the original surgery, so arthroplasty tends to be reserved for older patients who are less likely to require replacements.

1

Some time before surgery you will have a complete examination to make sure you are in good health for the operation and make some last minute checks. You may be asked to give blood so that your own blood will be on hand in case you need a transfusion during surgery.

One the day of the operation you'll be admitted to hospital. Before your operation begins the scrub nurse will check all the knee components. The nurse is responsible for making sure the surgeon gets the instruments at the right time during the operation.

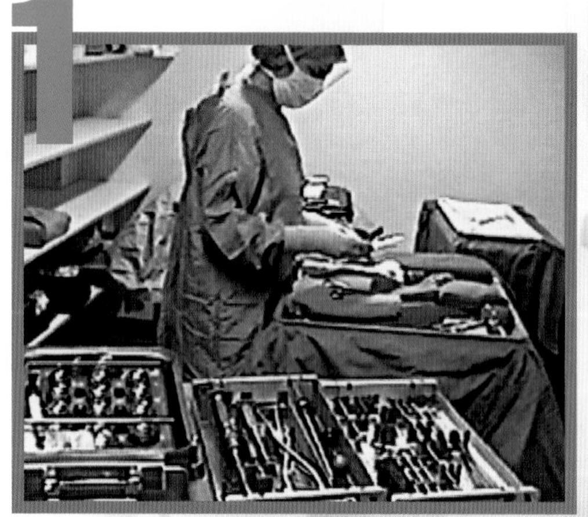

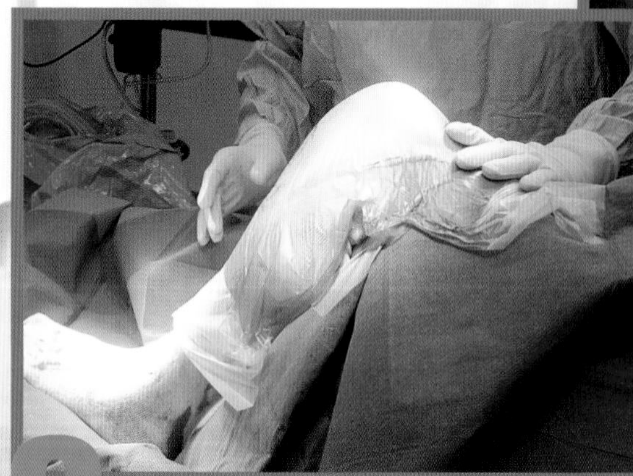

2

Knee arthroplasty is usually performed under general anaesthetic, although the anaesthetist may give you a spinal or epidural anaesthetic (when you stay awake but your leg is anaesthetised) instead. Once you are arranged on the operating table, the surgical staff will isolate your knee with sterile drapes and an iodine-impregnated stocking and draw the line of the incision on your knee.

The artificial joint...

Most joints consist of a strong metal 'femoral component' which attaches to your thigh bone; a 'tibial component' of a durable plastic (often held in a metal tray) which attaches to your shin bone; and the plastic 'patellar component' which fits under the kneecap. Some new types of joint use a ceramic alloy instead of plastic. The joint may be attached to your bones using an epoxy-type cement. Alternatively, it may have a fine mesh of holes so that your bone can grow into the mesh and fuse naturally.

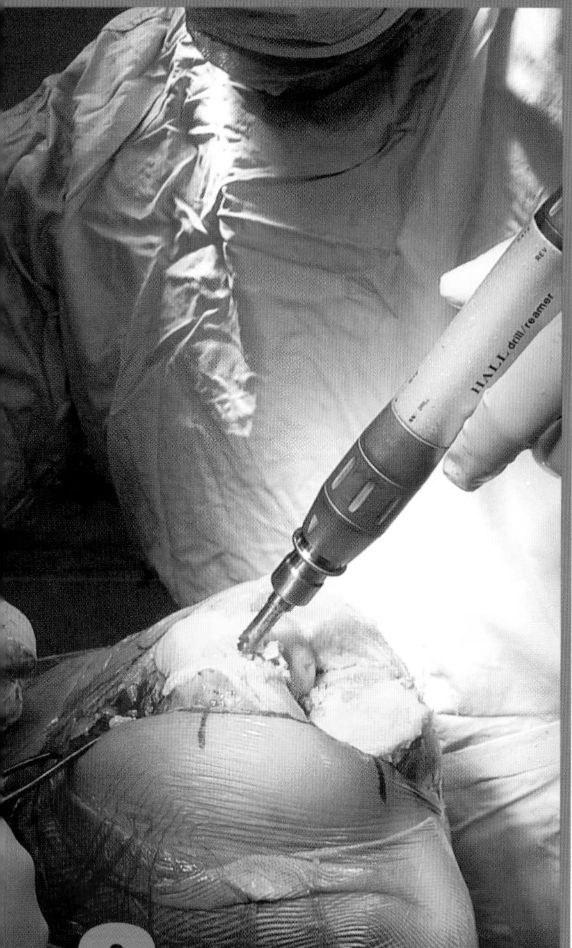

3 The operation itself should last 1–2 hours. Usually, the surgeon will make a 15–30cm (6–12in) incision down the front of your knee and move your kneecap to one side to reveal the joint. To control bleeding, most surgeons use an electric cautery device to seal the blood vessels around the incision. Worn or damaged joint surfaces are removed and the replacement joint components are attached to your bone ends, including your kneecap. In some types of knee replacement operations the surgeon replaces the entire kneecap.

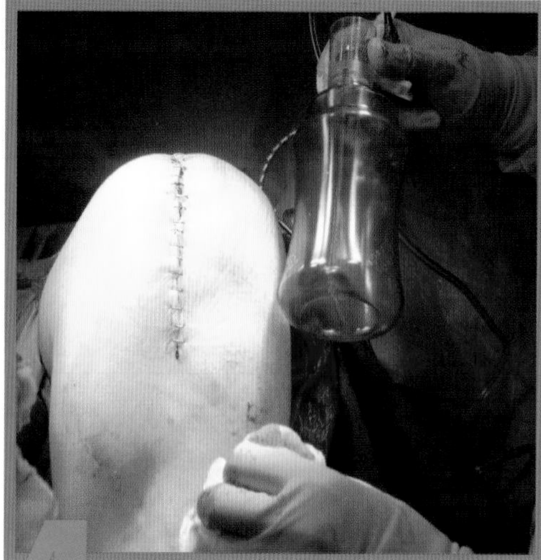

4 The surgeon closes the incision using stitches or clips. During the first 24 hours or so, you will be attached to tubes to remove fluid from your knee and a drip to supply you with fluids and pain-relieving drugs. Many hospitals now have patient controlled anaesthesia (PCA) – a button you can press to receive a fresh dose of painkillers when you feel you need relief. If everything goes smoothly, the tubes can be removed around 24–48 hours after the operation.

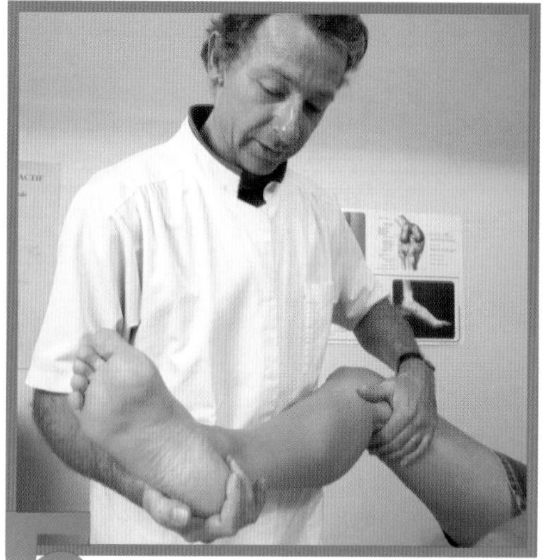

5 You will probably be able to start exercising your knee the day after surgery. The physiotherapist will show you specific exercises to strengthen your leg and restore movement. Recovery rates vary, but after 7–14 days – if you can get about on crutches and manage stairs – you should be able to go home. You will probably need crutches for another six weeks or so. It is vital to practise your exercises regularly. It will take at least six months for your knee to reach full function.

POSSIBLE COMPLICATIONS

Knee replacement surgery is relatively low-risk. Blood clots are common, affecting around half of patients, but are not usually serious. Very rarely a blood clot can travel to the lungs, which can be dangerous, so you should always follow your doctor's advice and take any measures necessary to avoid clots.

The most common major complication is infection, which occurs in 1–2 per cent of patients. An infection will prolong your recovery period, may mean the new joint has to be removed and can be life threatening. Complications such as heart attacks or strokes are rare, although certain medical conditions can make problems more likely. You should discuss any potential problems fully with your doctor before surgery.

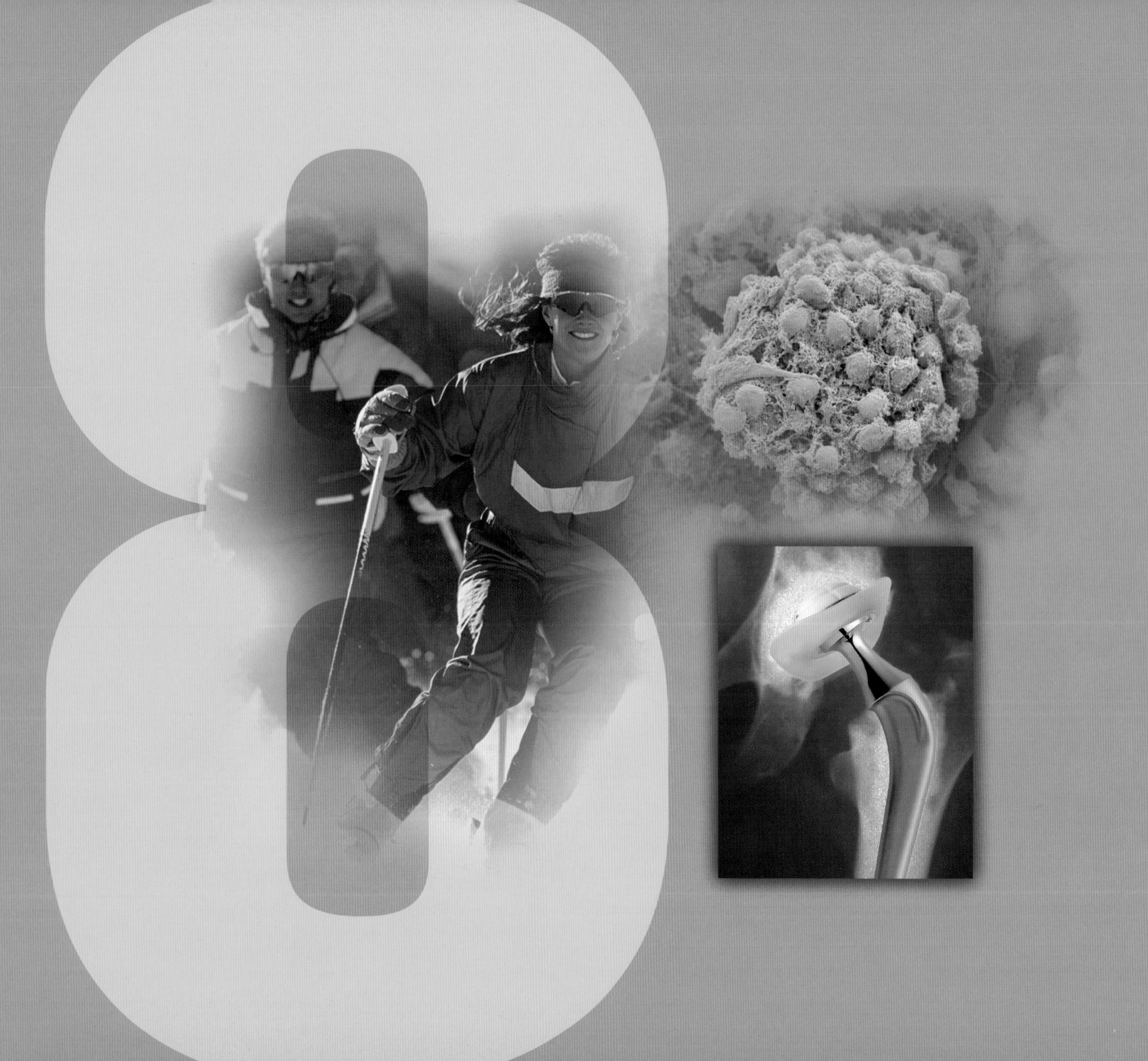

HIP HEALTH

The hips are subject to a great deal of strain, especially when weight is a problem, so it's important to understand how they work and what you can do to protect them. In these pages you will also find out how to keep your hips supple and pain free if damage has occurred, which exercises promote hip health and the self-help methods that can make life with hip problems a whole lot easier.

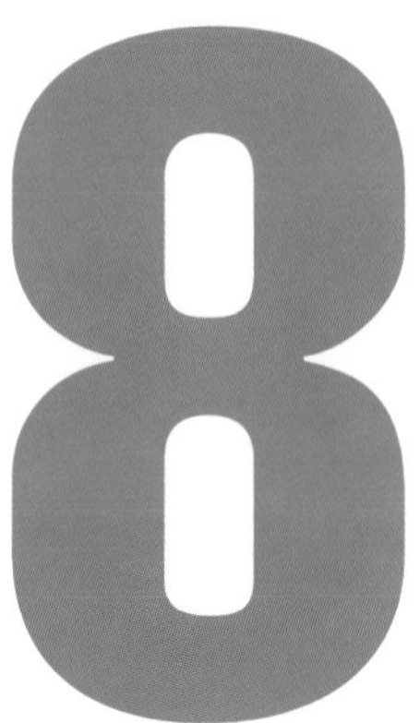

HIP HEALTH
How your hips work

Each of your hip joints is formed by the intersection of two bones, the thigh bone (femur) and your pelvis, the ring of flat bones that supports your spine and abdomen. Your hips are ball-and-socket joints, like your shoulders, so they let you move your legs in almost every direction – backwards and forwards, from side to side and in a circular motion.

14 The mechanics of movement

156 Avoiding falls and other problems

160 Improving your balance

Your thigh bones are the longest and strongest bones in your body, and the top end of each one narrows to form a 'neck' that slants inwards and ends in a round ball covered with slippery cartilage. This ball, the femoral head, fits snugly into a deep, dome-shaped, cartilage-lined socket (the acetabulum) at the side of the pelvis.

A ring of cartilage, the labrum, runs around the rim of the socket to increase its effective depth and help to keep the femoral head securely in place. In addition, the whole joint is enclosed by a fibrous membrane called the capsule, which extends from the hip socket to the neck of the thigh bone and is lined with a thin membrane. This membrane, the synovium, produces synovial fluid, a lubricant that keeps the joint operating smoothly.

The capsule consists of fibres reinforced by a number of ligaments – strong, flexible bands of fibrous tissue that anchor the thigh bone to the pelvis. The ligaments and capsule, together with the muscles of the hip, hold the femoral head tightly in its socket.

Hip stability

The mechanical demands on your hips are severe – hips must not only support the entire weight of your body but also securely transfer this weight from one leg to the other during walking, running and other movements. Despite this, dislocations of the hip are relatively rare compared to those of other joints such as the shoulder, knee and ankle.

The combination of a deep socket to securely hold the head of your thigh bone, a strong capsule and powerful ligaments and muscles means that it takes a fair amount of force to dislodge the femoral head from the socket. When hip dislocations do occur, they are usually the result of high-impact collisions: up to 70 per cent

DID YOU KNOW?

In an X-ray image of a healthy hip joint there appears to be a gap of about 6mm (¼in) between the femoral head and the socket. This is because the femoral head and the inner surface of the hip joint are both covered by a layer of cartilage that doesn't show up on the X-ray.

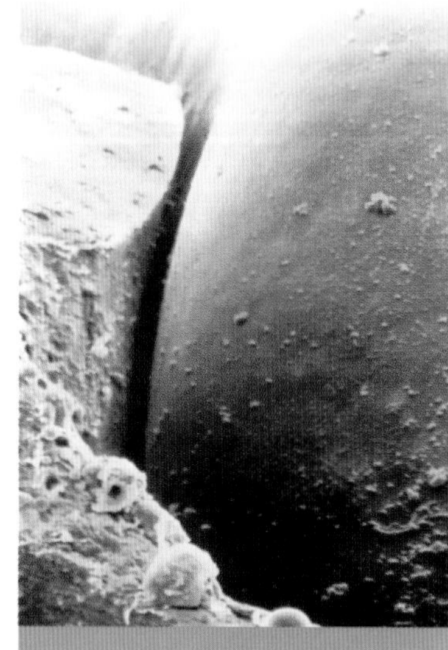

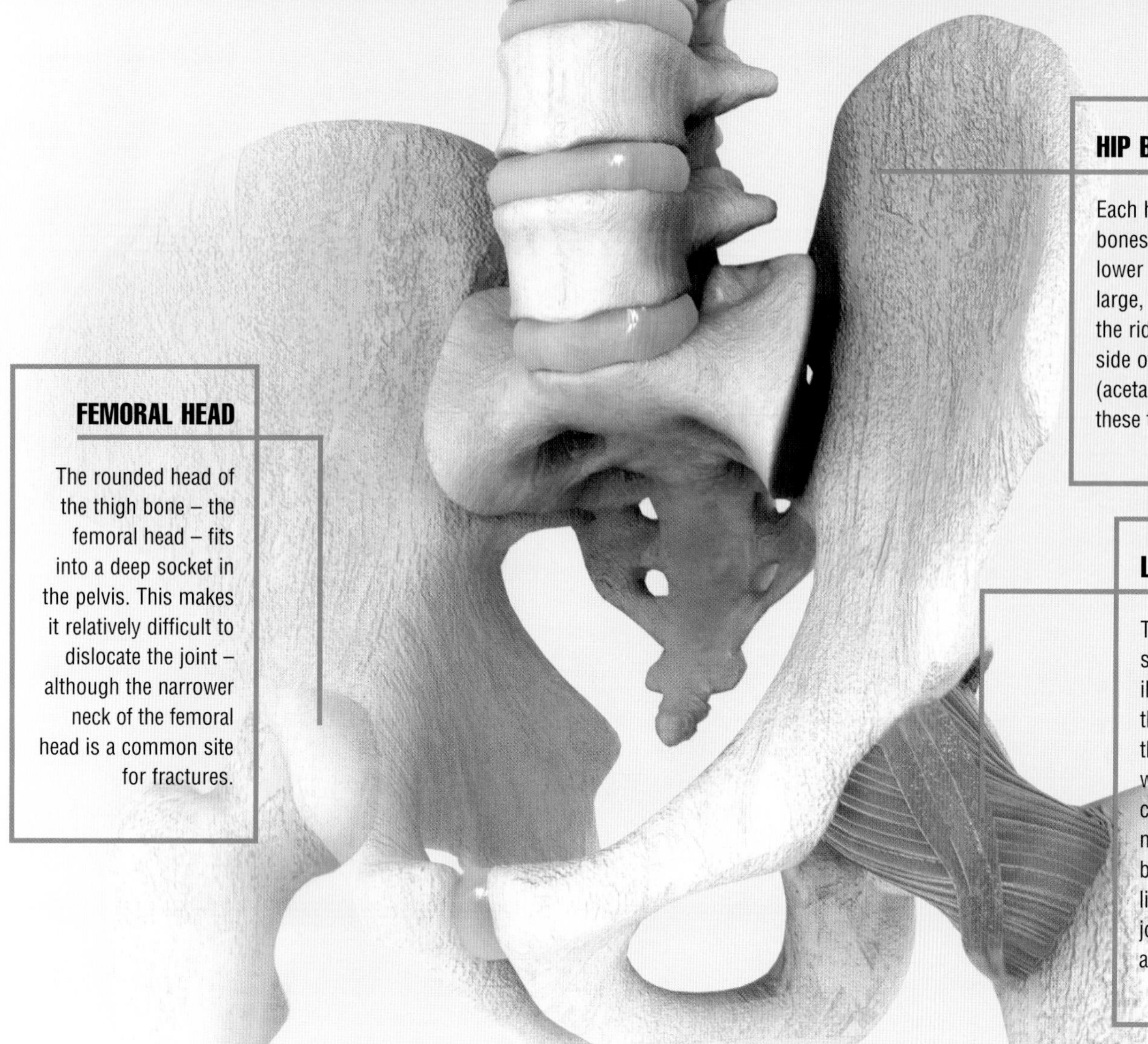

are due to road accidents. Falls from heights are another major cause, and in sport the highest numbers of hip dislocations occur in American football, rugby and skiing.

FEMORAL HEAD
The rounded head of the thigh bone – the femoral head – fits into a deep socket in the pelvis. This makes it relatively difficult to dislocate the joint – although the narrower neck of the femoral head is a common site for fractures.
HIP BONE
Each hip bone consists of three fused bones: the ischium and the pubis form the lower loop-shaped portion of the bone; the large, wing-shaped ilium juts out to form the ridge of bone that you can feel along the side of your waist. The cup-like hip socket (acetabulum) is formed at the intersection of these three bones.
LIGAMENTS
Three strong ligaments surround and support the hip joint. The Y-shaped iliofemoral ligament links the socket to the upper end of the femur. This screws the femur securely into place as you walk. The ischiofemoral ligament connects the rim of the socket to the neck of the femur and stops the hip bending too far back. The pubofemoral ligament links the pubic bone to the joint capsule and iliofemoral ligament and stops your leg moving sideways.

Hip muscles and movements

Because your hips are ball-and-socket joints, they allow movement in many different planes. The groups of muscles that encircle your hip joints enable you to move your legs forwards and backwards and from side to side, to swing them in circles and to rotate them (to point your feet towards or away from each other). These muscles are among the most powerful in your body and the main groups can be classified according to their function:

- **Hip abductors and adductors** move your legs sideways away from each other or in towards one another. The adductors also help to keep your pelvis level when you are walking or running.
- **Hip flexors and extensors** move your legs forwards and back. Tight flexors (your iliopsoas) or weak extensors (your gluteus maximus and hamstrings) can cause lower back pain by causing your pelvis to tilt forward.

- **Internal and external rotators** rotate your feet inwards (towards each other) and outwards (away from each other).

Each of these muscle groups consists of several different muscles, and muscles that have more than one function appear in more than one group. For example, the gluteus medius and gluteus minimus muscles (two of your buttock muscles) act both as internal rotators and as abductors.

The abductors

Your hip abductor muscles (primarily the gluteus medius) are very important for maintaining hip stability. The abductors are among the strongest of your hip muscles because, as well as pulling your legs outwards, they help to keep your pelvis level when you stand on one leg and when you are walking or running.

When you lift one of your feet from the ground, your pelvis tends to tilt downwards on that side, but the abductors on your stance side (the leg you are standing on) exert a powerful pull on your pelvis to keep it level. When you are walking, the abductors on the stance side pull down even harder to raise the other side of your pelvis slightly. This tilts your body towards the stance side and raises the leg that you are swinging forwards so that your toes don't drag along the ground.

Hip blood supply

Although your hips are very robust joints with strong ligaments and muscles, their blood supply is relatively fragile. Your hip socket receives blood from the arteries in your pelvis, which are well protected from damage. Unfortunately, the arteries that supply the neck of your thigh bone and the femoral head are more vulnerable to injury.

Bone cells, like other tissues such as muscle and skin, need a good supply of blood to bring the nutrients they need to stay alive and to carry away their waste products. If this flow of blood is restricted, the bone tissue in the head of your thigh bone would soon begin to die, a condition called osteonecrosis.

Vital link

The neck of your thigh bone and the femoral head get blood from two sources:

- **Circumflex arteries** This pair of arteries branches off from the profunda femoris, a large artery deep in your thigh, and passes through the hip joint capsule into the neck of the thigh bone. If you put your hand on the upper front part of your thigh, you can sometimes feel the pulse in this artery.
- **Femoral head artery** Another small artery runs through the ligament on the head of your thigh bone (the ligamentum teres femoris). This artery supplies only a very small amount of blood to the femur.

Although the blood supply through the ligament on the femoral head is limited, its contribution can be vital if something disrupts the flow of blood through the circumflex arteries. This can happen if the neck of your thigh bone is fractured or if stiffness or arthritis in your joint restricts the flow of blood from the circumflex arteries.

The small artery in the ligament can help to keep the femoral head alive until the fracture begins to heal and blood starts to flow through the circumflex arteries again.

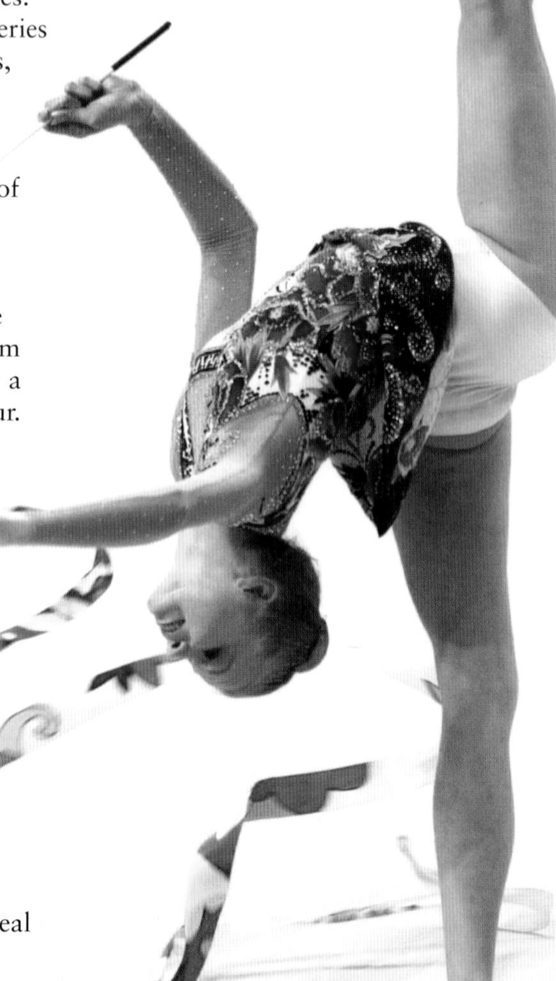

HIP SWINGS AND CIRCLES
The ball-and-socket joints of your hips allow a very wide range of movements – although only trained athletes such as gymnasts or dancers tend to have flexible enough muscles and ligaments to reach the full range of motion around the hips.

> ‘The annual incidence of hip fractures in the UK will rise from around 1.7 million to 6.3 million in 2050, say experts, unless aggressive preventative measures are taken’

The strains on your hips

Your hips are two of the hardest-working joints in your body. Everyday activities such as walking, running and even standing still will all subject them to enormous loads that can be many times your body weight.

The loads that your hip joints have to bear come not just from your body weight and the forces involved in movement, but also from the ways in which your hip muscles act to maintain your balance, even when you are standing still.

When you are standing up, your pelvis carries the weight of your body, arms and head and is in turn supported by your legs, via your hip joints. Each of your hip joints bears half of this weight, but because they are positioned towards the front of your pelvis, the weight tends to tilt your pelvis backwards. To counteract this, muscles at the front of each hip joint pull down on the front of your pelvis to keep it level, and the force of this pull creates an extra load on your hip joints.

Measuring the forces

Measuring the forces exerted on the hips can be quite difficult because they depend on so many different factors, such as body shape and thigh length. However, researchers can estimate the forces reasonably accurately with the help of a gait analysis system. This uses cameras to track the motion of reflective markers placed around the body of a volunteer. A computer system analyses the images from the cameras and combines this data with information from pressure-sensitive plates to measure the forces on the body over the course of various movements.

Standing on one leg

If you then lift one foot from the floor to take a step forwards or stand on one leg, the hip joint of the leg that remains on the ground has to support the whole weight of your body, arms and head plus the weight of the raised leg. The hip joint also has to cope with the forces needed to stop your pelvis from tilting backwards.

An even greater strain on your hip comes from the forces needed to stop your pelvis from tilting downwards on the raised-leg side. When you stand on one leg your pelvis acts a little like a seesaw, with its pivot point being the hip joint of the leg you are standing on. The abductor muscles of that hip, especially your gluteus medius and gluteus minimus, pull down on their end of your pelvis to stop the other end from dropping down. This process pulls your pelvis down hard against your thigh bone. This force, plus the weight that your hip is carrying, makes up the total load on your hip joint. This load can be up to twice your overall body weight.

DID YOU KNOW?

Measuring the loads on your hip joints is normally impossible but researchers at the Free University of Berlin fitted some hip replacement patients with artificial joints containing load-measuring sensors. The researchers found that:

- **Walking at a speed of 1km/h (0.6mph), the load on each hip joint was about 280 per cent of body weight. This increased to around 480 per cent at 4km/h (2.5mph) and 550 per cent during jogging.**
- **Stumbling increased the load dramatically: up to 870 per cent of the body weight in one case.**
- **Carrying a load equal to a quarter of the volunteer's body weight increased the forces on each hip by around 25 per cent. Carrying the load in just one hand, however, made the load on the opposite hip two-thirds greater than the load on the carrying side, due to the increased leverage.**

Hips in motion

When you are walking, your abductor muscles have to work even harder because they raise the end of your pelvis slightly each time you take a step. Because women tend to have slightly wider pelvises than men, the hip drop is more pronounced, one reason why women's hips tend to sway more as they walk.

A normal walking gait will produce a force on each hip joint of around two to three times your body weight, and climbing stairs will increase that to about four to six times your weight. Jumping and other vigorous athletic activities can increase the peak load on your hips to as much as 12 times your weight.

Common hip problems through life

Your risk of developing hip problems varies considerably at different times of life. Some conditions are more likely to occur during childhood, while the bones around the hips are still growing. Other problems are connected to age-related diseases and general wear-and-tear.

Childhood and adolescence

Occasionally, hip problems may be present at birth. The most common of these is a congenital dysplasia (dislocation) of the hip (CDH). The usual cause is a looseness of the joint capsule or ligaments that lets the hip become partially or fully dislocated.

CDH affects around 1 in 1,000 babies and is more common in girls than boys. If left untreated, it can lead to walking problems, chronic pain and osteoarthritis. However, the routine medical examination of newborns includes testing for CDH. The usual treatment is to immobilize the joint with a brace or cast to allow it to repair itself and develop normally.

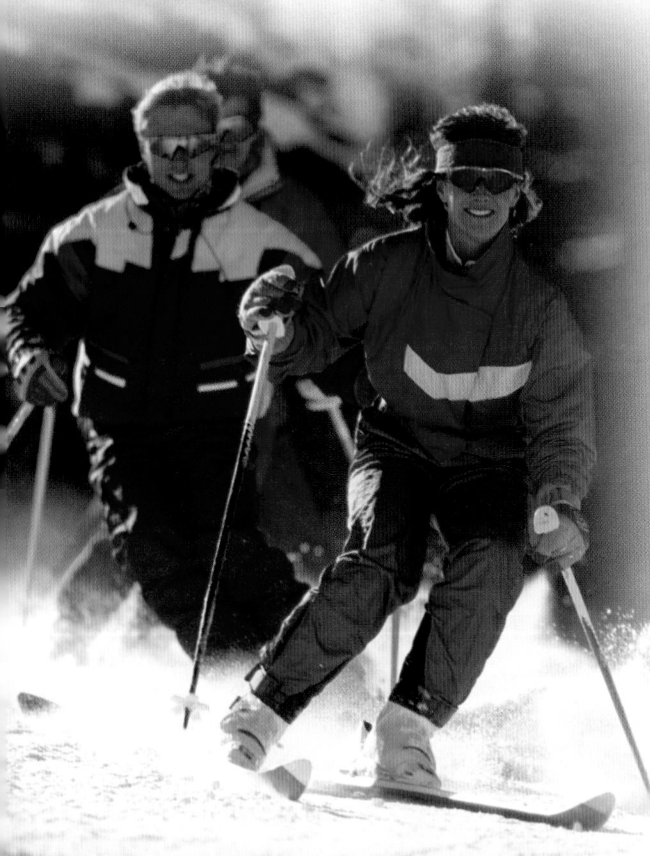

Legg-Calvé-Perthes

Between the ages of 5 and 11, the most common condition to affect the hip is juvenile osteonecrosis, or Legg-Calvé-Perthes' disease. This is a poorly understood disorder but its most likely cause is a shutdown of the blood supply to the head of the femur, which slowly dies and eventually becomes crushed by the child's own weight. Initial symptoms include pain or stiffness in the hip or knee and walking difficulties. The condition affects five times more boys than girls.

With early detection and treatment, which may involve resting or immobilizing the joint to allow the bone to regrow, it is usually possible to minimize bone damage. Even so, in the longer term the outcome is usually osteoarthritis with the need for early joint replacement. For more details >>299.

CRASH LANDING

Hip dislocations or fractures are most common in sports with the potential for high-impact falls or collisions, particularly where there are any existing weaknesses such as brittle bones.

Slipped femoral epiphysis

During puberty, the classic hip problem is slipped femoral epiphysis (SFE), which involves damage to the growth plate between the neck of the thigh bone and the femoral head. The body's long bones grow during childhood and adolescence as the thickness of the growth plates (the discs of cartilage at either end of the bone) increases. The cartilage cells in the growth plates are slowly replaced by bone cells, a process which continues until the bone is fully grown. In SFE, the growth plate slips (tears) and the femoral head comes away from the neck of the femur.

> **Slipped femoral epiphysis (SFE) is the most common non-traumatic hip problem in adolescents. It is particularly common among teenagers who are overweight**

This condition affects more boys than girls and overweight teenagers are at extra risk. Pain in the hip and knee, particularly if accompanied by stiffness, should alert parents to the problem. Early treatment, which consists of pinning the femoral head in place, is usually effective – but left untreated SFE can lead to deformity and osteoarthritis. For more information >>325.

Adulthood

Among adults, the most common hip problem is osteoarthritis >>228–247. This condition is often the result of years of normal wear-and-tear on the joint – over the years the cartilage in the joint slowly wears away. Without this protective covering, the bones in your hips start to rub directly against each other leading to stiffness and pain. Osteoarthritis is the most common reason for hip replacement surgery >>226–227.

Damage to the hip joints in adults can also result from inflammation-causing diseases such as rheumatoid arthritis (>>248–263), gout (>>294) and psoriasis. Methods for treating these diseases have greatly improved in recent years but some patients do not respond well and may eventually need a hip replacement.

Fractures

Hip fractures are relatively uncommon in younger adults and usually occur after a major trauma, such as a car crash. As you grow older, however, your bones start to lose density and you become more vulnerable to fractures after relatively minor knocks and falls. More than 90 per cent of hip fractures in people over the age of 65 occur after a fall. When a fracture is due to a fall, the part of the bone that breaks is usually the neck of the femur. Breakages of the main shaft of the bone are more likely to be the result of a high impact, such as that caused by a road accident. In both types of fracture, the broken bone ends are likely to be considerably displaced, causing severe pain and swelling.

The weaker your bones, the more vulnerable you are: around 90 per cent of hip fractures occur in people with osteoporosis (>>264–275). In women, who tend to have lower bone density following the menopause, the risk of hip fracture is equal to risk from breast, uterine and ovarian cancer combined. For more information on bone fractures >>291.

Do I need medical attention?

Most people occasionally get some discomfort or stiffness in one or both hips, but problems are usually harmless and short-lived. If you tick 'yes' to any of the following questions, however, you should consult your doctor.

YES	NO	
☐	☐	Do you have hip pain that makes you walk with a limp?
☐	☐	Do you have fever with hip pain?
☐	☐	Does your hip feel unstable or loose when you walk?
☐	☐	Do you have trouble moving, bending or straightening your leg?
☐	☐	Do you have persistent or unexplained pain in your groin?
☐	☐	Is there any visible deformity around your hip or groin?
☐	☐	Do you have a persistent numbness or tingling sensation in your hip, groin or leg?
☐	☐	Have you heard or felt a snapping, popping or grating in your hip when you move it?
☐	☐	Does your hip feel hot or swollen or do you have any signs of inflammation around your hip?
☐	☐	Is there any bleeding or significant bruising around your hip?
☐	☐	Did your hip pain begin after a fall or a blow?

QUESTIONNAIRE

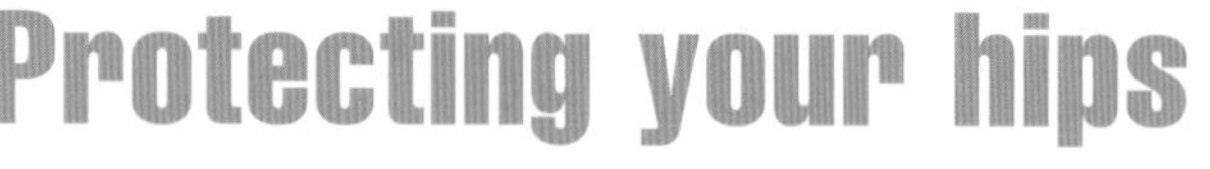

Protecting your hips

Some of the effects of ageing are inevitable and, of course, accidents do happen, but there are plenty of simple measures you can take to help protect your hips from their worst enemies – excessive wear and tear, lack of exercise and fractures.

One of the best ways to help your hips stay healthy is to keep your weight within the healthy range for your height. At any one time the points of contact between the bones in each hip can be just a few square millimetres in area, so the pressures within the joints can be high. Each extra kilo will add 2kg (4lb) to the force on your hips when walking, 5–6kg (11–13lb) when you are climbing stairs and as much as 10–12kg (22–26lb) when you are running or jumping.

These are heavy loads for your hips to bear, so any extra weight will significantly add to the daily wear-and-tear and increase your risk of osteoarthritis in later life. Losing excess weight will protect your hips from unnecessary wear. Aim for a body mass index of 18.5–25; for details of how to calculate your BMI >> 114–115.

Keeping moving

Your hip joints' main defences against early wear are the thick layers of cartilage that cover their load-bearing surfaces. Cartilage is very tough but also spongy, which allows it to absorb the synovial fluid produced in the lining of the joint capsules. When this fluid soaks into the cartilage, it brings with it vital oxygen and nutrients. Then, when your hip is under pressure, the fluid is squeezed out of the cartilage and into the joint space, where it acts as a lubricant and carries away waste materials and toxins.

Because your cartilage has no blood vessels to deliver nutrients and carry away waste, this process of absorbing synovial fluid and squeezing it out again is essential to prevent degradation and keep the cartilage supple and well fed. Without movement this fluid can't circulate, so your hips need regular exercise to stay healthy.

Helping damaged hips

If you have very painful or arthritic hips, it can be difficult to keep your joints moving. Nevertheless, frequent mild exercise such as walking is likely to be beneficial because it will help to keep your hips mobile. If walking is painful, try an exercise such as swimming or cycling in which your hips don't have to bear the full weight of your body. If you can't manage a full workout, the stretches shown on pages 220–221 will help to keep your hips supple.

If your hip needs to be immobilized for any length of time, after you've suffered a fracture for example, you may experience a significant degree of stiffness and muscle degeneration around the joint. As soon as you are able to move your hip again, start a programme of regular, gentle exercise to restore strength and flexibility.

Avoiding fractures

The older you get and the weaker your bones, the more likely you are to fracture your hip if you have a fall. Luckily there are plenty of steps you can take, whatever your age, to reduce your risk of fractures.

The most important thing is to help your bones stay strong and healthy by eating a healthy, balanced diet containing plenty of calcium. Most of the calcium in Western diets comes from dairy products, but good alternative sources include beans and pulses, some green vegetables, nuts, fruit and canned fish that is eaten with the bones such as salmon and sardines. If you don't get a lot of exposure to sunlight, you may also wish to consider vitamin D supplements. For more details about diet and supplements >>98–117.

Regular weight-bearing exercise such as walking or running will also help to strengthen your hip bones. If you already have weak bones or osteoporosis, weight-bearing exercise will still bring benefits. However, you will also need to take measures to avoid bumps and falls.

Reducing the risk of falls

The home can be a hazardous environment, particularly if you are not as sure-footed as you once were. In the UK, 46 per cent of the fatalities due to accidents in the home are the result of falls. Fortunately, there are some relatively simple measures that you can take to reduce your risk:

- Dizziness is one of the most frequent causes of falls. When you get out of bed, sit on the edge of the bed a moment to make sure you're not dizzy before you stand up and start walking. Don't skip breakfast: missing a meal could make you dizzy later.
- The kitchen and the bathroom are common places for people to have falls. Always try to keep the floors dry and watch out for slippery wet patches. If you are unsteady and prone to falls you should consider fitting a shower chair or proper handrails that will bear your weight.
- Take plenty of exercise to keep your muscles supple and improve your balance. If you are unsteady, you could use a pole or cane with a secure rubber tip for support.
- Reduced vision is one of the most common causes of falls. Make sure you wear glasses if you need them, remove reading glasses before you walk and make sure you have good lighting in your home.
- Be aware of any pets you have around the house – cats and dogs can easily get under your feet or jump up on you and knock you off balance.
- When using the stairs, never carry an object that obstructs your view of the next step. When possible, keep at least one hand on the handrail. Keep your stairs free from obstructions and secure loose carpeting on the stairs and elsewhere in the home.
- Don't let your clothing cause a fall. If a coat, pair of trousers, skirt or bathrobe is too long it may cause you to trip, so wear clothes that fit you properly.
- Don't leave clothes, newspapers or other items on the floor where you can trip over them. Close cabinet drawers and doors so that you won't stumble into them.

HIP PROTECTORS

These are light, tough convex shields that fit over your hips to absorb or deflect the impact of a fall. The soft fitted shields are usually held in place in pockets on undergarments but some are carried on special belts worn underneath or over your clothing.

If you are prone to falls or have weak bones, hip protectors may reduce your risk of fractures; a study carried out by Finnish researchers found that they can reduce the risk of a fracture by up to 80 per cent. Other studies have been slightly less encouraging, however. Shields certainly don't provide total protection, so you should still take care not to fall.

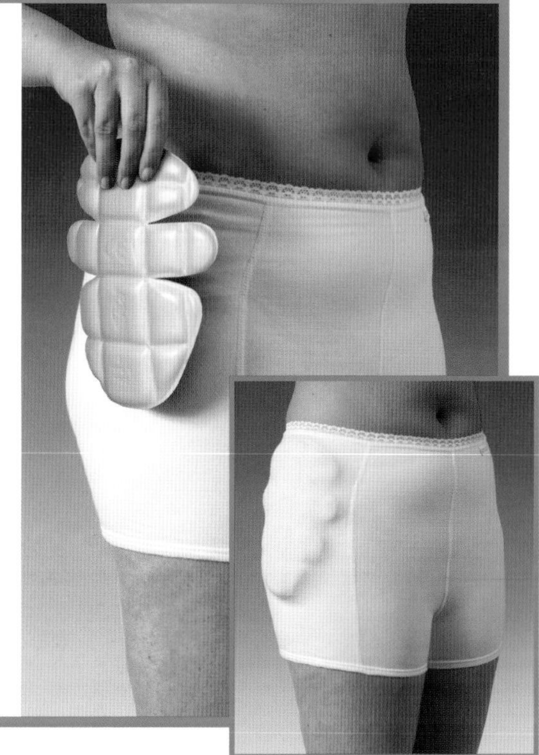

Exercises for hip flexibility

These simple stretching exercises don't involve any special equipment and take only a few minutes to complete, but they will help to keep your hips flexible and strengthen the muscles and ligaments around them.

You can use these exercises on their own to keep your hips supple or incorporate them into your stretch routine (>>66–67). Whichever way you use them, it's important to warm up first (>>64-65) to raise your body temperature, increase your blood flow and loosen your muscles before you stretch. Used as part of a pre-workout stretch routine, these exercises will help to maximize the range of motion of your hips, allowing you to contract the muscles around them fully and, by stretching the muscles and tendons, they will also reduce your risk of injuring them during your workout.

These exercises are designed to stretch your hamstrings, quadriceps and hip flexors, and they work best when you simply stretch the muscles slowly and hold the stretch – don't be tempted to make large numbers of rapid stretches.

Hip flexors

Your hip flexors (the iliopsoas and the rectus femoris) connect your pelvis to the front upper ends of your thighs. Your hip flexors are the muscles that trigger the forward movements of your legs when you are walking or running.

Hip flexor stretch

1 Kneel down with your right knee on a small cushion and your left leg bent out in front of you, foot flat on the floor.
2 Keeping your body upright, slowly move your hips forward until you feel a stretch in the muscles at the front of your right thigh. Hold this position for 30 to 60 seconds, then repeat using your left leg.

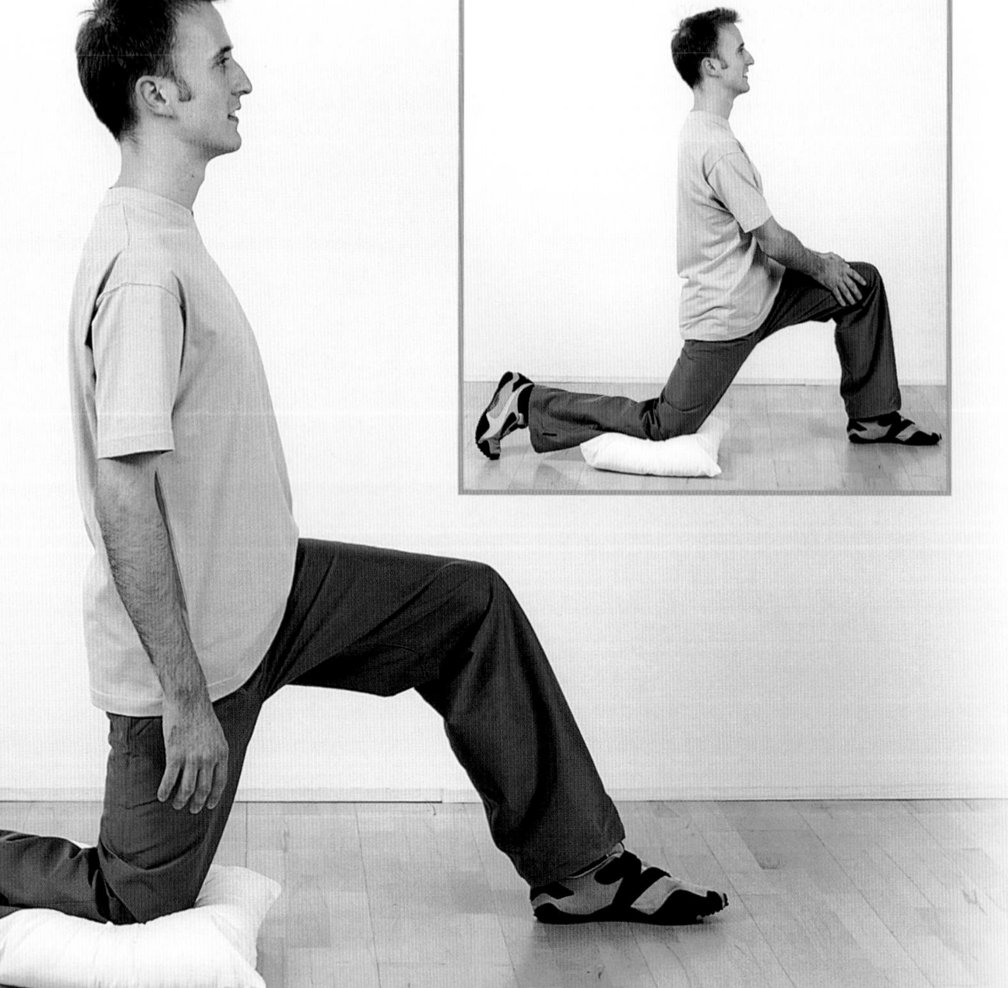

TAKE CARE

If you have had a hip replacement or are recovering from a hip injury, consult your doctor before attempting any of these exercises.

Hamstrings

Your hamstring muscles start at your pelvis, run down the back of your upper leg and end at a pair of tendons attached to your calf and shin bones, just below your knee. You use them to swing your leg backwards from the thigh and to bend your knee.

Quadriceps

The quadriceps is a group of four muscles at the front of your thigh, connecting your pelvis to the lower end of your thigh bone and your knee. The main role of the quadriceps is to straighten your leg at the knee, but you also use one of them – the rectus femoris – when you raise your thigh towards your pelvis.

Hamstring stretch

1 Sit sideways on a bench or on two chairs placed side by side, with your left leg flat along the bench and your right leg extended over the side with your foot flat on the floor.
2 Keep your back and shoulders straight and gently lean forwards from the hips until you feel a stretch along the back of your left thigh. Hold this position for 30 seconds, then repeat the exercise using your right leg.

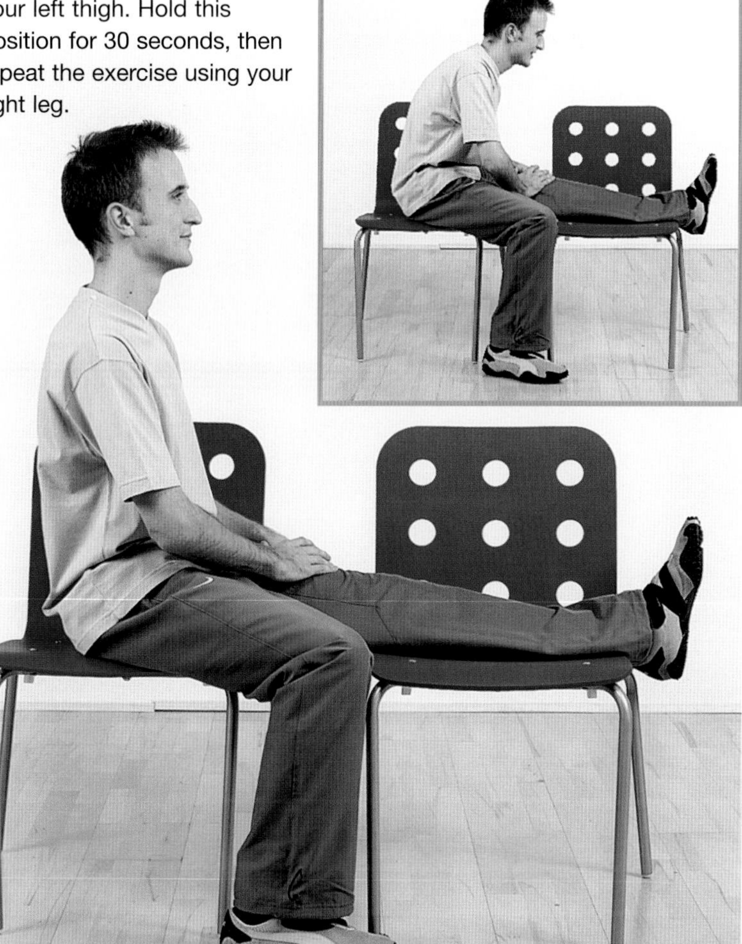

Quads stretch

1 Using a wall or the back of a chair for support, stand on your left leg and raise your right ankle until you can grasp it with your right hand.
2 Keeping your right knee close to your left, pull up gently on your ankle until you feel a slight stretch in the front of your thigh. Do not lean too far forward or back and pull just hard enough to maintain a constant, gentle stretch. Hold the position for 30 to 60 seconds, then repeat the exercise raising your right leg.

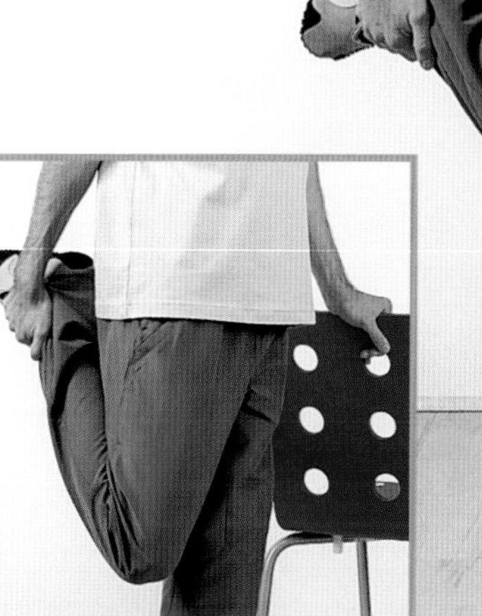

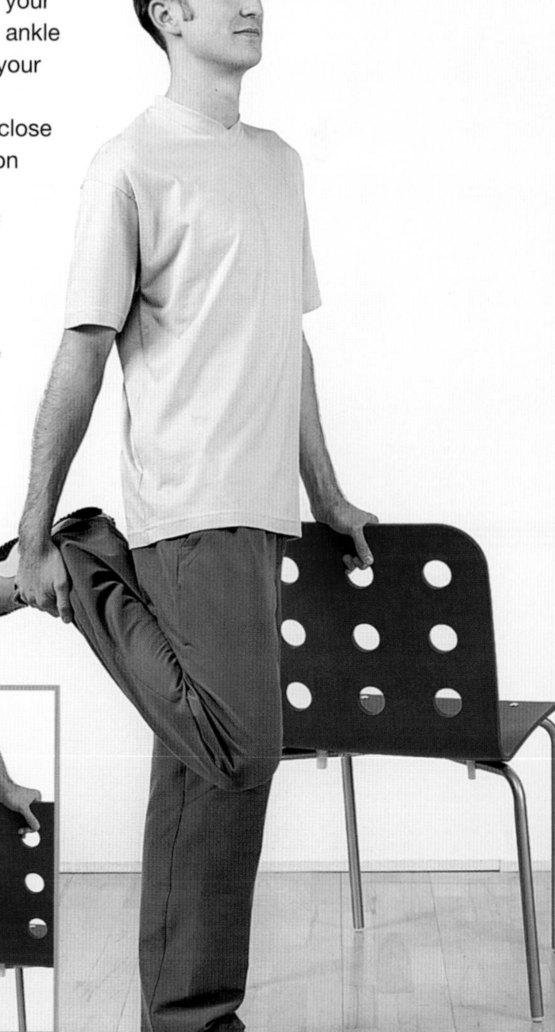

Alleviating pain and stiffness

Pain or stiffness in your hips can have many different causes and the ways in which you should treat it will depend on its cause. The remedies range from simple painkillers, ice packs and gentle exercise to powerful drugs that tackle joint diseases.

The first step in treating hip pain or stiffness is to find out what is causing it. Sometimes, the reason is obvious: perhaps you bruised your hip when you bumped into the edge of a table or strained your hip muscles in some way. In such cases, the problem will soon clear up on its own.

Mild painkillers such as ibuprofen or aspirin or heat treatments (warming packs or hot baths) will help to alleviate any discomfort.

The most frequent causes of serious hip pain and stiffness are various forms of inflammatory arthritis. If the problem persists or if your hip is stiff or sore for no obvious reason, you should consult your doctor for a proper diagnosis and advice on treatment. The more serious the symptoms, the sooner you should seek medical help >>217.

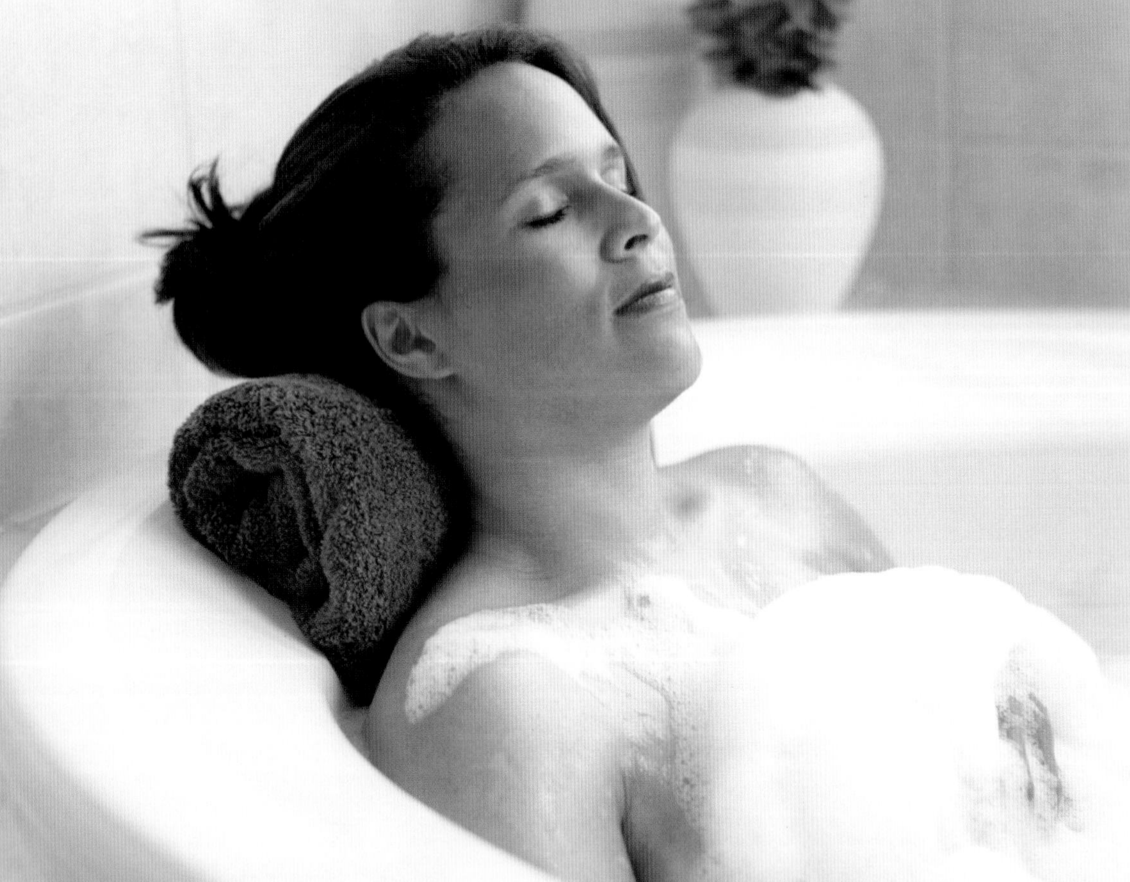

Relieving inflamed joints

If inflammatory arthritis is the cause of your hip problems, your doctor will recommend that you try one or more of several treatments that can alleviate the pain and stiffness or even halt the progression of the disease. These include a physical therapy programme to keep your hip joints mobile and drugs to reduce the inflammation and relieve pain and stiffness.

One consequence of arthritis is that it not only makes your joints stiff and painful but also limits how far you can move them. In the case of your hips, this limitation can make it increasingly difficult for you to walk or to get up and down stairs. Regular sessions with a physical therapist can bring big benefits because they can help you to increase the range of motion of your hip joints.

Exercising the muscles around your hips can also be very useful because it will strengthen them and increase or maintain their tone, which will help to overcome joint stiffness. Swimming is one of the best forms of exercise for this because it stretches and strengthens your muscles and gives your hip joints a good workout without placing any weight on them.

Non-steroidal anti-inflammatories

Of the many drugs that can help to relieve arthritic hip joints, the most frequently used are non-steroidal anti-inflammatories (NSAIDs) such as aspirin or ibuprofen. These reduce the inflammation effectively and are relatively safe, although there is a very small risk of intestinal bleeding or ulcers. However, some of these drugs have recently been linked to an increased risk of heart attacks >>box, 280. If you plan to use an NSAID for an extended period, talk to your doctor about the latest guidelines.

Corticosteroids

If your arthritis is particularly severe, your doctor may prescribe corticosteroids. These mimic the action of inflammation-reducing hormones produced by the cortexes (outer rims) of your adrenal glands. They are the most powerful of the anti-inflammatories and belong to a category of medications known as SMARDs (symptom-modifying anti-rheumatic drugs).

Corticosteroids come in various forms. Some you take by mouth, others come in creams that you apply to your skin and some need to be injected. Corticosteroids can have serious side effects, particularly if you take them for a prolonged period, so whichever form your doctor prescribes, you will require careful monitoring. When you stop taking them, you have to do so gradually and carefully because the withdrawal symptoms can be quite serious.

Disease modifying drugs

While corticosteroids and other SMARDs alleviate the symptoms of inflammatory arthritis, DMARDs (disease-modifying anti-rheumatic drugs) can effectively halt the progression of the disease and prevent the destruction of the joints. Methotrexate and sulfasalazine are the most frequently prescribed drugs but, like corticosteroids, may have serious side effects. Your doctor will need to monitor your use carefully. For more information about DMARDs to treat rheumatoid arthritis >>257.

Relieving osteoarthritis

Unfortunately, the drugs that are effective treatments for inflammatory arthritis are not particularly good at combating osteoarthritis. NSAIDs such as ibuprofen may help relieve pain but will not prevent the progression of the disease.

In the early stages of hip osteoarthritis, your doctor is likely to recommend that you rest your hip to avoid overuse and take some gentle physical therapy. This can include regular gentle exercise such as swimming, water aerobics or cycling to keep your hips functioning and improve their strength and range of motion.

If you are overweight, losing weight can be very beneficial because it reduces the load that your hip has to carry. The use of a cane when you are walking will also reduce the weight you apply to the joint.

Easing the load on your hip in this way should help to slow the degeneration of the joint. For more information on relieving the symptoms of osteoarthritis >>228–247.

Relieving tendon trouble

The tendons that connect your hip muscles to your thigh bone and pelvis can often be a source of pain. A tendon normally glides smoothly as the muscle it's attached to contracts and relaxes, but sometimes it becomes inflamed and causes pain every time you use the muscle. When this condition, called tendinitis, affects the tendons of your hip, it is usually caused by unaccustomed exercise. Tendinitis can also occur in later life as your tendons lose their elasticity and can no longer glide so easily.

Bursitis is another common tendon-related source of hip pain. A bursa is a fluid-filled sac that acts a shock-absorbing cushion between a tendon and a bone. The bursae in your hip can cause pain if they become swollen, perhaps because of too much exercise or a hard blow to the hip.

Effective treatments for tendinitis and bursitis include resting the hip as much as possible and applying an ice pack to the affected area for 15 to 20 minutes, three or four times a day. A mild painkiller such as aspirin or ibuprofen can help to relieve the pain, but if pain is severe or persistent you should consult your doctor.

OMEGA-3 FISH OILS

Your body uses omega-3 oils to produce the chemicals that reduce inflammation. Studies suggest that omega-3s can help to relieve stiff and swollen hips caused by rheumatoid arthritis and possibly also osteoarthritis. Your body cannot make the oils itself, so they must come from your diet: the best source is oily fish, particularly cold-water fish such as Atlantic mackerel or sockeye salmon.

OMEGA-3 CONTENTS OF FISH

- Mackerel: 2.5g omega-3/100g
- Herring: 1.6g omega-3/100g
- Salmon: 1.2g omega-3/100g
- Trout: 0.5g omega-3/100g
- Tuna: 0.4g omega-3/100g
- Cod: 0.3g omega-3/100g
- Shrimp: 0.2g omega-3/100g

Medical advances

The long-term success rate of hip replacements continues to rise, aided by the development of new materials and improvements in surgical techniques. Meanwhile, researchers are looking for alternatives to replacements and making steady progress in the fight against the joint diseases that make these transplants a necessity for so many people.

Mending damaged hips

The development of hip replacements was one of the great surgical advances of the 20th century but it is not the final answer to arthritis problems. Most artificial hips start to wear out after 15–20 years and may occasionally cause complications, such as inflammation from tiny particles worn away from the artificial joint that become embedded in the surrounding tissue.

Artificial hip joints usually consist of a metal ball that replaces the head of the femur and a polyethylene cup that replaces the socket. It may be possible to extend the lifespan of artificial joints by using tough ceramic components instead.

Another alternative that has recently been approved by the National Institute for Clinical Excellence (NICE) for use in younger, more active patients is a procedure called hip resurfacing. This is less invasive than a total hip replacement because less bone is removed – only a layer from the socket instead of a large chunk of the thigh bone. For more information >>226–227.

Growing new joints

A further line of research involves finding a biological rather than an engineering solution to damaged hip joints. The reason that our natural joints, when healthy, last so much longer than the artificial versions is that our bodies are in a constant state of self repair. In a process known as turnover, your body more or less continually removes damaged parts and replaces them with new tissue. Problems arise when the damage occurs faster than your body can repair it, as is the case with osteoarthritis.

In the near future it might be possible to boost the body's ability to repair itself by harvesting undeveloped bone and cartilage cells, multiplying them in cultures (nutrient solutions) and then reinserting them into the body to create new hip joint surfaces. A similar procedure has already proved effective for repairing joints in which only a small area of cartilage is damaged.

Bone grafts

Another alternative to hip replacement is to take a bone graft from another area of the body – usually the fibula. One of the hip's major design flaws is the poor blood supply: if the flow of blood from the main arteries to the femoral head is restricted, the bone can die, a condition known as osteonecrosis. Rather than replacing this dead bone with an artificial joint, doctors have developed a procedure known as a free vascular fibular graft.

In this operation, the surgeon removes some of the blood-starved bone from the hip bone. A section of bone is then harvested from the fibula with the blood

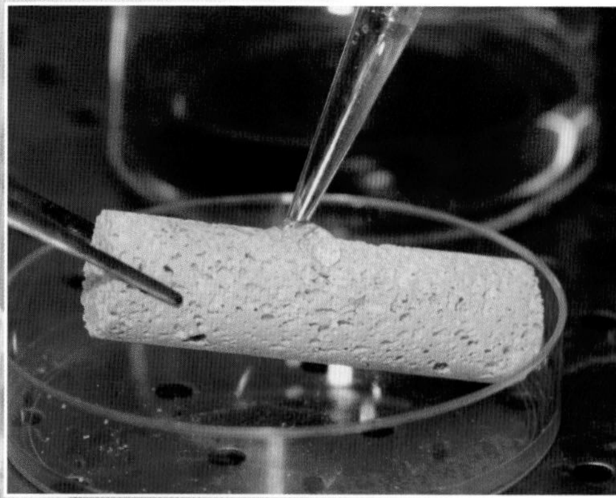

STEM CELLS AND BIOCERAMICS
Human stem cells (left) are undifferentiated cells that have the potential to mature into any of the 200 different cell types in the human body. In the future it may be possible to grow new hip bones or cartilage by harvesting stem cells from a patient's bone marrow and growing them within artificial materials that mimic the porous structure of bone, such as the calcium phosphate mineral complex above. This way the artificial material becomes living tissue, receiving nourishment from the body and able to heal from wear and injury.

vessels still attached. The surgeon implants this into the hip and attaches the blood vessels to the blood supply around the thigh bone. This living bone should then rejuvenate the femoral head.

Researchers are currently also looking into ways to improve this operation using substances called growth factors which encourage the spread of new blood vessels to nourish the regenerated bone.

Fighting arthritis

If scientists can find effective treatments for the various forms of arthritis – or perhaps even cures – the need for hip joint replacements will steadily decrease.

Preventing cartilage damage

Despite our incomplete picture of how and why arthritis develops, researchers are having some success in the search for drugs that will stop the degeneration of cartilage in the hip and even reverse the process.

- **Anti-TNF therapy** Some new types of DMARDs (disease-modifying anti-rheumatic drugs) work by blocking the action of tumour necrosis factor (TNF). This is a blood protein that attacks cancer cells but is also one of the substances that seems to cause inflammation in people with rheumatoid arthritis. It appears to make the body's immune system attack the synovial lining of the joints, causing swelling and pain. Unfortunately, blocking the action of TNF can occasionally cause serious side effects.
- **Glucosamine and chondroitin** Both of these substances occur naturally within the body as components of cartilage. The results of several small trials suggest that supplements of these substances may be as useful as non-steroidal anti-inflammatory drugs (NSAIDs) in suppressing pain in arthritic joints >>244.
- **S-adenosyl-methionine (SAM-e)** This compound occurs naturally in all living cells and is involved in many of the body's biochemical reactions. Among other roles, SAM-e contributes to the building blocks for cartilage. A number of recent studies suggest that supplements (available in the UK on prescription) may be as effective as NSAIDs for treating hip osteoarthritis, with fewer side effects.

DID YOU KNOW?

- **Many of the disease modifying anti-rheumatic drugs (DMARDs) in use today were originally developed for other purposes. Hydroxychloroquine, for example, is a malaria drug; azathioprine and cyclosporine started out as anti-rejection drugs for transplant patients and chlorambucil and methotrexate are cancer medications.**
- **Statins are another type of drug which was developed for other purposes but may have a role to play in hip health. Scientists in Cambridge are investigating whether these common cholesterol-lowering drugs could stimulate bone growth around hip implants and so make the connection between the new hip and existing bone more stable, improving the results of hip surgery.**

Lubricating the joints

Osteoarthritis involves not only damage to the cartilage and the underlying bone but also a partial breakdown of the synovial fluid that helps to lubricate and cushion the joint. Injecting an arthritic joint with hyaluronic acid (HA), a natural component of synovial fluid, increases the fluid's lubricating and shock-absorbing abilities.

This technique, which is called viscosupplementation, helps the joint to move more easily and reduces pain. It works very well in knee joints, but in hip joints the effect is short-lived and lasts for only a few hours or days. As a result, continuing relief requires repeated injections, which can lead to complications including infection. The research quest in this area is to find drugs that will both lubricate the hip joint and remain active for a prolonged period of time.

Hip replacement surgery

If one or both of your hip joints becomes damaged and you can no longer walk or even get in and out of a chair without pain and difficulty, your doctor may recommend hip replacement surgery. This involves replacing the damaged parts of the hip joint with metal, plastic or ceramic components.

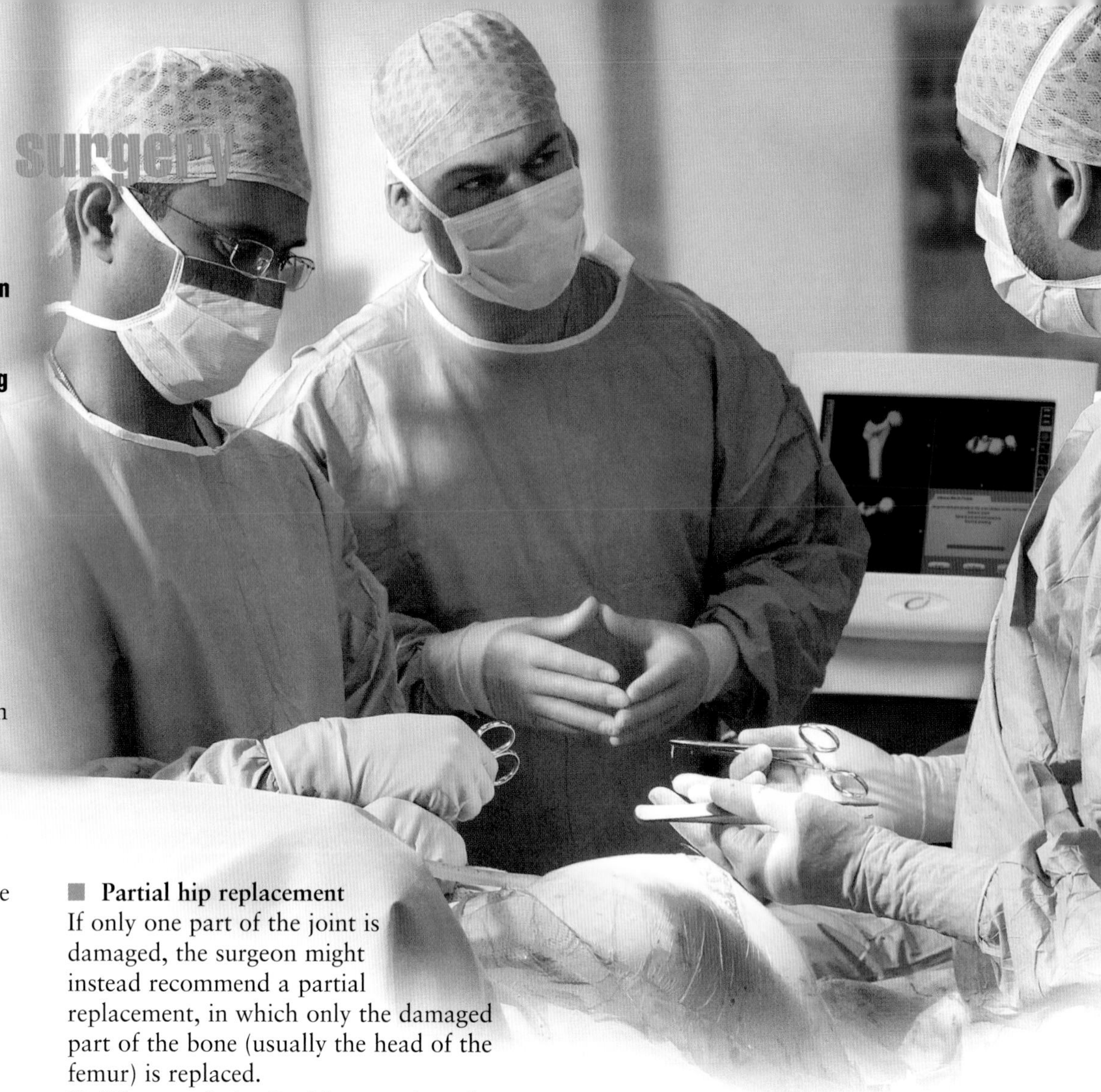

The most common reason for hip replacement is osteoarthritis – excessive wear and tear of the cartilage that covers and protects the working surfaces of the joint >>228–247. The cartilage normally cushions the joint and enables the ball-like head of the femur to move smoothly within its socket (the acetabulum). When the cartilage wears away, the joint becomes increasingly stiff and movement becomes more and more painful.

Apart from osteoarthritis, there are many other conditions that can damage the cartilage in your hip joints. These include inflammatory diseases such as rheumatoid arthritis and gout, infections and fractures affecting the surfaces of the joint.

Replacement options

If you need a hip replacement, your orthopaedic surgeon will have a number of options available – total replacement, partial replacement and resurfacing:

- **Total hip replacement** If both the ball and the socket of your hip joint are damaged, both parts of the joint will need to be replaced. Most hip replacements are of this type and 25–40 per cent of total hip replacements are performed on both hips.
- **Partial hip replacement** If only one part of the joint is damaged, the surgeon might instead recommend a partial replacement, in which only the damaged part of the bone (usually the head of the femur) is replaced.
- **Hip resurfacing** In this operation, the surgeon doesn't remove any bone from the femur but simply enlarges the hip socket slightly to make room for a metal cap over the femoral head.

Resurfacing doesn't substantially reduce the amount of existing bone, so if it wears out it is relatively easy for a surgeon to remove it and fit a total or partial replacement. This makes it a very good option for younger patients.

Total hip replacement

For a total hip replacement, the artificial joint consists of two implants: a plastic-lined metal shell that fits inside the joint socket and a tapering metal stem and ball that replaces the femoral head.

- First the surgeon makes an incision about 20–30cm (8–12in) long to gain access to your hip joint, then dislocates it to expose the femoral head and the socket.

DID YOU KNOW?

The first hip replacement operations were carried out over 80 years ago. In 1923 Marius Smith-Peterson at Massachusetts General Hospital, Boston, used a tough glass cup to cover a damaged femoral head.

Modern hip replacement surgery is largely based on the work of British surgeon Sir John Charnley, who pioneered the use of metal femoral implants and plastic acetabulum implants in 1961.

Today surgeons carry out more than 43,000 total hip replacement operations each year in the UK and over 172,000 in the USA.

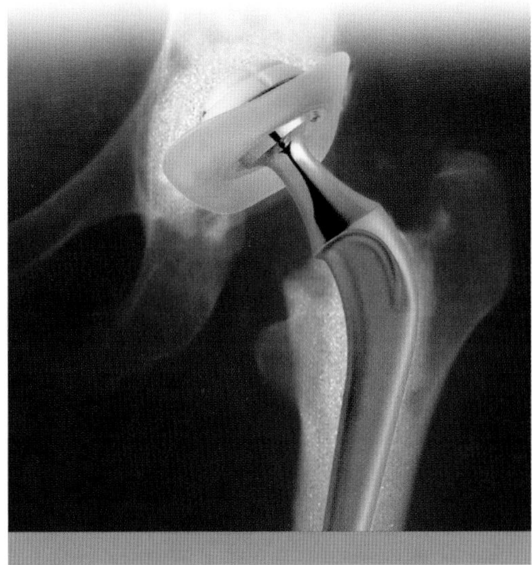

The surgeon uses a tool called a reamer to enlarge the joint socket before fitting the shell of the prosthesis into the cavity.

Next, the surgeon cuts off the femoral head at the base of the neck, using a power saw, cleans and enlarges the hollow central part of your thigh bone and pushes the stem of the artificial femoral head into it.

When both implants are in place, the surgeon carefully seats the ball within the socket and closes the incision.

With some designs of hip prosthesis, the two implants rely at first on tightness of fit to hold them into the bone cavities but have textured surfaces into which the bone eventually grows to keep them securely in place. Other designs rely on an acrylic cement to hold them in place.

Minimally invasive techniques

A recent innovation is the development of minimally invasive techniques. Instead of making a single long incision to expose the hip joint, surgeons make one or two short incisions and use specially designed instruments to prepare the bones and instal the implants. These techniques cause less blood loss and less damage to the surrounding soft tissue during the operation, so they heal and regain their strength more rapidly.

In a single-incision operation, the surgeon makes a cut less than 15cm (6in) long on the outside of the hip. In a two-incision operation, the surgeon makes one incision 5–8cm (2–3in) long in the groin to fit the socket implant and another one 3–5cm (1–2in) long in the buttock to fit the femoral implant. Instead of spending up to five days or more in hospital, as is usual with conventional surgery, most patients are able to go home within 24 hours.

Possible complications

Despite the progress in hip replacement surgery and the excellent results that it produces, there are still risks associated with it. The most common complications include dislocation, loosening of the implants and infection.

The most serious of these is infection and, although the risk of serious infection following joint replacement is not much greater than 1–2 per cent, when it does happen it can be devastating. The new joint may have to be removed and a new one fitted when all traces of the infection have gone, usually 6–12 weeks later. You should discuss any potential problems fully with your doctor before surgery.

After the operation

Following the operation, a physiotherapist will advise you on the type of activities you should or should not perform. Exercise is important to get your new hip working, but you should avoid squatting, sitting in a low chair or crossing your legs for some time after the operation.

It takes a little while to regain full function, but with proper care the vast majority of hip patients are left pain free for a great many years.

BIONIC GOLFERS

There are now so many people with successful hip replacements and other artificial hips that one US surgeon has started a golf tournament just for them. The 'Bionic Open' is a 9-hole golf tournament for 127 patients who've had total joint replacement surgery at Associated Orthopaedic Specialists in Florida.

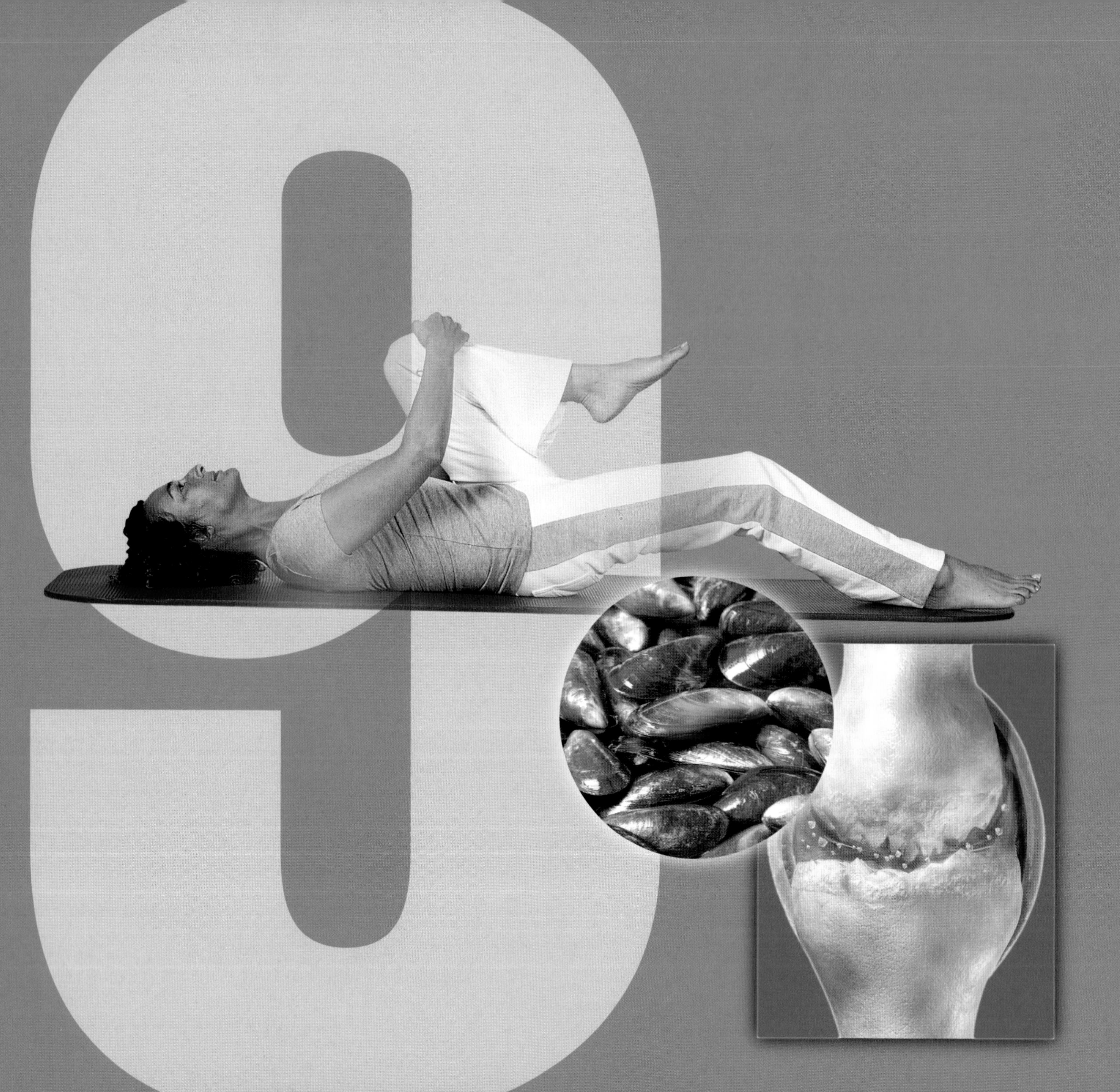

OSTEOARTHRITIS

The most common cause of bone and joint problems, osteoarthritis – the gradual thinning of the protective cartilage that cushions the ends of bones at the larger, weight-bearing joints – can be painful and debilitating. But, if you are susceptible to OA, there is much you can do to alleviate pain, promote flexibility and make life easier.

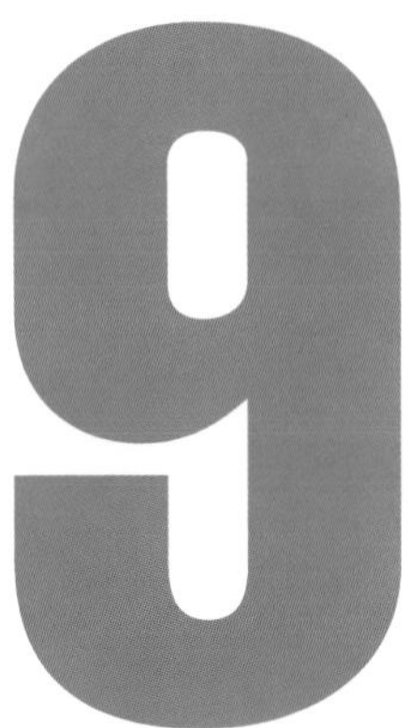

OSTEOARTHRITIS What is it?

By far the most common joint disease – especially in later life – osteoarthritis (OA) occurs when the cartilage that lines and cushions joints breaks down and the bones rub painfully against each other. It tends to affect the small joints of the fingers, the large weight-bearing joints of the hips and knees, or the vertebrae in the upper spine, a condition known as cervical spondylosis.

What happens?

Cartilage cushions many joints; it is very smooth, allowing the bone ends that form a joint to glide easily over each other. In osteoarthritis, the cartilage lining the affected joints becomes roughened and patches of it are destroyed. The underlying bone thickens in an attempt to repair the joint. Spurs of bone known as osteophytes form around the joint. Sometimes fluid collects within the joint, causing swelling.

Often, the joints repair themselves adequately with time and the pain may then settle. However, in some cases the damage is not successfully repaired, the pain becomes more persistent and the joint no longer works properly. Eventually, the joint may become deformed. The muscles around the joint also weaken, which may in turn affect the joint's stability.

In some cases, calcium crystals form within the cartilage of a joint affected by OA – the knee is particularly susceptible to this. The OA in such joints tends to be more severe and to worsen more quickly. In addition, periods of inflammation may occur causing increased pain and swelling of the joint. During these times, the joint may also feel hot to the touch. These flare-ups are similar to those that occur in gout, a condition caused by the deposition of urate crystals within joints. The condition is therefore known as pseudogout.

72

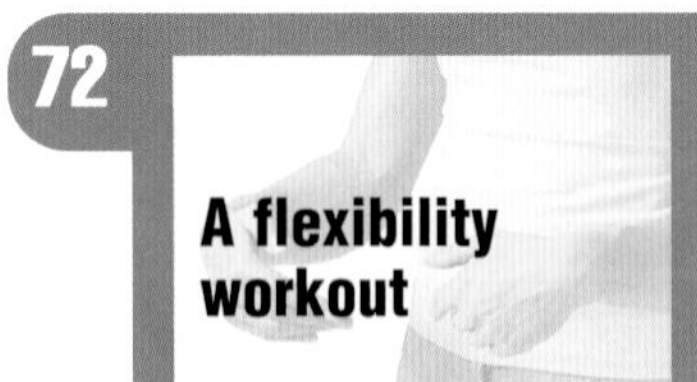

A flexibility workout

96

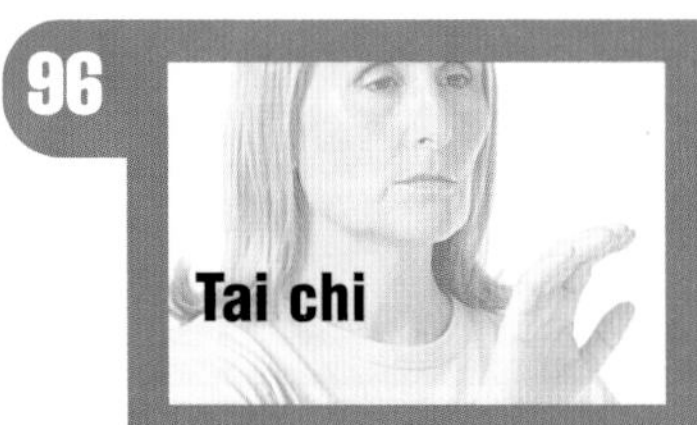

Tai chi

222

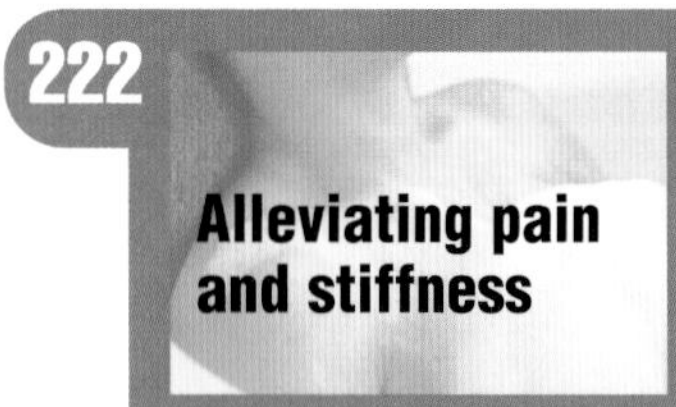

Alleviating pain and stiffness

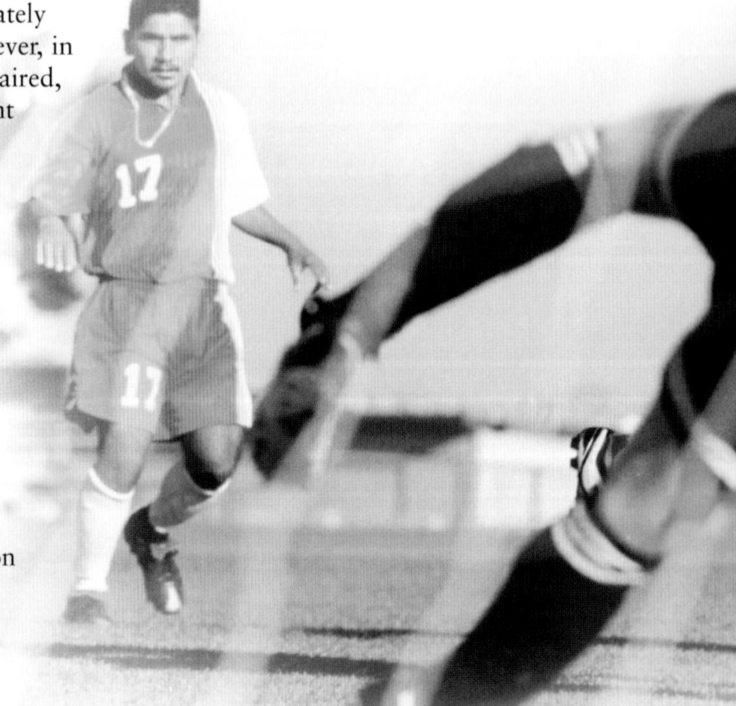

DID YOU KNOW?

- Osteoarthritis affects about eight million people in the UK. Some X-ray evidence of OA has been observed in as many as 80 per cent of people aged over 65, although only around 30 per cent of these people have any symptoms.
- Over the age of 65, more women than men suffer from OA and it is often more severe.
- The condition affects all races – but often differently. For instance, OA of the hips and hands is common in Europeans but far less common in Afro-Caribbean people. No-one knows why this is, but genes and environment may play a role.

What are the causes?

It is not completely understood how osteoarthritis develops and often no particular reason can be identified. Various factors that may play a role include:

- **Ageing** We are more likely to develop osteoarthritis as we get older; the condition usually begins to develop after the age of 40. OA is not an inevitable consequence of getting older but ageing does increase the effects of general wear and tear on joints.
- **Genetic factors** These are thought to play a role, although the specific genes responsible have not yet been identified. Nodal arthritis tends to run in families >>232.
- **Gender** For most joints – particularly the small joints in the hands – OA is more common in women.
- **Sex hormones** As the disease is more common in women after the menopause, falling levels of oestrogen may play a part.
- **Obesity** This is a major risk factor for developing OA later in life, particularly increasing the risk of OA of the knee.
- **Injuries** Serious damage or trauma to a joint, such as a fracture, can also increase the risk of OA, although the disease may not develop until many years later. Operations on joints can also make them vulnerable to OA.
- **Certain sports** Sports that inflict stress repeatedly on a joint can lead to OA. For example, football or rugby, if played frequently over long periods, can increase the risk of the condition developing in players as young as in their 30s.
- **Joint problems** Certain joint problems that are present from birth can result in OA later in life.
- **Certain joint diseases** Joint diseases that involve inflammation, such as rheumatoid arthritis (>>248–263) and gout (>>294) can predispose to OA.
- **Certain occupations** Jobs that put joints under particular strain can lead to the condition. For example, farming is associated with OA of the hip.

Some people with OA find their symptoms worsen in certain weathers, often when the atmosphere feels damp. However, it has not been shown that moving to a warmer climate will improve the condition in the long-term. OA occurs in all parts of the world, even when it is warm all year round.

Under the skin...

Osteoarthritis occurs when the protective layer of cartilage lining the joints breaks down, causing bones to rub painfully against one another. Bone spurs (osteophytes) gradually build up around the joints causing stiffness and impeding movement.

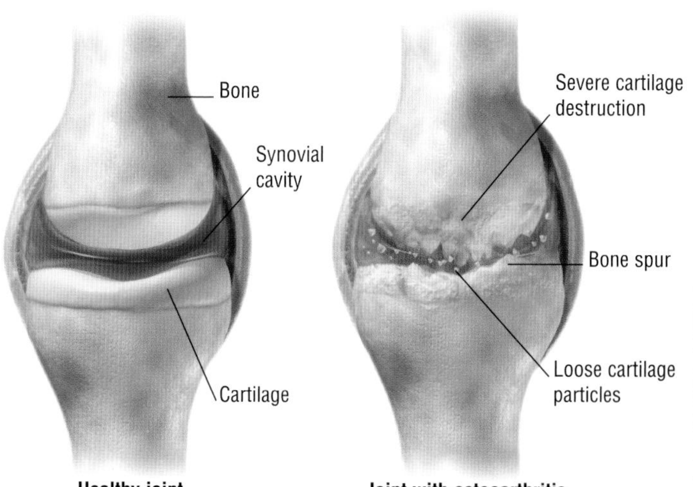

Which joints are affected?

Most joints can be affected but weight-bearing joints, such as the knees and hips, and the small joints of the hands and wrist are most commonly involved.

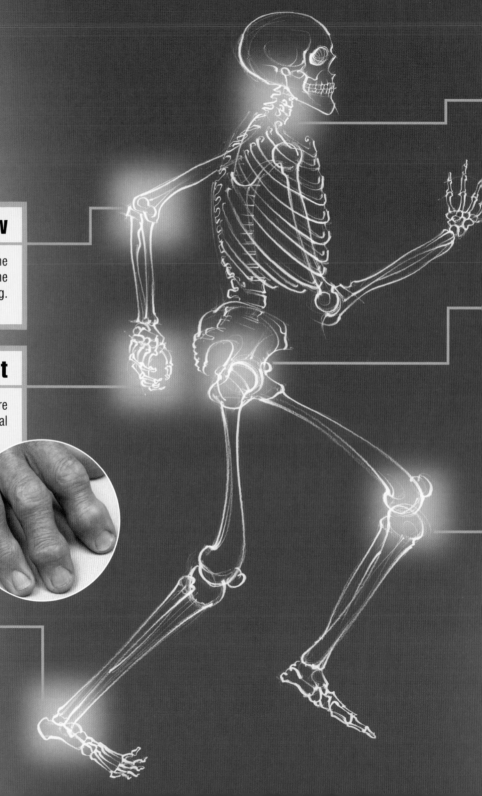

Shoulder and elbow

In osteoarthritis of the shoulder, pain restricts movement of the arm, particularly raising it to the side and to the front. OA of the elbow limits bending and straightening.

Hands and wrist

The joints of the fingers and the joint at the base of the thumb are particularly frequently affected, often as part of the condition nodal arthritis. More women than men have the disease which tends to start in middle age and often runs in families. The joints become painful and bony lumps slowly develop. In many cases the pain eventually improves but some degree of deformity and stiffness of the fingers can remain. There may be some impairment of hand function but this is usually mild. OA of the wrist usually develops years after an injury to the wrist.

Ankle

This results from damage to the joint, perhaps as a result of an injury or an infection. Stress placed upon the joint repeatedly, as may occur during jogging or running, is another cause. The main symptoms are pain, stiffness and limited movement in the joint.

Neck

X-rays of the neck and back in older people often show signs of osteoarthritis. However, many of these people have no obvious symptoms of the disease. OA of the upper spine, known as cervical spondylosis, tends to affect men more frequently than women. If symptoms do occur, they may include neck pain, restriction of neck movement and pains that spread down the arms from the shoulders. There may also be numbness and tingling in the arms and hands due to nerve compression in the neck.

Hip

Osteoarthritis of the hip is one of the most common causes of disability in the developed world, affecting men and women in roughly equal numbers. The condition may start as early as the 40s and one or both hips may be involved. A child with hip problems may go on to develop osteoarthritis later in life. However, often no cause is identified. The pain from OA of the hip tends to be felt in the groin or buttock area, but may also be felt around the thigh or extend down to the knee. Occasionally, pain extends to the lower back. Discomfort is generally related to activity. Bony osteophytes (outgrowths of bone) may form around the joint reducing hip movement, and a limp may develop.

Knee

About 40 per cent of people over the age of 75 are thought to have some degree of osteoarthritis of the knee. The condition affects women more than men and tends to involve both knees. Obesity is a particular risk factor. OA may develop in one knee years after an injury, but often no cause is found. The front and sides of the knee tend to be painful. Occasionally, the knees become deformed with bowing of the legs.

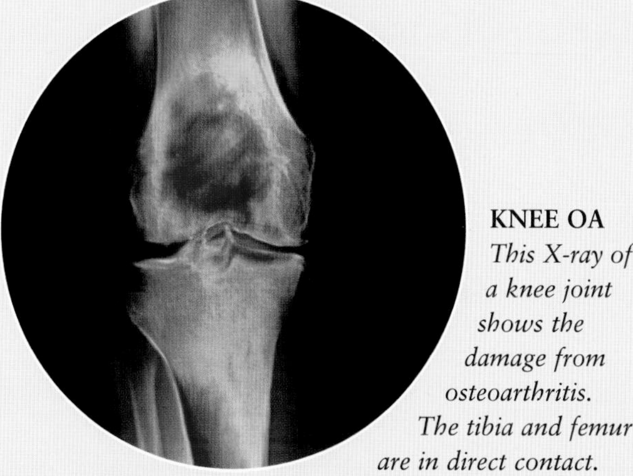

KNEE OA *This X-ray of a knee joint shows the damage from osteoarthritis. The tibia and femur are in direct contact.*

What are the symptoms?

Symptoms tend to come on gradually with the severity varying from day to day. The main symptoms of osteoarthritis are:

- Pain and tenderness
- Stiffness
- Restricted movement
- A creaking sensation as the joint moves
- Swelling of the joint (due to fluid collected within the joint capsule)
- Bony swellings (osteophytes) on the joint

Joints are often stiff in the morning or after rest but improve with movement. Joint pain tends to be worse when the joint is moved but improves with rest.

How is it diagnosed?

Osteoarthritis is usually diagnosed from a description of the symptoms and an examination. The doctor will check the affected joints for tenderness, restriction of movement, decreased stability, creaking and swelling.

There are no blood tests that can diagnose OA, but blood may be tested to rule out other conditions that produce similar symptoms. X-rays are often taken but may be of limited help as abnormalities often show only when the disease is severe.

Magnetic resonance imaging (MRI), in which a magnetic field and radio waves are used to create cross-sectional or three-dimensional images of the affected joint, may be arranged as it can show early damage to cartilage. Arthroscopy (>>206) in which a viewing instrument is passed through the skin and tissues into the joint cavity, may also be used to look for changes in the cartilage.

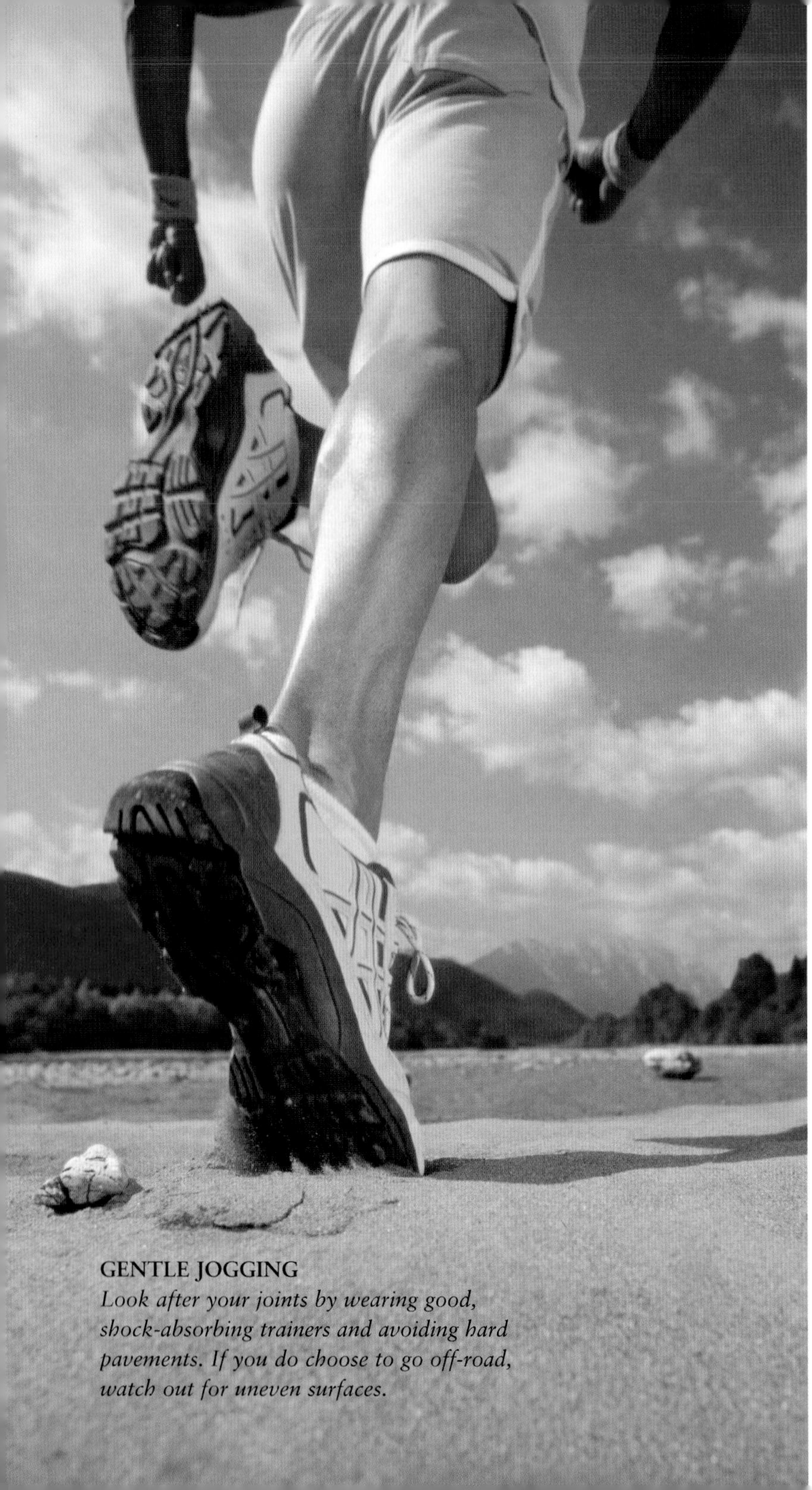

What can I do?

There are many things you can do to help to slow the progression of osteoarthritis and relieve pain. These include reducing the stress on joints and keeping active, which will also help those with healthy joints to reduce their risk of developing OA in the future.

Reduce stress on joints

It has been estimated that for every kilo over your ideal weight you increase your chance of developing osteoarthritis by 9–13 per cent. Losing weight therefore significantly reduces the stress placed on your weight-bearing joints. Aim for a gradual weight loss that can be sustained through a combination of a healthy diet and exercise. Regular exercise will not only help with weight loss, but will also strengthen bones and joints and keep them mobile. For information on finding your ideal weight >>114–115.

Wear appropriate footwear

Look for comfortable, well-fitting footwear to support your foot and prevent jarring. Most outdoor-clothing shops and many regular shoe shops now stock a good range of stylish, shock-absorbing footwear, designed for sport or off-road use but equally useful for pounding city streets. For more advice >>48–49.

If you are worried about your feet, it is worth contacting a chiropodist or podiatrist for advice. Feet affected by OA may change shape, making it difficult to find suitable footwear. Consider buying a pair of custom-made shoes – that way you can order the style and type you want, usually for a very reasonable price.

If your hips or knees are particularly painful, consider buying a stick or walking pole to reduce the weight on your joints. Most outdoor-equipment shops offer a wide range of modern, extendable models designed for Nordic and fitness walking.

Avoid prolonged bursts of repetitive movements

Repetitive activity can place joints under excessive stress. If the joints of your hands are affected by osteoarthritis, limit keyboard use to short periods with frequent breaks and rest your wrists on a sponge bar in front of the keyboard. If your hips or knees are affected, avoid standing for prolonged periods – try perching on a stool in the kitchen or workshop.

GENTLE JOGGING
Look after your joints by wearing good, shock-absorbing trainers and avoiding hard pavements. If you do choose to go off-road, watch out for uneven surfaces.

4 WAYS TO...

Alleviate joint pain

Although these measures do not affect the disease itself, you may find they help to relieve your symptoms:

1 **Local heat,** such as a heat lamp, a heat pad or a wrapped hot-water bottle held to the painful joint, may relieve pain and stiffness.

2 **Swimming** improves muscle strength, joint mobility and general fitness. It may also help to relieve painful joints.

3 **Non-steroidal** anti-inflammatory gels are available over the counter. Applying them regularly can help to relieve pain and stiffness. Side effects are limited as the drugs are only absorbed into the body in very small amounts.

4 **Massaging** the affected area can provide relief. Creams are available that create a soothing heat as they are rubbed on.

QUESTIONNAIRE

Could I be susceptible to OA?

Do any of the following risk factors apply to you? If so, you could be at increased risk of developing osteoarthritis.

YES	NO	
☐	☐	Are you overweight?
☐	☐	Do you have any family history of osteoarthritis?
☐	☐	If you are a woman, have you passed the menopause?
☐	☐	Have you suffered any previous damage to your joints, such as a fracture or an operation?
☐	☐	Do you practise an occupation or have a hobby known to increase the risk of OA, such as farming or football?
☐	☐	Do you suffer from any inflammatory joint diseases such as rheumatoid arthritis or gout?
☐	☐	Do you have any other joint abnormalities?

Keep active

Normal joint use does not cause damage – in fact appropriate exercise can strengthen joints and improve mobility. Ideally, an exercise programme should incorporate:

- **Strengthening exercises** designed to strengthen the muscles you use to move and keep your joints stable.
- **Aerobic exercises** to strengthen the heart and lungs and help with weight loss, taking pressure off painful knees and hips. The correct level of aerobic exercise depends on your general level of fitness and the severity of the osteoarthritis. Your doctor or physiotherapist can advise you on the appropriate level and explain how to build up gradually to avoid straining muscles.

In addition, stretching exercises may help to relieve pain and improve mobility. For more information on taking exercise to benefit not only your joints but also your whole body >>238-241.

Seek advice

Pain and stiffness can limit everyday activities and make simple tasks more difficult. There are many ways to make things easier, however, as well as handy aids to make your home more user-friendly.

Advice is available from many sources, including your GP, occupational therapists, physiotherapists, patient support groups and specialist shops. For more information on special aids and devices >>236-237.

MAKING LIFE EASIER IN THE HOME

Osteoarthritis and rheumatoid arthritis can make it a little more difficult to perform everyday tasks, especially if the small joints in your hands and fingers are affected. Although you may find fiddly tasks such as turning cooker knobs more tricky, arthritis needn't stop you living life as normal. There are lots of simple labour-saving measures you can take and a host of easily-available aids and gadgets. Here we describe just a few of them: for more detailed, tailor-made advice consult an occupational therapist.

You should be able to find all of these aids in any good high-street department store. The internet is another great place to shop for gadgets (for a list of useful websites >>336–9). Most of the measures shown below are simple and inexpensive, but if you need to make extensive changes to your home you may be eligible for a grant to help with the costs. A number of charities and other organizations also offer free products and services. Ask your social services department or occupational therapist for more details.

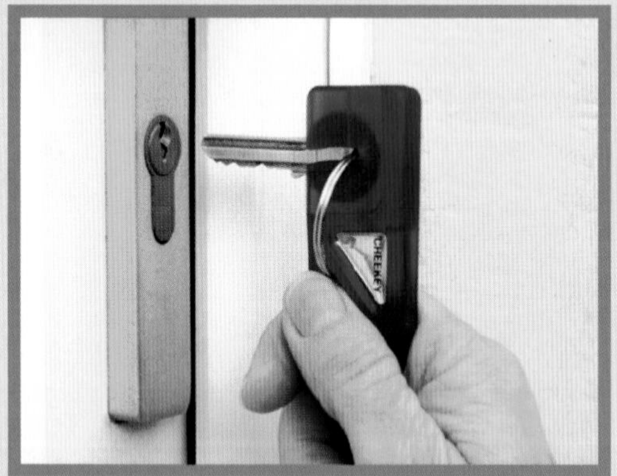

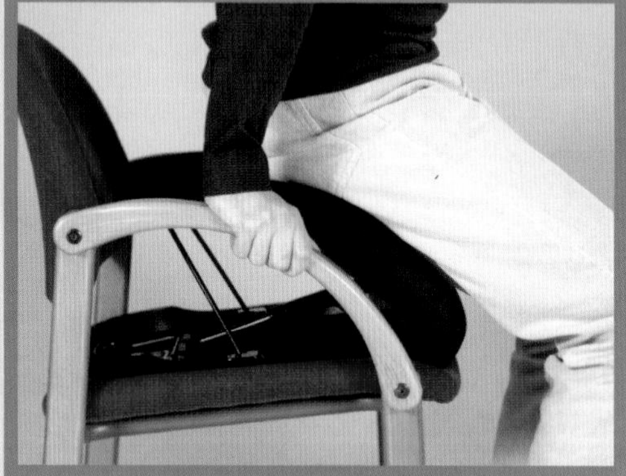

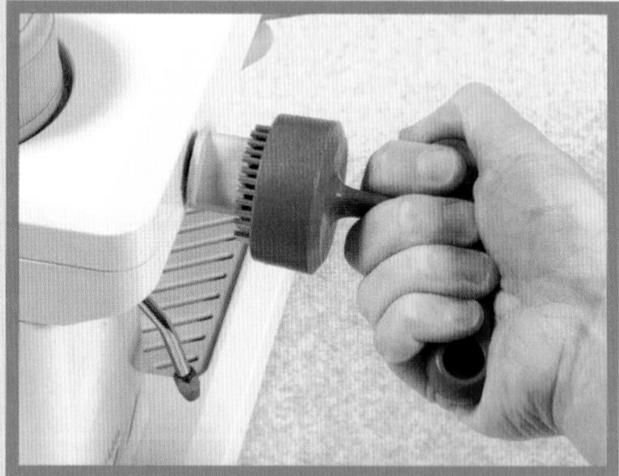

Adapting your home

- A basket on the inside of the letterbox means you don't need to bend to pick up letters
- Large handles attached to door keys makes them much more manageable
- Levers on door handles and special grips to door knobs make them easier to turn
- Special plugs with handles are much easier to plug in and pull out; alternatively, special grips can be fitted to regular plugs
- Touch or rocker-type light switches make house lights easier to use
- A hands-free phone avoids the need to hold the receiver for long periods

In the living room

- Adding cushions to a chair seat may make standing up easier
- Special blocks are available that can be placed under chair legs to raise the chair
- Riser-recliner chairs let you sit back in comfort and tilt to bring you to a standing position. You can adapt regular chairs using portable lifting cushions
- A reacher stick helps you to pick things up without needing to stand up or bend over

In the kitchen

- Placing frequently-used items in easily accessible cupboards and drawers reduces bending and stretching
- Knob turners give more leverage to turn small or fiddly knobs
- Lever taps on the kitchen sink are easier to use than regular taps; alternatively, special turners can be attached to the taps
- Special aids are available to help open jars and bottles and remove ring pulls
- A trolley to move things around helps avoid the need to carry heavy pans and plates

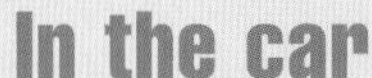

In the car

- A panoramic rear-view mirror and blind-spot mirrors give a better view if you have a stiff neck
- A swivelling seat can help you get in and out of the car
- Seat-belt fasteners and other adaptions are available to make fastening and wearing belts more comfortable
- If you are getting a new car, consider buying one with power steering and automatic gears

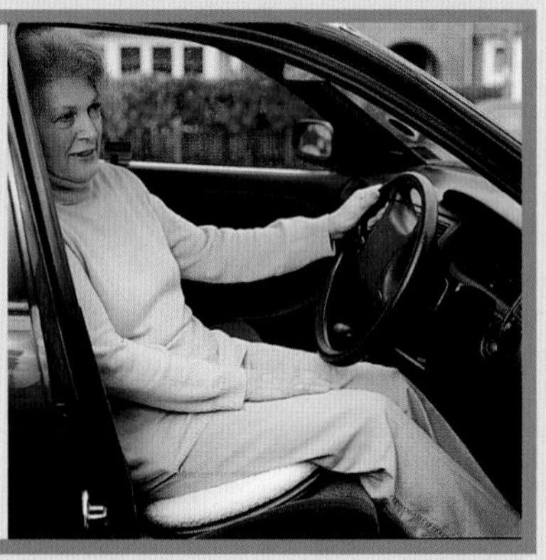

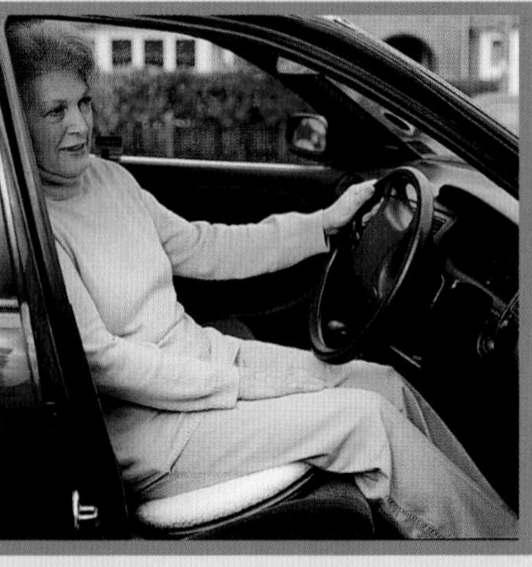

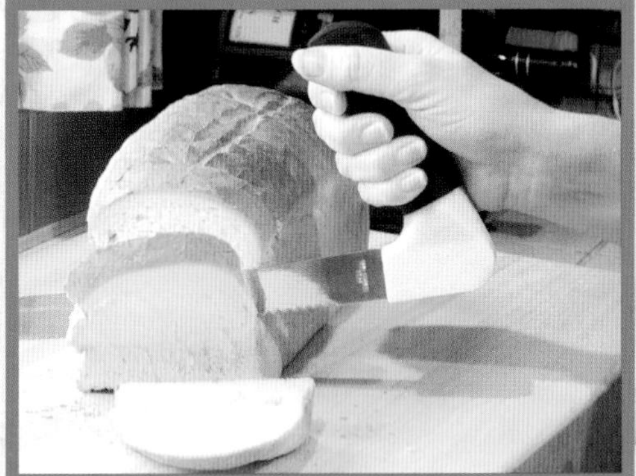

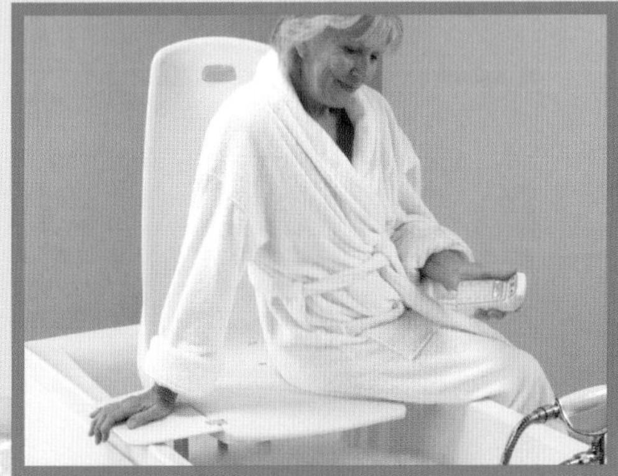

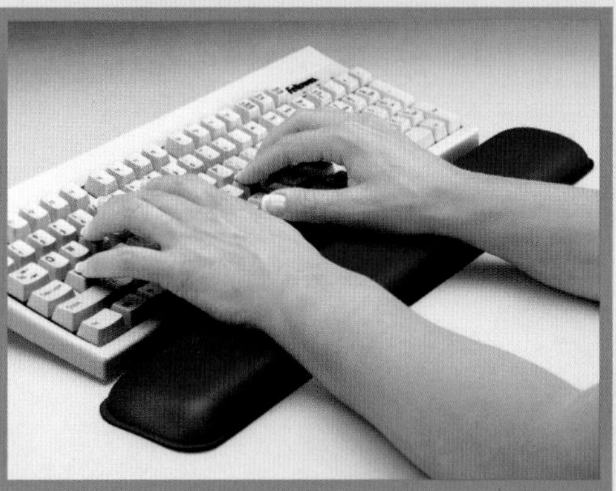

Cooking and eating

- Kitchen utensils with chunky or moulded handles are much easier on stiff fingers; rocker knives help with cutting and chopping
- Cutlery is available with large or curved handles; lightweight crockery and cups with large handles can be held more safely
- Light pans with two handles are easier to lift without dropping or spilling the contents
- Spike boards can be used to hold vegetables still while cutting them

In the bathroom

- Lever taps can be fitted to wash basins
- Long-handled sponges and hairbrushes help those with stiff arms and shoulders
- A thick towelling dressing gown helps with drying off after a bath or shower
- A grab-rail next to the toilet and the bath makes it easier to manoeuver
- Walk-in baths are very helpful for those who cannot climb in and out of the bath, although fitting is expensive; another option is a powered lift in the bath

In the study

- Wrist splints or a sponge bar in front of the keyboard are easier on your wrists
- Frequent breaks reduce the strain placed on your hand and wrist joints
- If your hands are severely affected, voice-activated software can make using the computer much easier and less painful

Keeping active

Studies have shown that regular exercise relieves pain and increases mobility in people with osteoarthritis of the knees. This may well be true for other joints too, so exercise is considered an important part of the treatment programme. Exercise also improves balance, helping to prevent falls and subsequent fractures.

A suitable exercise programme should not place excessive stress on joints. Some forms of exercise are particularly suitable for osteoarthritis sufferers. Swimming, for example, is a low-impact exercise that keeps the joints moving while improving general fitness. Both aerobic and strengthening exercises are recommended for people with OA and stretching exercises are also likely to be beneficial. Before starting any exercise programme, however, you should always seek advice from your doctor or physiotherapist who can suggest what type of exercise is most suitable for your condition.

Aerobic exercise

This increases the heart rate, improving general fitness and increasing energy levels. The most suitable type of exercise for you depends on your own tastes – swimming, walking or cycling are all good options. If you prefer organized activities, you should be able to find an aerobics class to suit your fitness level.

4 WAYS TO...

Build up your fitness

1 Exercise frequently but only for short periods to start with. Initially you should work out for just a few minutes a few times a day.

2 Build up slowly. If possible, increase the length of your exercise sessions by about 10 per cent every week.

3 Don't overdo it. Aerobic exercise should increase your heart rate, but if you are too breathless to talk you may be exercising too hard and should slow things down.

4 Set realistic goals. Ideally, you should aim to do 30 minutes of exercise on most days. This is only a guide – your doctor or physiotherapist will advise you on your limits depending on your level of fitness, the severity of your arthritis and any other medical conditions you may have.

TAKE CARE

Whether you are doing aerobic, strengthening or stretching exercises, always listen to your body. If exercise causes discomfort or swelling, or increases pain, this may be a sign that you're putting too much stress on your joints. Stop and get medical advice.

Strengthening exercises

Try these exercises to strengthen the muscles that move and support affected joints. If possible, perform each exercise five times and repeat twice a day.

Knees

1 Sit on the edge of your bed and cross your legs at the ankle.
2 Straighten your legs from the knee, lifting your feet off the floor. Push your top leg downwards and your bottom leg upwards so that they press against each other and you can feel the muscles at the front of your thighs contract. Count to 10 and relax.
3 Change the legs over and repeat.

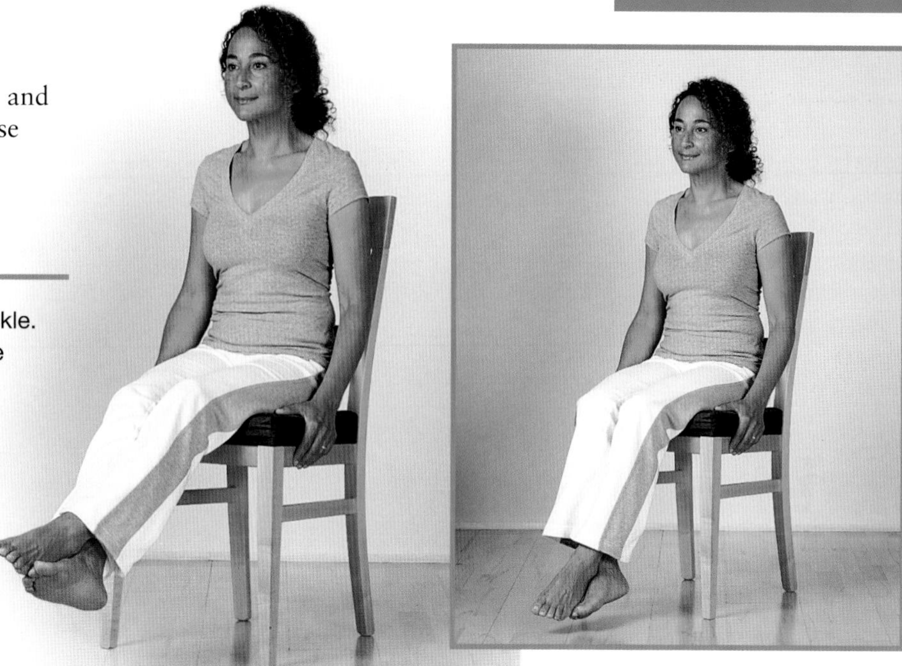

Hips

1 Lie flat on your front.
2 Raise one leg a little way off the ground and hold it there for a count of three before lowering it slowly. Repeat with your other leg.
3 Lie on your side.
4 Raise your upper leg slowly to a count of three, hold it in the raised position for a moment and then lower it to a count of three. Turn onto your other side and repeat.

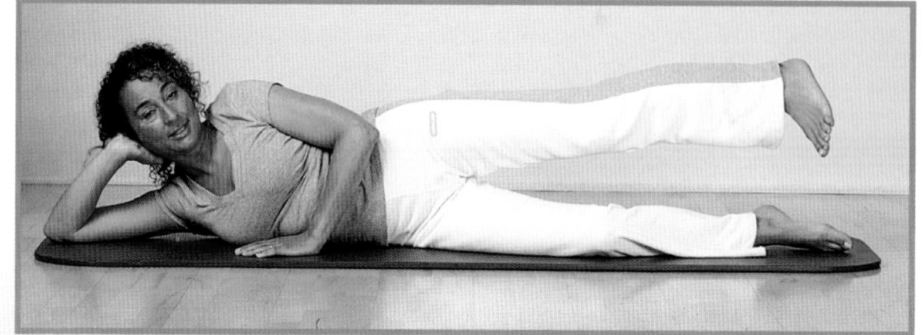

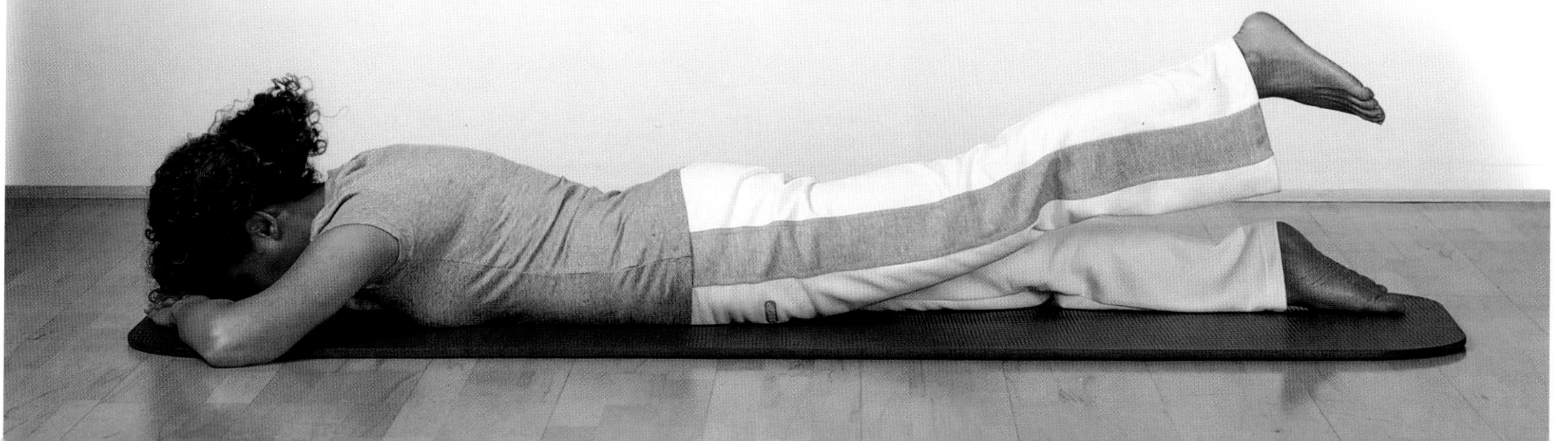

Stretching exercises

It is important to move affected joints through their full range of movements every day to keep stiffness to a minimum. Stretching exercises can help to ease the pain of osteoarthritis as well as reducing stiffness and improving joint mobility. They may also help you to relax. If possible, perform appropriate exercises five times and repeat twice a day.

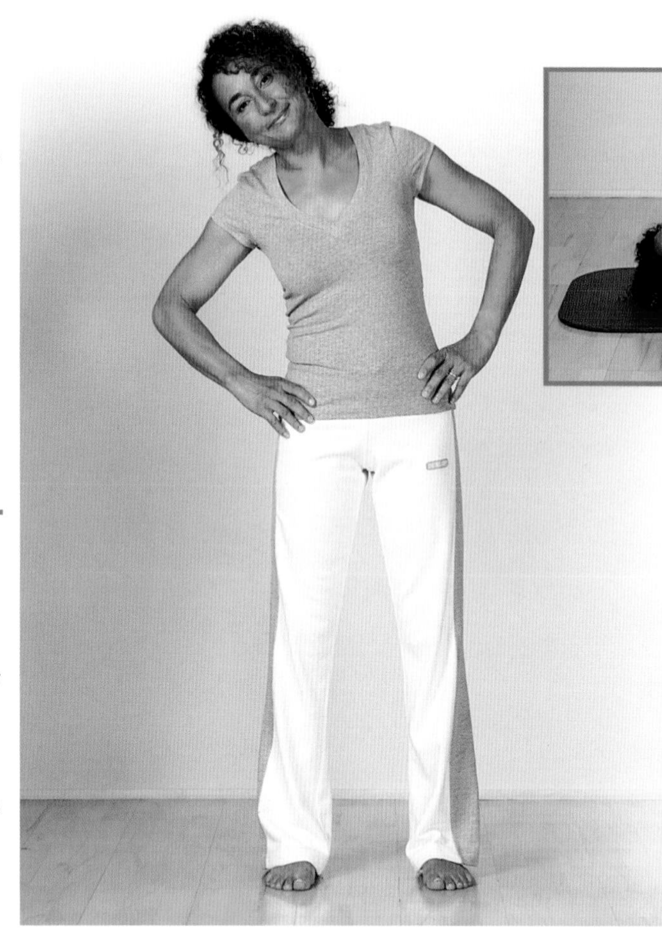

Back stretches

1 Stand with your hands on your hips.
2 Keeping your hips facing forwards, slowly bend to one side and then to the other.
3 Lie flat on your back with your arms by your sides and bend your knees.
4 Keeping your shoulders on the floor, roll your knees to one side and count to 10. Then roll your knees to the other side and count to 10.

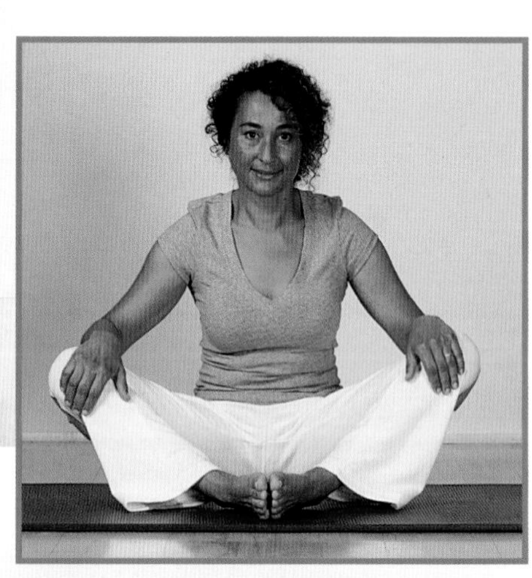

Hip stretches

1 Lie on your back and pull one knee slowly up to your chest. Keep your other leg as straight as you can. Repeat with your other leg.
2 Press the small of your back into the floor to stretch your back.

3 Sit up straight and draw the soles of your feet together so that your knees are bent and flop apart. Then gently press your knees further apart.

Relaxation exercises

Everyone can benefit from taking time to relax each day. As well as promoting general well-being, people with osteoarthritis may find relaxation exercises help them to cope with the stress of chronic pain. There are many different relaxation techniques; you may like to try the exercise on the right to start with.

Relaxation exercise

1 Lie on your back. Try to focus your mind on the muscles in your toes. Tense your toes, slowly count to 5 and then relax.

2 Working up from your toes, focus your mind on each part of your body in turn. Tense each group of muscles, count to 5 and relax. Work your way all the way up to your eyes – open them wide, raise your eyebrows and then relax.

3 Lie still, breathing slowly and enjoying the state of relaxation.

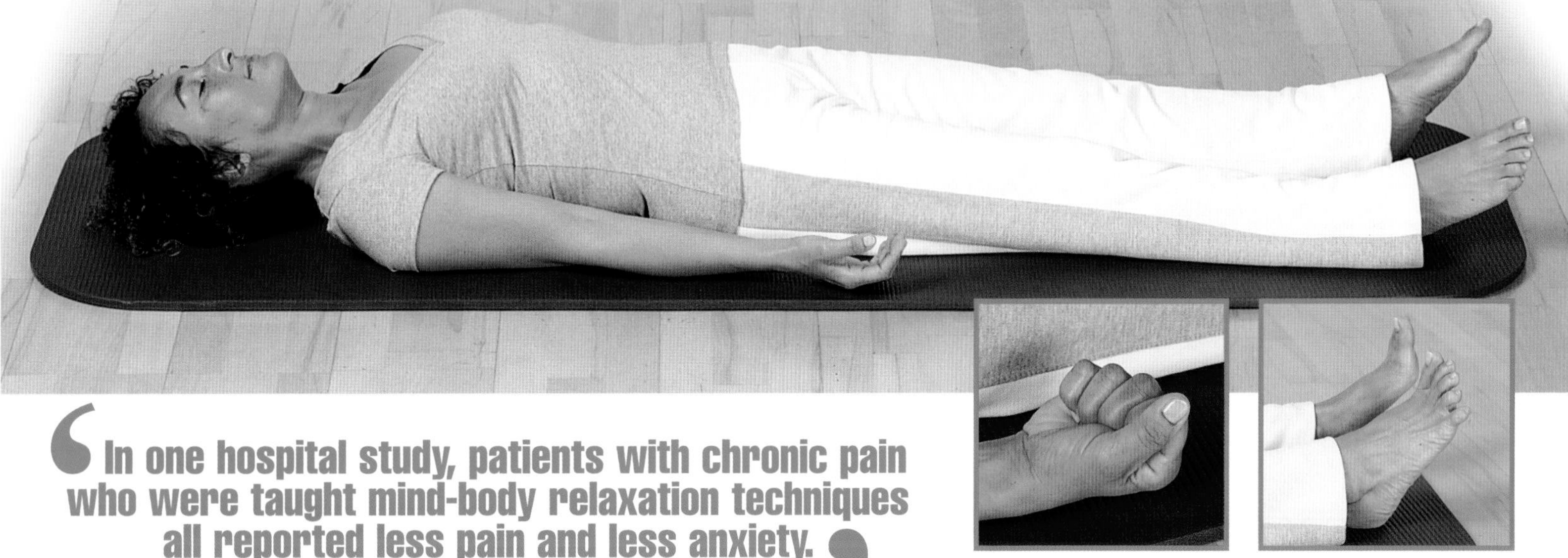

‘In one hospital study, patients with chronic pain who were taught mind-body relaxation techniques all reported less pain and less anxiety.’

HYDROTHERAPY

Water-based exercises are particularly beneficial for people with joint problems because the water provides support for the joints while the muscles are strengthened and flexibility improved. Aerobic fitness will also be improved.

Hydrotherapy involves a regime of special exercises in a specially heated pool. The warmth of the water relaxes muscles and so can help to ease painful joints. Hydrotherapy is often given in hospital as part of a physiotherapy treatment programme. A course of six sessions or so may be recommended and each session is likely to last for around 30 minutes.

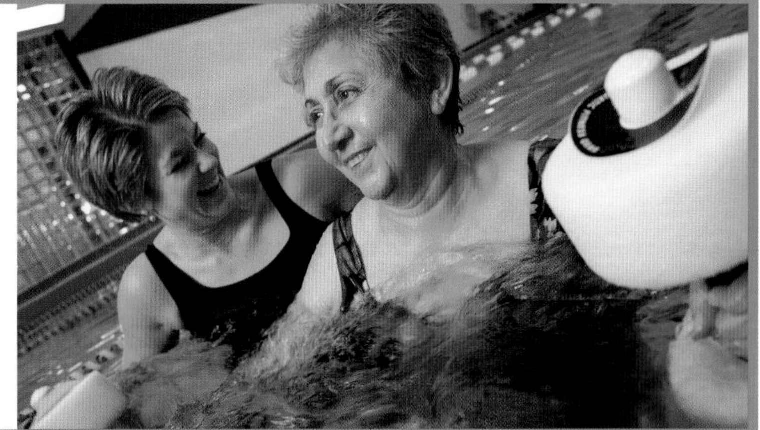

Conventional treatments

A wide range of treatments are available to relieve your symptoms. These are sometimes used alone and sometimes in combination.

Gels and creams

Non-steroidal anti-inflammatory gels are available over the counter. These can be rubbed over the affected joint to relieve mild symptoms. Side-effects are unlikely as only a very small amount of drug is absorbed into the body through the skin. Capsaicin cream, derived from chillies, is sometimes used for pain relief. It may initially cause a burning sensation but this should soon wear off.

Oral treatments

- **Analgesics** such as paracetamol or co-dydramol may be useful in the short term to relieve pain.
- **Non-steroidal anti-inflammatory drugs** (NSAIDs) such as ibuprofen, naproxen and diclofenac can reduce pain, swelling and stiffness. They may be used on a temporary basis for severe symptoms and are sometimes taken in combination with analgesics. They may also be given rectally as a suppository, as this form is tolerated better by some people. NSAIDs may cause a number of side effects, some of which can be serious (see caution box).

CAUTION

Around 15–20 per cent of patients find that NSAIDs cause stomach or intestinal ulcers. 2–4 per cent suffer serious complications such as bleeding in the digestive tract; women over 70 with heart disease or a history of ulcers are at greatest risk. NSAIDs have also been linked to an increased risk of heart attack. People who have heart problems or suffer from asthma and certain other conditions should not take NSAIDs unless otherwise advised by their doctor.

Injections

- **Corticosteroid injections** can help to ease particularly painful joints. As with the other treatments for osteoarthritis, steroid injections cannot repair the damage caused by the disease but may provide pain relief.
- **Hyaluronic acid** may be injected into a knee joint to supplement the hyaluronic acid that is present naturally in the fluid of the joint. This treatment may relieve pain over a period of up to six months, though it can initially worsen symptoms. Research is currently looking into hyaluronic acid's effect on the progression of osteoarthritis.

Surgical treatments

Surgery may be considered if symptoms are very severe and if there is a marked limitation of movement and severe pain even after trying other treatments.

Joint replacement

Arthroplasty, or joint replacement, aims to relieve pain and improve mobility. Many joints can now be replaced, the most common being the hip and knee.

- **Hip replacement** The upper part of the thigh bone including the head (the ball that fits into the socket of the pelvis) is removed and replaced by an artificial ball. Many types of replacement hip last for 20 years or longer. For more details about hip replacement surgery >>226–227.
- **Knee replacement** The ends of the bones that form the knee joint are removed and replaced by plastic and metal. A full knee replacement may be performed or alternatively only parts of the joint are replaced. The success of this operation varies from person to person; some find walking much easier but others still have some difficulty. Most artificial knees last at least 10 years. For more details about knee replacement surgery >>208–209.

Other surgical options

Various other options exist. All have their own potential benefits and risks, which should be discussed with the orthopaedic surgeon. Other operations include:

- **Removal of osteophytes** The bony growths around affected joints can seriously limit movement, in which case surgical removal may be helpful.
- **Fusion of the joint** Known as arthrodesis, this procedure relieves pain but leaves the treated joint immobile. For those who have very severe pain this limitation may be worthwhile, particularly in the small joints of the hands or toes.
- **Osteotomy** This procedure involves cutting bones, often with the aim of re-aligning them and reducing abnormal stresses on them. Osteotomy may slow the deterioration in a joint and sometimes reduce pain a little.

a visit to

THE PHYSIOTHERAPIST

Physiotherapists use physical methods, rather than surgical or drug-based treatments, to increase the mobility of joints and help ease pain and discomfort in the affected area.

You will usually need a referral from your GP to make an appointment with a chartered physiotherapist – the therapist will want to keep your GP or consultant closely informed over the course of your treatment.

At your first appointment, the physiotherapist will examine you to assess your problem and decide how physiotherapy can help you. Appointments may take place in a hospital physiotherapy department or at your home and treatment is usually given as a course of sessions, each one lasting around 45 minutes.

The physiotherapist may show you particular exercises to improve the movement in your joints, strengthen your supporting muscles and help you to relax. The therapist is also likely to draw up an exercise programme to help you to increase your range of movement and the stability of the affected joint. Other treatments include hydrotherapy, electro-heat treatment and ultrasound, massage and manipulation.

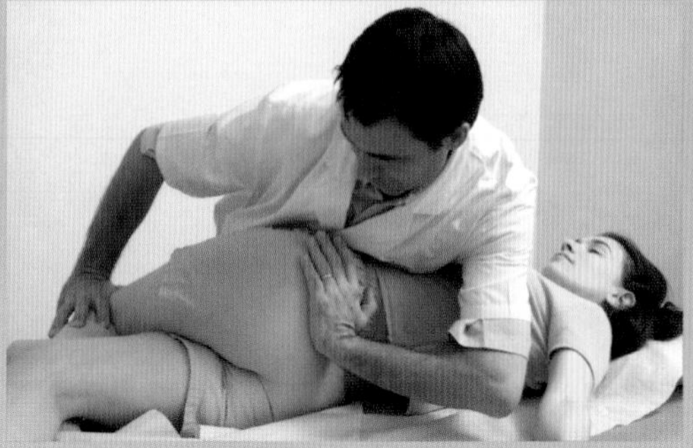

Manual therapy The physiotherapist may use a number of hands-on techniques to stretch joints and muscles, provide pain relief and improve joint range-of-motion. Techniques include passive exercise and manipulation, where the physiotherapist adjusts limbs and joints without your active assistance. Massage may help to relieve muscle spasm, stimulate blood flow and relieve inflammation.

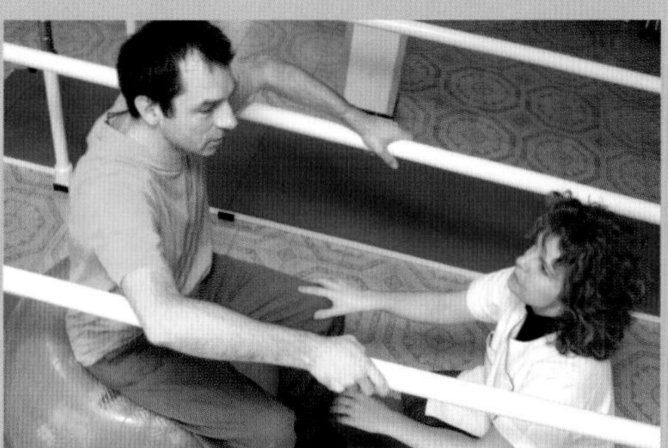

Exercise The physiotherapist will show you how to perform active exercises to work your joints and muscles and may draw up a tailored exercise programme for you to follow at home or under supervision. The therapist may recommend hydrotherapy, where exercises are performed in water to support your body weight and take pressure off your joints.

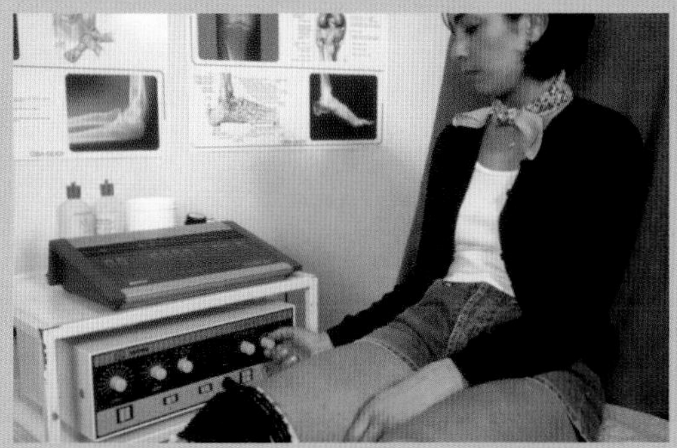

Electrotherapy and heat treatment Methods include applying heat packs, passing a small electrical current through pads on the skin (diathermy), and using high-energy ultrasonic waves delivered by a probe moved over the affected area. These treatments may help to relieve muscle tension, pain and stiffness.

>> **Hydrotherapy:** page 258 >> **Massage:** page 245

Other treatment options

Diet and supplements

No studies have found hard evidence of foods that cause or worsen osteoarthritis, but some people find that certain foods do make their symptoms worse. Examples of such foods include cheese, tomatoes, red meat and wine. Review your diet to see whether any foods affect your symptoms.

A substance called solanine, found in foods including potatoes, tomatoes and peppers, may play a role in the development of OA. Avoiding such foods may bring about an improvement in symptoms after a period of several months.

Many supplements have been recommended for OA, but only a few are likely to have a significant beneficial effect. The most important are listed below. If you are considering taking supplements or making dietary changes always talk to your GP first.

Essential fatty acids

Your body uses essential fatty acids (EFAs) to produce chemicals that reduce inflammation. Your body cannot make them itself, so EFAs must come from your diet.

- **Omega-3** is found in oily fishes, such as mackerel, herring, sardines and salmon. You can buy fish-oil capsules at health food stores and chemists. Fish liver oil, which contains both EFAs and vitamin D (to help the body absorb calcium) also contains a large amount of vitamin A which is harmful if taken in excess. As with other supplements, take care not to exceed the recommended dose. A number of new omega-3 fortified milks have recently been developed for the UK market.
- **Omega-6** may also be beneficial. This EFA is found in nuts and seeds and in evening primrose oil and blackcurrant seed oil supplements.

Glucosamine and chondroitin sulphate

Glucosamine and chondroitin are naturally occurring compounds in the human body. Glucosamine is an amino sugar believed to play a role in cartilage formation and chondroitin is a protein molecule and a key component of cartilage.

People with osteoarthritis may benefit from taking additional amounts of these substances. Dietary supplements containing versions derived from crab and lobster shells and animal cartilage are widely available from health food shops and chemists. Glucosamine supplements are claimed to relieve osteoarthritis symptoms and may even encourage cartilage repair. Chondroitin sulphate is believed to draw water into cartilage, making it more spongy. Some people find this relieves pain and improves joint movement.

More studies are needed before any definite conclusions can be drawn but these substances are unlikely to cause any serious side effects. Children and pregnant women should not take the supplements.

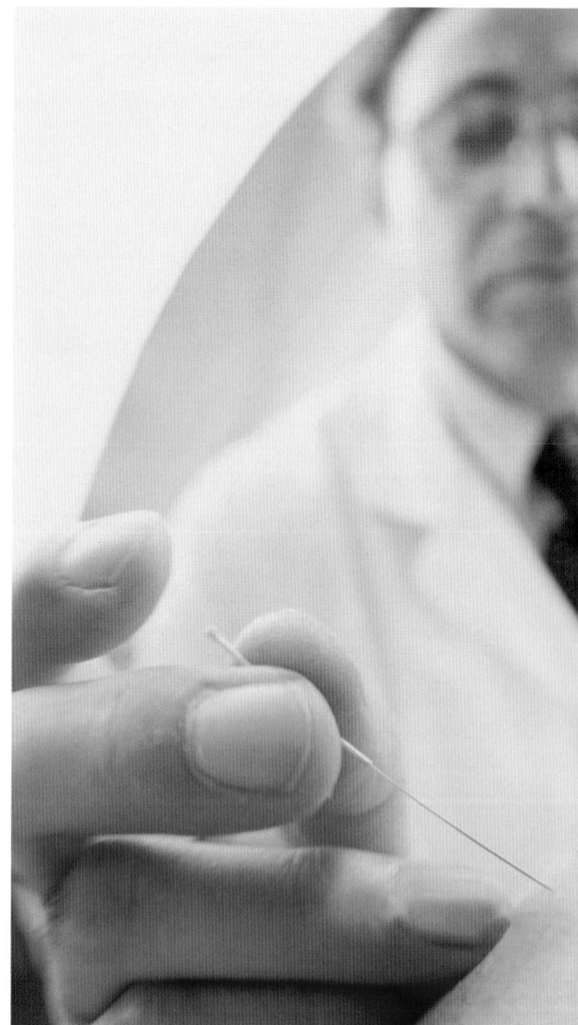

DID YOU KNOW?

A traditional remedy for the symptoms of arthritis has received a timely boost by the *British Medical Journal* (BMJ). According to a report in 2003, a cool cabbage leaf held against a painful joint may have a beneficial anti-inflammatory effect. It's also the perfect shape for fitting around a kneecap!

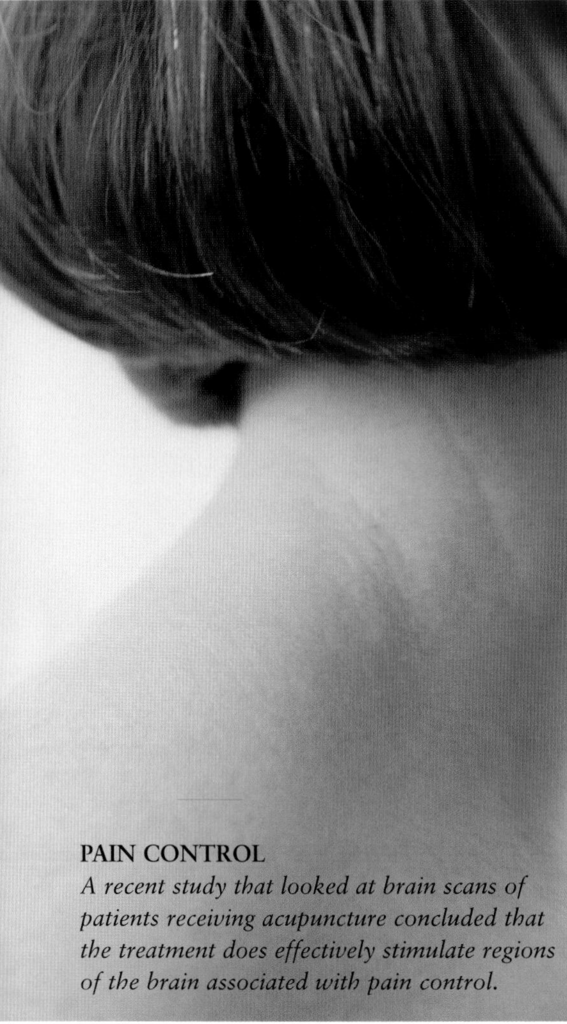

PAIN CONTROL
A recent study that looked at brain scans of patients receiving acupuncture concluded that the treatment does effectively stimulate regions of the brain associated with pain control.

Complementary medicine

Opinions differ as to the role that complementary therapies play in the treatment of osteoarthritis. Some people choose to use these treatments alone while others take them alongside their conventional medical treatments. If you are considering complementary medicine, it is important first to seek a medical opinion to confirm your diagnosis and give you informed advice.

There are a wide variety of therapies to consider, from acupuncture to herbal medicine. Whichever form of therapy you choose, be sure that you find a reputable practitioner who is registered with an appropriate professional body. Your doctor may be able to advise you.

Acupuncture

A number of studies have suggested that acupuncture can be helpful in relieving the pain of osteoarthritis, particularly if the condition affects the knee or the hip. Research published in the BMJ in 2004 showed that patients with OA of the knee who received acupuncture as well as an anti-inflammatory painkiller suffered less pain and stiffness than those who received the drug plus sham acupuncture, where the needle did not puncture the skin.

Many NHS pain clinics and some physiotherapists now offer acupuncture and may recommend a course of regular sessions followed by maintenance sessions, perhaps once a month, to keep your symptoms under control.

Homeopathy

Some people believe homeopathy to be beneficial in relieving their symptoms. This has been backed up to a certain extent by research although more studies are needed.

> **‘I find that massage really helps me cope with the pain. I'm not sure that it has any effect on my arthritis but it certainly puts me in a more positive state of mind’**

Homeopaths may prescribe a number of remedies together, depending on a patient's general health and the nature of their symptoms. Examples of remedies used include rhus toxicodendron, causticum and calcarea fluorica.

Western herbal medicine

Many herbal remedies are used for the treatment of osteoarthritis. They include anti-inflammatory substances such as meadowsweet, birch leaves and willow bark, all of which contain salicylate, a substance found in aspirin. Some treatments may be applied directly to the affected area, such as seaweed plasters for painful or swollen joints. Creams and lotions containing substances including lavender, rosemary and menthol may also be used for mild symptoms.

When considering herbal remedies, it is important to seek advice from a reputable supplier. People who have other diseases or who are taking conventional drugs must take particular care and should always check with a doctor first.

Manipulation

Performed by a registered osteopath or chiropractor, manipulation may help to relieve pain affecting the neck and back. It has not been found to offer much help in treating osteoarthritis in other joints. Joints that are swollen and inflamed should not be manipulated.

Massage

Effects from massage may include relief from muscle tension and joint pain, as well as a reduction in stress levels. There are many different types of massage available, so you should check with the therapist to find out what is involved.

Looking to the future

The majority of people diagnosed with osteoarthritis find it a nuisance rather than a debilitating disease. As our understanding of OA and of the different ways to treat and manage the disease improves, life for sufferers is also likely to get easier. One day it may be possible to halt or even reverse the damage that OA causes to joints.

The outlook

Often, the symptoms of osteoarthritis seem to worsen over a period of time before stabilizing or even improving. In only a relatively small number of cases, symptoms continue to worsen and the function of the affected joint is impaired.

There is much that affected individuals can do to take control of the disease. Many people with OA require no medical treatment but rather rely on simple self-help measures such as weight-loss, exercise and supplements to deal with their symptoms. Surgery should be considered only when severe symptoms persist despite trying the more moderate treatment options.

Hope for the future

Research is constantly improving our understanding of how and why osteoarthritis develops. This increasing knowledge should lead to the development of new treatments and may one day help doctors to achieve the ultimate aims of reversing or even preventing the disease. Areas currently under research include:

Making new cartilage

- **Stimulating cartilage cell repair** New research is focusing on changing cartilage cells so that they can be stimulated to repair themselves.
- **Growing new cells** Research is also ongoing into growing new cartilage cells from existing ones removed from a joint, a process known as autologous chondrocyte implementation (ACI). Cells are removed from an area of the joint that is only minimally load bearing and grown as a tissue culture before being injected back into the joint. Initial trials are encouraging and researchers are currently examining how well the implanted cartilage integrates with existing tissues over the longer term.
- **Using stem cells** Another option could be to use mesenchymal stem cells (MSCs) found in bone marrow. These cells are capable of becoming an array of tissue types, including cartilage. The advantage of this process over ACI is that stem cells are better able to recreate the structure and organization of the original tissue.

Preventing damage to cartilage

- **Drugs** Certain chemicals in the body, notably enzymes called metalloproteinases, are thought to play a key role in cartilage break down. Drugs may be available in the future that block their action.
- **Genetic engineering** One day, cells may be taken from the body and their genes altered so that they are able to prevent the action of the chemicals. The genetically engineered cells would then be injected into the joint to prevent further damage.

4 WAYS TO...

Cope with your emotions

Chronic pain is not only physically tiring, it can be emotionally draining too. As well as taking steps to deal with the physical symptoms of osteoarthritis, it is important to learn how to manage the emotions created by the disease.

Research has shown that people who understand their disease and who have support are likely to experience less severe pain and need less medication. The following are likely to help you cope with the condition:

1 **Understand OA** Make sure you understand what your condition involves so that you feel more in control of what is happening to your body and you don't panic.

2 **Rest and relax** Set aside time to rest and relax every day. Stress may exacerbate symptoms and make it harder to cope mentally with your condition. Try the relaxation exercise shown on page 241.

3 **Share your feelings** Talk to your GP, occupational therapist, physiotherapist, family or friends about how you feel. Consider getting help from a counsellor or psychotherapist if you feel things are getting on top of you.

4 **Find a support group** People who have undergone common experiences can offer reassurance, inspiration and advice. For some useful contact addresses >>336-339.

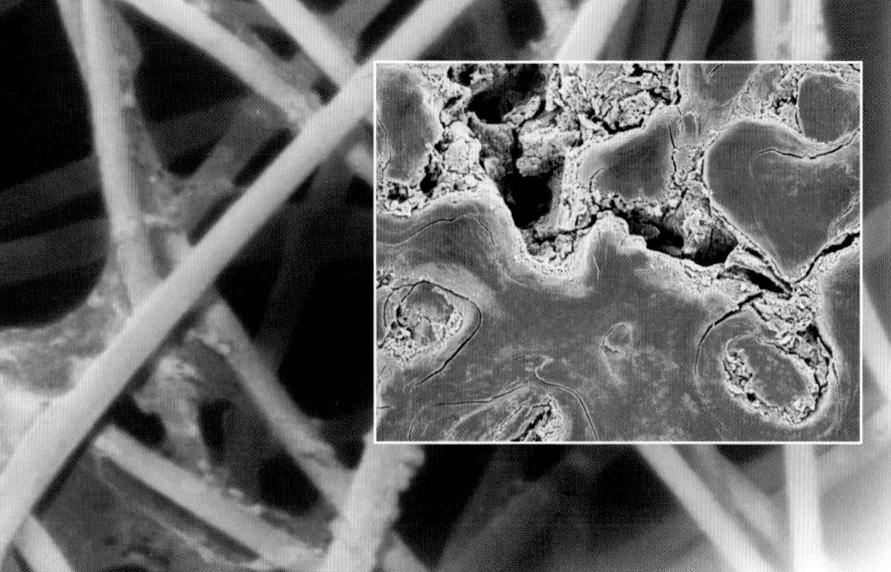

REPLACING DAMAGED CARTILAGE
The electron micrograph seen on the left shows cracked, damaged cartilage on the head of a femur removed during a hip replacement operation. Rather than having to resort to this type of surgery, however, it is now possible to inject artificially-grown cartilage into a joint. The electron micrograph far left shows new cartilage cells growing on pink strands of synthetic fibres. Once the cartilage is implanted into a damaged joint, the fibres safely break down in the body.

Identifying abnormal genes

In about a quarter of cases, abnormal genes may play a part in the development of osteoarthritis. Using data from the Human Genome Project, scientists at Oxford's Institute of Molecular Medicine believe that they have narrowed down the search for the genes responsible to five areas of chromosomes. Meanwhile a Japanese study, published in the journal *Nature Genetics* in 2005, pinpointed a mutant form of a gene called asporin as more common in osteoarthritis patients.

Eventually, it may be possible to find those people at increased risk of developing OA by testing for the presence of the abnormal genes. They can then be shown how to make the lifestyle changes necessary to reduce this risk. It may even one day be possible to change the abnormal genes and so prevent the condition from developing.

Research into existing treatments

Studies are assessing the impact that regular exercise has on joints affected by osteoarthritis and what exercises are the most beneficial. Research continues on non-steroidal anti-inflammatory drugs (NSAIDs) to develop new ones that are less likely to cause side effects, particularly the problems in the upper digestive tract.

Research also continues into the use of supplements, particularly glucosamine and chondroitin sulphate (>>244). Exciting results from a three-year Belgian study, reported in *The Lancet* in January 2001, show that glucosamine can actually prevent the knee joints from narrowing, suggesting the supplement has the potential to stop OA in its tracks. It takes many years to assess the impact of treatments on the damage that occurs in OA but our understanding of the effects of such supplements is improving all the time.

DID YOU KNOW?

Researchers in Korea have recently confirmed that extracts from New Zealand green-lipped mussel (*Perna canaliculus*) can significantly reduce the symptoms of knee and hip osteoarthritis, apparently without causing other side effects. American researchers have shown that this extract can work in dogs too. This treatment could be one to watch for the future.

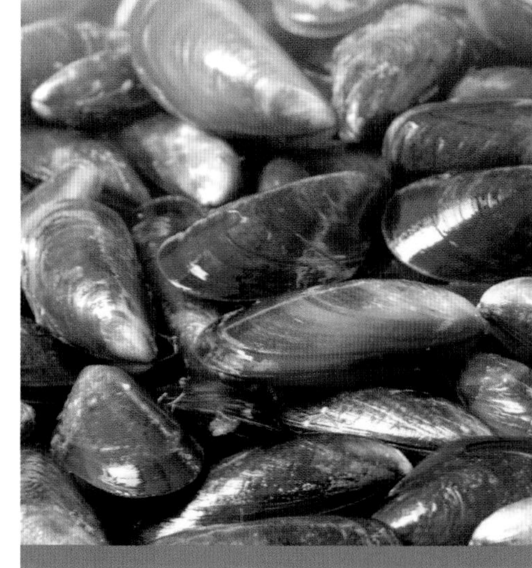

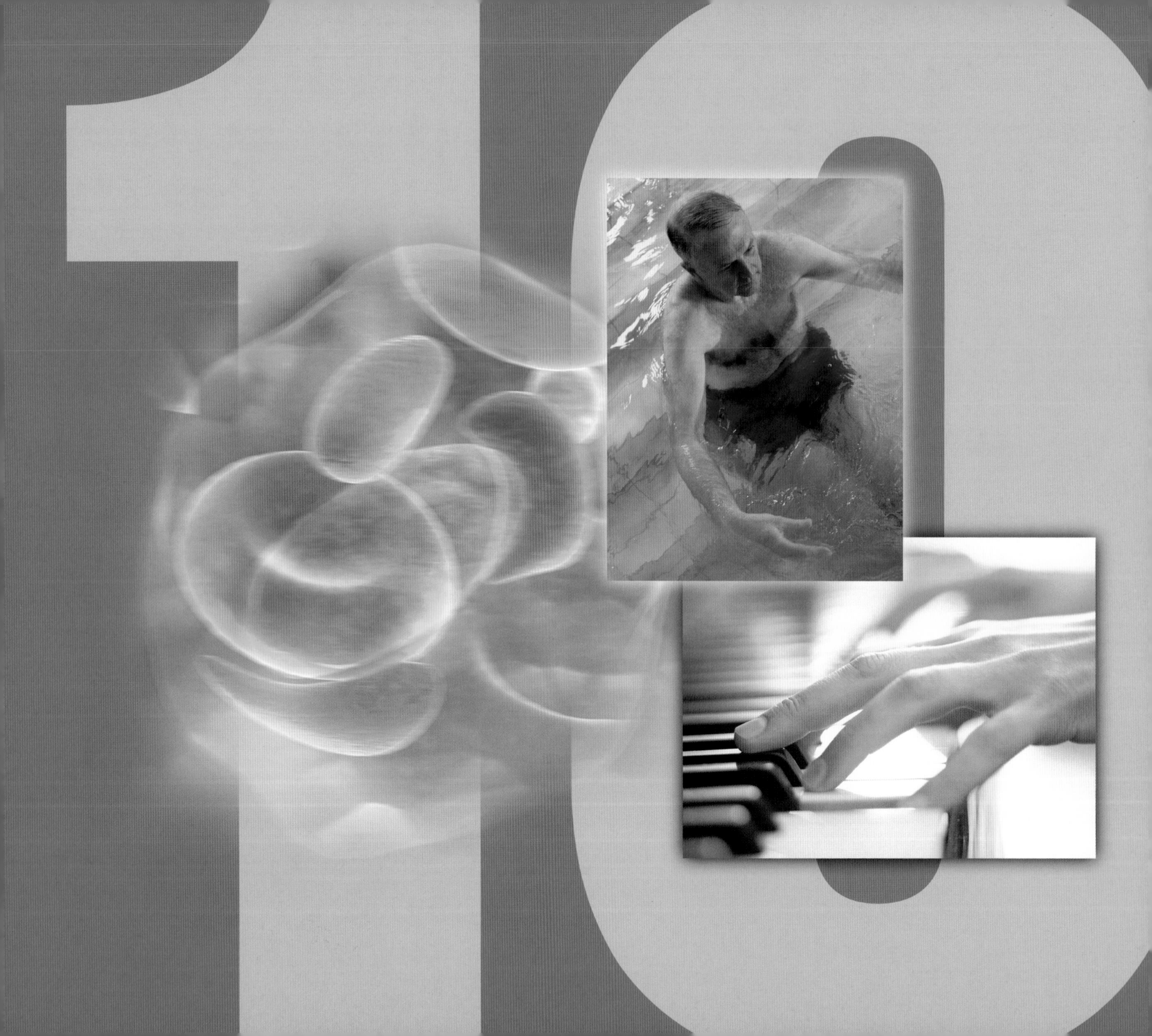

RHEUMATOID ARTHRITIS

An autoimmune disease that can strike individuals of any age, rheumatoid arthritis often affects the smaller joints, causing pain and inflammation. With both hereditary and non-hereditary risk factors, it's a complex condition but one that does respond to changes in diet and to modern medicines. In these pages you will find the latest information and proven techniques for combating pain, swelling and stiffness, and for alleviating other symptoms.

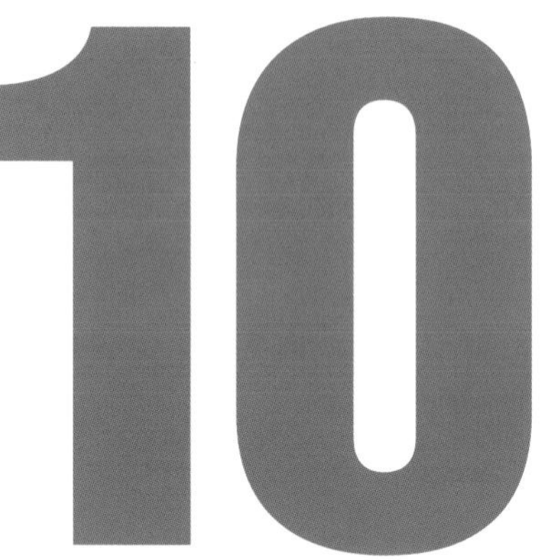

RHEUMATOID ARTHRITIS What is it?

This painful autoimmune disorder occurs when the immune system forms antibodies against the body's own cells – specifically the cells of the synovium, the thin layer of tissue that lines the joints. Unlike osteoarthritis, body tissues outside the joints are sometimes also affected, causing problems in other body systems.

What happens?

As the synovial lining of the joints becomes inflamed (synovitis), the tissues swell and produce more than the usual amount of fluid needed to lubricate the movements of the bones within the joint. This irritates nearby nerves and stretches the capsule surrounding the joint. The cartilage covering the bone ends and eventually the bone itself may also be damaged.

Rheumatoid arthritis (RA) can also cause inflammation in the heart, lungs, blood vessels and eyes. Anaemia – a deficiency of the oxygen-carrying haemoglobin in blood – is a common feature.

DID YOU KNOW?

- Rheumatoid arthritis affects more than 350,000 people in the UK. The disease often develops between the ages of 30 and 50, although it can occur at any age.
- For reasons not yet fully understood it is least common in black African and Chinese people.
- RA affects two to three times more women than men. The higher risk in women is increased further in the weeks after giving birth and when breast-feeding.
- Cigarette smoking is associated with an increased risk of RA.

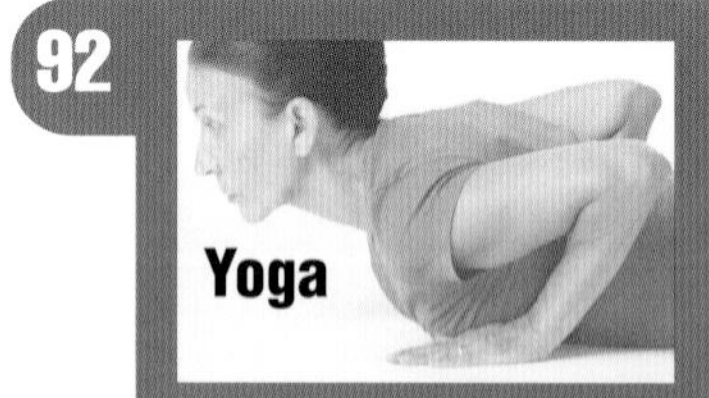
92 Yoga

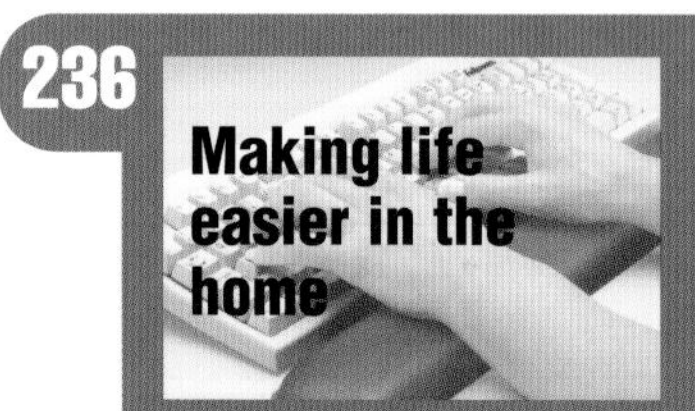
236 Making life easier in the home

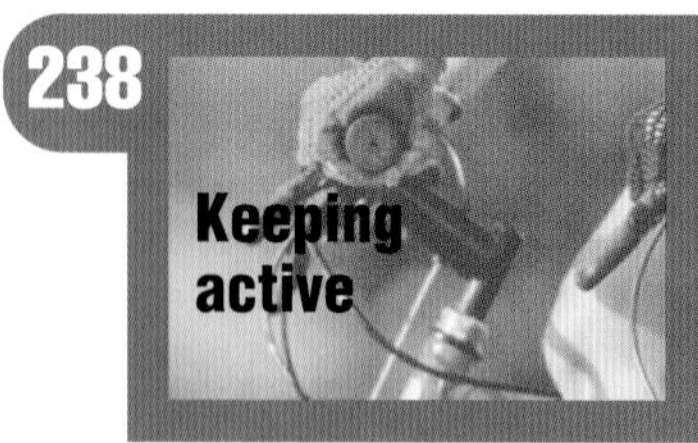
238 Keeping active

Under the skin...

The capsule around our joints consists of a tough fibrous membrane on the outside and a thin synovial membrane, or synovium, on the inside. Rheumatoid arthritis occurs when the synovium is invaded by white blood cells, causing inflammation and swelling in the joint capsule. This may also cause damage to cartilage and bones.

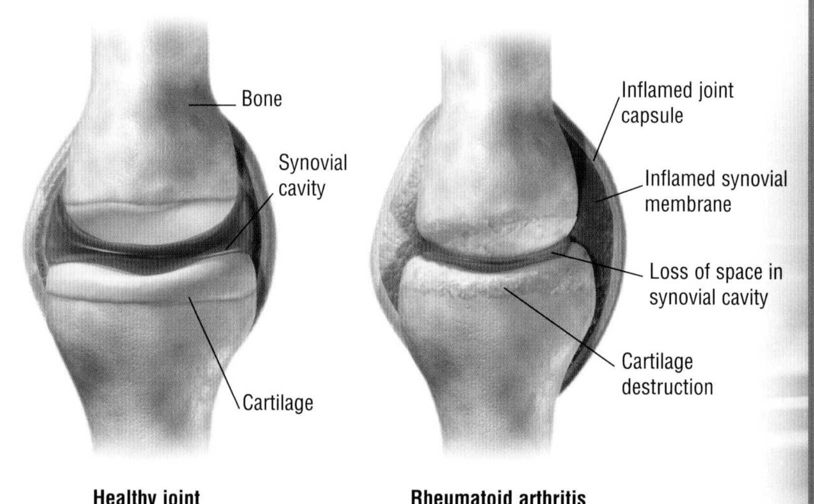

Rheumatoid arthritis tends to begin between the ages of 30 and 50, but it may occur later in life and occasionally in early childhood. In most cases, several joints are involved and it usually affects the same type of joint on each side of the body. The small joints in the hand tend to become inflamed first, but it may start in any joint. Sometimes the inflammation occurs in just one joint, often the shoulder or the knee.

How the disease develops varies. Some people have the disease for less than 12 months after which the joints return to normal; in some cases it stops after several years leaving only slight joint damage; in other cases the damage progresses rapidly and is severe after only a few years.

In most cases the disease persists for many years and it can be life-long with a pattern of relapses, in which the symptoms flare-up for weeks or months, interspersed with periods of remission. What triggers a relapse is not always clear; it may be set off by another illness or by emotional stress. Often, there will be no apparent reason.

Some people believe that RA occurs particularly in cold climates, but the disease affects people in every part of the world. Moving to a different climate does not change the way the disease develops, but it may influence the symptoms.

What are the causes?

The causes of rheumatoid arthritis are not fully understood, but a number of factors may play a part in its development. There is no evidence that the disease is triggered by an infection.

- **Female sex hormones** Around three times more premenopausal women are affected than men; after the menopause men and women are affected equally. This suggests that female sex hormones such as oestrogen and progesterone, the levels of which fall at the menopause, play a role.
- **Genetic factors** RA sometimes runs in families and genes may be a factor in around 60 per cent of cases.
- **Human leukocyte antigens (HLA)** These proteins are found on the surface of most body cells. Our immune system uses them to distinguish between normal cells and foreign invaders, such as cancer cells or bacteria, that it needs to attack. Many different types of HLA are present in the body; each of us inherits a personal set from our parents.

Some HLAs are linked to certain autoimmune disorders – the presence of these types may indicate an increased risk from rheumatoid arthritis. But because these HLAs are not always present, and also may occur in people without arthritis, the presence of a certain HLA cannot be used alone to diagnose the disease.

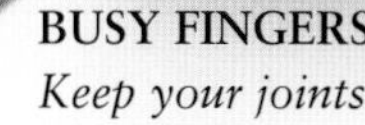

BUSY FINGERS
Keep your joints mobile to prevent stiffness, especially the small joints in your hands and fingers.

What are the symptoms?

In most people, the condition develops over weeks or months. In some cases, inflammation develops rapidly over a period of only a few days. The symptoms tend to include:

- Pain and stiffness in affected joints
- Joints that feel warm to the touch
- Swollen joints due to the accumulation of synovial fluid
- Thinning and weakening of the muscles around affected joints
- Painless lumps called nodules on pressure areas such as the elbows
- A general feeling of malaise
- Eventually there may be deformity of affected joints

The joint pain is usually at its worse in the morning. Stiffness is also worse in the morning and generally lasts for more than an hour, although it may improve as you use the joints. RA usually develops in a symmetrical pattern, so both hands or both knees are likely to be affected together.

If you think you may have rheumatoid arthritis you should make an appointment to see your doctor – it is important to start treatment as soon as possible.

Which body parts are affected?

The small joints of the hands are the most common area for inflammation but various other joints may also be affected, including the wrists, elbows, shoulders, ankles and knees. The hips are sometimes also involved, but less often. The lymph nodes around an affected joint may be swollen and the disease occasionally causes inflammation in other body systems including the lungs and blood vessels. There may also be weight loss.

Shoulder and elbow

The shoulders are often affected by rheumatoid arthritis. Typically, sufferers experience pain in the upper arm at night and difficulty lifting the arm. Eventually, stiffness may limit arm movements making it difficult to wash, dress and perform other activities. Nodules often develop under the skin on the elbows.

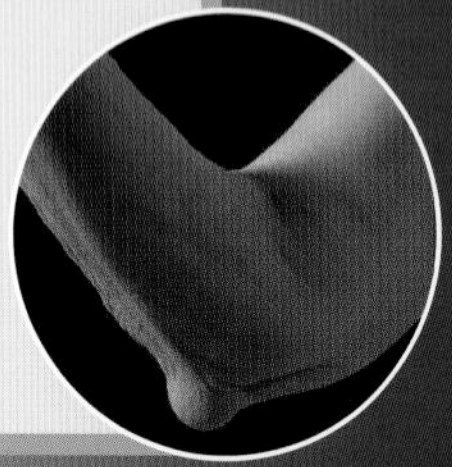

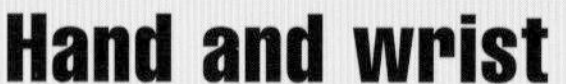

Hand and wrist

Rheumatoid arthritis in the hands can be severe, with pain, swelling and stiffness of the joints. Deformities can develop, although hand function often remains good. RA in the wrist can cause carpal tunnel syndrome, a condition in which compression of a nerve at the wrist results in tingling, pain and later weakening in the hand.

Knees

Inflammation of the knee joints can be severe and is often associated with marked swelling due to the accumulation of a large amount of synovial fluid in the joint. Knocked knees or bowing of the legs at the knees may eventually develop.

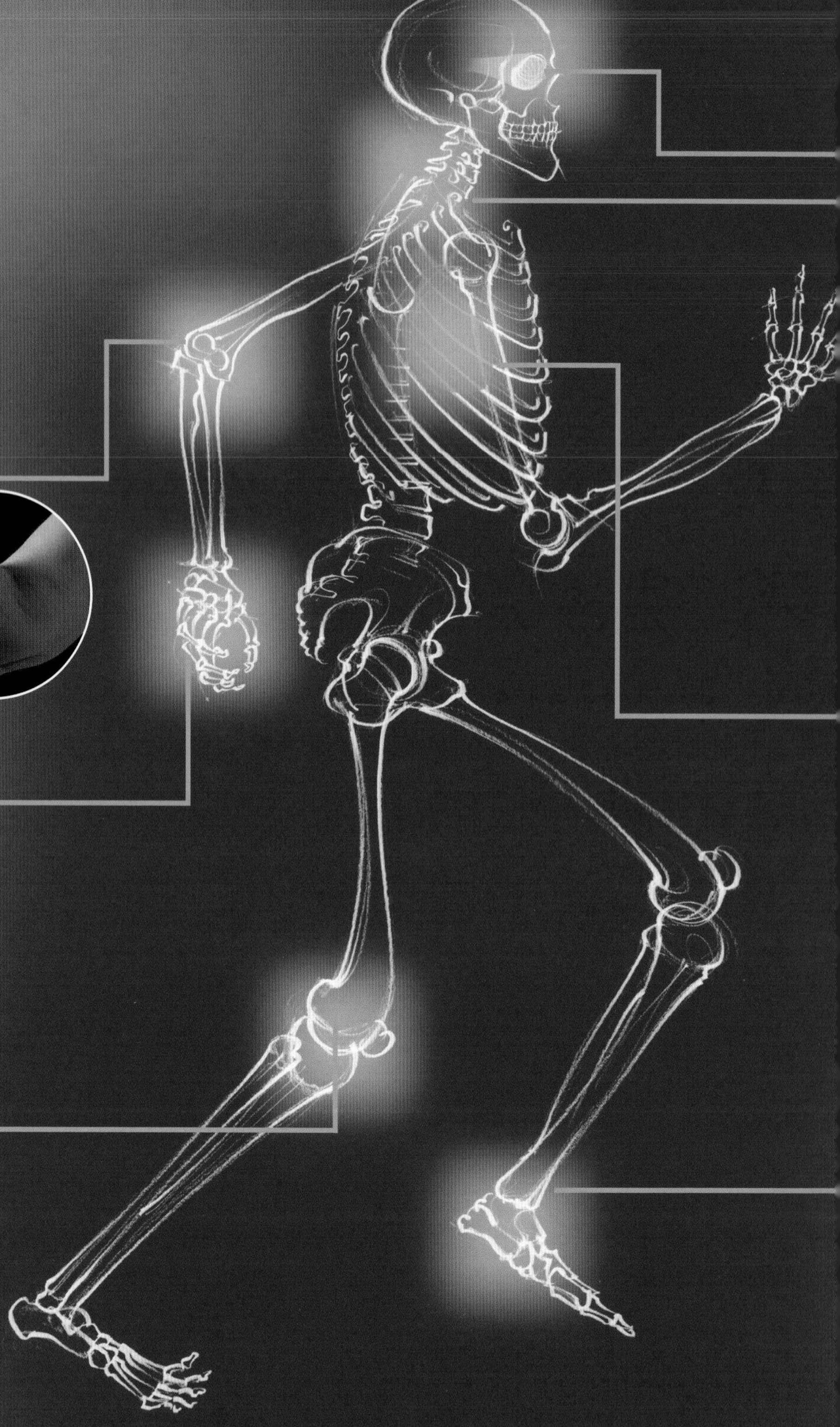

Eyes

Around 25 per cent of people with RA suffer from dry eyes. Other eye problems include inflammation of the cornea (keratitis) and inflammation of the blood vessels in the whites of the eyes (scleritis). Inflammation may leave red painful lesions.

Neck and jaw

Other joints that may be affected include the vertebrae of the spine in the neck and the temporomandibular joint, which connects the lower to the upper jaw.

Lungs, heart and circulation

Tiredness caused by anaemia, in which the amount of oxygen-carrying haemoglobin in the blood falls, is a feature in about 80 per cent of cases. Lung disorders may develop, including fibrosing alveolitis, a long-term condition which affects the walls of the air sacs within the lungs. In a few cases, the membrane that surrounds the heart may become inflamed in a condition known as pericarditis. The walls of small blood vessels around the body may also become inflamed, affecting blood supply to the bowel. Another possible feature is Raynaud's phenomenon, in which the arteries supplying blood to the hands narrow when they are cold, causing tingling and numbness.

In addition to these possible cardiovascular problems, RA often causes weight loss.

Feet and ankles

Rheumatoid arthritis affects the feet and ankles almost as frequently as it does the hands. The feet are often affected early on in the disease. They widen and may be painful, often making walking difficult.

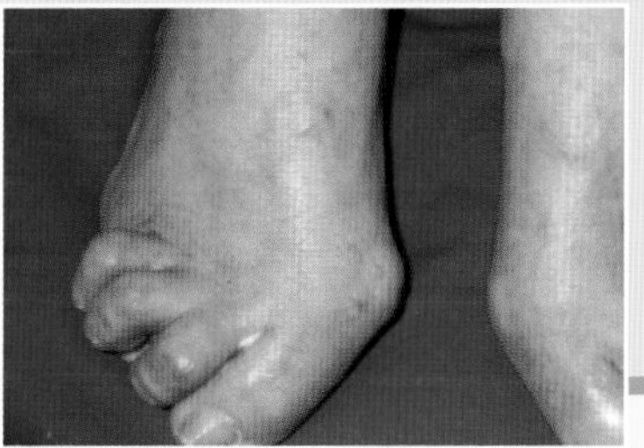

How is it diagnosed?

Rheumatoid arthritis is usually diagnosed from a description of the symptoms and from an examination the joints involved, although a few tests will be performed to back up the findings.

Around 80 per cent of people with rheumatoid arthritis are also anaemic, so a blood sample will be taken to check for a low red blood-cell count. Your blood may also be tested generally for signs of inflammation as well as for Rheumatoid factor (RF), an antibody often found in people with RA. Unfortunately this cannot be used to make the diagnosis on its own: although the antibody is present in 60–80 per cent of those affected, it is also present in around 10 per cent of the population without the disease.

X-rays may show changes that are suggestive of rheumatoid arthritis, such as a narrowing of the spaces between the joints or erosion of bone or cartilage. However, X-rays often appear normal during the first 3–6 months of the disease.

Your doctor may also insert a needle into an affected joint and withdraw a sample of the synovial fluid which can be examined under a microscope for signs of inflammation. He or she may also remove a small tissue sample, called a biopsy, of any rheumatoid nodules.

A specialist may arrange magnetic resonance imaging (MRI) or ultrasound scanning, although these tests are of limited use in the diagnosis of RA at present. They may become more widespread as their ability to pick up changes improves.

What can I do?

In most cases, rheumatoid arthritis is a long-term illness. Often flare-ups seem to arise for no apparent reason. There are many things you can do to help reduce the severity of your symptoms and improve your general well-being. Taking such positive actions will help you to feel more in control of your condition.

Take good care of your joints

The mechanical arrangement of your joints means that any excess weight can place four or five times more pressure on certain parts of the joints than it does elsewhere in your body – so even small amounts of weight loss can make a big difference to the load your joints carry. If you are overweight and have rheumatoid arthritis of the weight-bearing joints (the knees or hips) it will be worth losing weight to reduce the pressure placed upon these joints. Regular exercise combined with a healthy diet will help you achieve this.

An occupational therapist (>>259) can provide advice on how best to perform daily tasks without putting too much pressure on your joints. There are also lots of gadgets and devices available that can help in your day-to-day life. For more advice on making everyday tasks easier, and for a run down on some of the different products available >>236-237.

Wear appropriate footwear

As with osteoarthritis, it is important to wear comfortable and supportive footwear (>>48–49). Feet affected by rheumatoid arthritis can change in shape and tend to broaden, so wide shoes may be needed. If you have problems finding the right footwear it is worth seeking advice from a podiatrist (>>w53); you may need shoes that are tailor-made to suit your feet. Supportive footwear is particularly important when exercising; you should wear sports shoes with shock-absorbing soles to protect your knees.

Support your joints when necessary

During serious flare-ups you may find it helps to use a walking stick or frame to take weight off painful hips and knees. Splints and braces may help by limiting movement of joints when they are particularly painful. Seek advice from a physiotherapist or occupational therapist.

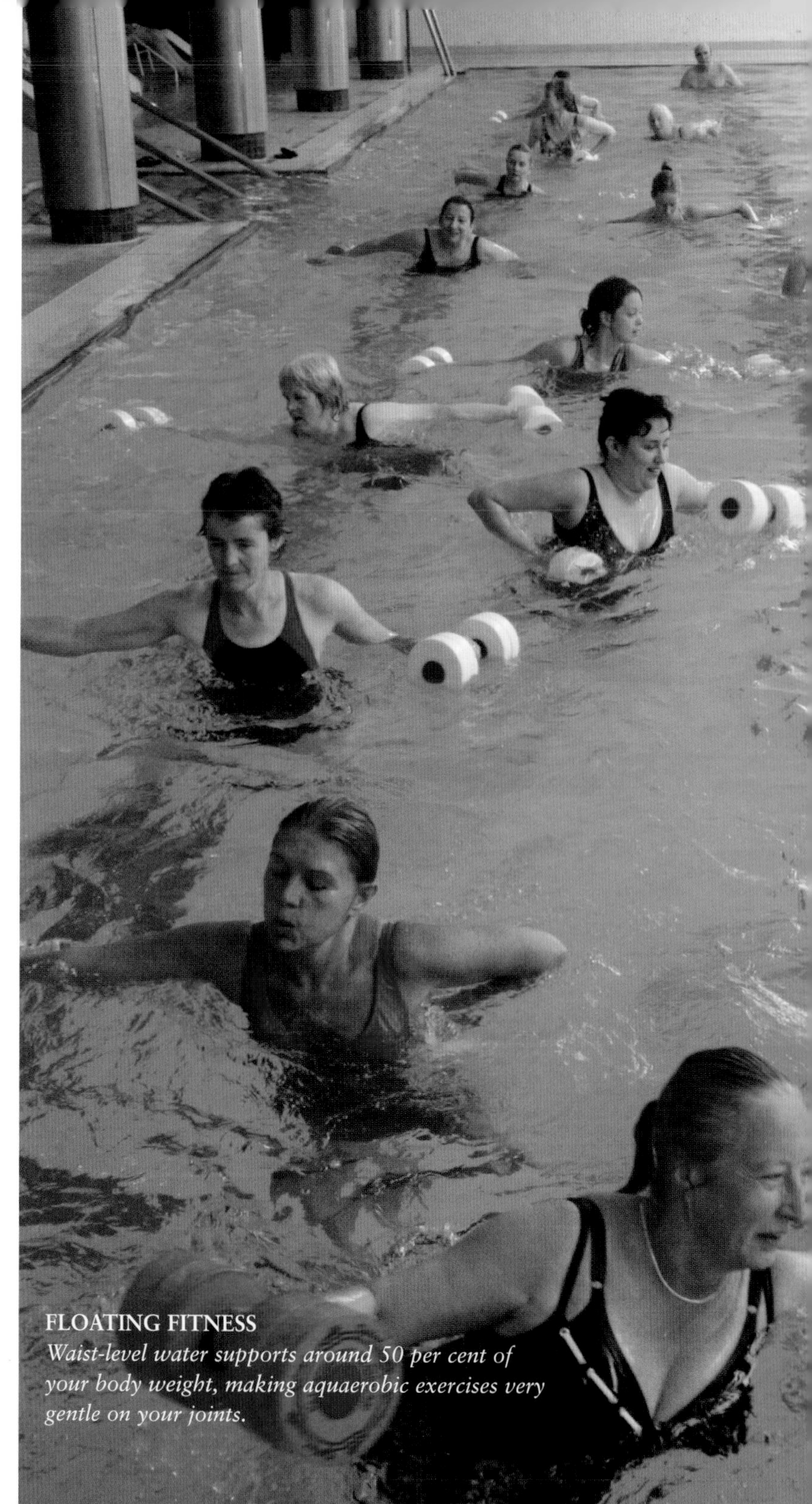

FLOATING FITNESS
Waist-level water supports around 50 per cent of your body weight, making aquaerobic exercises very gentle on your joints.

Rest when necessary

Periods of rest are important during flare-ups when your joints are very painful and swollen. Resting affected joints may help to bring on a period of remission. Your physiotherapist will be able to advise on activity levels during and after attacks.

Keep active

When your joints are painful the very idea of exercise can seem overwhelming but it is important to keep the joints mobile, reduce stiffness and maintain the strength of your muscles. Exercise also stimulates the release of endorphins, chemicals which can help block pain signals. But because joints affected by rheumatoid arthritis need rest as well as activity, a good balance between the two must be found.

As the severity of symptoms varies between individuals and from day to day, you will need to find an exercise level that keeps you active without worsening the disease. Before starting an exercise programme ask your doctor and, if possible, your physiotherapist for advice. Your physiotherapist will be able to design a tailor-made exercise programme that will help your joints as well as improving your stamina and general fitness. He or she will also suggest ways to work specific joints if necessary, although many specialists believe that whole-body exercises are more beneficial than joint-specific ones.

Doctors generally recommend that people with RA avoid violent or high-impact sports such as rugby. Walking is a great form of exercise that can be started gently and built up gradually. Swimming and aquaerobics are particularly good ways to exercise your muscles and move your joints without placing them under any added strain. They are also good aerobic activities that benefit the heart and lungs and help burn body fat.

4 WAYS TO...

Exercise safely

1 **Always warm up** properly before an exercise session to prepare your body for the stress of exercise. Cool down at the end.

2 **Exercise your whole body** rather than focusing on just one area – swimming is a great way to do this.

3 **Avoid contact sports** or high-impact sports such as football or squash and always wear supportive, shock-absorbing trainers.

4 **Reduce exercise** during flare-ups. If your joints become very painful, swell or feel warm, you should stop exercise immediately.

Take good care of yourself

It is worthwhile trying to remove stress from your life and taking time to relax and rest when necessary. Some people believe that stress may contribute to the development of rheumatoid arthritis. While this has not been clearly proven, it is likely that relaxation techniques and other mind-body therapies such as yoga or tai chi have a beneficial effect and reduce the severity of pain experienced. Certainly they should help you to maintain a positive outlook. Yoga and tai chi should also improve your balance and posture, which may help to alleviate some of the stress on your joints.

As with other chronic illnesses, it can be hard at times to cope with rheumatoid arthritis. The unpredictability of the flare-ups can make the disease particularly stressful and it can be difficult having to wait to find out how effective medications will be. The period following the diagnosis tends to be the most difficult.

A good GP is the first port of call; he or she should understand the problems of coping with a chronic illness and be able to give advice and support. Contacting local patient groups and talking to other people with the disease is likely to help you to maintain a positive outlook and to find the information you need to live with RA.

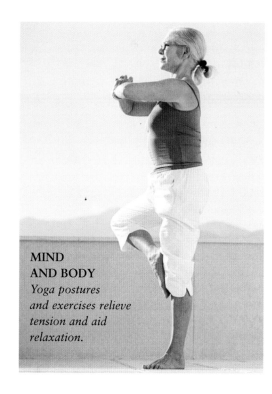

MIND AND BODY *Yoga postures and exercises relieve tension and aid relaxation.*

Conventional treatments

There is as yet no cure for rheumatoid arthritis. Drugs and other measures can relieve symptoms and slow its progress. The earlier treatment begins, the more effective it is.

Two basic classes of medication are used to treat RA: fast-acting 'first-line' drugs designed to reduce pain and inflammation in the short-term and slower-acting medicines (known as disease modifying anti-rheumatic drugs, or DMARDs) that help delay the progress of the disease.

In addition to joint problems, some patients with RA may need treatments for problems affecting other parts of the body. Depression may also be a feature so it is important to seek advice from your doctor should this develop. A team of healthcare professionals, including doctors, specialist nurses, physiotherapists and occupational therapists, are available. They will be able to answer questions as well as offering personal advice and support.

Short-term relief

Oral analgesics may help during flare-ups when the pain from joints is particularly bad. Over-the-counter drugs such as paracetamol may be sufficient in some cases but for severe symptoms doctors will prescribe stronger drugs. The most common side effect is constipation.

Painkillers are often used to complement the analgesic effects of non-steroidal anti-inflammatory drugs (NSAIDs). Painkillers may also be used alongside DMARDs, whose painkilling and anti-inflammatory effects take time to develop and usually offer only partial relief.

Non-steroidal anti-inflammatories

Drugs such as ibuprofen, naproxen or diclofenac reduce stiffness and pain by relieving inflammation in the joints. These non-steroidal anti-inflammatory drugs (NSAIDs) may cause a number of side effects: in particular, they can cause ulcers in the stomach or duodenum which may lead to internal bleeding. A new generation of NSAIDs, the Cox-2 inhibitors, target a different enzyme and are easier on the stomach. Unfortunately, recent research suggests that both classes of NSAID increase the risk of heart attacks. For more information on NSAIDs >>280.

Oral corticosteroids

Steroid drugs similar to the natural hormones produced by the adrenal glands help relieve inflammation in the joints and

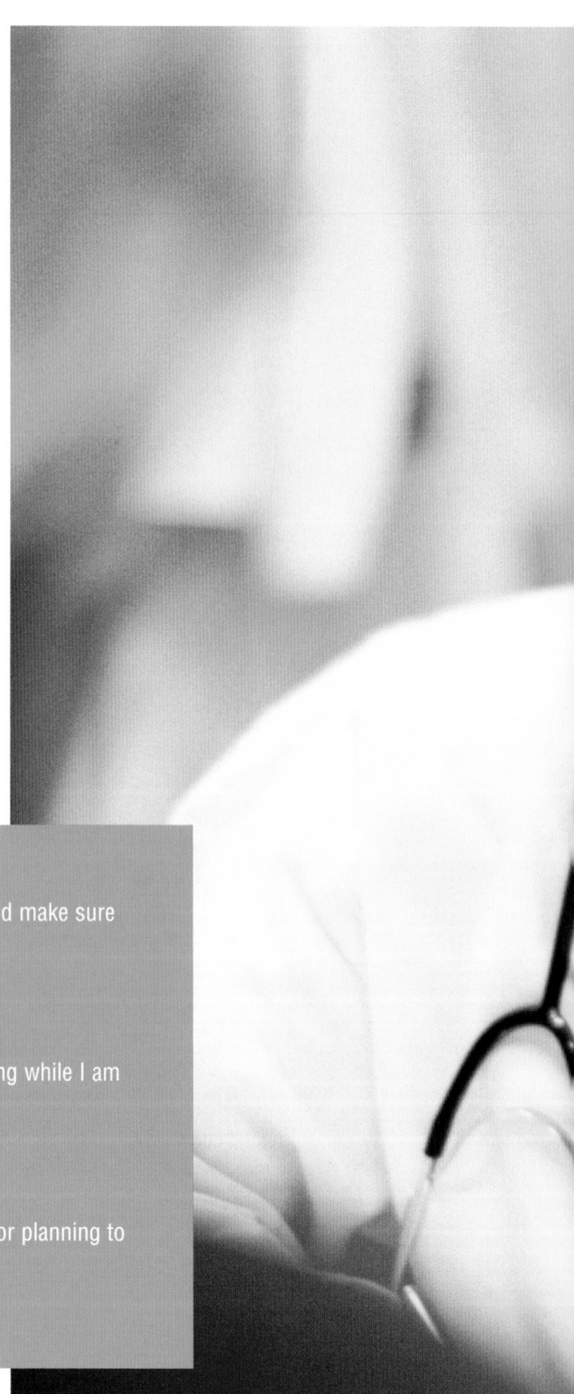

What to ask your doctor

If your doctor recommends a particular drug, you should make sure that you know the answers to the following questions:

- Should I take the drug before or after meals?
- How long should the drug take to start working?
- What side effects may occur?
- Will I need any blood tests or other special monitoring while I am taking the drug?
- Can I take the drug with my other medicines?
- Does it matter if I stop taking the drug suddenly?
- Can I drink alcohol while taking the drug?
- Can I take the drug if I am breast-feeding, pregnant or planning to have a baby?

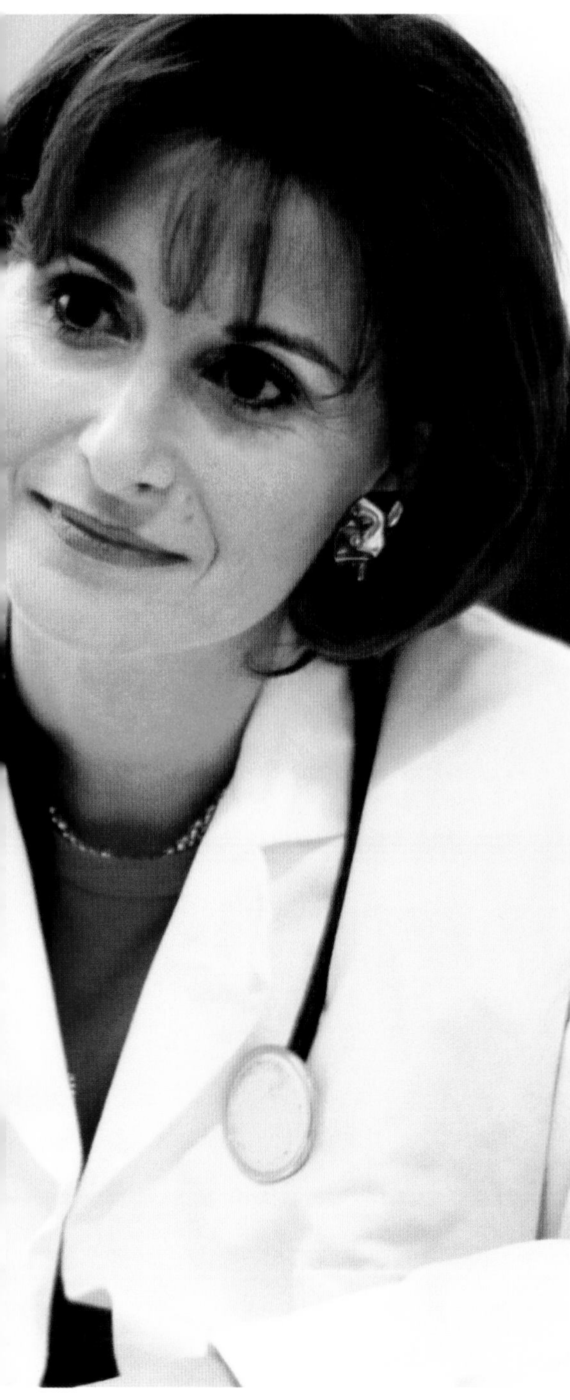

so reduce symptoms. They may be prescribed in low doses for a few weeks; long-term high doses can cause serious side effects. Corticosteroids are injected directly into affected joints for short-term pain relief and occasionally into a muscle during a severe flare-up.

Longer-term options

Disease modifying anti-rheumatic drugs (DMARDs) target inflammation and the progress of the disease. They work by suppressing the body's inflammatory system and not only relieve the symptoms of pain and stiffness but can also slow the rate at which damage occurs. These drugs work slowly and may be taken for years.

All of these drugs can have significant side effects and require close monitoring. See caution box, right, for more details.

- **Sulfasalazine** This drug is usually taken orally in a coated form that is broken down into its active form in the colon. Around 50 per cent of people treated with this drug find some improvement in their symptoms in the first six months.
- **Methotrexate** This drug inhibits the immune system, reducing inflammation and slowing the rate at which joint damage occurs. It is usually taken orally, in weekly doses, but can be given as an injection. If the drug works, patients usually start to notice the benefits after about six weeks.
- **Antimalarials** Some drugs used to treat malaria, such as hydroxychloraquine and chloraquine, also benefit people with rheumatoid arthritis. These drugs are usually used for up to a year, during which time they can produce a significant reduction in inflammation, although the reasons for this are not fully understood. Side effects are generally minor.
- **Gold** The gold preparation sodium aurothiomalate is given by injection into a muscle to help modify the abnormal immune response that causes RA. The drug is given on a weekly basis until there is a response; this usually takes about three months. If an improvement occurs, the injections are then given less frequently – usually once a month – for up to five years.
- **D-penicillamine** Any improvement with this penicillin-derived drug is likely to take about three months or longer to appear. D-penicillamine is taken before meals.
- **Leflunomide** This is a newer anti-inflammatory drug that, if it is effective, begins to relieve symptoms after about four weeks. It is taken orally once a day and may also be combined with methotrexate therapy. Side effects including stomach pain, sickness and diarrhoea are common.

CAUTION

Disease modifying anti-rheumatic drugs (DMARDs) work by suppressing the body's immune or inflammatory system and in rare cases this can affect blood cell production or cause liver problems or lung disease. Most DMARDs therefore require close monitoring, sometimes with regular blood and urine tests.

Some DMARDs should not be taken during pregnancy or by women who are trying to conceive or their partners. This restriction may apply for some time after the drug is stopped. Leflunamide, for example, needs to be stopped up to two years before a woman becomes pregnant.

ANTI-TNF THERAPY

A number of newer drugs are available that work by blocking the action of tumour necrosis factor alpha (TNF alpha), a protein involved in the body's inflammatory response. Anti-TNF drugs slow or halt joint damage in many patients and even cause damage to heal in a few; they may also relieve feelings of tiredness and malaise. They have only been in use for a few years and are currently prescribed by specialist centres only if other drugs have not proved satisfactory.

- ***Etanercept*** **is given twice weekly as an injection under the skin. Patients often learn to inject themselves for convenience.**
- ***Infliximab*** **is given by a drip into a vein every 6 weeks. It is combined with methotrexate, which blocks the formation of antibodies against it.**

Physiotherapy

Like other joint conditions, rheumatoid arthritis can benefit greatly from a programme of physiotherapy to keep joints moving and maintain strength. Possible physiotherapy treatments include:

- **Hydrotherapy** This treatment, which involves exercising in a specially heated pool, has been found to help rheumatoid and other forms of arthritis. The warm water soothes painful joints while the exercises help to improve flexibility and muscle strength.
- **Ultrasound therapy** High-energy sound waves delivered by a probe can relieve pain and stiffness in a joint.
- **Low-level laser therapy (lllt)** This differs from laser treatment used in surgery in that it does not damage the tissues. A probe placed on the skin delivers light of a specific wavelength to the affected area. This produces an anti-inflammatory effect for short-term relief from pain and stiffness. Lllt is provided by some physiotherapists as well as being available in some pain clinics.

Surgery

If other medical treatments fail to provide relief, surgery may be considered. Three main types of surgery are used:

- **Removal of inflamed synovium**
If synovial swelling persists despite medical treatment, removal of the synovium (synovectomy) may make the joint less prone to flare-ups. The surgeon may use keyhole surgery or more traditional methods to remove the synovium.
- **Repair of damaged tissue**
If tendons around the joint rupture, surgery may help to repair the damaged tissue. Other procedures are used to remove troublesome knots of tissue called rheumatoid nodules.
- **Repair of damaged joints**
Procedures may be carried out to salvage severely damaged joints and in some cases to replace them. The hip and knee are the most commonly replaced joints, but the shoulder and elbow are now replaced in some cases. The wrists and other joints of the arm may be fused together to make them less painful and more stable.

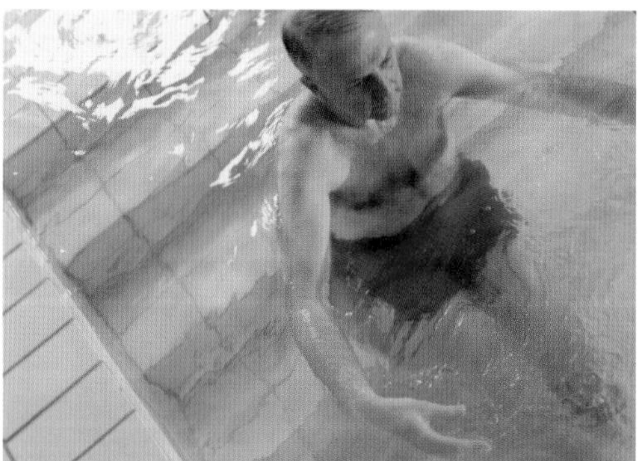

HYDROTHERAPY
The soothing warmth and buoyancy of water makes it invaluable for treating joint injuries.

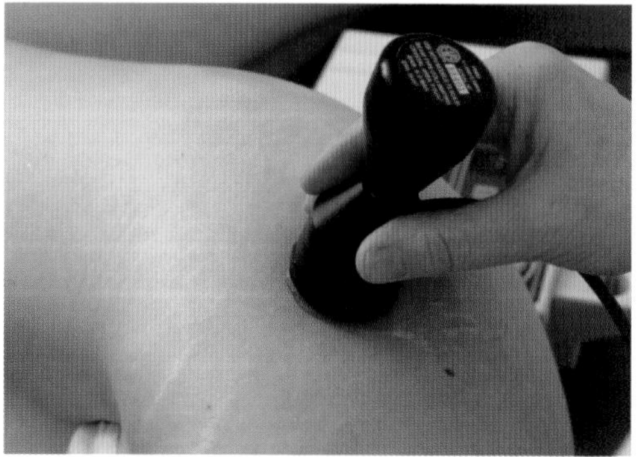

ULTRASOUND THERAPY
High-frequency sound waves reduce symptoms and improve mobility in rheumatic joints.

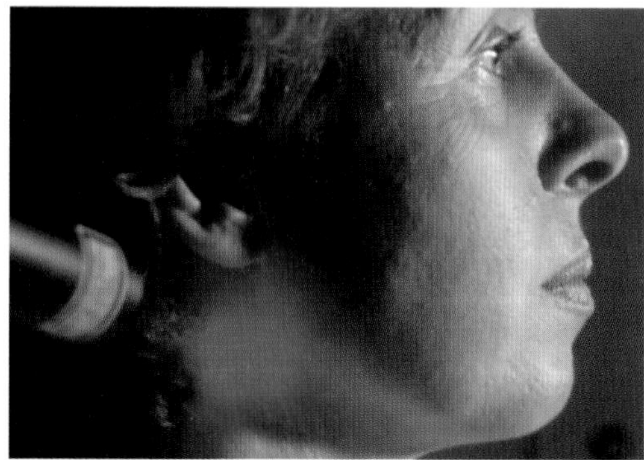

LOW-LEVEL LASER THERAPY
Low-intensity light beams produce chemical responses in cells without damaging tissues.

a visit to

THE OCCUPATIONAL THERAPIST

An occupational therapist will work closely with you to evaluate your personal needs, help you adapt your living or working environment and show you how to approach everyday tasks.

Arthritis can make performing even routine tasks more difficult – if you find that arthritis (or any other type of disease or injury) interferes with your daily life and activities, you should ask you GP to refer you to an occupational therapist. Alternatively, you can approach social services yourself.

Occupational therapists are often attached to a hospital or social services department. and will usually see you in an occupational therapy department, outpatient clinic or at your home. The length of treatment varies but a course will usually begin with a thorough assessment of your lifestyle and your individual needs.

The therapist will show you how to adapt your home or working environment to your particular needs and may be able to teach you techniques to improve your strength and mobility or manage your pain. You can talk through any practical or emotional difficulties that you may be experiencing and explore coping strategies. The therapist should also be able to tell you about any financial benefits or assistance that are available.

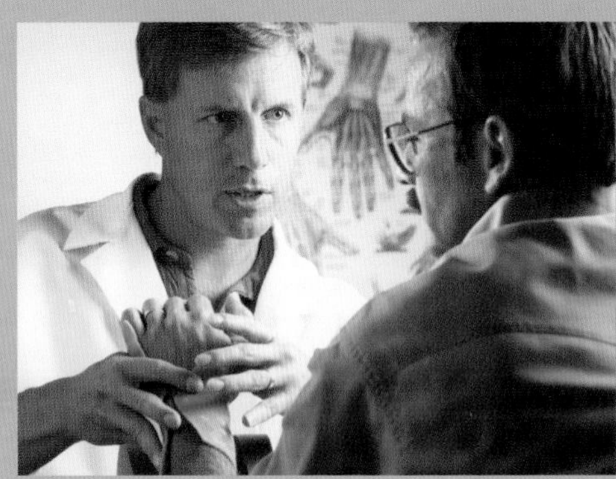

Assessing your needs An occupational therapist offers tailor-made advice. The therapist will make a complete assessment of your condition, noting which joints are affected, where it is most painful, and what range of motion you have in your joints.

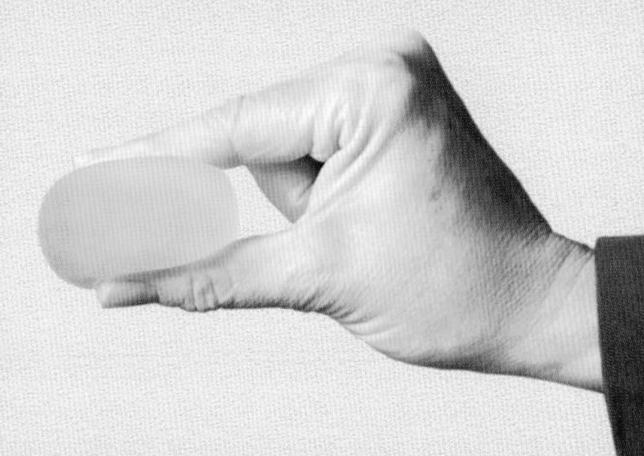

Building strength and mobility Your therapist may be able to show you therapeutic activities to improve your joint function and mobility and recommend simple ways to help you to manage your pain, such as splints or warming packs. If you require physical, hands-on therapy or extensive treatment, you may need to visit a physiotherapist.

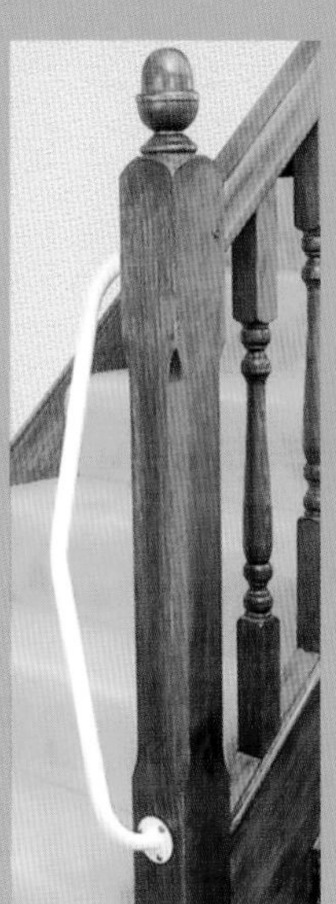

Adapting your environment The therapist may suggest simple adjustments to make to your home or your working environment, such as repositioning furniture or installing specialist equipment. The therapist may also recommend aids and assistive devices to make your life easier and increase your independence. For information on some of the aids and equipment available >>236–237.

>> **Making life easier:** page 236 >> **A visit to the physiotherapist:** page 243

Other treatment options

Diet and supplements

The role of food in the development of rheumatoid arthritis remains a subject of debate. There is some evidence that foods such avocados (see box, right) and oily fish bring benefits, but most specialists simply recommend that their patients eat a balanced diet to stay as healthy as possible. A survey of over 46,000 people in Italy, for example, showed that simply eating more vegetables significantly reduces your risk.

Some studies have suggested that the condition may be related to certain foods such as milk, nuts, grains and eggs, or to foods containing colouring. However, it may be that avoiding these foods has only limited and short-term benefits, reducing the severity of the symptoms temporarily rather than influencing the course of the disease in the long-term. If you do wish to try eliminating certain foods from your diet, it is important that you do not omit whole food groups or a large number of foods as this may disrupt your dietary balance. A nutritionist or dietician will be able to advise you how to get all the nutrients your body needs.

Essential fatty acids (EFAs)

Omega-3 and omega-6 fatty acids may help relieve the symptoms of rheumatoid arthritis. Good dietary sources include oily fish, such as salmon and sardines, extra-virgin olive oil and sunflower seeds.

If you wish to take EFA supplements, cod liver oil is a good source of omega-3 and evening primrose oil a good source of omega-6 EFAs. Omega-3 fortified milks are also now available. Remember to talk to your doctor if you are considering taking these supplements, particularly if you are already taking other medications.

DID YOU KNOW?

■ Drinking decaffeinated coffee – but not ordinary coffee – may increase your risk of developing rheumatoid arthritis. Among over 31,000 women in the Iowa Women's Health Study, those who drank four or more cups of decaffeinated coffee per day had a more than doubled risk of developing rheumatoid arthritis.

■ Drinking tea, however, may protect you; the same study showed that women drinking three or more cups of tea had a 60 per cent lower risk.

■ Meanwhile Japanese scientists have shown that green tea has anti-inflammatory effects that can help to prevent not only rheumatoid arthritis, but also heart disease and cancer.

Complementary medicines

Some people with rheumatoid arthritis find that certain complementary therapies do offer symptomatic relief. It is important to speak to your doctor or specialist before taking any complementary medicines to ensure that they can be taken safely with existing treatments. It is important that you do not neglect regular medications.

Acupuncture

There is a long tradition of using acupuncture to treat inflammatory conditions and reduce pain and swelling;

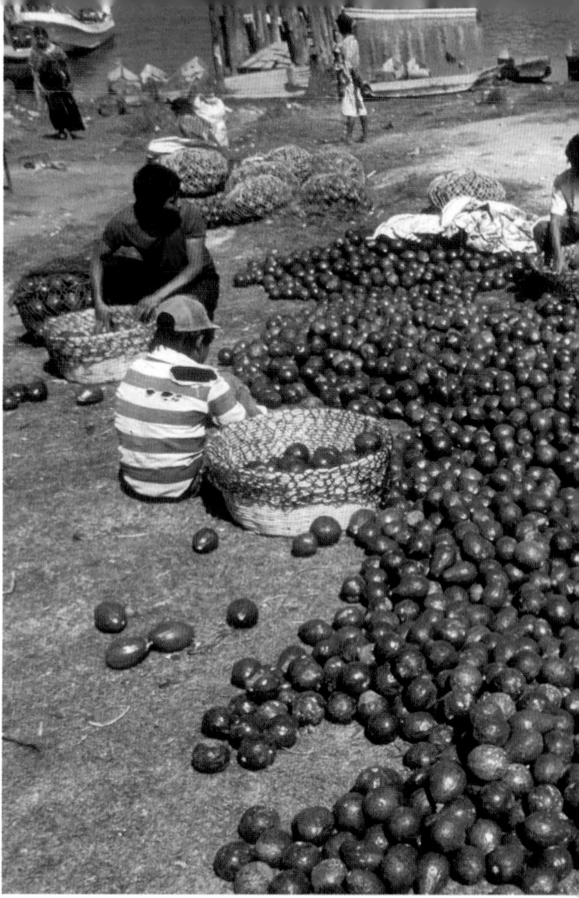

AVOCADO PEARS

Some years ago, Dr John Heinerman, a medical anthropologist, reported that the Mayan Indians of the Yucatan Peninsula and Guatemala – whose diet includes large quantities of avocado pears – do not suffer greatly from rheumatoid arthritis. Neither do tribes in the North-west Amazon region – where large quantities of avocados grow wild – unless they give up their native diet and start to eat Westernized foods. Studies have subsequently shown that avocado and soya bean extracts can help relieve the symptoms of arthritis.

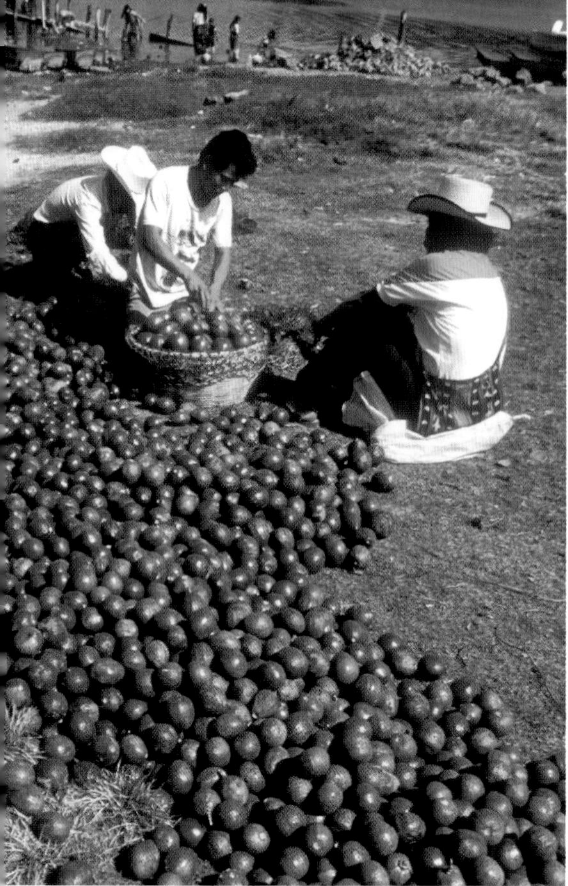

practitioners believe it helps to re-establish the energy balance within the body's organs. In April 2005, researchers at University College, London and Southampton University conducted brain scans on patients receiving acupuncture that may shed light on how this effect works. The scans showed that treatment activated the opiate centre and the ipsilateral insular – two regions of the brain known to be involved in pain modulation.

Although acupuncture involves inserting fine needles into specific points of the body, it is not painful. The therapy is now available in many NHS pain clinics and your GP can put you in touch with other qualified practitioners in your area.

Homeopathy

A homeopath is likely to prescribe a combination of medicines that are tailored to the individual, taking account of factors such as the pattern of the disease and individual personality traits. Medicines that are commonly used include Rhus toxicodendron, which tends to help those who suffer particularly from morning stiffness, Pulsatilla and Lycopodium. Apis mellifica may also be recommended for warm, swollen joints. Rheumatoid arthritis is a complex disease; consult an experienced homeopath rather than attempt to treat symptoms yourself.

Herbalism

There are no standard herbal remedies for rheumatoid or other forms of arthritis. The herbalist will recommend individual therapies depending on various factors including general health and symptoms.

Anti-inflammatory remedies are often recommended during flare-ups. These may include willow, poplar, meadowsweet, birch and feverfew. Rheumatoid arthritis is often associated with low mood and general malaise so herbalists also suggest preparations that they believe boost the immune system and improve general well-being. These include ginseng and astralagus. Certain herbs, such as motherwort and Chinese angelica, are also thought to help relieve anaemia, a common feature of rheumatoid arthritis.

Those taking herbal remedies need close monitoring by an experienced herbalist. Remedies may have unpleasant side effects and may also interact with certain medical drugs. It is important that both your doctor and your herbalist know exactly what you are taking. Always buy herbs from a reputable manufacturer.

Massage

This can provide benefits in terms of relaxation and so may help to relieve pain, although special massage oils and creams do not seem to provide any additional benefits. Your physiotherapist may practise massage together with other techniques such as manipulation and stretching. If you wish to try further massage you should visit a qualified practitioner, preferably with the guidance of your doctor or physiotherapist.

FEVERFEW

The herb feverfew has a very similar pain-relieving and anti-inflammatory action to aspirin and can be a good way to treat mild rheumatoid arthritis symptoms. To be effective, however, the active ingredient parthenolide must be present in a concentration of at least 0.4 per cent. One study of 35 commercially available feverfew preparations found that few had sufficient levels to be effective.

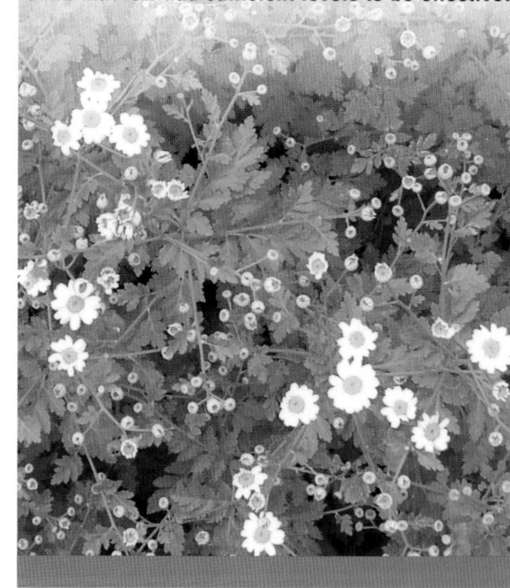

Looking to the future

The majority of people with rheumatoid arthritis can lead a perfectly normal and active life. Modern treatments and medications can greatly ease the symptoms and can slow the progression of the disease. For those with more severe disability there are many effective ways to manage the disease and make day-to-day living easier.

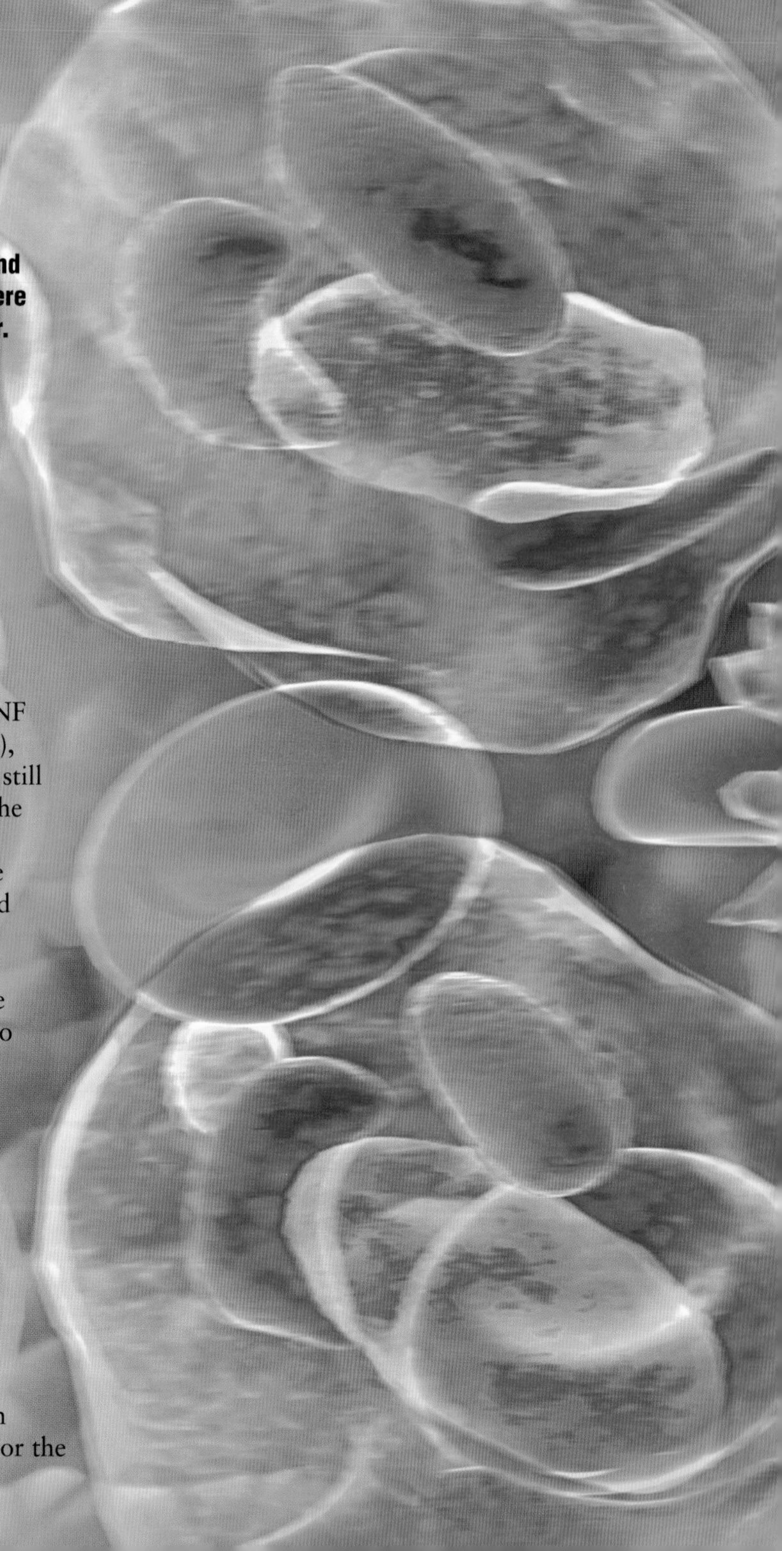

The outlook

Although there is no cure available for rheumatoid arthritis at present, the disease can sometimes stop spontaneously for no apparent reason. Around 25 per cent of people with RA make a complete recovery. Recent studies also suggest that the number of new cases of RA may be going down. Only a minority of people become severely disabled. Most people will have to modify their lifestyle to some extent but can expect to lead a full life.

Hope for the future

A huge amount of research is currently taking place into why and how rheumatoid arthritis develops. As our understanding of RA improves, it may be possible to find new ways to prevent the disease developing or even find a cure. Some potentially very productive avenues for research include:

The autoimmune process

Scientists are trying to improve our understanding of the abnormalities found in the immune systems of those affected by rheumatoid arthritis. There may also be significant differences in the way that a woman's immune system functions during pregnancy that makes her less vulnerable. A fuller understanding of the autoimmune process would help in the development of treatments to target these abnormalities and halt the inflammatory process.

Researchers are trying to find new drugs to suppress the inflammation that underlies rheumatoid arthritis while producing minimal side effects. The most effective current therapies target the TNF alpha protein (see box, >>258), although many of these drugs still have significant drawbacks. The compound Interleukin-10, for example, suppresses the whole immune system when delivered intravenously; scientists are developing a nasal spray that they hope will produce a more targeted effect. Research is also underway into other possible targets including neutrophil white blood cells.

The role of infections

Scientists have long suspected that infections by bacteria, viruses or fungi may sometimes play a role in the development of rheumatoid arthritis. If researchers can discover which infectious agents are involved or the

AUTOIMMUNE RESEARCH
White blood cells (such as the neutrophil, monocyte and eosinophil cells pictured here) perform a vital role in your immune system. Unfortunately, antibodies produced in these cells sometimes attack the body's own tissues, causing autoimmune disorders such as rheumatoid arthritis. It may be possible to suppress inflammation by developing drugs that target these cells and antibodies.

mechanism by which the disease is triggered, it may be possible to take preventative action to limit flare-ups or even stop the disease from developing.

The role of hormones

Research into the possible role of sex hormones and their interaction with the immune system may offer further avenues for treatment. We already know that women are more likely than men to develop rheumatoid arthritis before the menopause, but that the risk is equal after the menopause when levels of oestrogen and progesterone fall.

Susceptibility varies throughout a woman's reproductive life at times when hormone levels fluctuate significantly – the risk appears to be higher after having a baby and when breast-feeding. Fluctuations in hormones also seem to influence the timing and severity of flare-ups – the disease often improves during pregnancy. Male sex hormones may also play a role in arthritis, perhaps a protective one.

The role of genes

Genetic abnormalities may play a role in around 60 per cent of cases of rheumatoid arthritis. As well as putting some people at increased risk of developing RA, abnormal genes may also play a part in determining the severity of the disease. Research centres across the United States are now working together to collect information and genetic material from around 1000 families in which two or more brothers and sisters have the disease. This information will help form a picture of the role of genes in RA and may pave the way for new treatments. Eventually it may be possible to test for the presence of RA-specific genes or even to repair or replace such genes to prevent the disease developing.

Emotional well-being

The importance of a positive mindset should not be underestimated. Studies allied with clinical experience show that people who are happier and have a more positive outlook are likely to cope better with rheumatoid arthritis and experience symptoms that are less severe. Researchers are examining why this should work and the best ways to help patients achieve good emotional health.

CAUTION

- People with rheumatoid arthritis are at increased risk of osteoporosis. This particularly applies to women, who have a higher risk after the menopause in any case. Calcium and vitamin D supplements may be helpful. In some cases, other treatments for osteoporosis are required.
- People with arthritis also have greater risk of heart disease, probably because they have higher rates of cardiovascular risk factors such as diabetes, high blood pressure and high cholesterol levels. The link between these risk factors may provide new avenues for research.

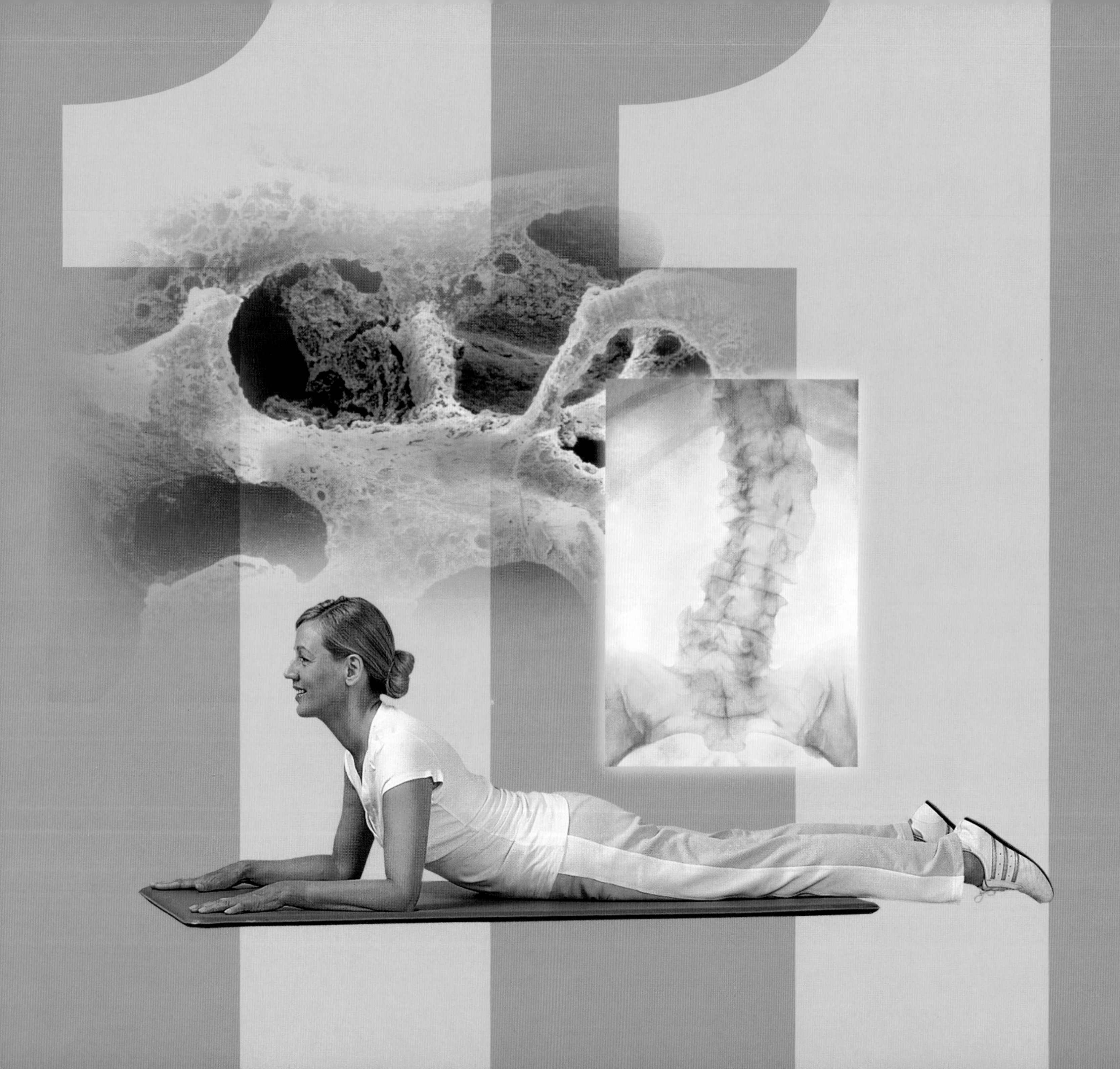

OSTEOPOROSIS

The older we get, the greater our risk of bone loss and related fractures. Osteoporosis is largely irreversible, but there are ways you can help prevent or reduce your rate of bone loss. In these pages you'll find the tools to help you assess your risk of developing the disease and ways of lessening that risk. Also, if you have already been diagnosed, you'll find information on treatments and techniques that can make a real difference.

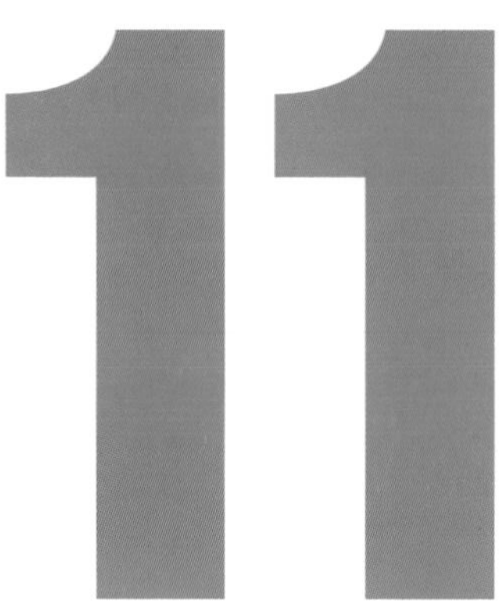

OSTEOPOROSIS
What is it?

Everyone's bones start to lose tissue and become less dense as they grow older. In some people, this loss of bone tissue is particularly severe and associated with an increased tendency to bone fractures – a condition known as osteoporosis, meaning porous bones. Around one in three women and one in twelve men over the age of 50 suffer from osteoporosis in the UK.

What happens?

Throughout life the tissue making up our bones is constantly broken down and replaced – a process known as bone turnover. Bone mass reaches its peak around the age of 25 and then gradually decreases throughout life as new bone formation fails to keep pace with bone breakdown. This is a normal part of ageing and bone mass usually stays within the acceptable range for the age group.

Sometimes, however, bone mass falls below this normal range. As bone becomes more porous it weakens and tends to fracture more easily, often after minor knocks and falls. Common sites for bone fractures are the wrists, spine and hips. Around three million people in the UK are estimated to suffer from osteoporosis.

What are the causes?

We are all more likely to develop osteoporosis as we grow older and our bone mass decreases. Around 55 per cent of people over the age of 50 have low bone mass, putting them at increased risk of developing the condition and related fractures. A number of factors can increase your chances of getting osteoporosis.

- **Genetics** Osteoporosis often runs in families. Genes are thought to play a role in determining the peak bone mass achieved and the risk of getting osteoporosis later in life. Family history does not mean that the condition is inevitable, however, particularly if those at risk take preventative measures.
- **Hormones** Women can lose up to 20 per cent of their bone mass in the five to seven years following menopause. This increased rate of depletion is associated with lower oestrogen levels. Women

34 The structure of bones

76 A strength-training workout

219 Protecting your hips

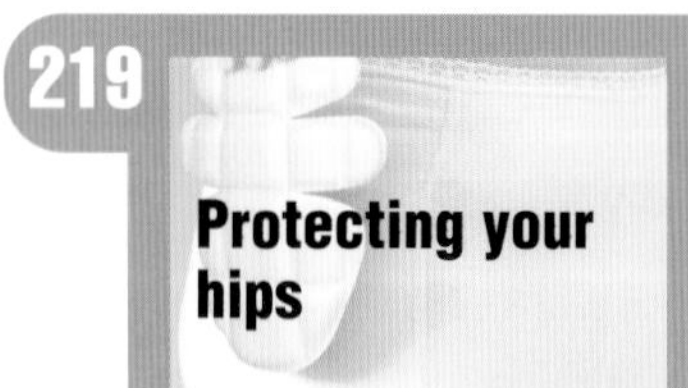

DID YOU KNOW?

- **A 50 year old woman has a 40 per cent chance of having a hip fracture at some point during the rest of her life; for men the risk is around 13 per cent.**
- **By the age of 80, one woman in three compared to one man in five can expect to have a hip fracture.**
- **Differences occur because bone loss in women increases as levels of oestrogen fall after menopause. The drop off in male bone density as testosterone declines occurs later.**

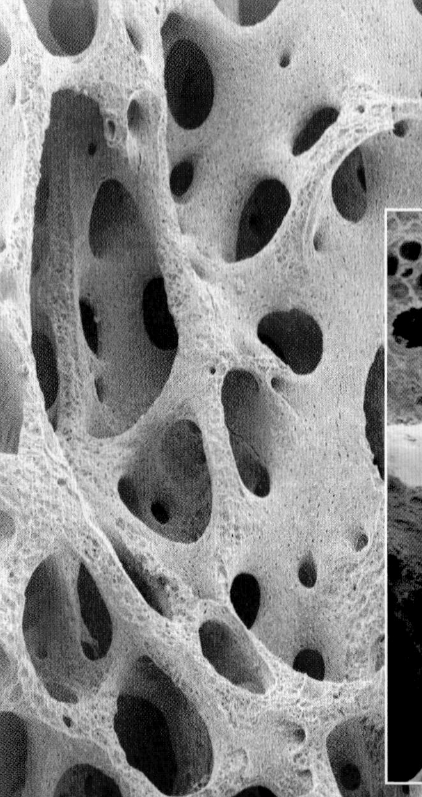

who have an early menopause have a greater risk of developing the condition later in life because they spend more years with low oestrogen levels.

Women with anorexia nervosa may also have reduced oestrogen production and are at increased risk of osteoporosis. A study published in 1996 in the *Journal of the American Medical Association* found that 50 per cent of young patients with anorexia also had osteoporosis. Men with particularly low levels of testosterone are also at greater risk.

■ **Medical conditions and medications** Rheumatoid arthritis and some other joint disorders are associated with an increased risk of osteoporosis. The disease has also been linked to various other medical diseases, including Type 1 diabetes mellitus, an overactive thyroid gland and chronic liver disease. Bowel disorders such as coeliac disease, in which absorption of nutrients is impaired, may also increase the risk. Corticosteroids and some other drugs can cause the condition if taken long-term.

■ **Diet and lifestyle** Lack of calcium in the diet, particularly during childhood and adolescence, can significantly affect maximum bone density. The body also needs the full range of vitamins and minerals, including vitamin D to help absorb calcium. Regular exercise is vital in order to maintain bone strength and lack of exercise or long-term immobility is a serious risk factor. Smoking and excessive drinking can also increase the chance of suffering from osteoporosis.

BONE DENSITY

Normal, healthy bone (left) has a dense honeycomb structure – the spaces in between contain bone marrow. Osteoporotic bone (below) is more porous and brittle than healthy bone and fractures more easily.

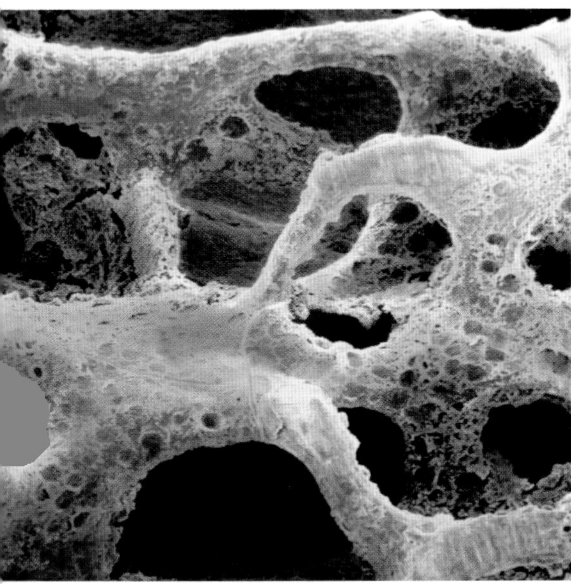

What are the symptoms?

Most people are unaware that they have osteoporosis until a minor injury causes a bone fracture. Osteoporosis usually affects all the bones in the skeleton, but the most common sites for fractures are the wrists, hips and spine. As well as the pain associated with acute fractures, the condition may cause rounding of the back or a gradual loss of height due to fractures of the vertebrae in the spine.

How is it diagnosed?

If you are worried that you may be suffering from osteoporosis, your doctor can arrange for a bone densitometry test, sometimes called dual X-ray absorptiometry (DXA). Densitometry can also give an indication of the severity of the disease and the likelihood of bone fractures occurring. People treated for osteoporosis may have regular bone densitometry to monitor the progress of their treatment.

Taking the test

During a bone densitometry test the patient lies on a padded examination table. X-ray beams pass up through the body and a detector arm moving over the body takes measurements for analysis. The test usually takes around 20 minutes.

Bone density measurements are most often taken from the lower spinal column and the hip. Following this, additional tests may be carried out to identify problematic areas or to look for an underlying cause. Sometimes smaller machines are used to screen for osteoporosis by assessing the density of bones in other areas, such as the forearm or the heel.

Results

The results of bone densitometry are made up of two scores:

■ **The T-score** indicates bone density compared to a reference group of young healthy adults with average bone density. This gives an indication of an individual's risk of having a fracture.

A T-score score above –1 is normal, between –1 and –2.5 indicates that significant bone thinning, known as osteopenia, has occurred, below –2.5 is classed as osteoporosis.

■ **The Z-score** gives an indication of the bone density when compared to other people of a similar age. A very high or very low Z-score may indicate that further investigation is required. The Z-score may also be used to monitor the progress of osteoporosis treatment.

What can I do?

While you can't completely reverse bone loss from osteoporosis, there are a number of simple measures you can take to conserve bone mass and maintain your health. These are also good preventative measures for those with healthy bones who wish to avoid osteoporosis in the future.

Diet and supplements

A healthy, balanced diet with a good range of vitamins and minerals is essential for maintaining healthy bones – as well as being important for general health and well-being. Certain foods and nutrients also have a more specific role in the prevention and control of osteoporosis.

Calcium

It is particularly important to have a diet rich in calcium, found in milk and other dairy products. Non-dairy sources of calcium include green leafy vegetables, baked beans and bony fish. Studies have shown that calcium, as a daily supplement or in the diet, plays an important part in achieving a high peak bone mass at the age of 25 and preventing osteoporosis in later life. A good calcium intake for a healthy adult is thought to be around 700–1000mg per day – a 1998 survey found that a quarter of men and half of women had calcium intakes below 700mg.

People who already suffer from osteoporosis or are at particular risk of thinning bones (such as pregnant women) may need to up their intake. The National Osteoporosis Society recommends that people with osteoporosis have an overall calcium intake of at least 1200mg per day, since sufficient calcium must be present in the body to enable other drugs to work properly. It may be difficult to achieve this intake through diet alone, so doctors often recommend calcium supplements. Adults with osteoporosis are generally prescribed 500-1000mg of calcium per day together with their osteoporosis treatment to supplement their regular calcium intake from other dietary sources.

Calcium can interfere with the absorption of some drugs, so supplements should be taken at a different time to other medications, usually with or after food. The maximum recommended limit for calcium intake is 2000–2500mg per day, including calcium derived from the diet. For more information about supplements >>104–106.

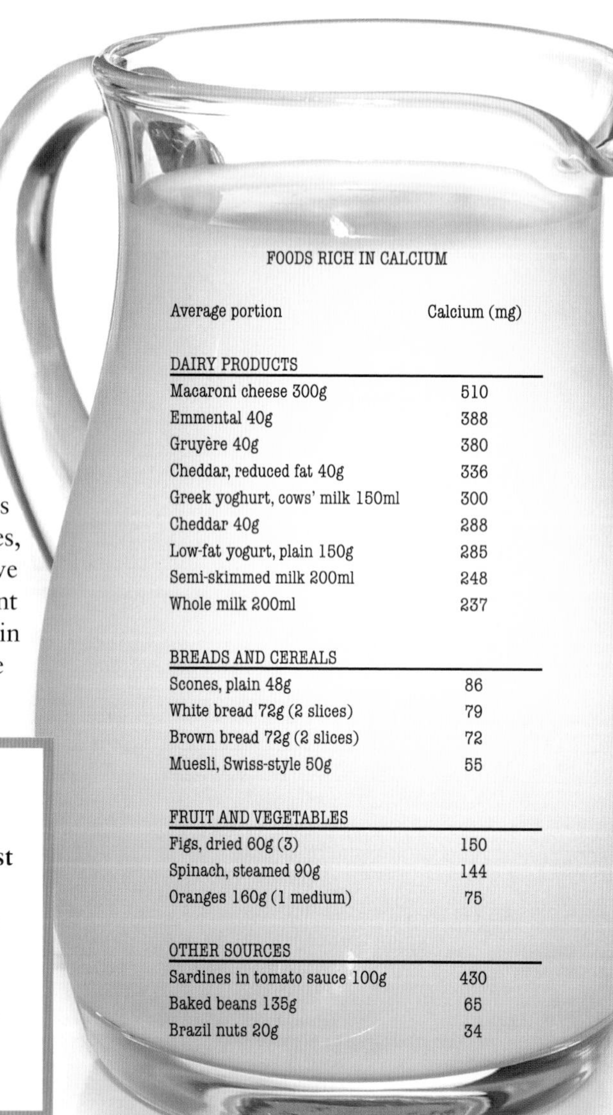

FOODS RICH IN CALCIUM

Average portion	Calcium (mg)
DAIRY PRODUCTS	
Macaroni cheese 300g	510
Emmental 40g	388
Gruyère 40g	380
Cheddar, reduced fat 40g	336
Greek yoghurt, cows' milk 150ml	300
Cheddar 40g	288
Low-fat yogurt, plain 150g	285
Semi-skimmed milk 200ml	248
Whole milk 200ml	237
BREADS AND CEREALS	
Scones, plain 48g	86
White bread 72g (2 slices)	79
Brown bread 72g (2 slices)	72
Muesli, Swiss-style 50g	55
FRUIT AND VEGETABLES	
Figs, dried 60g (3)	150
Spinach, steamed 90g	144
Oranges 160g (1 medium)	75
OTHER SOURCES	
Sardines in tomato sauce 100g	430
Baked beans 135g	65
Brazil nuts 20g	34

CALCIUM ABSORPTION

Calcium supplements are not all readily absorbed by the body. To test how well your calcium supplement is absorbed, place a tablet in a glass of warm water or vinegar. If it dissolves entirely within 30 minutes your body should be able to absorb the calcium properly.

GUM DISEASE

If you're losing teeth through gum disease, you could be losing bone density too. Researchers have uncovered a strong correlation between tooth and bone loss. Dental X-rays could be a useful way to screen for osteoporosis.

Vitamin D

This vitamin controls the absorption of calcium from food in the gut. Most of our vitamin D is made by the action of the sun on our skin. This may explain why vitamin D supplements help to reduce bone loss in postmenopausal women, as the amount of time many elderly people spend out in the sun is limited. Try to get at least 15 minutes sunshine daily when possible and include vitamin-D rich foods such as fish-liver oils, eggs, fortified margarines, tuna, salmon or sardines in your diet.

Vitamin D may also help to promote muscle strength. A study of elderly people with low vitamin D levels found that those who took 800mg of vitamin D and 1200mg of calcium daily for 12 weeks had a 49 per cent reduction in falls compared with those taking calcium alone.

Other substances

- **Magnesium** Magnesium encourages calcium uptake by bones and may help to reduce bone loss. Dietary sources of magnesium include nuts and pulses, seafood and green vegetables. Some nutritionists recommend a magnesium supplement at a dose of 500mg per day.
- **Phytoestrogens** These substances, which are derived from plants, are similar to naturally occurring oestrogens in the body although their actions are weaker. Some evidence suggests that phytoestrogen-rich foods such as tofu, chickpeas or lentils, may help to protect against osteoporosis.
- **Multivitamins** Certain other vitamins and minerals are believed to be good for bones, including vitamin C, vitamin K, potassium, copper and zinc. A high vitamin C intake, for example, is associated with a threefold reduction in the progression of knee osteoarthritis. You may wish to consider taking a daily multivitamin that contains these substances. If you already take calcium or vitamin D supplements, you should be aware that a multivitamin may contribute to your intake.

Smoking

Smoking has a detrimental effect on bones in men and women. It also affects oestrogen production, which may cause an early menopause and further increase the risk of osteoporosis in women. Giving up smoking will not only benefit your bones but also your general health, reducing the risk of various serious diseases such as cancer, heart disease and strokes.

Alcohol

Excessive alcohol consumption can affect normal bone turnover and increase your risk of osteoporosis. Moderate drinking should not be a problem; a study in 1999 showed that women who consumed the equivalent of one glass of wine per day actually had higher bone density in the lumbar spine than non-drinkers. However, alcohol intake should stay within the recommended range of 14 units per week for women and 21 units for men (one unit is equal to one small glass of wine or half a pint of normal strength lager).

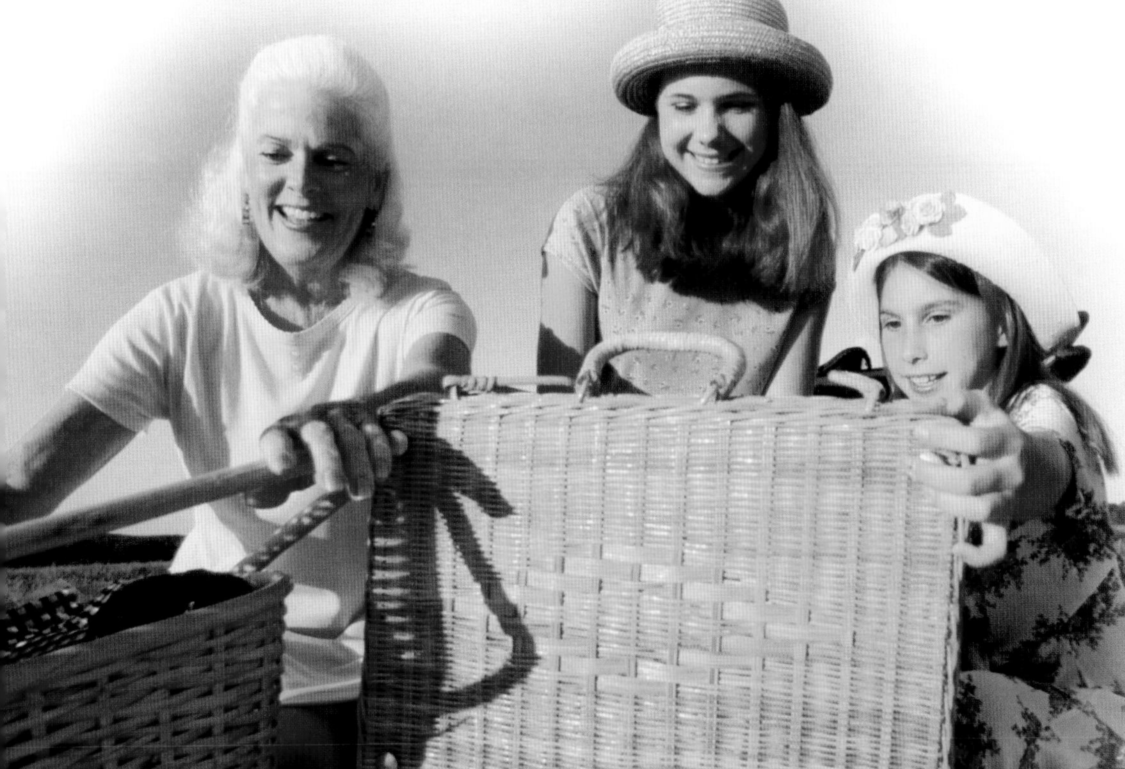

GETTING YOUR VITAMINS
Your body needs moderate amounts of sunshine to make vitamin D – around 30 minutes most days from April to October should be sufficient to store enough for the winter. Other vital nutrients come from a healthy, balanced diet.

?

Could I be susceptible to osteoporosis?

Often, osteoporosis is not picked up until after a fracture occurs, but it is much better to catch the problem at an early stage and take steps to prevent further deterioration. If you answer yes to any of the following questions, you could be at risk of developing osteoporosis. Your doctor may wish to arrange a bone densitometry test to determine whether treatment is needed.

YES	NO	
☐	☐	Have you ever had a hip fracture or a vertebral fracture or a fracture caused by a minor bump or fall?
☐	☐	Have either of your parents suffered from osteoporosis or broken a hip after a minor bump or fall?
☐	☐	Have you every suffered from osteoarthritis or rheumatoid arthritis?
☐	☐	Have you ever had anorexia nervosa or a bowel disorder such as coeliac disease, or have you ever suffered from kidney failure, cancers, liver disease, Paget's disease, Type 1 diabetes mellitus, or endocrine or glandular disorders?
☐	☐	Have you ever taken oral corticosteroids, seizure drugs or blood thinners on a long-term basis?
☐	☐	Are you, or have you ever been, a heavy smoker or drinker?
☐	☐	Do you lead a particularly sedentary lifestyle?
☐	☐	If you are a woman, were you aged less than 45 when you had the menopause or when you had a hysterectomy?
☐	☐	If you are a woman, have your periods ever stopped for a period of 12 months of longer, other than during pregnancy?
☐	☐	If you are a man, have you ever suffered from problems connected to low testosterone such as impotence or loss of libido?

Exercise

Weight-bearing exercise in childhood and early adulthood plays an important role in determining peak bone mass and therefore the risk of developing osteoporosis in later life. Like muscle, bone soon deteriorates with inactivity – regular weight-bearing exercise builds and maintains density. The benefits are not limited to the young: even in middle age weight-bearing exercise may produce a small increase in bone density. In older people, exercise remains important in order to conserve bone density.

Weight-bearing exercise strengthens bones by 'loading' the skeleton. This load may be provided by the pull of gravity on your body mass or on extra resistance from strap-on weights, dumb-bells or resistance bands. The key is to provide a short, sharp load that is more challenging for your bones than your normal activities.

Although swimming is an excellent form of exercise in most respects, it is not weight bearing because the water supports your weight. Endurance activities such as cycling are also of limited benefit. Suitable exercises to maintain strong bones include running, aerobics and weight-training.

Exercise for osteoporosis sufferers

Weight-bearing exercise is not only important to prevent osteoporosis developing, it should also be included as part of the treatment programme for people already affected by the condition. For these people, the aim is to maintain existing bone density and improve balance, reducing the risk of falls and fractures. Your doctor or physio will be able to give you advice on exercise that is appropriate for your condition, but walking, moderate strength training or yoga are all suitable. The strengthening exercises shown over the following pages target the wrist, hips and spine, the areas most likely to fracture due to osteoporosis. Also included is an exercise to improve your balance.

PREVENTING FRACTURES

- Take exercise to improve your strength and balance, reducing the risk of falls and fractures
- Wear supportive shoes with shock-absorbing soles
- Adapt your home to avoid falls by removing loose carpets and clearing away excess clutter
- Wear hip pads to absorb and deflect impact away from your hips, particularly during exercise

EXERCISE AND BONE DENSITY

This chart shows how bone mineral density (given as a T-score) falls with age. The middle line shows how the bone density of an average person declines over time. The upper and lower lines show the bone densities of an active and a sedentary person, respectively. When a person's bone density falls below the fracture threshold (a T-score of below –2.5) fractures become more likely and a diagnosis of osteoporosis is made. The graph shows that this tends to happen at a much earlier age in sedentary people than in active ones.

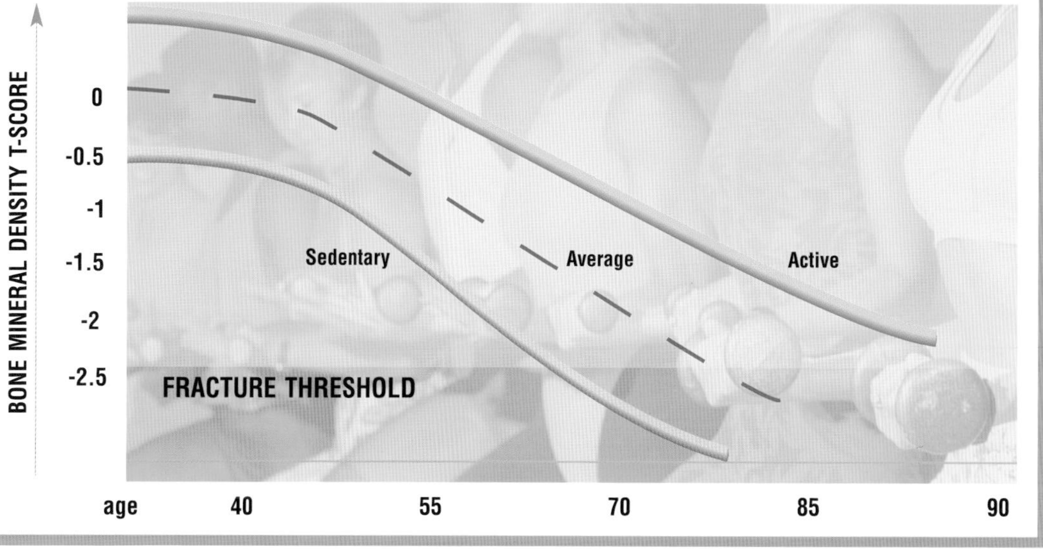

The hips

This exercise will strengthen the bones in your hips and your outer thigh muscles. If you are unable to get down to the floor safely, you can do this exercise in bed.

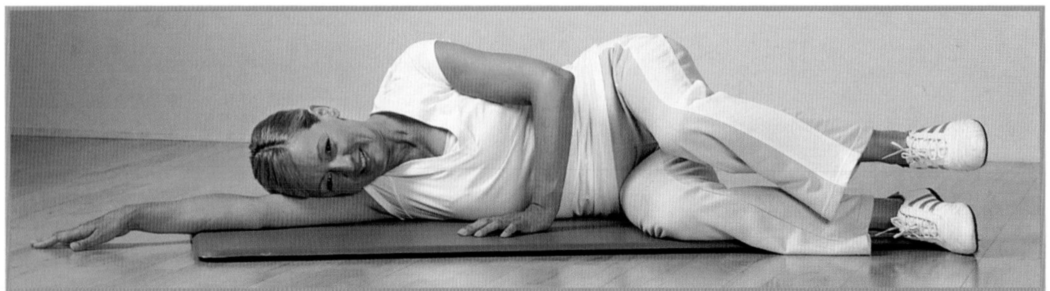

1 Lie on your side with your hips and knees at right angles. Rest your head on your lower arm for comfort and place your other hand on the mat for support.

2 Slowly raise your top leg about 10cm. Hold it there for a moment and then slowly lower it again. Turn onto your other side and repeat.

- To increase the resistance, add a light weight to your ankle or perform the lift with your top leg straight.

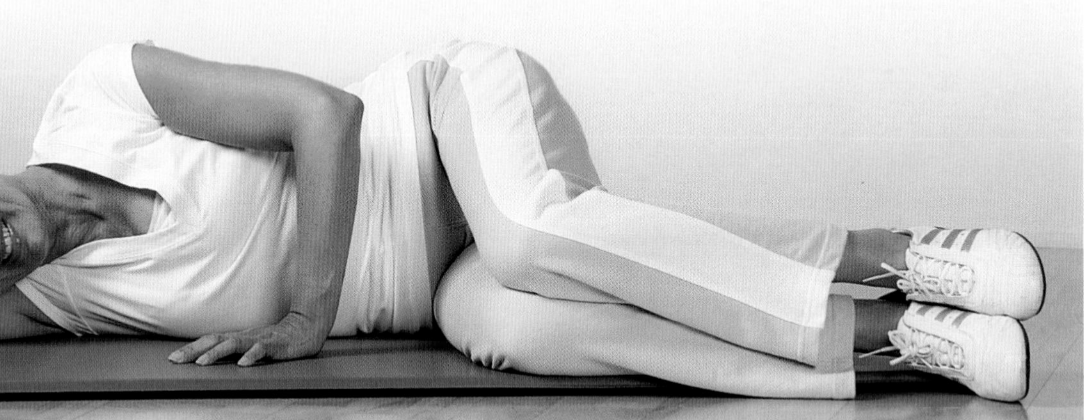

The spine

This exercise strengthens the muscles that support your spine and improves spinal alignment, reducing the risk of vertebral fracture. If you are unable to get down to the floor safely, you can do this exercise in bed.

1 Lie face down on a mat with your legs together. Place your hands, palms down, underneath your forehead.

2 Slowly lift your head and shoulders off the floor. Hold for a moment and slowly lower yourself back onto the mat.

- To increase the resistance, place your arms by your side with your palms down.

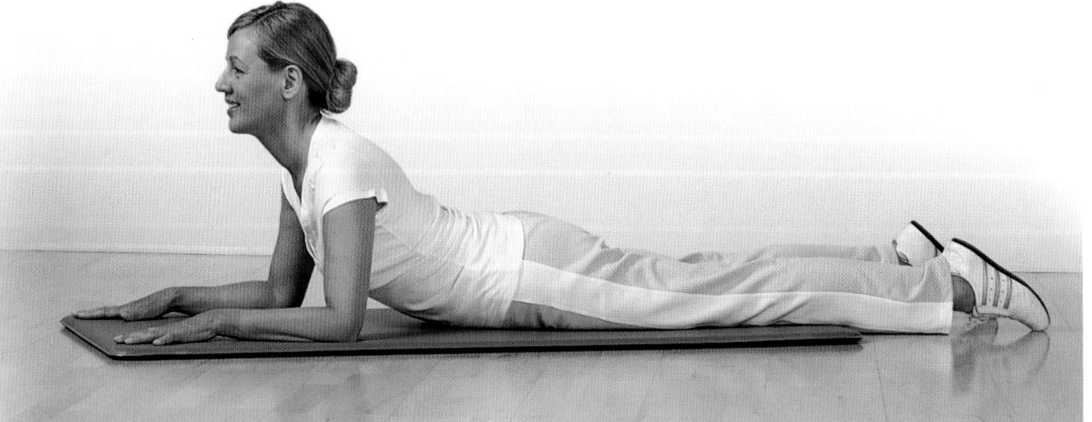

The wrists

This exercise improves bone density in your wrist and forearm and strengthens your wrist flexor muscles.

1 Sit towards the front of a chair with your feet hip-width apart and your knees over your ankles. Hold a light dumb-bell in one hand and rest your forearm on your thigh. Use your other hand to support your forearm.
2 Slowly curl the dumb-bell upwards, hold for a moment and slowly lower it back down as far down as possible. Hold and bring your wrist back to its initial position. Repeat with your hand palm down. Then repeat with your other arm.

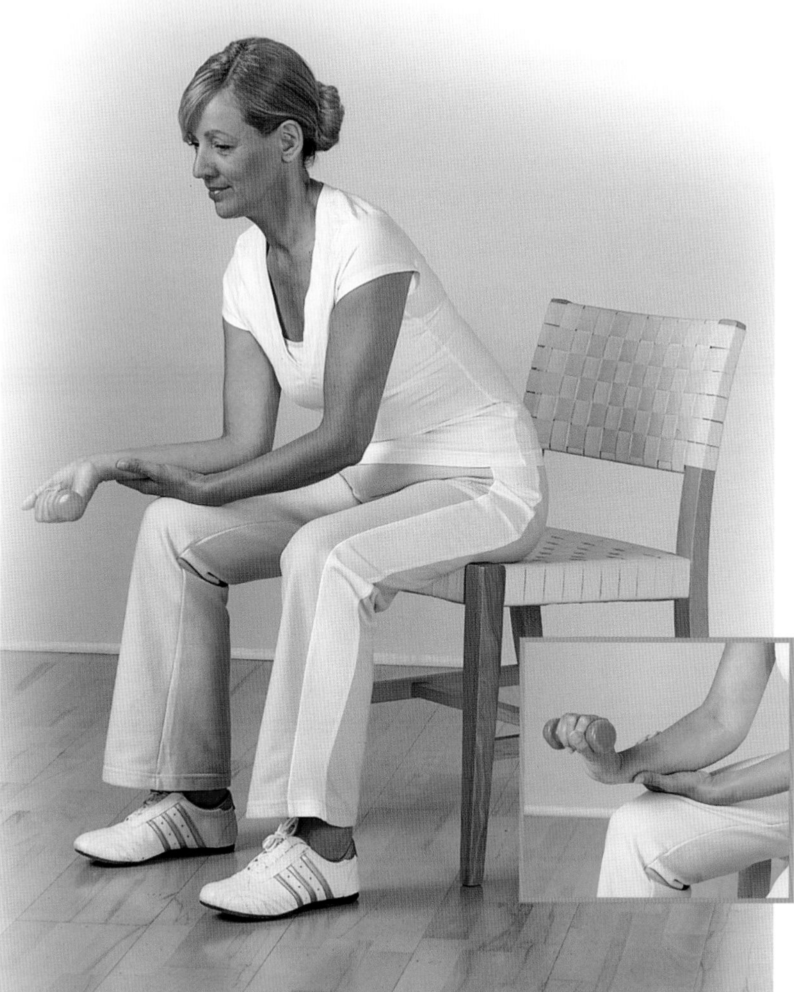

Balance

This exercise aims to work your stabilizing muscles and improve your general sense of balance – vital to prevent falls and subsequent risk of bone fractures and other injuries.

1 Place two stable chairs back to back, with half-a-metre space in between. Stand between the chairs. Rest your hands on the chair backs in case you lose your balance, but don't use them for support unless you need to.
2 Transfer your weight onto one leg. Slide your other foot forwards, keeping your toes in contact with the floor. Lift the extended leg about 5cm off the floor. Hold your foot in the air for as long as you feel comfortable or until you start to lose your balance. Then repeat with your other leg.

• To increase the resistance, secure a weight across the top of your thigh before lifting.

Conventional treatments

There are a range of drugs available to help treat osteoporosis, most of which work by slowing the rate of bone loss. Drugs should always be used alongside general lifestyle measures, such as eating a healthy diet and taking regular weight-bearing exercise. People who are at risk of osteoporosis but have not yet developed the disease should concentrate on these preventative measures rather than drugs.

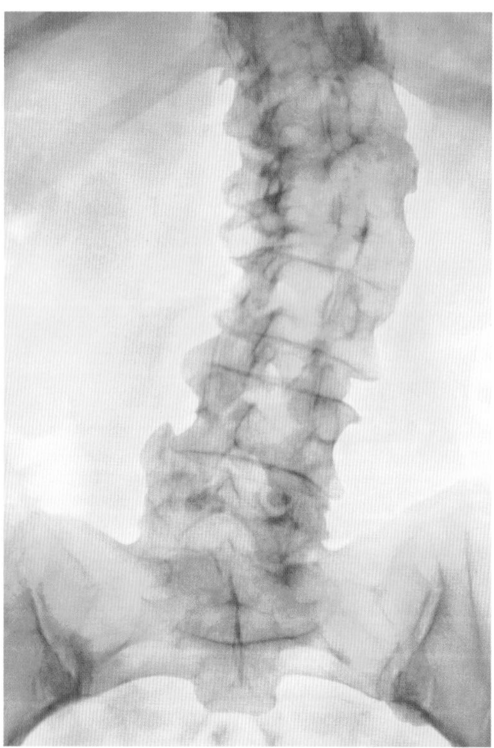

CURVED SPINE

This coloured MRI scan shows how vertebrae weakened by osteoporosis can compress under pressure, hunching the spine.

You may wish to make an appointment with a physiotherapist (>>243) who can suggest treatments and exercises to conserve bone density and improve mobility. A physiotherapist will also be able to recommend an exercise programme that is tailored to your individual needs.

Bisphosphonates

Drugs such as etidronate, alendronate and risedronate help to reduce the rate of bone loss by binding to the surface of bone and slowing the action of osteoclasts (the cells that break down bone). Long-term use may also produce an increase in bone density.

Bisphosphonates have few serious side effects, although they can cause digestion problems and more rarely inflammation in the oesophagus. Although you should continue to take calcium supplements while using bisphosphonates, calcium can interfere with the absorption of the drug – wait at least 30 minutes after using bisphosphonates before taking calcium containing foods or supplements.

Hormone replacement therapy (HRT)

There is a close connection between osteoporosis in women and the hormonal changes that take place at the menopause. Hormone replacement therapy (HRT) counteracts these changes by replacing lost oestrogen. HRT reduces the risk of fractures and the rate of bone loss after the menopause, although it must be taken for five or more years to be effective.

Once considered a front-line treatment, HRT is now reserved for treating women who have tried other drugs but have found them ineffective or hard to tolerate. This change in prescribing practice is the result of better knowledge about the potential side effects of HRT, including strokes, heart disease and breast or uterine cancer. For more advice about the menopause and HRT, >>148–149.

Calcitonin

This hormone prevents bone loss in women after the menopause by suppressing the action of the bone-reducing osteoclast cells. The drug also helps to reduce the risk of fractures of the vertebrae of the spine in women affected by osteoporosis. Once only given by injection, calcitonin is now available in the form of a nasal spray. Side effects are usually mild.

Raloxifene

This is one of a class of drugs known as selective oestrogen receptor modulators (SERMs). These drugs mimic the effects of oestrogen in one or more target tissues, while blocking its effects in others. Given with calcium and vitamin D supplements, raloxifene has been found to increase bone mass and reduce the risk of fractures of the spine vertebrae in postmenopausal women affected by osteoporosis.

Testosterone

Testosterone has a protective effect on bone density in men which is similar to that of oestrogen in women. There is some evidence that testosterone replacement therapy may be helpful for men with very low levels of the hormone, although more research needs to be done. It is not recommended for treating osteoporosis in men with normal levels of testosterone.

Hope for the future

So long as osteoporosis is diagnosed in its early stages, it is usually possible to conserve bone mass using simple self-help measures and medical treatments. Early diagnosis is also key to avoiding fractures. For this reason, it is important to identify those at risk and encourage them to adopt an appropriate lifestyle as early as possible.

Hope for the future

As research into osteoporosis continues and our understanding improves of how and why the condition occurs, new ways to treat and prevent the disease may emerge. Potentially productive areas for research and development include:

The role of genes

According to a report in the *Journal of the American Medical Association* in 2004, researchers have identified certain gene mutations that make people with osteoporosis less susceptible to fractures. Although the mutations do not appear to have a direct effect on bone density, they are associated with a 20–40 per cent reduction in the risk of fracture. It is still not completely clear why these mutations should have this effect; a more detailed knowledge of the role that genes play in bone density and fractures could offer new ways to treat and prevent osteoporosis.

Bone turnover

Research continues to look into how the cells that break down and form bone are controlled. There are already a number of drugs available to suppress the action of the bone-reducing osteoclast cells. It may one day be possible to actually reverse the effects of osteoporosis by promoting the action of the bone-forming osteoblast cells.

Bone cement

Further research is taking place into a method, first developed several years ago, to inject a type of bone cement into damaged spine vertebrae. Researchers hope it may eventually be possible to use special cements that encourage the bone around them to grow.

New drugs

A number of drugs are under development or undergoing clinical trials. New bone-forming drugs such as strontium ranelate and parathyroid hormone (PTH) may offer the chance to rebuild weak bones. A recent study showed that PTH reduced the risk of fractures in postmenopausal women by about 70 per cent within 18 months.

Another potentially exciting group of drugs is the selective oestrogen receptor modulators (SERMs). These drugs mimic the effects of oestrogen on bones, helping to conserve bone tissue and reducing fractures without causing some of the unwanted effects of natural oestrogens. Raloxifene is currently available on prescription in the UK and there are other types of SERM undergoing trials.

A study funded by the Arthritis Research Campaign is testing the theory that a class of drugs used to treat high blood pressure, thiazide diuretics, may also increase bone formation.

GENETIC DEFENDERS
The body's ageing process is closely linked to the built-up damage to cells from molecules such as free radicals. It may one day be possible to alter or control the genes that protect against these molecules, reducing some of the harmful effects of ageing on the bones.

DID YOU KNOW?

- **Scientists at the University of Limerick have developed a new way to test for osteoporosis by scanning patients' fingernails. Low levels of disulphide, a substance used to bind proteins in collagen, indicate low levels of the substance in bone. The scanner was nominated for the 2005 Medical Futures Innovation Awards.**
- **A prototype ultrasound scanner, which can be mounted on a car dashboard, has recently been designed by a UK safety research centre. The scanner measures bone density and adjusts the tension of the seatbelt and force of the airbags accordingly. Researchers believe it could cut chest injuries in older drivers by as much as 20 per cent.**

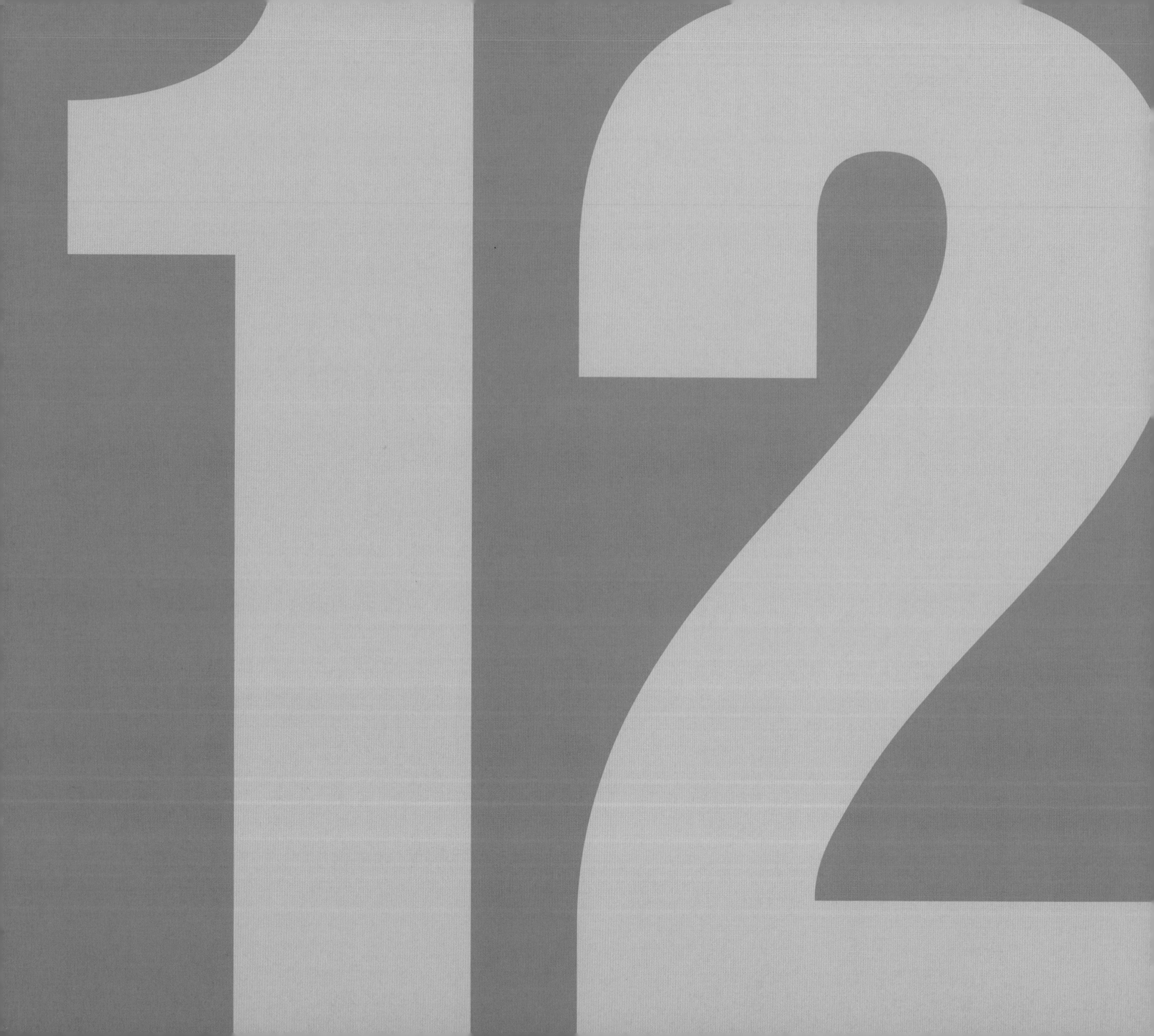
12

DIRECTORY OF DISORDERS

The following pages provide comprehensive and up-to-date information on the other main medical conditions that can affect your bones, muscles and joints, as well as extra detail on some of the disorders mentioned earlier in the book. This section also includes brief descriptions of some of the most common tests and techniques used to help diagnose musculoskeletal disorders.

12 DIRECTORY OF DISORDERS

The following A-Z section provides up-to-date information on many of the other medical conditions affecting bones, muscles and joints, and also includes extra detail on disorders touched on earlier in the book. Each entry describes the condition, its causes, symptoms and how it is diagnosed, and outlines the latest tests and treatment options available.

ACHONDROPLASIA

A congenital growth defect that causes abnormal body proportions.

Achondroplasia is present in around one in every 25,000 births. The condition affects the rate at which the bone growth plates produce cartilage and consequently the rate at which this cartilage develops into bone. The result is a form of dwarfism with stunted growth and short limbs.

What are the causes?

The condition is caused by a genetic abnormality. In most cases this gene mutation occurs in the sperm or egg but in around 20 per cent of cases the condition is inherited from a parent who also has the disorder. The faulty gene is one that usually helps to produce proteins called fibroblast growth factor receptors. Without these receptors, the body cannot produce cartilage normally.

What are the symptoms?

At birth, babies with achondroplasia tend to have a relatively long, narrow torso and short arms and legs, particularly in the upper arms and thighs. Most babies have a large head, prominent forehead and low nasal bridge. Fingers are stubby with a separation between ring and middle fingers. Most joints can extend further than normal, although the elbows and hips have more limited movement. There is often a small hump in the middle to lower back, although this usually disappears around the time the child learns to walk.

As children with achondroplasia develop, their abnormal proportions and low muscle tone means that they tend to have delayed motor skills, although the condition does not affect intelligence. The structural abnormalities also mean children are more likely to suffer ear infections and breathing problems. Children with achondroplasia can expect to reach a height of around 120cm (4ft). Adults often also suffer from low back pain and leg pain due to pressure on the spine.

How is it diagnosed?

Prenatal tests can check for the gene mutation – these tests are often performed if one or both or the parents also have achondroplasia. Otherwise, the condition is usually diagnosed at birth based on the baby's physical appearance and is then confirmed using X-rays (>>319).

What are the treatment options?

There is no cure although there is also no reason why people affected by the condition should not lead otherwise normal lives. Human growth hormone may lead to modest height increases, although how this affects adult height is not clear. Another option is leg lengthening surgery. Both options can cause complications.

Treatment tends to focus on managing associated problems such as ear infections. Babies and children should be monitored for hydrocephalus (fluid on the brain) which can be drained if necessary.

ANKYLOSING SPONDYLITIS

An inflammatory disease that typically involves the joints of the back and mainly affects young adults.

This disease is characterized by inflammation of the spinal column and the sacro-iliac joints that connect the spinal

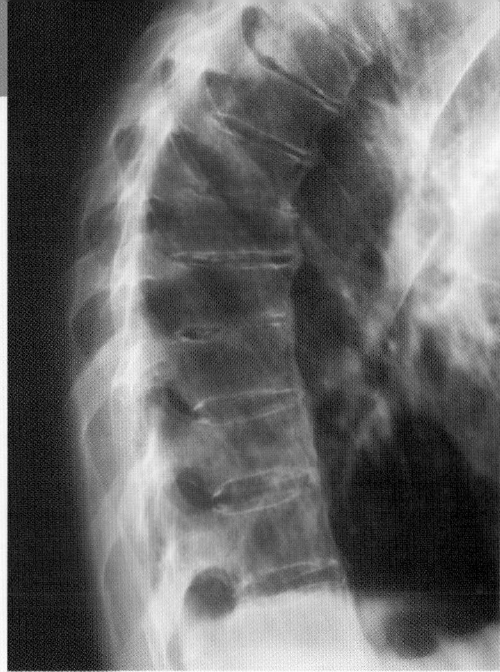

ANKYLOSING SPONDYLITIS
This coloured X-ray shows ankylosing spondylitis in the lower back. This patient has developed a particularly severe fixed kyphosis – an outward curvature of the spine – but for the vast majority of cases, with the right exercise programme, the outlook is good.

column to the hips but other joints can be affected. The disease most commonly starts in the teens or early twenties. About one in 200 people in the general population are affected, although it is about three times more common in men than in women.

What are the causes?

The cause remains unknown, but the disorder often runs in families, suggesting that genes play an important role. Some believe it may be triggered by an infection, but no infective cause has yet been found.

In Europe, around 90 per cent of people with ankylosing spondylitis also test positive for HLA-B27, an antigen which is closely associated with a number of related rheumatic diseases (>>box, right). There are several types of HLA-B27, some of which increase the chances of getting ankylosing spondylitis and others that may reduce the risk. However, HLA-B27 is not specific to the disease and may also be found in people who are never affected.

What are the symptoms?

Ankylosing spondylitis comes on slowly over months or even years, with episodes of pain and stiffness in the lower back. These symptoms tend to be at their worst in the morning and following periods of rest; they often improve with movement. Less commonly, the symptoms begin in the upper back or the neck area.

The disease can spread gradually up from the lower spine until, in some cases, the whole spine is involved and becomes increasingly rigid, with restriction of movement. Without the right treatment, the spine may become curved and the back muscles weakened.

In around 40 per cent of those affected other joints in addition to those of the spine are involved. These may include the hips (most commonly), knees or shoulders. Pain in the chest can occur, resulting from inflammation of the joints of the rib cage.

In some cases other parts of the body are affected, the most common complication being acute anterior uveitis, an inflammation of the eye that requires urgent treatment. Eye pain, blurred vision or an aversion to bright light are all signs that medical attention should be sought.

How is it diagnosed?

The diagnosis is largely made from a description of the symptoms. Tests may be used to help confirm it but these tests are not specific to the disease, so cannot be used solely to make the diagnosis. Blood may be taken to look for HLA-B27 antigens but, again, this is not specific to ankylosing spondylitis. X-rays of the sacro-iliac joints and spine may show signs of the disease. However, in the early stages X-rays may be normal, even when symptoms are severe.

What are the treatment options?

The aims of treatment are to relieve the pain and stiffness, to keep all affected joints as mobile as possible and to avoid the development of spinal curvature.

Exercise is the key to achieving these aims and those affected are given advice on daily back exercises and good posture. They should also avoid staying sedentary for

HUMAN LEUKOCYTE ANTIGENS (HLAs)

HLAs are proteins that are present on the cell membranes of nearly all the cells in the body. They are used by the immune system to distinguish between cells that are meant to be present and foreign cells such as cancers or infective organisms that need to be attacked.

There are many different types of human leukocyte antigens, but certain HLAs are of particular interest because they are frequently found in people who have some autoimmune disorders. HLA-B27, for example, is present in up to 90 per cent of people with ankylosing spondylitis, 80 per cent of people with reactive arthritis and around 50 per cent of people with psoriatic arthritis. However, this antigen is also present in around 5 per cent of people without any type of autoimmune disease, so the presence of HLA-B27 cannot be used to confirm a diagnosis of a disease.

long periods. Regular swimming will help to maintain mobility and flexibility of the spinal column.

Non-steroidal anti-inflammatory drugs (NSAIDs >>box, below) are often prescribed when the disease flares up. Although they help to relieve the symptoms, they do not affect the progress of the disease or the long-term outcome and may have serious side effects. A long-acting preparation taken at night may help to reduce morning stiffness so that an exercise programme can be continued even when the symptoms are severe. Certain anti-rheumatic drugs including sulfasalazine may help if joints outside the spinal column are affected.

Surgery is sometimes recommended when movement of the hip, knee or shoulder is severely limited.

What is the outlook?

As long as the diagnosis is made early and the recommended exercise programme is followed, the disease has a good prognosis. Back stiffness may be a problem but is unlikely to cause disability; mobility tends to be worse if the hips are affected. Overall, around 80 per cent of those affected can work and have a good quality of life.

BLOUNT'S DISEASE

A growth disorder of the tibia (shin bone) that causes the lower leg to angle inwards.

This rare condition affects the growth plate on the upper shine bone. This means that bone growth at the top of the shin bone is asymmetrical (more bone is produced at one side than the other) causing the lower leg to angle inwards. This can produce a bow-leg appearance but, unlike regular bow legs, Blount's disease grows progressively worse.

Blount's disease usually occurs in young children but can affect adolescents, particularly overweight adolescents. In around 60 per cent of cases both legs are involved. It may eventually lead to early osteoarthritis due to uneven wear on knees.

What are the causes?

Doctors do not fully understand why Blount's disease occurs. It is much more common among black children but does not appear to have an obvious genetic cause. It is closely associated with obesity and with early walking, so it may be due to excess weight on the growth plate.

How is it diagnosed and treated?

In children below the age of three, Blount's disease can be hard to distinguish from regular bow legs. In most toddlers bow legs start to correct themselves between three or four years of age. Bowing that grows progressively worse, occurs from below the knees or appears asymmetrical (one leg is more affected than the other) should be checked out by a doctor who will take an X-ray to check the angle of the knee. If the angle is more than 10–12 degrees, corrective treatment may be necessary.

The earlier that treatment can be started, the more effective it will generally be. If the condition is spotted in time, a brace can be used to correct bone growth and straighten the leg. If it is more advanced, surgery may be necessary.

NON-STEROIDAL ANTI-INFLAMMATORY DRUGS (NSAIDs)

Known for their inflammation and pain-relieving properties, these drugs are used extensively in treating muscle and joint problems. Examples include ibuprofen, diclofenac and indomethacin. NSAIDs may be used in a gel form applied to the skin but more commonly they are taken by mouth. Some NSAIDs are also available as injections or suppositories to be used rectally.

NSAIDs may cause a variety of side effects, including nausea and diarrhoea. They can lead to the formation of ulcers and bleeding in the stomach and intestines and they have recently been linked to an increased risk of heart attack. Newer NSAIDs which target an enzyme called Cox-2 carry a lower risk of ulcers and bleeding but are also associated with an increased risk of heart attack.

People who have heart problems, asthma and certain other conditions should not take NSAIDs unless otherwise advised by their doctor. The risk of bleeding and heart attacks increases with long-term use, stronger medications or large doses – anyone who needs to use an NSAID for more than a few days should talk to their doctor about the latest guidelines.

BONE TUMOURS

An abnormal growth of cells within the bone tissue that may be benign (non-cancerous) or malignant (cancerous).

Cancerous tumours can be further divided into those that originate within the bone (primary tumours) and those that spread to the bone from elsewhere in the body (secondary tumours or metastases). Occasionally infections, fractures and other conditions can resemble tumours. Most bone tumours are benign.

BENIGN BONE TUMOURS

Some benign tumours cause deformities or pain but most can be left untreated.

The most common benign bone tumours are bony outgrowths called exostoses, which often develop on the heel, but may grow on the ends of long bones like the femur (thigh bone), where they can interfere with muscle contraction. Other benign tumours include osteoblastomas and osteoid osteomas, which can be painful. Rarely, some benign tumours can develop into cancerous tumours.

The tumour may be diagnosed using X-rays or MRI (>>319, 297), or by using radionuclide scanning (>>box, right). A biopsy (a small tissue sample) may be taken and examined to confirm that the tumour is benign. In many cases no treatment is required but if the tumour causes pain or deformity it may need to be removed. This is usually successful, though benign tumours can occasionally recur.

PRIMARY BONE TUMOURS

A primary bone tumour is one that starts in the bone rather than spreading to the bone from elsewhere.

Primary bone tumours are rare. In the UK, only around 500 people are diagnosed with primary bone tumours each year:

- **Osteosarcomas** are the most common form of primary tumour and can occur in any bone, although they usually involve bones in the legs and arms and tend to affect teenagers and young adults.
- **Fibrosarcomas** tend to occur in thigh bones, usually in middle-aged patients.
- **Chondrosarcomas** also tend to affect middle-aged people. They originate in cartilage cells and are most common in sites such as the pelvis and the ribs.

WHAT IS RADIONUCLIDE SCANNING?

Also known as isotope bone scanning, this test uses low-dose radioactivity to look for abnormal areas of bone. A radioactive substance – called a tracer – is given by injection into a vein and a scan is taken up to three hours later, when the tracer has been distributed around the skeleton. Abnormal areas of bone take up more of the tracer than normal bone, causing bright areas known as 'hot spots'. However, it is not always clear that the hot spots are due to cancer, as other conditions, such as arthritis, can cause a similar appearance. Further tests may be necessary to look at the areas in more detail.

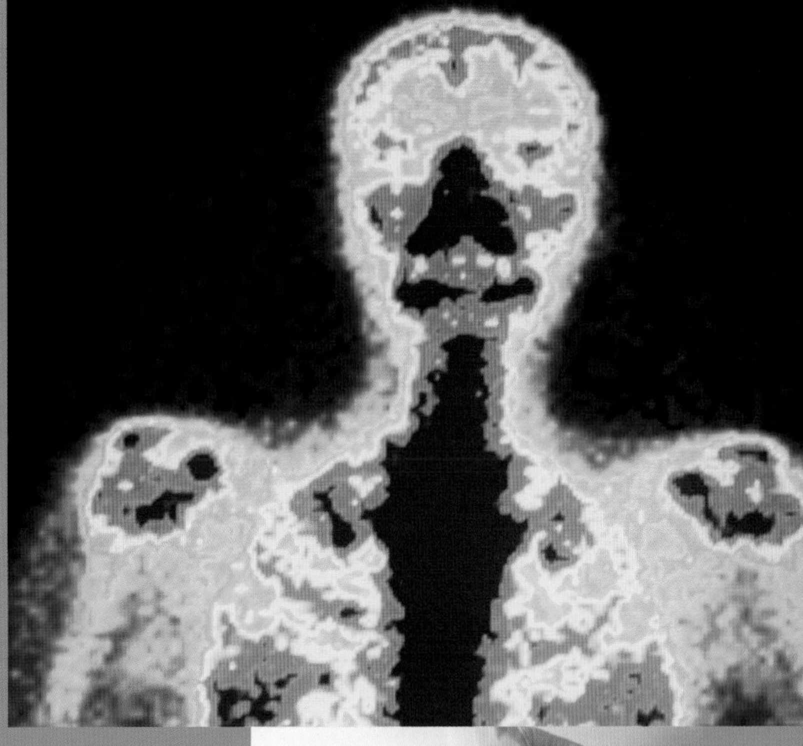

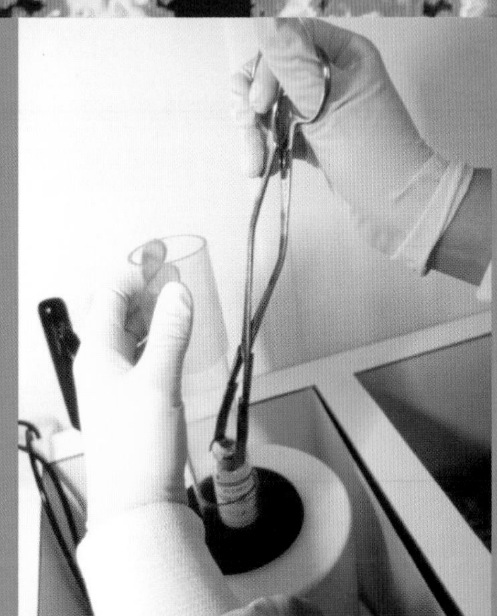

RADIONUCLIDE BONE SCANNING

The bone scan of the upper body (top) shows hot spots in bones that have absorbed the radioactive tracer – though not all of the red areas indicated will necessarily be cancerous. The isotopes used in a bone scan are safe and leave the body quickly – the level of radiation involved is lower than in some conventional X-rays. However the isotopes used to make the tracer have to be handled very carefully. When not in use, they are kept in a thick container made of materials which absorb gamma rays.

The causes of primary bone cancer have not yet been discovered. Treatment of cancer with high-dose radiotherapy may slightly increase the risk, as does the chronic bone condition Paget's disease (>>313). Some rare hereditary conditions are also associated with an increased risk and certain types of benign bone tumour very occasionally become cancerous.

What are the symptoms?

Symptoms vary depending on the size and site of the tumour. There may be pain and swelling. Walking can be affected if there is a tumour in one of the leg bones. If a tumour develops in the bones of the spinal column, it may compress the spine and the nerves that spread from it, causing weakness and tingling or numbness. A bone affected by cancer may also be more prone to fracture; sometimes bone cancer is detected when a fracture occurs. Non-specific symptoms may also be present, such as tiredness, fever or weight loss.

How is it diagnosed and treated?

Various tests are used to make a diagnosis. Blood calcium levels may be checked as they are elevated in some people with bone tumours. The levels of another substance, alkaline phosphatase, may also be raised. X-rays often reveal changes suggestive of a tumour. CT or MRI scans (>>301, 297) can then be used to examine areas of bone in detail. A sample of bone tissue (a biopsy) may be taken to confirm the diagnosis and to identify the type of tumour. This will guide the specialist towards the most suitable treatments.

Analgesics and NSAIDs (>>280) may be taken for pain. Primary bone tumours can be treated with anticancer drugs as well as radiotherapy, and in some cases surgery, to remove the tumour. The outlook varies between individuals and is determined by factors such as how early and at what stage the diagnosis is made, as well as the type of tumour.

SECONDARY BONE TUMOURS

Also known as bone metastases, secondary bone tumours spread to bone from primary tumours at other sites in the body.

Secondary bone tumours are much more common than primary tumours. They most commonly spread to bone from the lungs, breasts, prostate gland, thyroid or kidney.

What are the symptoms?

Bone metastases can cause dull, persistent pain. There may also be swelling. Like primary bone cancer, bone metastases can cause weakness and may make bones more liable to fracture. If the bones of the spinal column are affected, nerve tissue may be compressed, causing weakness, tingling or numbness. If the tumour affects the bone marrow, where blood cells are formed, there may be anaemia, an impaired ability to fight infections or a tendency to bleed more easily than usual.

How are they diagnosed and treated?

Blood tests may be arranged to check calcium levels and look for evidence of cancer. X-rays may be performed as well as radionuclide scanning (>>281), which shows very bright areas if secondary tumours are present. These scans don't always give a definite diagnosis and CT or MRI (>>301, 297) scanning may be used to examine abnormal areas closely. If secondary bone cancer is diagnosed before a primary tumour is found, tests may be arranged to look for the original tumour.

Generally, the aim of secondary bone cancer treatment is to relieve the symptoms and reduce the number of cancer cells. It may also lessen the likelihood of fractures occurring. Bone metastases are often treated with radiotherapy; treatment may also be needed for the primary tumour. The outlook varies depending on the type of primary tumour and how well it can be treated.

BRITTLE BONE DISEASE

>>osteogenesis imperfecta

BUNIONS

A swelling next to the big toe joint.

Strictly speaking, a bunion consists of a fluid-filled sac next to a deformed big toe joint. But the term is usually used to describe any of various conditions that involve swelling around the big toe. Women are affected more commonly than men.

What are the causes?

Bunions can be caused by friction from shoes rubbing over a big toe joint that is misshapen in some way, perhaps by hallux valgus (>>box, right) or by a benign growth called an exostosis on the first metatarsal bone (the bone of the foot that connects to the big toe). Women are often affected by bunions because they are more likely to wear tight, narrow shoes or high heeled shoes that put pressure on the toes. Tight shoes can also cause other foot problems such as corns and calluses.

What are the symptoms?

Bunions can be red and painful, which may affect walking. If this irritation is ignored, hardening of the skin takes place. Bunions

WHAT IS HALLUX VALGUS?

This is a deformity of the big toe joint that causes the joint to project outwards and the toe to point inwards. A hallux valgus is not the same as a bunion (which is a fluid-filled sac) but bunions often develop as a result of a hallux valgus. Contrary to popular belief, there is no evidence that pointed or badly fitting shoes are the cause. The condition sometimes runs in families and may develop in young people for no apparent reason. Hallux valgus can also affect the elderly, particularly elderly women – in these cases osteoarthritis is often the underlying cause. A bony lump on top of the toe joint is usually due to a different condition, hallux rigidus.

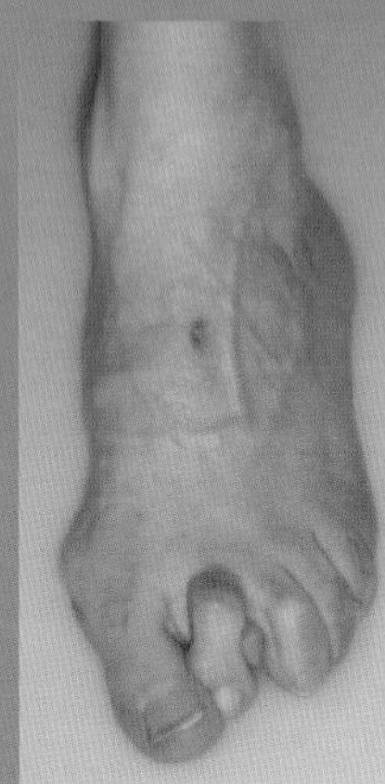

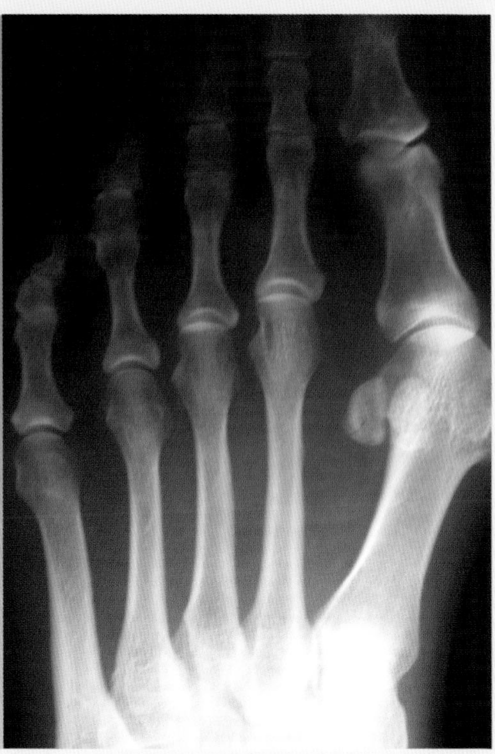

can become infected and this infection can spread into the big toe joint. Bunions can indicate a predisposition to osteoarthritis of the big toe >>228–247.

What are the treatment options?

Many people choose to cushion the bunion and wear comfortable, roomy shoes; this usually provides some relief from pain and discomfort. Surgery – which is successful in most cases – may be considered if there is severe discomfort or if walking is affected. Most bunion operations are done on a same-day basis although a long recovery is common and may include persistent swelling and stiffness. If there is hallux valgus present (>>box, above) this must be treated before the bunion is removed.

BURSITIS

Inflammation of a bursa resulting in pain and swelling.

Bursae are fluid-filled sacs located around joints which act as cushions and prevent friction between tendons, ligaments and bones. Inflammation of these sacs is called bursitis. There are more than 150 bursae located around the body, but common sites for bursitis include the knee and elbow.

What are the causes?

The most common cause of inflammation is repeated friction or prolonged pressure over a bursa but it may also be caused by an infection or an injury. Inflammatory joint conditions such as gout (>>294) and rheumatoid arthritis (>>248–263) increase the risk from some types of bursitis. Sometimes the cause cannot be determined.

What are the symptoms?

The bursa may be red, swollen and painful. Sometimes movement of the nearby joint is limited. Common types of bursitis include:

- **Prepatellar bursitis** The prepatellar bursa is located over the patella (kneecap) to help skin move freely over the bone when the knee bends. If the bursa becomes inflamed, a swelling will develop in front of the kneecap. Some people find that they also have severe pain when kneeling.

  Prepatellar bursitis is sometimes known as housemaid's knee, although nowadays it is more likely to affect gardeners, tilers and carpet-layers. People who need to kneel for long periods should wear protective knee pads and change position regularly.
- **Infrapatellar bursitis** The infrapatellar bursa lies below the kneecap and over the upper shin bone (tibia). Infrapatellar bursitis is also known as clergyman's knee because the type of kneeling position used by clergymen during prayer can place pressure on this area.
- **Olecranon bursitis** The olecranon bursa lies over the point of the elbow and performs a similar role to the prepatellar bursa in the knee. Long periods spent resting on the elbows may aggravate this bursa, making elbows feel hot and painful.

What are the treatment options?

The swelling will often go down following a period of rest. Non-steroidal anti-inflammatory drugs (NSAIDs >>280) may help to relieve the inflammation. Sometimes a corticosteroid injection is given directly into the joint to relieve the inflammation. In a few cases, when the problem persists or recurs, the bursa may be removed surgically. Infected bursae will require antibiotic treatment and possible drainage if pus accumulates.

CARPAL TUNNEL SYNDROME

Tingling and pain in the hand due to nerve compression.

The carpal tunnel is a narrow space in the wrist enclosed by the bones of the wrist (the carpal bones) and the fibrous band that overlies them. The tissues that travel through this space include the median nerve and the tendons that extend from the forearm to the fingers.

The median nerve controls the movements of specific muscles in the hand and relays sensory information between certain areas of the hand (most of the palm, the thumb, forefinger, middle finger and part of the ring finger) and the brain.

Carpal tunnel syndrome occurs when the median nerve is compressed within the carpal tunnel, impairing its function and causing altered sensations in the hand and weakness of the hand muscles that are supplied by the median nerve.

Carpal tunnel syndrome tends to develop between the ages of 40 and 60 years and women are affected more frequently than men.

What are the causes?

Exactly why carpal tunnel syndrome develops cannot always be identified. It is often associated with conditions including diabetes mellitus, an underactive thyroid gland (hypothyroidism), pregnancy, obesity, rheumatoid arthritis and acromegaly, a rare disorder in which excessive production of growth hormone leads to enlargement of certain bones and organs. In some cases, the reason for this association is clear: during pregnancy, for example, fluid retention causes pressure on the carpal nerve. With other conditions the connection is not fully understood.

Carpal tunnel syndrome is also associated with typing and other activities that involve repeated movements of the hands, causing inflammation of the tendons at the wrist (RSI >>321).

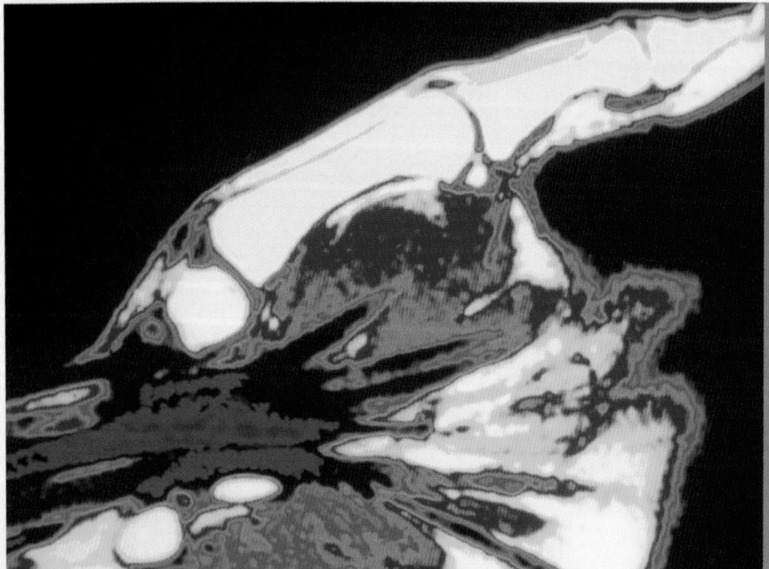

CARPAL TUNNEL *This coloured MRI scan of a hand affected by carpal tunnel syndrome shows the bones of the thumb and the wrist in white and the tendons and ligaments that pass through the carpal tunnel in pink and blue. The median nerve, which passes under these ligaments, is compressed by the bones of the wrist.*

What are the symptoms?

Symptoms vary between individuals but pain and tingling in the palm, the thumb, the second and third fingers, and the side of the fourth finger is common. This sensation sometimes extends up into the forearm. The tingling and pain tend to be worse at night and may be relieved briefly if the arm is shaken. Over time the thumb muscles and the other muscles in the hand may grow weaker causing a weakened grip. Eventually the hand may grow numb.

How is it diagnosed?

A diagnosis can usually be made from a description of the symptoms and an examination. The doctor will look for changes in sensation and weakness in the parts of the hand that are supplied by the median nerve. Tapping over the wrist may bring on the tingling and pain – this is known as Tinel's sign.

If the symptoms and examination findings are not typical of carpal tunnel syndrome, the doctor may arrange nerve conduction studies to assess how well the nerve is transmitting impulses.

What are the treatment options?

Where possible the underlying cause of the problem should be addressed: if any of the conditions mentioned above are present, for example, treatment for that problem may remove pressure on the nerve.

Another way to reduce pressure on the median nerve is to splint the wrist so that the carpal tunnel is held in a position that doesn't obstruct the nerve. The splint can be worn at night or during activities that particularly tend to bring on symptoms. Non-steroidal anti-inflammatories (NSAIDs >>280) may be helpful in some cases and corticosteroid injections directly into the wrist may provide relief. Some studies suggest that vitamin B_6 (pyridoxine) supplements may ease the symptoms of carpal tunnel syndrome.

In some persistent or recurrent cases, surgery may be carried out to relieve pressure on the nerve. In a carpal tunnel release, a cut is made in the fibrous tissue that overlies the carpal tunnel. This usually takes about 15 minutes and is performed under general or local anaesthetic.

CEREBRAL PALSY

Damage to the area of the brain controlling muscle tone and coordination.

Cerebral palsy is an umbrella term for a variety of muscular disorders that are caused by the faulty development of, or damage to, the motor areas of the brain – the parts of the brain that control movement and posture. Cerebral palsy does not affect intelligence.

Around two children out of every thousand have some degree of cerebral palsy, although the symptoms and severity of the condition vary considerably. There are three basic forms of cerebral palsy:

- **Spastic cerebral palsy** This is the most common form of the condition, affecting 70–80 per cent of patients, and impedes the ability to relax muscles, causing stiff or difficult movement.
- **Athetoid cerebral palsy** This form affects the ability to control muscles, meaning limbs flutter and move suddenly.
- **Ataxic cerebral palsy** This form affects balance and depth perception.

It is not unusual for patients to have symptoms of more than one of these forms: the most common combination is spasticity and athetoid movements.

What are the causes?

Cerebral palsy is usually a congenital disorder, in that it commonly develops before birth. Many different factors can affect brain development in the womb including infections, exposure to certain chemicals, alcohol or drugs, physical trauma and malnutrition – in most cases doctors are never able to identify exactly why the problem occurs.

Premature babies, very small babies who do not cry in the first five minutes after delivery and babies who need to be on a ventilator for more than four weeks after birth are known to be at particular risk, probably because all of these factors indicate wider problems with development. However, even a small premature baby has a very low risk of also having cerebral palsy. Babies who have congenital malformations of the heart, kidneys, or spine are also more likely to develop the condition.

Occasionally, the condition may be acquired during the birthing process or in early childhood. Lack of oxygen to the brain due to factors such as choking, infections such meningitis or encephalitis, or physical trauma such as shaking may all be responsible for damage to the brain.

What are the symptoms?

Depending on which areas of the brain have been damaged, symptoms may include muscle tightness or spasm, involuntary movement, disturbances in gait and mobility, abnormal sensation and perception, impairment of sight, hearing or speech, seizures and excessive drooling.

The extent of these symptoms can also vary considerably: children with very mild cerebral palsy sometimes recover by the time they are four or five but for most patients cerebral palsy is a lifelong disability. Some people with cerebral palsy may need to use a wheelchair. Others may be able to walk in an unsteady way with the help of crutches or braces. In some cases, speech is affected or the patient cannot speak at all.

How is it diagnosed?

Cerebral palsy may be suspected if the child is slow to achieve the normal developmental milestones such as reaching for toys (3–4 months), sitting (6–7 months), and walking (10–14 months). These delays can be signs of other developmental problems so a child may be up to 18 months old before cerebral palsy can be diagnosed with any degree of certainty.

The condition is not progressive; it is unlikely that cerebral palsy will cause the loss of motor skills once they have developed. If a child loses the ability to perform a skill that has already been mastered, doctors should consider other possible problems.

A diagnosis of cerebral palsy cannot be made on the basis of an X-ray or blood test alone, although the doctor may order these tests to exclude other neurological diseases. As a group, children with cerebral palsy are more likely to have scars, cysts and other changes affecting the motor area of the brain so an MRI or CT scan may be of help (>>297, 301). These tests can also look for hydrocephalus (fluid on the brain).

What are the treatment options?

Cerebral palsy cannot be cured but it is almost always possible to improve physical capabilities and independence.

Therapy usually forms the foundation of cerebral palsy treatment: physical, occupational and behavioural therapists can help the child to learn how best to manage the condition and perform tasks. Physiotherapy exercises, for example, will help to prevent weakening and contracture of muscles, will improve voluntary control and help to develop skills such as walking, sitting, swallowing and hand control.

Mechanical aids may help to overcome specific physical limitations. These aids can range from basic adjustments to everyday objects (such as velcro shoes that are easier to take on and off) through to sophisticated computers or voice synthesizers to assist with communication.

Drugs can help to control muscle spasms and prevent seizures. Common medications are diazepam, which acts as a general relaxant; baclofen, which blocks signals to contract the muscles; and dantrolene, which interferes with the process of muscle contraction. In some cases surgery may be helpful, either to lengthen excessively contracted muscles or to cut overactive nerves.

What is the outlook?

The damage to the brain that causes cerebral palsy will not get any worse as the child gets older: a child whose condition only affects the legs, for example, will not develop cerebral palsy affecting the arms or difficulties speaking later on in life. However, some people do develop further complications as a result of the condition, such as dislocated hips or scoliosis (curvature of the spine).

CERVICAL SPONDYLOSIS

Degenerative disease of the spinal column in the neck causing neck pain and stiffness.

This term is usually used to describe osteoarthritis (>>228–247) of the cervical spine – the portion of the spine in the neck. Although the effects of general wear-and-tear mean that most people develop a degree of cervical spondylosis as they get older, many people have no symptoms of the condition. Men tend to be affected more than women.

What are the symptoms?

As cartilage between vertebrae starts to break down and the spaces between vertebrae narrow, neck pain may develop. Bony outgrowths called osteophytes may form on the vertebrae, restricting head movements and causing stiffness.

If the head is turned suddenly, the bony spurs may press against nerves or blood vessels in the neck causing shooting pains and aches down the arms or numbness and tingling in the arms and hands. This may cause transient faintness, dizziness or double vision.

How is it diagnosed and treated?

X-rays can identify signs of the disease such as narrowing spaces between vertebrae. A CT or MRI scan (>>301, 297) may be used to look at the spinal column in greater detail. The doctor may arrange special tests to assess how well the nerves supplying the arms and the hands are transmitting impulses.

Painkillers, heat packs and non-steroidal anti-inflammatories (NSAIDs >>280) may help to relieve any painful symptoms. Exercises and physiotherapy can help with pain relief, improve neck mobility and strengthen the muscles that move and support the spinal column. Relaxation techniques can help to relieve the tension that neck pain can cause throughout the body.

Surgery is seldom used to treat cervical spondylosis. In severe cases, doctors may consider cervical fusion to fix the affected vertebrae rigidly in place, making the spine more stable and preventing friction between vertebrae. However, this operation entails considerable loss of mobility.

CHONDROMALACIA PATELLAE

Softening of the cartilage where the kneecap (patella) meets the thigh bone. Associated with pain in the front of the knee.

This condition occurs when the cartilage on the underside of the kneecap softens and swells because of excessive pressure on the knee. Eventually, the surface of the cartilage cracks and becomes deformed. In its early stages the condition is usually reversible but if the damage persists it can increase the risk of knee osteoarthritis.

The condition may result from recurrent injuries to the knee joint or from chronic stress caused by frequent episodes of a strenuous exercise such as running, over a long period. It most commonly affects sporty adolescents.

What are the symptoms?

The most obvious symptoms will be knee pain and restricted movement of the knee. Pain may be worse while walking up and down stairs. In more severe cases there may be a creaking sensation (crepitus) caused by the bone and damaged cartilage rubbing together or clicking as the knee is bent and straightened.

To make a diagnosis, the doctor will thoroughly examine the knee and may then arrange an X-ray (>>319) and sometimes an MRI scan (>>297) to look at the structures of the knee joint in more detail.

What are the treatment options?

Painkillers and certain non-steroidal anti-inflammatory drugs (NSAIDs >>280) may help to relieve the pain and swelling. In mild cases, where the condition is likely to resolve itself over time, it may be sufficient to follow a very conservative treatment plan, with a check-up every six months or so to ensure that the condition does not deteriorate further.

Chondromalacia patellae is often caused by overuse, so strenuous or prolonged exercise involving the knees should be avoided. The doctor or physiotherapist may provide information on exercises that aim to strengthen the muscles that support and move the knee joint. If crepitus or clicking are present or the imaging tests suggest that the condition is severe, it may be possible to smooth down the irregular surface of the cartilage surgically using an arthroscope (>>206).

COCCYDYNIA

Pain in the region of the coccyx (tail bone) which may have a number of causes.

The coccyx is the small, triangular bone at the bottom of the spinal column. Pain in this area can occur for a variety of reasons and it is not always possible to identify exactly why coccydynia develops. Women are affected more often than men.

Possible underlying causes include falls, damage caused as a result of sitting down hard on the base of the spinal column, or repetitive strain due to poor sitting posture, often at work. Coccydynia may be brought on by a prolapsed disc in the spine >>317.

If pain occurs during childbirth it may be caused by the baby pushing against the mother's coccyx. Very rarely, pain in the coccyx is caused by a tumour of the uterus or the rectum.

How is it diagnosed and treated?

Diagnosis is usually made from a description of the problem and a physical examination. Sometimes the spinal column is X-rayed to look for damage.

Painkillers and non-steroidal anti-inflammatory drugs (NSAIDs >>280) may help to relieve the pain. Heat and cold packs applied to the painful area can also provide relief. Sitting on a rubber ring will relieve pressure on the coccyx and so help the condition to resolve.

CONGENITAL HIP DISLOCATION

A condition present at birth in which the upper end of the thigh bone is outside its normal position in the hip socket.

The incidence of congenital hip dislocation varies around the world but the condition occurs in about 1 in every 1000 babies in Europe. Girls are more likely to be affected than boys and the left hip tends to be involved more frequently than the right.

What are the causes?

Congenital hip dislocation occurs when the hip socket develops abnormally and is unable to hold the femoral head (the rounded head of the thigh bone) securely. Certain conditions increase the risk of dislocation. These include having a family member with the condition and being born in breech position (when the baby is born bottom first rather than head first). Hip dislocation is often associated with congenital torticollis (twisted neck).

How is it diagnosed and treated?

All newborn babies have their hips routinely checked for abnormalities. If a problem is suspected, an ultrasound scan of the hips is used to confirm diagnosis.

Congenital hip dislocation should be treated as early as possible. If it is diagnosed at birth, a harness or splints are used to hold the hips in the correct position for about 12 weeks. Treated at this early stage, the hip should develop virtually normally, although the child will need regular check-ups.

If the problem is not spotted at birth, it may be picked up at the eight-week check. At this stage, treatment may involve wearing a brace or the hips being held in position with a plaster cast for up to six months. If this treatment is unsuccessful, surgery may be required.

CONGENITAL HIP DYSPLASIA

This term covers a range of problems affecting the hip from mild abnormalities in which the head of the femur is loose in the socket to severe problems in which the hip is permanently dislocated. The mild cases result from weakness of the supporting ligaments; in severe cases, the acetabulum (socket) may have developed abnormally. Between these two extremes are the cases in which the hip dislocates but the head of the femur can be manipulated back into place.

If the condition is not picked up at any of the early checks, it may not become apparent until the child begins to walk at 12–18 months. One leg will appear shortened and the skin creases on the back of the baby's legs will be asymmetric. An abnormal gait and a limp will be present. At this stage several operations may be needed to correct the problem and replace the femoral head in the socket.

What is the outlook?

If the condition is treated early enough, the prognosis is generally very good. Without treatment, however, the hip will develop abnormally causing a permanent limp or a side-to-side gait. Osteoarthritis (>>228–247) may develop early in life.

CRAMP

A sudden, involuntary contraction of the muscle fibres causing muscle pain.

These painful muscle contractions usually affect a single muscle group, such as the calf muscles or the hamstrings. As the muscle contracts it becomes tight, hard and tender to the touch. Sometimes muscles also twitch or spasm. In most cases episodes of cramp last only for a few minutes. Cramps can happen to anyone and are rarely a sign of any underlying muscle problem or disorder.

Cramps often develop during or just after exercise. This may be due to muscle fatigue and over-exertion, a build-up of lactic acid and other waste substances, or an insufficient oxygen supply to muscle cells. They may occur during vigorous exercise in hot weather as a result of dehydration or loss of mineral salts in sweat – drinking water during exercise replenishes lost fluid but does not replace the lost salts.

During exercise, cramp often affects the muscles of the abdomen – this is also known as a stitch. Cramp can also occur in bed at night, when it particularly tends to affect the calves. Prolonged activities, such as long periods spent gripping a pen while writing, can also bring on cramp.

> ‘To check if you are at risk of writer's cramp, try to pull the pen from your writing hand with your other hand. If it doesn't slide out easily, you may be gripping too tightly’

> **CAUTION**
>
> Recurrent episodes of pain in the calves when walking may be caused by an inadequate blood supply to the calf muscles due to peripheral vascular disease (narrowing of the arteries in the calf). This needs to be checked out by a doctor.

What are the treatment options?

To avoid cramp, warm up thoroughly before exercise and drink plenty of fluids. If exercising in hot weather, eat something salty or drink an isotonic sports drink.

Cramp can be relieved by stretching and massaging the affected muscles. A heat pad may help to relieve spasm. Tonic water is also recommended as it contains quinine, which has been shown to reduce cramp. The drug quinine sulphate may be prescribed for persistent night cramp.

DISLOCATED JOINT

An injury in which the bones in a joint are forced out of position so that the joint surfaces are no longer in contact.

In a full dislocation the bones that would normally meet to form the joint no longer touch. If the joint is only partially dislocated (subluxation) there will still be some contact between joint surfaces.

When a dislocation occurs, the tissues that surround and support the joint (the ligaments and the joint capsule) may also be damaged. In addition, the impact or trauma that caused the dislocation may cause a fracture close to the joint. This is known as a fracture-dislocation.

What are the causes?

Dislocation usually results from a strong force applied to a joint. This may be caused by a knock or fall or it may be because the joint has been tugged out of position. Dislocations are common in contact sports such as rugby and sports that involve hard falls, such as skiing. Very occasionally, dislocation may occur after minor trauma because of abnormally lax ligaments.

Dislocations can occur in almost any joint, but the shoulders, elbows and fingers are the joints most commonly affected. Dislocated shoulders account for around half of all dislocations treated in hospitals; this is because the shoulder has a very wide range of motion, making it less stable than most other joints. Dislocated elbows can occur after a fall onto an outstretched hand.

What are the symptoms?
The joint may have an abnormal shape and there will probably be severe pain. There may be swelling and joint movement will be limited. The skin around the joint may be bruised and tender.

How is it diagnosed and treated?
The diagnosis is usually made from an examination of the joint. X-rays may help to confirm the diagnosis and reveal any accompanying fractures.

Painkillers will help to relieve the pain of a dislocated joint. No other treatment is usually required for a subluxed (partially dislocated) joint, as stability is usually restored when the tissues that support the joint heal. In a fully dislocated joint, the doctor will often be able to return the bones to their correct position (a process called reduction) by manually manipulating the joint or using traction – the application of a force in order to stretch a certain part of the body in a specific direction. If this is not possible or not successful, surgery may be needed to reposition the bones.

Following reduction, the joint must be kept immobile to give the surrounding tissues time to heal. This usually takes about six weeks. After the tissues have healed, physiotherapy can help to rebuild the strength of the muscles around the affected joint and restore mobility.

What is the outlook?
Dislocations are usually treated very successfully although some joints, such as the shoulder and the joint around the kneecap, may be liable to dislocate again. Fracture-dislocations usually heal well too, although treatment may initially be more difficult if there are any bone fragments lodged inside the joint.

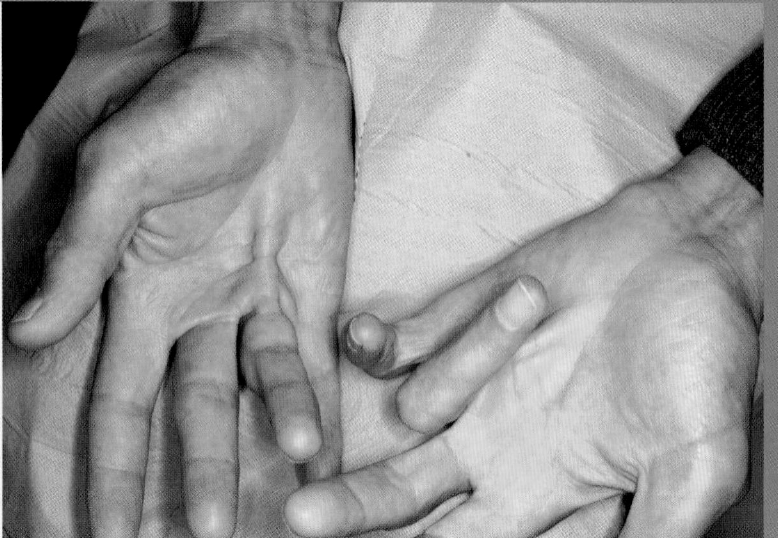

DUPUYTREN'S CONTRACTURE
These hands show the effects of Dupuytren's contracture. As the skin on the palms of the hands thickens, the tendons gradually pull the ring and little fingers in towards the palm.

DUPUYTREN'S CONTRACTURE
A thickening of the tissues in the palm of the hand that eventually causes the fingers to be drawn in towards the palm.

The palmar fascia is the layer of fibrous tissue in the palm of the hand. This tissue is attached to the skin above it and to the tendons of the fingers below. Dupuytren's contracture occurs when this tissue thickens, making it contract and gradually pulling one or more fingers in towards the palm.

Eventually, in severe cases, the fingers cannot be straightened at all. Often, both hands are involved and occasionally the soles of the feet. The condition affects men more than women and is more common in people over the age of 50. In the UK around 20 per cent of men over the age of 60 have some degree of contracture.

What are the causes?
The exact cause is unknown but since it often runs in families (with up to 70 per cent of those affected having a family history of the disease) there is probably a genetic factor involved. It is most common in people of Northern European or Scandinavian ancestry. Dupuytren's is also associated with conditions including diabetes mellitus, epilepsy and alcoholism.

It has been suggested that chronic trauma to the palm, such as may occur during manual labour or prolonged use of machinery such as pneumatic drills, is a factor in some cases. But there is no conclusive evidence for this and no particular occupations have been shown to be associated with the condition.

What are the symptoms?
Dupuytren's contracture usually develops very gradually. Early symptoms may include small painless lumps in the hand, thickening in the palm and puckering of the skin. In many cases symptoms remain mild but if the condition progresses it may be difficult to straighten the fingers and there may be problems with hand movements and gripping objects.

What are the treatment options?

Mild cases are usually left untreated and simply monitored. Often, the condition develops very slowly and never reaches a point where it becomes troublesome.

If the fingers are bent and hand function is affected, surgery may be considered to remove pieces of the thickened fascia. This can be a long procedure as the thickened tissue needs to be carefully removed from around the small nerves in the hand. Sometimes deformity returns after surgery.

FIBROMYALGIA

A common condition characterized by muscle pains all over the body and general tiredness and fatigue.

About 2 per cent of the population are thought to be affected by fibromyalgia. It is more common with age and is most common among women over the age of 70.

People with fibromyalgia suffer from widespread muscular pain and tenderness, tend to tire easily and often have broken sleep at night. The symptoms may settle down after a few weeks but the condition can last months or even years. Because there are no obvious outward signs, and the causes are still not fully understood, people do not always appreciate the distress that fibromyalgia can cause to sufferers. It is, however, a recognized medical condition.

What are the causes?

No one knows exactly what causes fibromyalgia but it may be connected to disrupted sleep patterns. Brain wave studies of fibromyalgia sufferers show that periods of deep sleep tend to be disturbed by periods of lighter 'REM' sleep. This may cause the muscle pains, which can in turn make the sleep problems worse.

Stress is also thought to be a key factor: experiencing stressful events, such as divorce or assault, is known to increase the risk of developing the condition.

What are the symptoms?

Symptoms tend to come on slowly over several weeks. The persistent muscle aches often start in the neck and back but later occur in all areas of the body. Other common symptoms include broken sleep, feelings of depression, anxiety or irritability and difficulty concentrating. As a result of tiredness, particularly in the morning, people with fibromyalgia may find it harder than normal to perform daily tasks.

Tension-type headaches, swollen hands, abdominal discomfort and bloating are also quite common. All of these symptoms may become worse if stress levels increase and may be influenced by factors such as the weather, infections, allergies, hormonal fluctuations, depression and over-exertion.

DID YOU KNOW?

- **Fibromyalgia is around ten times more common in women than in men. Women are at greater risk than men of many rheumatic diseases, possibly due to the effects of female hormones.**
- **Nine out of ten people with lupus are women.**
- **Rheumatoid arthritis is two to three times more common in women than in men.**
- **Polymyalgia rheumatica occurs around twice as often in women as it does in men.**
- **However, both gout and ankylosing spondylitis occur more frequently in men than in women.**

How is it diagnosed and treated?

There are no specific investigations for fibromyalgia; diagnosis is usually based on the description of the symptoms and an examination. Tests, such as blood tests to check the function of the thyroid gland, may be used to rule out other conditions that could be responsible for the symptoms.

Painkillers and other non-steroidal anti-inflammatory drugs (NSAIDs >>280) may help to relieve the muscle pain in some cases. Low doses of certain types of antidepressants, prescribed for their pain-relieving properties, may be given on a trial basis for two to three weeks.

Aerobic exercise and relaxation techniques may help to improve general well-being and aid sleep. The doctor may also recommend certain lifestyle changes, such as reducing caffeine intake to see if it is contributing to sleep problems. Cognitive behavioural therapy (CBT) can help sufferers to devise coping strategies and change perceptions of the illness.

FLAT FEET

A deformity of the feet that can affect both children and adults.

Most people's feet have a raised arch along the inner edge of the sole between the heel and the ball of the foot. This arch usually develops between the ages of three and ten. If it is absent, the term flat foot is used.

CHILDHOOD FLAT FEET

Flat feet are very common in childhood but usually disappear as the child grows older.

The most common type of flat foot in children is flexible flat foot. This is when the arches of the foot are visible when the foot is lifted, but disappear when the child is standing up. Flexible flat foot is usually caused by loose joint ligaments (children naturally have looser ligaments than adults). This type of flat foot nearly always resolves as the child gets older and the ligaments tighten. Treatment is not usually required, although shoes with supports under the arches are sometimes worn until the deformity is corrected. A child with flexible flat feet will not experience any limitations in sports or physical activities.

More rarely a child may have rigid flat foot, where the arches are flat whatever the position of the foot. This is caused by abnormalities of the joints in the foot and spasms of the muscles around them. Sometimes it may result from abnormal development of the foot in the womb. Special shoes may help to correct the underlying abnormalities and in severe case surgery may be an option.

FOOT AND ANKLE MECHANICS

The foot on the left is an example of a very flat foot with no visible arch, which causes the foot and ankle to roll inwards (over-pronation). The foot on the right has a normal arch that spreads the weight of the body over the whole foot.

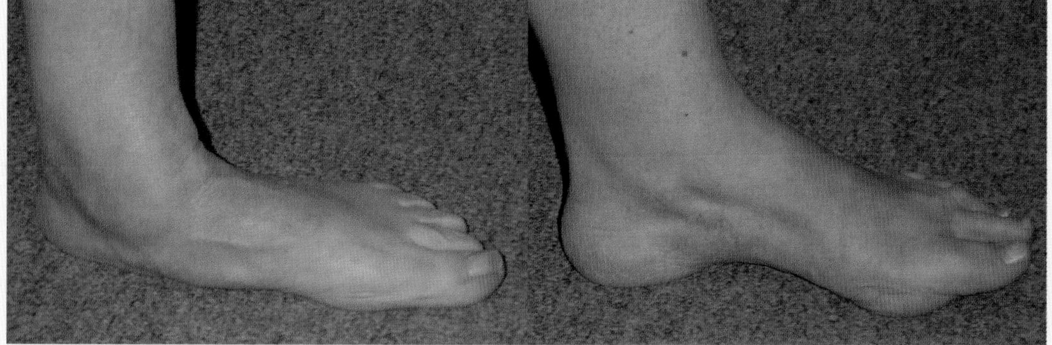

ADULT FLAT FEET

Around 20 per cent of adults have flat feet.

Sometimes flexible flat feet last into adulthood, usually because the shape of the feet is naturally flat; adults with flexible flat feet often have lax ligaments in other joints. The condition may run in families. Occasionally, the condition develops later in life, perhaps due to a ruptured tendon or an injury to the foot. Flat feet may also be caused by osteoarthritis, which can affect certain joints of the foot >>228–247.

Flat feet in adulthood can cause over-pronation – an excessive inward roll of the feet during walking or running. This increases the strain on feet and calves and over time may contribute to a range of other musculoskeletal problems. Other symptoms of overpronation include shoes that are particularly worn along the inside edges of the soles.

Often no treatment is required other than a comfortable pair of shoes, perhaps with supports for the arches (medial supports); older patients may wear shoes that are specially made to suit their feet. In severe cases, surgery may be used to correct the deformity. A podiatrist (>>53) can recommend the most suitable treatment.

FRACTURES

Breaks in bones, usually as a result of trauma such as a knock or a fall.

Broken bones are very common, particularly in older people with weak or osteoporotic bones. Bone fractures often also cause damage to muscles, ligaments, blood vessels and nerves around them.

What are the causes?

Fractures are caused by trauma in the form of either a sudden injury such as a direct blow, a twisting injury, or repeated stress on a bone. A stress or fatigue fracture, for example, might occur in the shin bone of a long distance runner – most stress fractures occur in the lower leg.

Certain conditions can weaken bone tissue making bones more likely to fracture. These include osteoporosis (>>264–275) and bone tumours (>>280).

What are the symptoms?

The symptoms of a bone fracture depend on where the fracture occurs, the severity of the fracture and whether any nearby tissues are damaged. The site of the fracture is likely to feel painful and tender to the touch. There may be swelling and bruising around the affected area and it may be difficult or painful to move. Depending on the site of the fracture and the type and severity of the break, there may be a grinding sensation as broken bone ends rub together.

Fragments of broken bone can sometimes damage nearby tissues and organs. A broken rib, for example, may puncture a lung. Tissue damage can cause bleeding and infections may develop. If bone fragments are pushed out of position there may also be visible deformities.

CLASSIFYING FRACTURES

Fractures can be classified in a number of ways, such as whether the wound is open or closed, the line of the break and the shape of the bone fragments at the fracture site. They include:

- **Closed fractures** when the skin covering the broken bone remains intact.
- **Open or compound fractures** when the tissue beneath the skin and sometimes the bone itself are visible through a break in the skin.
- **Spiral fractures** caused by twisting injuries and have a spiral fracture line along the bone.
- **Oblique fractures** which have a slanted fracture line similar to spiral fractures but along to one plane.
- **Transverse fractures** which have a fracture line across the width of the bone .
- **Comminuted fractures** when there are two or more fragments of bone broken off.
- **Crush fractures** when an area of bone is completely crushed and leaves no pieces to join back together. These tend to occur in the spine, often as a result of osteoporosis.
- **Greenstick fractures** when only the inner part of the bone is broken and the outer layers stay intact. These fractures particularly affect children.
- **Hairline fractures** where there is minimal trauma to the bone and surrounding tissues. The crack does not extend past the outer layer of bone.

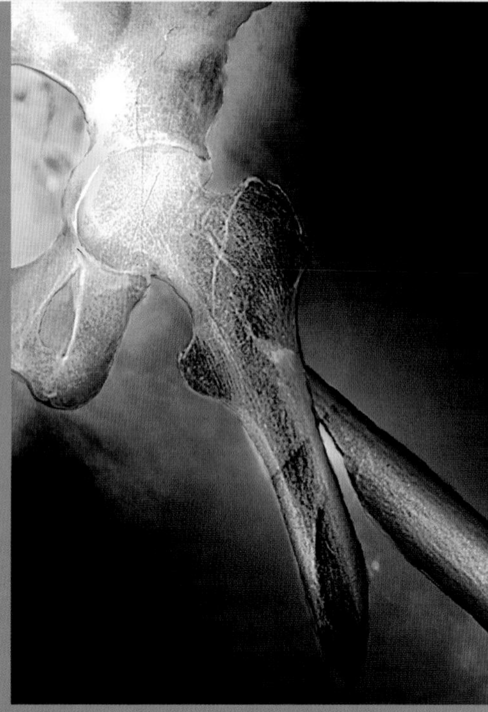

COMPOUND FRACTURE
This coloured X-ray shows a fractured thigh bone with an oblique fracture line. The sharp ends of the bone may have penetrated the skin, causing a compound fracture and increasing the risk of infection.

How are they diagnosed and treated?

Broken bones are usually confirmed by X-rays >>319. Fractures can cause severe pain and effective pain relief may be needed, particularly during the first few days after the break. Any open wounds will need to be cleaned carefully.

Treatment aims to return the bone fragments as closely as possible to their original position and to help them to heal, hopefully making the bone as strong as it was before the fracture. The process by which bone fragments are returned to their original position is known as fracture reduction. Closed reduction refers to bone realignment without breaking the skin – this is usually achieved by manual manipulation, generally with an anaesthetic. Open fracture reduction refers to use of surgery to reset the bones.

After reduction, the fragments are immobilized using plaster casts, metal plates and screws or by traction. The goal is to fix the fragments in position until they re-unite and are strong enough to hold together without support. Immobilization is not always required – fractured ribs, for example, are usually left to heal naturally. Because immobilization can cause muscle wastage, patients often need physiotherapy exercises afterwards to restore the range of movements and strengthen muscles.

What is the outlook?

The time taken to heal depends on a number of factors, including the site of the fracture, the age of the patient and how well the fragments can be repositioned. Fractured leg bones usually take around four months to heal; some smaller bones take only two months. Children's bones tend to take around half as long to heal as adults' bones. For more details about the healing process itself >>36. Complications such as infections may slow healing.

Although relatively uncommon, there may occasionally be problems with the way the broken bone heals. Bone fragments that heal together strongly but in the wrong position (mal-union) can cause bone deformity. Occasionally bone fragments fail to knit together at all (non-union). This may result from a serious long-term condition known as aseptic necrosis, which occurs when the fracture severs the blood supply to an area of bone causing the tissue to die off gradually.

In the long-term, fractures that fail to heal properly put additional strain on nearby joints and may increase the risk of later developing osteoarthritis (>>228–247). Fractures that involve joint surfaces also increase the risk.

FROZEN SHOULDER

A common disorder, also called adhesive capsulitis, in which shoulder pain is followed by stiffness and restricted movement of the shoulder joint.

Normally the anatomy of the shoulder joint allows a wide range of movements: when a frozen shoulder develops, the lining of the fibrous capsule that surrounds the joint becomes inflamed and thickened and scar-like tissue forms limiting shoulder movements. Often no cause can be found. In some cases, an injury to the shoulder (particularly repetitive or overuse injuries) may trigger the problem; in others, a period of immobility may be the cause. The condition affects more women than men and is most common in people over 40.

What are the symptoms?

There are usually three basic stages in the development of a frozen shoulder:

- **Phase one** usually lasts up to six months. During this phase it is the pain, which may be severe, that limits the movements of the joint in all directions.
- **Phase two** is characterized by painless restriction of shoulder movements as the stiffness takes over. This stage can last for six months to a year.
- **Phase three,** the recovery phase, may last another six months. The range of movement of the joint gradually increases as the stiffness resolves.

CORTICOSTEROID INJECTIONS

Corticosteroids are powerful anti-inflammatory medications. Synthetic corticosteroids are most effective when injected directly into the area of inflammation, such as a frozen shoulder joint, rather than being carried in the bloodstream.

How is it diagnosed and treated?

A frozen shoulder is usually diagnosed from the patient's description of the symptoms and an examination of the shoulder joint. The doctor may arrange for investigations such as X-rays to look for other conditions that may account for the symptoms. Non-steroidal anti-inflammatories (NSAIDs >>280) are often recommended to relieve pain and inflammation. Ice packs and heat treatments may help to reduce the pain. In severe cases, corticosteroids may be injected directly into the joint.

Physiotherapy can help to relieve stiffness and improve the range of motion in the joint. The physiotherapist will move the arm through a range of movements to stretch the capsule and will recommend exercises to keep the joint as mobile as possible and maintain muscle strength around the shoulder.

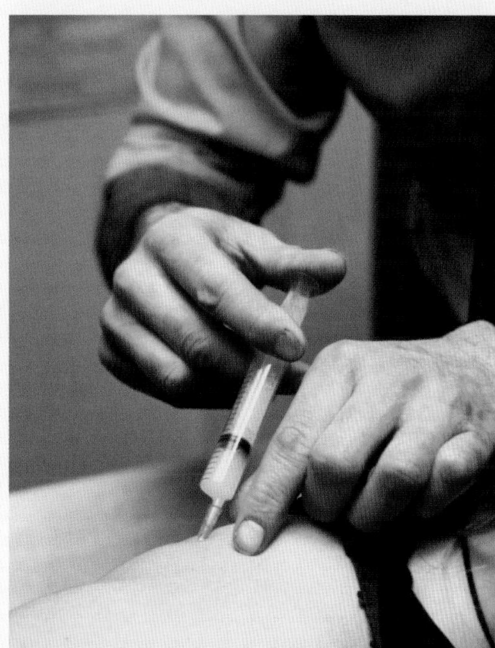

In some cases the joint is manipulated under a general anaesthetic. Occasionally, surgery may be used to cut through the adhesions (the scar-type tissue that will have formed in the joint). This can be achieved using a viewing instrument known as an arthroscope (>>206) and surgical instruments inserted through small incisions made in the skin. Surgery must be followed by physiotherapy to ensure that the frozen shoulder does not return.

What is the outlook?

A frozen shoulder lasts for about a year on average. The recovery process may be very slow and some degree of movement restriction may persist in the longer-term. People who have had a frozen shoulder once have a greater risk of getting the condition again in the future.

GANGLION

A swelling which develops in the sheath surrounding a tendon or in the tissues around a joint.

A ganglion develops when some of the jelly-like synovial fluid present within joints is released into the tissues around a joint. It is not known why this occurs. Common sites for ganglia are the wrist and the back of the hand but they may also develop on the foot. The swellings usually develop in early adulthood and are uncommon in later life. Ganglia are three times more common in women than in men.

What are the symptoms?

The swellings are usually painless although they sometimes ache and can eventually become painful. Occasionally a swelling can cause pressure on nerves although this is uncommon. Ganglia vary in size; they may grow to 1–2cm (3–5in) or more. A large ganglion on the hand can affect regular hand movements.

What are the treatment options?

Ganglia may disappear without treatment, sometimes as the result of the swelling being banged accidentally. It may be possible to withdraw fluid from a ganglion with a needle and syringe but this leaves the wall of the swelling present and the ganglion is likely to recur.

Often no treatment is required, particularly for small swellings. If a ganglion interferes with movement or is pressing on a nerve, surgical removal is likely to be recommended. This involves making a cut over the swelling and then carefully shelling it out. This may be done under local anaesthetic. Removal may cause further swelling in the area – often as large as the ganglion itself – and this may take as long as six months to go down. Ganglia often return, even after surgery.

GOUT

A condition in which crystals formed from uric acid are deposited in a joint causing inflammation and severe pain.

Uric acid is a normal by-product of the body's metabolism, produced when cells and proteins are broken down. Normally, uric acid dissolves in the blood, is passed through the kidneys and then removed from the body in urine. People with gout have high concentrations of uric acid in their blood (hyperuricaemia) meaning that crystals are more likely to develop. However, not everyone with high uric acid levels will develop gout.

PURINE-CONTAINING FOODS

Certain foods contain high levels of substances called purines, which are broken down into uric acid in the body. Cutting down on these foods may reduce the frequency or severity of gout.

High levels	Moderate levels
Alcohol, especially beer	Asparagus
Anchovies	Beef
Bacon	Chicken
Herrings	Crab
Kidney	Duck
Liver	Ham
Mackerel	Kidney beans
Mussels	Lobster
Sardines	Oyster
Sweetbread	Pork
Veal	Shrimp
Venison	Spinach

What are the causes?

Factors that are associated with increased blood uric acid levels include increasing age, a high-protein diet, obesity, high blood lipid levels and certain medical conditions including high blood pressure, ischaemic heart disease and diabetes mellitus.

An episode of gout may be triggered by excessive eating or certain types of foods, too much alcohol, some types of medications (such as diuretics, aspirin, cyclosporine or levodopa) or dehydration, which may result from taking diuretics. Cell breakdown resulting from certain types of cancer treatment may trigger the onset of gout. Minor injuries to joints may also trigger an attack.

Often there is no obvious reason why gout develops. The condition often runs in families so genetic factors may be involved, possibly a hereditary abnormality in the system that changes the nucleic acid into uric acid. Pseudogout is a similar condition but it is caused by deposits of a different substance (calcium pyrophosphate crystals). Unlike gout, more women than men are affected by pseudogout >>318.

What are the symptoms?

Symptoms usually develop suddenly. Pain is often first noticed during the night and is immediately severe. There is also redness and swelling around the affected joint, which in 75 per cent of cases is the big toe. Other joints that may be affected include the elbow, wrist or knee. Layers of skin are often lost from the area around the joint.

This first acute phase usually resolves within around seven days – but most sufferers will go on to experience more frequent and longer lasting attacks. Roughly 60 per cent of sufferers experience another episode of gout within a year. Left untreated, this acute form may eventually develop into chronic tophaceous gout. In

DID YOU KNOW?

- **Gout is rare before puberty when levels of uric acid start to rise. Men are around ten times more likely to be affected than women.**
- **About 5 in 100 people have high uric acid levels in their blood but not all of these people develop gout. About 2 in 1000 people are affected by gout at any one time in the UK, although the incidence is on the increase. High uric acid levels may also cause kidney stones to develop.**

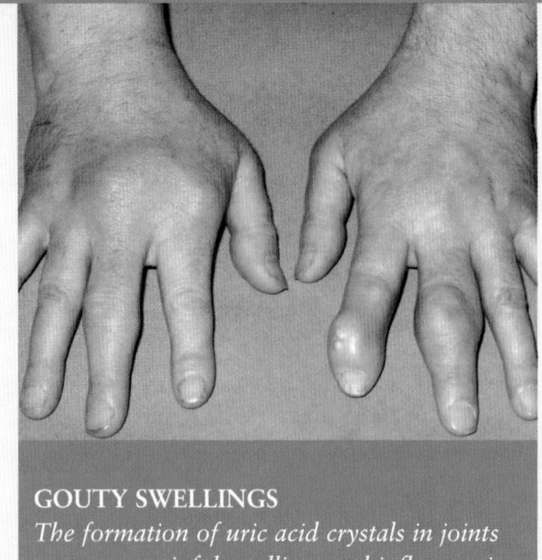

GOUTY SWELLINGS
The formation of uric acid crystals in joints can cause painful swellings and inflammation as well as small whitish lumps called tophi on the skin of the fingers or ear lobes.

this condition, uric crystal deposits cause small whitish lumps called tophi in the skin and around the joints. Common sites for tophi are the ear lobes and the fingers. The symptoms are more persistent with intermittent flare-ups.

How is it diagnosed?

If the symptoms suggest gout, the doctor will take a blood sample to measure uric acid levels. A high concentration of uric acid is not sufficient for diagnosis on its own – uric acid can be raised in other conditions and in people who do not have gout. Also, uric acid levels in the blood are occasionally normal despite a flare-up of the condition. In this case a sample of fluid may be withdrawn from the joint and examined for uric acid crystals.

Sometimes a joint infection needs to be ruled out and blood samples may be tested for signs of an infection. Blood will also be tested to check the function of the kidneys. X-rays of the joint are sometimes taken to look for the presence of joint damage and to assess its severity (>>319).

What are the treatment options?

Non-steroidal anti-inflammatories (NSAIDs >>280) may help to relieve the pain and swelling. These are initially given in high doses for about two days then as a reduced dose for a further week or so. A course of corticosteroids may be needed for people who do not respond to non-steroidal drugs. Additional drugs, such as colchicine, are used for individuals who are unable to take NSAIDs, perhaps because they have impaired kidney function or have had a peptic ulcer in the past.

If the condition recurs and the symptoms are severe, drugs that lower uric acid levels may be prescribed to help limit further attacks. Allopurinol reduces the production of uric acid while probenecid increases its excretion by the kidneys. These drugs should not be taken until at least four weeks after the last attack and should be taken together with NSAIDs for the first few weeks of treatment.

In all cases, dietary changes will be recommended. Drinking plenty of water and cutting down on alcohol intake ensures more effective removal of uric acid from the body, reducing the risk of crystals forming in the joints. It also makes sense to maintain a healthy body weight – according to a 12-year study published in 2005, being overweight almost doubles the risk of developing gout. Weight loss must be gradual, however, as rapid weight loss can cause uric acid levels to rise.

Finally, it may help to cut down on foods containing high levels of purines, organic substances that are broken down into uric acid inside the body's cells. Although purines also occur naturally within the body, high-purine foods such as offal and seafood can raise uric acid levels significantly. For further details >>box, left.

GUILLAIN-BARRE SYNDROME

An inflammatory disorder of the peripheral nerves causing muscle weakness, numbness and often paralysis.

The peripheral nervous system is the portion of the nervous system outside the brain and the spinal cord. The peripheral nerves convey motor signals from the brain to the body, telling muscles when to contract, and send sensory information from the body back to the brain.

Guillain-Barré syndrome is a rare disorder that affects one or two people per 100,000 and causes inflammation in these peripheral nerves, leading to numbness, muscular weakness and possibly paralysis.

What are the causes?

Guillain-Barré syndrome affects the myelin sheath, a fatty substance that surrounds the nerves and increases the speed with which signals can travel along the nerves.

The causes of the disease are very poorly understood. In around half of cases, Guillain-Barré develops after a bacterial or viral infection such as a fever or diarrhoea, suggesting that it may be an autoimmune disorder. In these disorders the body's immune system mistakenly attacks the body's own tissues – in this case the nerves.

What are the symptoms?

The initial symptoms are usually numbness and tingling in the fingers and toes. Muscle weakness in the arms and legs will start to develop over the next few days or weeks causing difficulty walking and performing simple tasks. Other possible symptoms include blurred vision, clumsiness, heart palpitations and muscle contractions.

In many cases the symptoms remain mild. In severe cases, however, the disease rapidly starts to worsen and in a matter of hours may lead to complete paralysis in the arms and legs. In around 25 per cent of cases paralysis also affects the muscles that control breathing or swallowing.

Severe symptoms may last for around three weeks with a recovery period of several months. In around 5 per cent of cases the respiratory or cardiovascular complications prove fatal, although prompt hospital treatment considerably improves the chances of recovery.

How is it diagnosed?

If the symptoms suggest Guillain-Barré, the hospital will organize tests such as a lumbar puncture, where a sample of cerebrospinal fluid is taken to check for elevated protein levels; an electromyogram (EMG) to check for loss of muscle reflexes; or a nerve conduction velocity test (NCV), which records the speed at which signals travel along the nerves.

What are the treatment options?

Patients will need to be admitted to intensive care for treatment. Some patients respond well to blood plasma exchange (plasmapheresis), a procedure in which the blood is filtered to remove the plasma, the fluid part of blood that contains the antibodies believed to be responsible for Guillain-Barré. The blood cells are then returned to the body together with antibody-free synthetic or donor plasma. A plasmapheresis treatment takes several hours but is not normally painful. An average course of plasma exchanges is six to ten treatments over two to ten weeks.

Large doses of immunoglobulin can help to suppress the immune response and other medications may be prescribed to reduce pain and muscle spasm. Corticosteroids should not be used as they can make Guillain-Barré syndrome worse.

Patients may need to stay in the hospital for several months – and complete recovery may take a year or more – but the long-term prognosis is good. A few patients will experience residual weakness, numbness and occasional pain.

INFECTIVE ARTHRITIS

>> septic arthritis

JUVENILE IDIOPATHIC ARTHRITIS

Persistent inflammation of one or more joints in children under 16. Also called Still's disease, juvenile chronic arthritis or, in the USA, juvenile rheumatoid arthritis.

There are three main types of juvenile idiopathic arthritis: pauciarticular arthritis (or oligoarthritis) involves four or fewer joints; polyarticular arthritis involves many joints; while systemic arthritis can also affect many other parts of the body.

This disease can begin at any age during childhood but it particularly affects younger children. Its causes are unknown, but it seems to have a genetic basis and is possibly triggered by an infection.

What are the symptoms?

Each type of chronic juvenile arthritis has its own pattern of signs and symptoms but they all affect the joints in a similar way with pain and swelling, stiffness (which is particularly bad in the mornings) and restriction of movement. In some cases, walking and other activities may be affected.

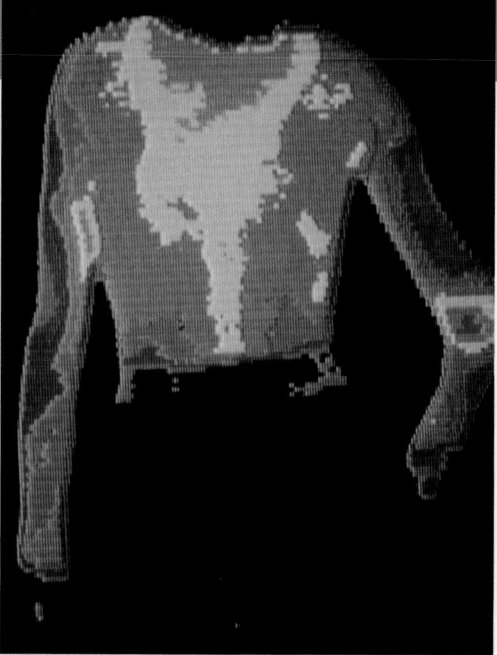

JUVENILE IDIOPATHIC ARTHRITIS
The thermogram of the back of a young boy suffering from the pauciarticular form of juvenile arthritis shows marked heat and inflammation in the right elbow.

■ **Pauciarticular arthritis** is diagnosed if fewer than five joints are affected in the first six months of the disease. It is the most common and usually the mildest form of the disease. It tends to affect girls under the age of five, involving the joints of the wrists, ankles or knees and sometimes the hands. Young children may find it difficult to put their symptoms into words but will often seem unhappy and irritable and can have problems walking.

Children with pauciarticular arthritis are at particular risk of developing uveitis (eye inflammation). Initially uveitis does not always cause any symptoms, so children with arthritis will need regular eye checks to look for signs of inflammation. Uveitis is a serious eye disorder that may lead to loss of sight so treatment should start early.

The majority of children with pauciarticular arthritis will fully recover after a few years. In others, however, the arthritis may develop in other joints after about six months.

■ **Polyarticular arthritis** In this type of arthritis, five or more joints are affected in the first six months. Like pauciarticular arthritis, it is more common in girls than boys. The children affected can be divided into those who have rheumatoid factor – an antibody often found in the blood of children and adults with rheumatoid arthritis – and those who do not. A simple blood test can be used to detect the presence of rheumatoid factor.

Most children with polyarticular arthritis do not have rheumatoid factor; the children in this group may be affected at any age. The disease usually involves the joints of the hands and feet, and sometimes also the hips, knees and shoulders. In some children the inflammation seems to move from one joint to another; in others more than one joint is affected at the same time. The disease varies from mild to severe – which may cause difficulties with walking and during other activities – and some children develop a mild fever when the joint symptoms flare up. Overall, in about one in four of those affected the symptoms disappear by about 16 years of age. In the others the joint symptoms persist.

About one in ten children with polyarticular arthritis, particularly girls, have rheumatoid factor. Left untreated, this form of the arthritis may go on to cause persistent joint damage.

WHAT IS MAGNETIC RESONANCE IMAGING (MRI)?

This type of scanner provides detailed two and three-dimensional images of organs and tissues. The images are generated by a computer which analyses the effects of radio waves and a strong magnetic field on atoms within the body area to be investigated.

MRI can be used to investigate various parts of the body, including the brain and large blood vessels, as well as some parts of the musculoskeletal system. It provides detailed images of soft tissues, such as muscles and tendons and can be used to diagnose the cause of back pain. The joints most often examined by MRI are the knees and shoulders, but it is also very useful in the examination of the intervertebral discs of the spine, in particular to look for a prolapsed disc (>>317).

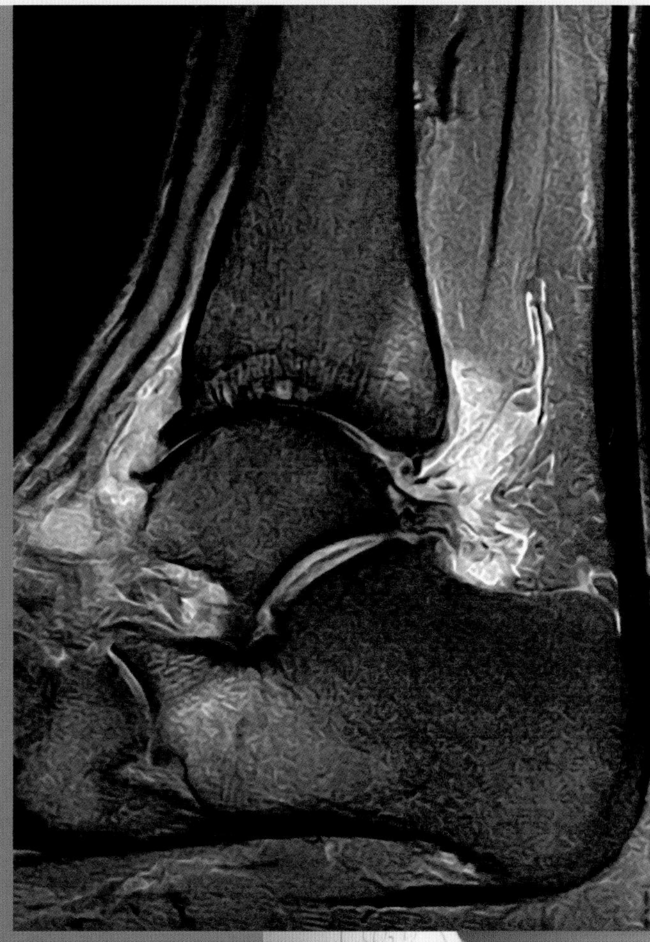

■ The patient lies on a movable table which slides into a cylindrical compartment. In most machines this compartment is closed and so may cause some people to feel claustrophobic. A sedative can be given if this is likely to be the case. New and more open scanners are becoming available although the image quality may not be as good. In some cases, a contrast fluid will be given intravenously which will pass through the tissues and enhance the images produced.

■ Movement can blur the image so it is important to lie still. The machine will make clicking or clanging sounds throughout the test. MRI is relatively quick – it usually takes no more than an hour, is painless and does not involve the use of radiation. It usually takes a couple of weeks for the results to come through, depending on the reasons for the scan.

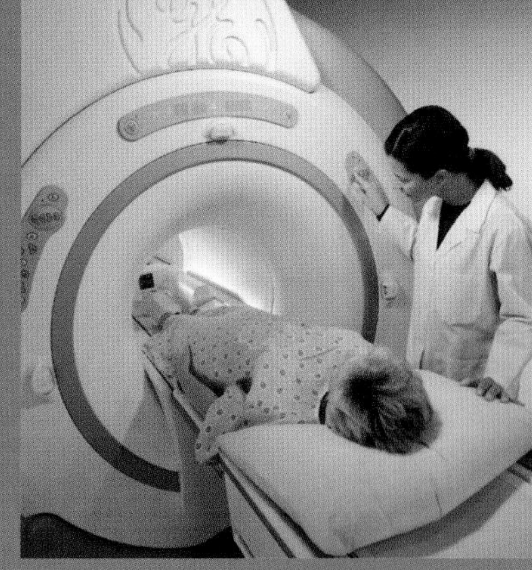

BLOOD ANTIBODY TESTS

Antibodies are a special kind of blood protein produced by the body in order to attack and neutralize substances that the body finds dangerous, such as toxins or bacteria. The presence of antibodies in the blood plasma can therefore suggest exposure to an infection or other antigen. Different antibodies are produced in response to different types of stimuli so they can often be used to identify a particular type of infection. In an ELISA test (enzyme-linked immunosorbent assay) specific types of antibody are mixed with blood samples to identify any antigens present in the blood that are sensitive to the antibodies.

Sometimes antibodies are targeted against the body's own tissues – these are called autoantibodies. The presence of certain types of autoantibodies in the blood plasma can provide evidence of autoimmune disorders such as lupus or myasthenia gravis. In the muscle-weakening condition myasthenia gravis, for example, antibodies known as acetylocholine receptor antibodies attack receptors on the muscle fibres and block messages from the motor nerves. If a patient is suspected of having this conditions, a blood test to look for the presence of these antibodies may help to confirm the diagnosis.

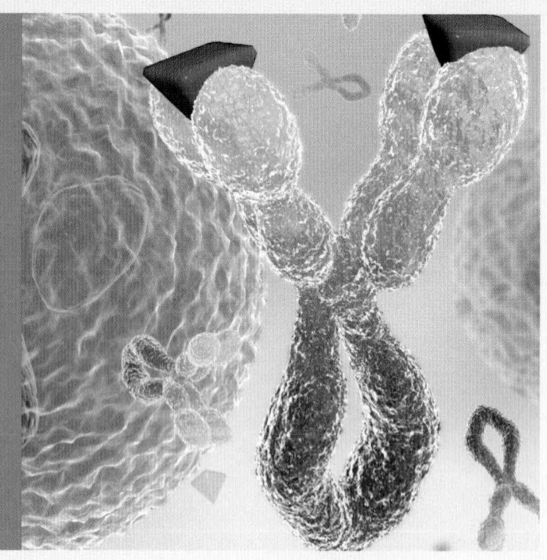

- **Systemic arthritis** This is the least common form of juvenile arthritis, affecting around 20 per cent of children with the condition. As well as affecting the joints, the disease can involve other parts of the body, such as the heart and spleen: in fact joint problems are not always present from the start, which can make the disease difficult to diagnose in its early stages. It commonly starts before the age of five and affects boys and girls in equal numbers.

The first sign of systemic arthritis is often a high fever once or twice a day, sometimes accompanied by a salmon-pink rash that tends to come on as body temperature rises. Other possible symptoms include swollen glands, pain in the abdomen and weight loss. Symptoms of joint inflammation often do not become apparent until later on in the disease. In some cases, the disease quite quickly clears up completely. In others, there will be recurrent episodes of the disease over a number of years. Some children go on to develop polyarticular arthritis.

How is it diagnosed?

To diagnose any of these types, the doctor will listen carefully to a description of the symptoms and will examine the child. Tests may be arranged to look for signs that are suggestive of the arthritis and to rule out other diseases. Blood will be checked to look for signs of inflammation and for the presence of antibodies such as rheumatoid factor or antinuclear antibody (>>box, above). Up to 80 per cent of children with uveitis and pauciarticular arthritis test positive for antinuclear antibody.

The doctor may also arrange to have the child's joints X-rayed and an MRI scan (>>297) will be needed to assess the extent of any joint damage. In addition, the child's eyes will need to be checked regularly for signs of inflammation.

What are the treatment options?

The usual treatment programme for juvenile idiopathic arthritis combines drugs, exercise and physiotherapy. Surgery is uncommon but in a few advanced cases, where joints have been severely damaged and are extremely painful, joint replacement may be considered. This will not take place until the child is fully grown.

A course of medication should begin as soon as possible to reduce the risk of long-term damage to the joints. Non-steroidal anti-inflammatory drugs (NSAIDs >>280) are often prescribed because they help to relieve the pain, stiffness and swelling. Disease-modifying anti-rheumatic drugs (DMARDs), such as methotrexate or sulfasalazine, may be prescribed on a long-term basis to reduce inflammation and slow the damage to the joints.

Corticosteroid drugs are sometimes prescribed because they can very effectively relieve inflammation. They may be injected into the joints or taken orally – oral corticosteroids are usually given as short courses because they can have harmful side-effects (>>320). Intravenous steroids may be necessary for very severe arthritis.

In some cases the doctor might prescribe one of the new drugs, such as etanercept, that have been developed to suppress the immune response by blocking the action of tumour necrosis factor alpha (TNF alpha). These can slow or even halt joint damage.

Daily exercises will strengthen the muscles that move and support the joints and may help to relieve pain and stiffness. A physiotherapist will advise on these and on other beneficial forms of exercise, such as swimming, and can design an appropriate exercise programme.

What is the outlook?

The treatments for juvenile idiopathic arthritis are constantly improving and most children can now live an active life. The outlook varies from one child to another, however, and even those with the same type of arthritis will respond differently to the treatments prescribed.

At present there is no cure for the disease, but in most children the problems clear up completely with no long-term damage and no problems in adulthood. For others there may be persistent problems that in some cases affect walking or other activities. Some children may also be at increased risk of developing osteoporosis (>>264–275) in later life.

LEGG-CALVE-PERTHES' DISEASE

A disease of childhood in which the head of the femur (the upper end of the thigh bone) becomes softened and then re-forms.

About 5 in every 100,000 children are affected by this condition, often simply called Perthes' disease. It is more common in boys than in girls by a ratio of about five to one. The disease occurs between the ages of 2 and 15 years. In most cases only one hip is affected but in around 10–20 per cent of cases both hips are involved. Perthes' disease should be treated early to avoid the development of osteoarthritis later in life (>>228–247).

What are the causes?

The condition results from a temporary loss of the blood supply to the head of the femur (thigh bone) causing osteonecrosis (bone death). Exactly why this interruption to the blood supply occurs is not understood, though it is probably connected to physical changes that occur as the child's bones and tissues grow. Children who are small for their age and very active are known to be at particular risk.

Without a proper blood supply the bone cells on the femoral head start to die. Then, when the blood supply returns, soft new bone is formed to replace the damaged tissue. Once softened, however, the femoral head can take 18–24 months to re-form and harden. During this period the soft bone is liable to collapse or fracture under pressure and may re-form in the wrong shape.

What are the symptoms?

The symptoms come on gradually and may include a limp as well as hip, knee or groin pain, particularly after exercise. Movement around the hip may be restricted. Later there may be thinning and weakening of the muscles around the affected hip.

Early symptoms of the disease are often mild and are sometimes ignored completely. Young children may also find it difficult to describe the sensation, especially if it seems to come from the knee, so if a child seems to limp after exercise but cannot explain why, Perthes' disease should be considered. Some patients are not diagnosed until many years later when, as young adults, they need to be treated for osteoarthritis.

How is it diagnosed and treated?

Perthes' disease can be difficult to diagnose. X-rays may show increased density of the head of the femur, although in the early stages of the disease the X-rays may look normal. An isotope bone scan (>>281) or an MRI scan (>>297 may help to confirm the diagnosis. The doctor may also want to test the hip's range of motion.

Treatment focuses on preventing collapse and ensuring that the femoral head reshapes well. Splints may be used to keep the femoral head in the socket so that it re-forms with as little deformity as possible. In some cases surgery is required to correct a deformity and reposition the femoral head inside the socket.

What is the outlook?

With early detection and treatment, it is usually possible to prevent or minimize bone damage. The prognosis is particularly good for children under five years – older children have less chance of a full recovery and there may be some residual deformity of the femoral head. This can increase the risk of later developing degenerative problems such as osteoarthritis >>228–247.

LIGAMENT INJURY (SPRAIN)

Damage to the ligaments of a joint.

Ligaments are tough, slightly elastic bands of fibrous connective tissue that hold bones together and keep joints stable. If a ligament is stretched too far (more than about 5 per cent of its regular length) it may be damaged – this is called a sprain.

Ligament sprains vary in severity. Normally the sprain is only partial, so that the internal structure is damaged but the ligament remains intact. Occasionally the

6 WAYS TO...

Avoid low back pain

The way that you hold your body in your daily life and during everyday tasks can have a significant impact on your risk of back pain.

1 Stay fit and flexible Strong, well-balanced back and stomach muscles and a flexible spine will help to maintain your back's natural curves and avoid injury.

2 Check your hamstrings Tight hamstrings are a common cause of low back pain. Always stretch your hamstrings after exercise to avoid putting pressure on your back or pulling your body out of alignment.

3 Watch your step Wear supportive, comfortable shoes. High heels throw the body off balance and increase the stress on your knees, ankle and lower back.

4 Squat don't bend Bend your knees, not your back, when you pick up heavy objects and keep the object close to your body. Make your legs do the work.

5 Push don't pull You are much more likely to slip and strain the muscles or ligaments in your back when you are pulling a heavy object than when you are pushing it.

6 Don't do too much Combinations of physical movements – such as bending and twisting or lifting and turning – can put even greater pressure on your spine, particularly if you are lifting or carrying a heavy object.

ligament is actually torn or ruptured. When a rupture occurs, the joint becomes unstable because the torn ligament is no longer able to help support it.

What are the causes?

Anything that pushes, pulls, knocks or twists a bone – and therefore the attached ligaments – further than its regular range risks causing a sprain. For this reason sprains often occur during strenuous sporting activities, such as contact sports or exercises involving sudden changes of direction. Cold ligaments cannot stretch quite as far as when warm, so not warming up properly increases the risk of a sprain. It is also possible to sprain a ligament by lifting something heavy.

Particularly risky are sudden, forced, twisting motions, which often occur in sports such as basketball or squash where one foot is planted on the ground while the rest of the body rotates clockwise and back. A sudden knock or a fall can also cause a ligament tear.

Certain ligaments are more likely to be injured because they are found in joints that are exposed to greater forces or are inherently less stable. The most common sites for ligament sprains are the ankles, knees, fingers, thumbs and shoulders. The cruciate ligaments inside the knee are very often damaged during sports such as football, as a result of either direct impact or twisting the knee. For more details >>197.

What are the symptoms?

The symptoms of ligament injuries come on suddenly. There may be a ripping sensation in the affected joint or a popping sound. This may be followed by joint pain that is worse on movement, swelling and possibly bruising in the affected area and restriction of movement in the joint. The pain will seem to come from inside the joint rather than from the surface of the knee. The joint may give way or feel unstable if weight is put on it.

How is it diagnosed?

The doctor will usually be able to diagnose a ligament injury from a description of the symptoms and a thorough examination of the affected joint. Sometimes an X-ray or a CT scan (>>box, right) may be used to make sure that none of the bones are fractured. Knee injuries sometimes require more detailed examinations – an arthroscope (a narrow fibre-optic tube inserted into a small incision in the knee >>206) or an MRI scan (>>297) may be needed to check whether there is a ligament tear or another problem such as damage to the meniscus (>>303).

What are the treatment options?

The usual way to treat a ligament injury is to follow the RICE procedure (rest, ice, compression, elevation >>204). This will reduce pain, bruising and swelling over the first 48–72 hours. Painkillers or heat treatment (such as heat packs, ultrasound therapy or hot baths) can also be useful. It is important not to put too much stress on the joint while it is healing; in some cases a brace or a plaster cast may be used to immobilize the joint. If a complete rupture occurs, it may require surgery.

Ligament sprains usually heal well, but the affected ligaments are at increased risk of sprains in the future. A complete rupture may cause permanent weakness of the ligament. Physiotherapy is recommended in all cases in order to build up the strength of the muscles around the joint and restore the joint's range of movements.

LOW BACK PAIN

A common problem that affects most of the population at some time and may have a variety of causes.

In most cases, this is a transient problem that will resolve over the course of a few days. This temporary low back pain is often the result of a muscle or ligament strain. However pain in the lower back sometimes results from a more serious underlying disorder, such as a prolapsed disc (>>317) or damage to vertebrae.

What are the causes?

Poor posture or a sedentary lifestyle are common in people affected by low back pain. Sudden movements, even small ones, can trigger muscle and ligament strains. Lifting heavy objects with an incorrect technique and exercising without warming up first are also common causes. For more information on posture, lifting technique and avoiding back problems >>176–179.

Pregnant women also tend to get low back pain – the weight of the baby and subsequent postural changes can place considerable strain on the back muscles and ligaments. For more details >>136.

A prolapsed disc can result in low back pain: this pain often comes on suddenly and is usually severe >>317. Chronic diseases such as osteoarthritis can also cause pain >>228–247. Less common causes include ankylosing spondylitis >>278. Occasionally, secondary bone tumours that have spread from a primary tumour in another part of the body can be responsible >>280.

What are the symptoms?

The nature of low back pain varies depending on the individual and the cause. It may come on suddenly, as often occurs

WHAT IS CT SCANNING?

A CT (computed tomography) machine uses X-rays to take multiple images of the body from many different angles. Instead of photographic film, the CT scanner uses an array of detectors. This information is then analysed by a computer to produce detailed two or three-dimensional and cross-sectional images on screen. The images are often clearer and more detailed than conventional X-rays and allow close examination of many parts of the body, including the brain and lungs as well as muscles, joints and bones.

■ The CT machine is a large, rectangular or doughnut-shaped machine with a hole in the centre. The patient lies on a movable table and passes slowly through the centre. At the same time a scanner inside the machine rotates making a rapid clicking noise. The scan takes from 5 minutes to half an hour to complete.

■ Each time the scanner makes a 360-degree rotation it records around a thousand images of a thin cross-sectional 'slice' through the body. The computer then reconstructs these into a two-dimensional image. As the patient moves through, multiple cross-sectional slices are captured in this way and reconstructed into a three-dimensional image of the body's interior.

■ Different organs and tissues absorb the X-rays to different degrees and therefore look different on the images. Dense tissues such bone appear white, for example, while the spinal cord appears grey. Sometimes a contrast fluid is injected into a vein so that the area under investigation can be viewed more clearly as the fluid passes through.

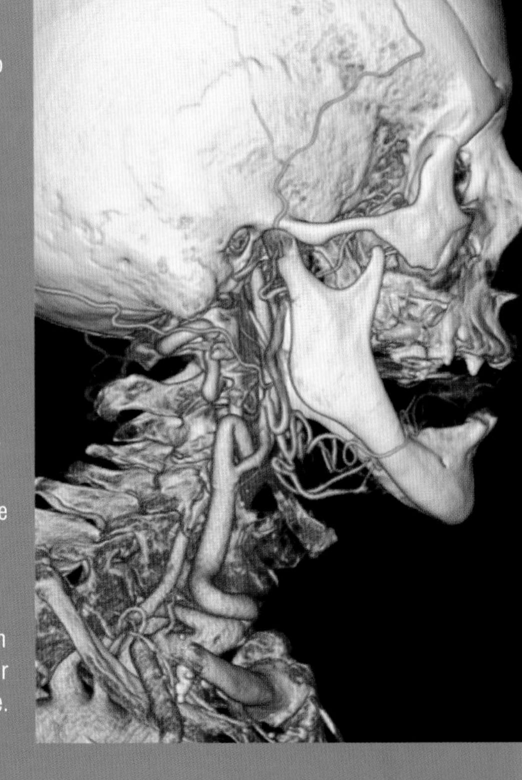

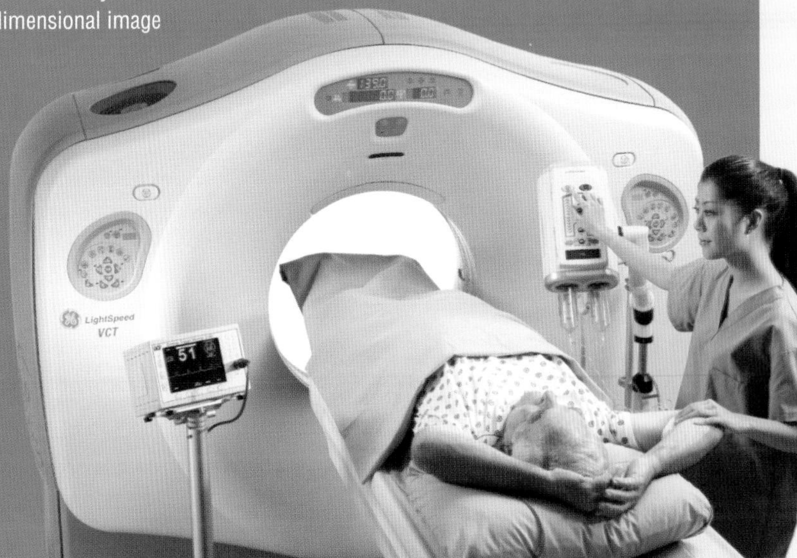

with muscle strains, or gradually, as it tends to do in pregnancy. It may be restricted to the area around the spine or may spread across the back. The muscles in the affected area may go into spasm and the back may become stiff with its movements restricted. Low back pain may also extend down into one or both legs, a condition known as sciatica (>>322).

A prolapsed disc may put pressure on nerves emanating from the spinal cord, causing pain, tingling, numbness and weakness of the legs. Occasionally, bladder and bowel control may be affected. These kinds of neurological symptoms require urgent medical treatment.

How is it diagnosed?

Muscle and ligament strains are usually diagnosed from a description of the symptoms and an examination. An X-ray may be arranged to check the position of the vertebrae, although problems affecting soft tissues such as muscles and ligaments do not show clearly on X-rays (>>319). A CT or MRI scan (>>301, 297) may reveal prolapsed discs or other possible causes and can assess pressure on nerves.

> **'In one study following candidates for back surgery, over 80 per cent of patients who completed a ten-week back-strengthening programme were still managing without surgery 16 months later'**

What are the treatment options?

In general, bed rest should be avoided unless the pain is very severe and even then should be limited to no more than 48 hours. It is important to get back to normal activities so that the back doesn't stiffen or the muscles of the back weaken. In most cases, the aim should be to return to work as soon as possible. Physiotherapy may be helpful, particularly during the acute phase. The physiotherapist will be able to recommend exercises to relieve pain, strengthen the back and improve flexibility. Manipulation or massage may also help to relieve low back pain.

Painkillers and other non-steroidal anti-inflammatory drugs (NSAIDs >>280) may give some relief. A heat pad or a wrapped hot-water bottle held against the affected area can also relieve symptoms. As well as specific back exercises, general physical activity is recommended to promote good health and well-being. Some exercises are particularly beneficial for problem backs: swimming takes weight off the joints and prevents jarring; exercise balls help to strengthen the core muscles that support the lower back; tai chi, yoga and Pilates improve posture and flexibility. It is important to advise instructors of any history of back problems so that they can tailor the exercise programme accordingly.

If low back pain is severe, persists for more than two days or if signs of nerve pressure are present you should seek medical advice immediately.

What is the outlook?

In most cases, low back pain will be a temporary problem. However each episode of back pain increases the risk of having another and subsequent episodes may be more severe and prolonged. Individuals who are particular at risk of problems should take special care of their backs with good posture, good lifting techniques and regular exercise. A few people find that pain persists and is a long-term problem that affects their daily life. In such cases, a management programme may be needed to help them to cope with the pain and to find ways to live the fullest possible life.

LUMBAGO >>low back pain

LUPUS >>systemic lupus

LYME DISEASE

A bacterial infection spread by ticks and causing inflammation of the joints and other body systems.

Lyme disease is a significant health problem in some areas of the USA and Scandinavia; it is less common elsewhere but remains a potential problem. Lyme disease is most prevalent in children under 15 years and adults older than 29. Left untreated, Lyme disease may develop over months or years causing rash, fever, arthritis and meningitis symptoms, or nervous system abnormalities such as numbness, pain and facial muscle paralysis.

What are the causes?

Lyme disease is caused by the borrelia burgdorferi bacterium. The infection is spread to humans through the bite of the deer tick – a small spider-like creature found in many areas of woodland, scrub or long grass. As humans and other mammals walk through tick-infested areas, the ticks attach themselves to an area of exposed skin and start to feed. Not all ticks carry these bacteria so tick bites do not necessarily lead to Lyme disease.

What are the symptoms?

The first symptom of the disease is usually a red, circular rash (erythema migrans) in the area of the bite – common sites are the thigh, groin, trunk and armpits. This rash usually develops 3–30 days after the bite. As the rash expands, the centre may clear giving it a bull's-eye appearance. Other early signs include fever, swollen glands and muscle and joint pain.

Symptoms of a more serious, persistent infection may not appear until weeks, months or years later. At this point there may be bouts of joint pain and swelling, usually in one or more large joints, especially the knees. There may also be nervous system problems including muscle weakness or pain, tingling or numbness in the arms and legs, and sometimes Bell's palsy (paralysis of the facial muscles).

How is it diagnosed?

Lyme disease can be hard to diagnose because symptoms vary considerably and mimic other diseases including rheumatoid arthritis, influenza and meningitis. The doctor will probably base his diagnosis on symptoms and any history of possible exposure to tick bites, especially in areas where Lyme disease is prevalent.

It is also possible to test for antibodies produced by the body as a reaction to the bacteria, although these antibodies are unlikely to be present in the early stage of the disease and when they are present do not always indicate infection. The blood test is usually positive in people who have been sick for over four weeks and haven't taken antibiotics.

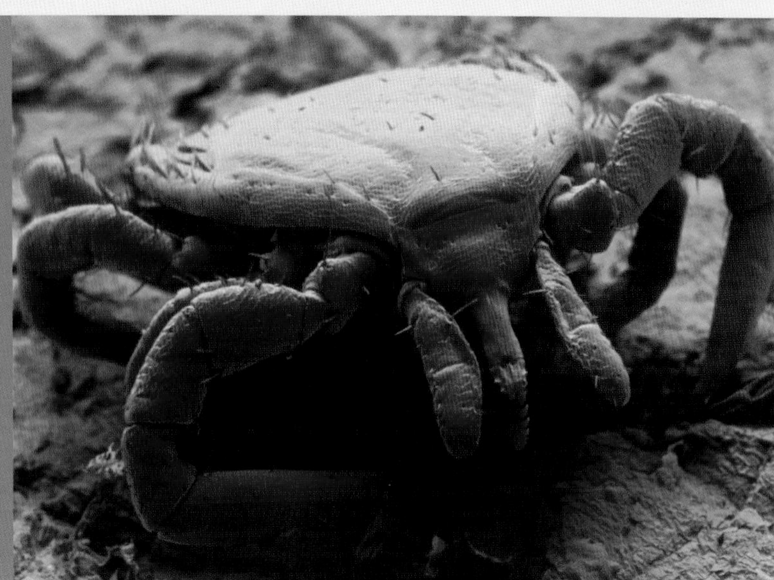

LYME DISEASE TICK
This tiny spider-like parasite is responsible for the spread of the bacteria that cause Lyme disease. The tick has three life stages: larva, nymph and adult: the nymph stage (right) is responsible for most cases of the disease. It is much smaller than the adult – around the size of a poppy seed – making it harder to spot.

What are the treatment options?

In most cases, especially when diagnosed early enough, Lyme disease is easily treatable with antibiotics. Occasionally symptoms persist or recur, and further antibiotic therapy is required. Left untreated, the joint inflammation can cause permanent bone or cartilage damage.

MENISCAL TEARS

Damage to the discs of cartilage that help the knees to carry their heavy load and act as shock absorbers.

The menisci are crescent-shaped discs of cartilage found in some joints, including the wrists and the knees (there are two in each knee). They help to reduce friction, stabilize the joints and absorb much of the force of impact during walking or running. The menisci in the knees are particularly susceptible to tears >>196–197.

Various injuries, including relatively minor ones, can cause meniscal tears in the knee. Sportsmen such as footballers and basketball players are at particular risk because the tears are often caused by sudden twisting or pivoting motions.

As the menisci age they become weaker and less elastic and degenerative tears can be caused by something as simple as turning over in bed and moving the knee awkwardly. Sometimes, an individual may not be aware of the injury until pain and swelling start to develop.

What are the symptoms?

If the tear occurs suddenly, as may occur with a twisting injury, there will probably be a sharp pain and the knee may swell up. In some cases, a flap or a ring of cartilage may float loose inside the joint, locking the knee completely. It may be difficult to stand properly on the affected leg if the knee cannot take the body's full weight.

How is it diagnosed?

A doctor may suspect a meniscal tear from a description of the symptoms or a physical examination of the joint. The diagnosis may be then confirmed using an arthroscope (a narrow fibre-optic tube that can be inserted into a small incision in the knee >>206) or an MRI scan >>297.

What are the treatment options?

Minor tears along the outside edge of the cartilage, where the blood supply is good, often heal by themselves after a period of rest. Major tears, or tears along the inner edge of the meniscus, heal slowly or not at all and often require surgery.

An operation called a meniscectomy may be arranged to remove any loose pieces of cartilage. This may be carried out using an arthroscope or, more occasionally, using open surgery. As much of the damaged meniscus as possible will be left in place so that it can continue to protect the joint from wear and impact.

A programme of physiotherapy after the operation will help to rebuild the strength of the muscles around the knee. Heavy work can often be resumed a couple of weeks after arthroscopic surgery or after several months following open surgery.

What is the outlook?

Surgical repair of a torn meniscus is very likely to be successful. Unfortunately the removal of meniscal tissue means that more pressure is placed on the joint, increasing the likelihood that osteoarthritis of the knee will develop later on in life >>228–247.

Several less drastic techniques of repair and transplant have also been developed, with varying degrees of success. These include meniscal repair, where the surgeon attaches sutures to hold the edges together.

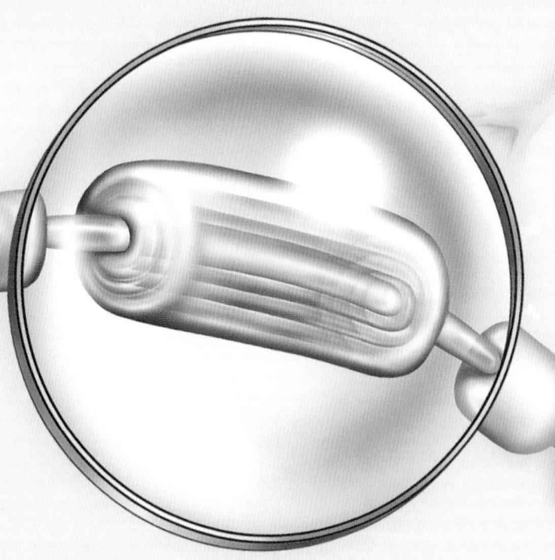

THE MYELIN SHEATH

This layer of fatty insulation speeds the transmission of nerve signals along the nerve pathways. Multiple sclerosis is believed to occur when the body's immune system attacks these sheaths, blocking signals to muscles.

MOTOR NEURONE DISEASE

A group of conditions characterized by progressive degeneration of the motor nerves causing muscle weakness and other neurological problems.

In the UK around 5,000 people suffer from motor neurone disease. It tends to affect 50–70 year olds and slightly more men than women. In many cases there is no obvious cause but in 5–10 per cent of cases there is some family history of the disease, suggesting that genetics may play a role.

The most common type of motor neurone disease is amyotrophic lateral sclerosis which damages the neurones that carry messages between brain and spinal cord and the spinal cord and muscles. This accounts for around 80 per cent of cases.

What are the symptoms?

Although the symptoms vary depending on the type of condition, there is often muscle weakness, cramps, stiffness and twitching, atrophied muscles, tiredness and possibly problems with speech and chewing. Patients usually maintain control of eye muscles and bladder and bowel function

How is it treated?

There is no cure for motor neurone disease, so treatment focuses on relieving symptoms. Muscle relaxant drugs and physiotherapy can help to improve muscle function and painkillers can help to relieve discomfort.

Patients may be prescribed a drug called Riluzole which inhibits the release of glutamate, a nerve transmitter that excites motor neurones. Excessive stimulation of glutamate receptors is thought to play a key role in the nerve damage.

Motor neurone disease is often fatal within around two to five years, although some sufferers live for ten years or longer.

MULTIPLE SCLEROSIS

Damage to nerve fibres causing numbness, muscle weakness and other symptoms.

Multiple sclerosis (MS) is caused by damage to the sheath of tissue that insulates the nerve fibres in the brain and spinal cord. It is usually diagnosed during the late 20s or early 30s and affects more women than men. There are four possible forms:

- **Benign MS** In around 20 per cent of cases, multiple sclerosis involves only a small number of mild attacks and no permanent disability.

- **Relapsing-remitting MS** In around 25 per cent of cases there are more severe attacks lasting 24-48 hours followed by a period of recovery. Attacks recur but do not grow worse
- **Primary progressive MS** In around 15 per cent of cases the disease grows progressively worse. Symptoms sometimes stabilize but do not permanently recover.
- **Secondary MS** In about 40 per cent of cases there is a period of intermittent attacks (similar to relapsing-remitting MS) that do not grow worse, followed by a progressive worsening of the condition.

What are the causes?

Multiple sclerosis is believed to be an autoimmune disease, when the immune system attacks the body's own cells. This causes inflammation that damages the myelin sheath around nerve cells, resulting in hardening (sclerosis) of the nerves and slowing down of nerve impulses to muscles.

It is not known exactly what causes this reaction – although it may be triggered by an infection such as a virus – or why some people are more susceptible than others. People who have a family history of the disease and people who live in northern Europe, the northern United States, southern Australia or New Zealand are more likely to be affected, so genetic and environmental factors probably play a role.

What are the symptoms?

The disease usually begins with numbness, tingling and muscle weakness. These symptoms may initially last for only a few days before improving. As the disease progresses it may cause blurred vision, loss of balance and coordination, muscle weakness, difficulty speaking, fatigue, loss of bladder and bowel control, or confusion.

How is it diagnosed and treated?

If the symptoms suggest multiple sclerosis, the doctor may organize neurological tests, including an MRI scan, to check for inflammation and damaged nerves.

A number of drugs are available that may help to delay the progression of the disease. These include beta interferon, a drug believed to inhibit the action of white blood cells called T-lymphocytes which are involved in the inflammatory immune reaction that causes multiple sclerosis. This drug may reduce the incidence of relapses in the relapsing-remitting and secondary progressive forms of the disease. Another drug, glatiramer acetate, can also inhibit the action of the T-lymphocytes. In some cases, though, these drugs have no effect.

Other treatments are intended to help sufferers handle their symptoms: these include physiotherapy and occupational therapy to strengthen and relax muscles and improve mobility, pain-relieving and muscle relaxant drugs and possibly corticosteroids to reduce inflammation.

The prognosis depends on the type of multiple sclerosis, the rate of progression and the response to treatment. Most people with MS continue to walk and function with the disability for 20 years or more. The disease has no effect on life expectancy.

MUSCULAR DYSTROPHY

A group of inherited muscular disorders characterized by progressive muscle weakness and degeneration.

Muscular dystrophy disorders result from faulty genes, which may be inherited or may in some cases occur spontaneously. Many of the most common types of muscular dystrophy, such as Duchenne's and Becker's muscular dystrophy, are caused by mutations in the gene for the muscle protein dystrophin.

DUCHENNE'S MUSCULAR DYSTROPHY

A severe form of muscular dystrophy occurring in early childhood

In this condition, a gene defect on the X chromosome (the female sex chromosome) results in the absence or severe abnormality of the protein dystrophin. The abnormal gene is inherited in an X-linked recessive pattern – this means that the condition affects boys who inherit the gene but almost never affects girls.

Around 1 in 3000 males are born with the disease although the signs and symptoms usually take a few years to develop. The skeletal muscles that move the bones of the skeleton are always affected but in some cases the muscles of the heart are also involved.

Symptoms usually become apparent by the fourth year and include difficulty running, climbing stairs and standing up from a sitting position. By the age of 10, most affected boys have become severely disabled. The condition may be fatal from around the age of 20 years.

How is it diagnosed and treated?

A diagnosis of Duchenne's can be made from a description of the symptoms and confirmed by measuring the blood level of the enzyme creatinine kinase, which is high in those affected. Gene analysis may also be arranged and in some cases tiny samples of muscle tissue (biopsies) may be examined for the characteristic changes.

If a positive diagnosis is made, other boys in the family can also be tested for muscular dystrophy by checking their

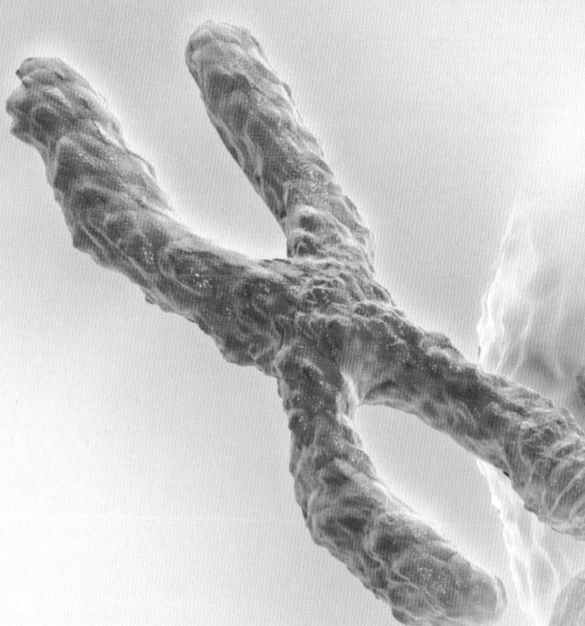

INHERITING DUCHENNE'S MD

In Duchenne's muscular dystrophy, the abnormal gene is found on the X chromosome. We all have two sex chromosomes: males have an X and a Y; females have two X chromosomes. For this reason women almost never have the condition – the normal version of the gene on the second X chromosome makes up for the abnormal gene. However, they can be carriers of the abnormal gene and pass it on to their offspring. Boys do not have a second version of the gene to protect them and therefore develop the condition if they have the abnormal gene. The son of a carrier has a 50 per cent chance of being affected by the disorder.

creatinine kinase levels. If the parents wish to have further children, prenatal diagnosis is available using tiny samples taken from the placenta (chorionic villus biopsy).

There is no cure for the condition and treatment aims to maintain independence for as long as possible and to help sufferers achieve the best possible quality of life. Close support for the patient and his family from a team of specialists is an important part of the treatment programme: physiotherapists, in particular, play a key role in helping to reduce the rate at which muscles shorten over time. Patients are also closely monitored for heart problems.

BECKER'S MUSCULAR DYSTROPHY

A condition similar to Duchenne's but milder and with a slower progression. It often develops during adolescence.

Like Duchenne's, Becker's muscular dystrophy results from a defect in the gene responsible for making the muscle protein dystrophin, so that the protein is either abnormal in structure or present in reduced amounts. As with Duchenne's, the pattern of inheritance is X-linked recessive and affects males almost exclusively.

Early symptoms may be apparent from around the age of 10 and include cramping of the muscles, which may be brought on by exercise. Very often, however, the symptoms first become apparent in the late teens or early twenties. Becker's affects primarily the legs and pelvis, although it can also spread to the arms and neck, and may include problems with running or walking upstairs. These symptoms become progressively more severe and, by middle age, patients may be unable to walk. However, the pattern of symptoms varies and walking may become a significant problem earlier or later than this. In some cases the heart muscles are also affected.

How is it diagnosed and treated?

If Becker's is suspected, diagnosis can be confirmed using a simple blood test to check for elevated creatinine kinase levels.

Daily exercise is important to strengthen the muscles as much as possible. Cramps in the calves may be helped by calf massage. As with Duchenne's, patients with Becker's will be carefully monitored to track the progression of the disease.

MYASTHENIA GRAVIS

An uncommon condition in which muscles weaken and tire with use.

Myasthenia gravis most commonly develops between the ages of 15 and 50 but can begin at any age. The condition affects about 15 in every 100,000 people and is more common in women than in men.

What are the causes?

Muscle contractions are triggered by chemicals called neurotransmitters which are delivered to the muscle fibres by nerves. Neurotransmitters are released from nerve endings at the neuromuscular junction and received by trigger receptors on the muscle.

Myasthenia gravis is an autoimmune condition in which the body's immune system forms antibodies against its own tissues, in this case the receptors on the muscle fibres. These antibodies block the receptors so that less of the neurotransmitter acetylcholine can become attached. This interferes with muscle contractions.

Although myasthenia gravis is not inherited, genes may play a role in determining who develops the condition. It is often associated with abnormalities of the thymus gland in the chest which plays an important role in the development of the immune system in early life. Such abnormalities could prevent the immune cells developing properly, causing them to attack the muscle receptors.

What are the symptoms?

The main symptom of myasthenia gravis is muscle weakness. This tends to worsen with use so that muscles are initially strong but weaken as the day goes on. Symptoms may also be worse during hot weather.

The muscles that move the eyes and eyelids are usually the first to be involved, causing drooping eyelids and double vision. In most cases the disease then goes on to affect other muscles. This can lead to difficulty smiling, swallowing or speaking, problems holding up the head or the arms or breathlessness when exercising.

The severity of the symptoms varies from person to person. Some people find they have periods when the condition seems to improve for a while.

How is it diagnosed?

An initial diagnosis may be based on symptoms and an examination, then confirmed by various tests. These include electromyography testing to measure the response in a muscle when a nerve that supplies it is stimulated and determine whether the neurotransmitters are reaching the receptors. Alternatively, an injection of a drug that prevents the breakdown of the neurotransmitter acetylcholine may be given to see if this relieves the symptoms. The majority of people who suffer from myasthenia gravis have acetylcholine receptor antibodies, so this can be checked using a blood test.

What are the treatment options?

Anticholinesterase drugs prevent the breakdown of the neurotransmitter and so make more acetylcholine available to attach itself to the receptors, improving muscle function. Removal of the thymus gland may be beneficial for some people, though symptoms can take a few years to improve. Corticosteroid drugs (>>320) may be prescribed to suppress the immune system and limit the production of the abnormal antibodies. The symptoms may worsen initially but when they improve the steroid dose will be reduced to the lowest possible amount in order to keep the side effects to a minimum. To allow the doctor to reduce the dose of steroids still further or even to stop the drugs, other drugs that suppress the immune system may be prescribed. For very severe symptoms, a patient may be admitted to hospital for intravenous drugs.

What is the outlook?

The condition is potentially life-threatening but in about nine out of ten people the symptoms will be controlled effectively with medical treatment. This is usually a life-long condition although in a few cases it clears up without treatment.

MYOSITIS

The general term for swelling of the muscles due to injury, infection or disease.

Swollen muscles due to exercise, injury or infection are usually temporary and will return to normal with rest or when the injury or infection is treated. However, certain autoimmune diseases are characterized by longer-lasting myositis.

These diseases occur when the immune system reacts to a perceived threat by attacking the body's own muscle tissue, causing inflammation, swelling and weakness. These diseases include:

- **Polymyositis** This condition usually occurs in people over the age of 20 and affects more women than men. Muscle weakness develops over days, weeks or months and begins in the muscles closest to the torso, such as the neck, hip, back or shoulders. Some people also suffer from aching, tender muscles, an irregular heartbeat or breathing problems.
- **Dermatomyositis** This is characterized by a rash as well as muscle weakness. It can occur at any age, but affects more women than men. It is the most common type of myositis in children. Because the immune response irritates blood vessels as well as muscle fibres, the first symptom is usually a patchy reddish-purple skin rash. Muscle weakness, caused by the swollen muscles, usually follows after a period of days, weeks or months, starting with muscles close to the torso.
- **Inclusion-body myositis** (IBM) This form of myositis progresses more slowly than other types and affects more men than women. It usually begins after the age of 50. Muscle weakness develops over months or years rather than weeks and involves most muscles. As the muscles grow weaker, they may shrink in size.

How is it diagnosed?

Diagnosis of autoimmune myositis is usually made on the basis of the symptoms and may be confirmed using blood tests to check for autoantibodies or enzymes (>>329). An MRI scan (>>297) may identify where muscle is inflamed and an electromyogram (EMG) can measure unusual patterns of muscle contraction.

What are the treatment options?

The sooner treatment begins, the better the results. Most types of myositis respond well to steroids such as prednisone, disease modifying anti-rheumatics (DMARDs >>257), or intravenous immunoglobulin. These all work by suppressing the unwanted immune response. Inclusion-body mysotis does not always respond as well as other types of myositis to these treatments, so exercise to maintain strong muscles and physiotherapy to rehabilitate weak muscles is particularly important.

OSGOOD-SCHLATTER DISEASE

A condition of childhood in which the front of the shin bone becomes inflamed.

This condition tends to occur between the ages of 11–13 and in boys more commonly than in girls. The disease is one example of a condition known as traction apophysitis where the surface of a bone is pulled away from the bone itself at the site of the tendon attachment. It usually occurs during the adolescent growth spurt when the muscles enlarge and strengthen before the bones themselves have fully matured.

In Osgood-Schlatter disease, bone fragments are loosened from the front of the shin just below the knee when the large quadriceps muscle (the muscle used to straighten the knee) pulls on the tendon attaching it to the shin bone. Sports that involve vigorous and repetitive kicking, jumping or running actions often contribute to the development of the condition.

What are the symptoms?

The symptoms usually come on gradually over a period of weeks or months. The main symptom is pain just below the kneecap, which is often made worse by strenuous exercise and relieved by rest. In addition a small swelling may develop just below the kneecap where the tendon attaches to the tibia. In most cases only one leg is involved but occasionally both legs are affected.

How is it diagnosed and treated?

The doctor may arrange for an X-ray to check the condition of the bone. Treatment usually consists of rest and painkillers – sport can be continued but vigorous exercise should be avoided to allow the area to heal. With time the fragments will usually reattach to the tibia. The condition may take a few months to clear and in a few cases persists until growth has stopped.

The outlook is good in most cases: once it has been cured the condition does not usually return. In a few cases a splinter of bone remains detached and may cause persistent pain. If this occurs, steroid injections may be given and occasionally the splinter of bone is surgically removed.

OSTEITIS DEFORMANS

>>Paget's disease

OSTEOARTHRITIS >>228–247

OSTEOCHONDRITIS DISSECANS

A disorder in which a fragment of bone and cartilage dies and may become loose inside a joint.

Osteochondritis dissecans is believed to be caused by a disruption of the blood supply to a section of bone inside a joint. The cartilage overlying the bone receives nourishment from the synovial fluid and remains alive but the bone underneath the cartilage starts to die and is gradually reabsorbed. As a result the cartilage loses its supporting structure and a bony fragment becomes detached. The fragment may eventually break off completely, making the joint unstable.

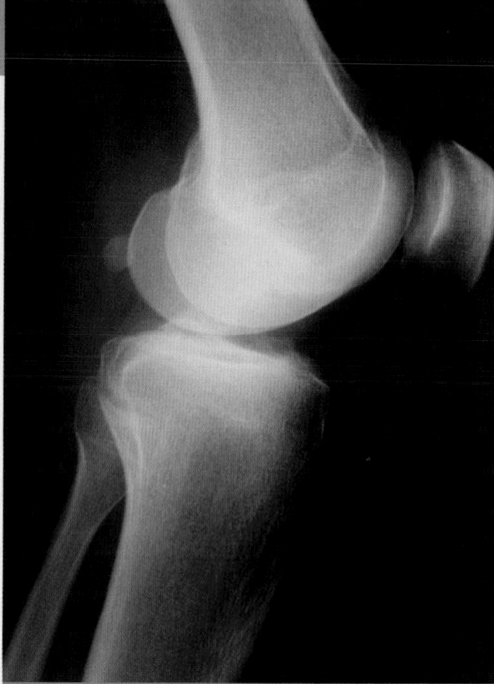

OSTEOCHONDRITIS DISSECANS
In this X-ray of a knee with osteochondritis dissecans it is possible to see a fragment of detached bone to the left of the joint and a small gap (in grey) in the bottom of the thigh bone, where the bone has degenerated.

In contrast to most types of osteonecrosis (bone death >>311) only a small section of bone is affected. The underlying bone generally retains a normal blood supply. Doctors still do not understand exactly why this disruption to the blood supply occurs but since the condition is more likely to occur in athletes, it may be a result of repeated microtrauma. One study of osteochondritis dissecans in the elbow found that repeated throwing actions or racket sports were often involved.

The disorder is most common in males aged 10–20 years, although it is becoming more common in women as they become more involved in sports. It usually occurs in growing bone but it can involve mature bone. The knee is the most commonly damaged joint, usually at the femur (thigh bone) – this accounts for around 75 per cent of cases. Another 10 per cent of cases involve the ankle or the elbow.

How is it diagnosed?

The joint may be painful and swollen and may seem to lock, catch or give way as it is used. Because these symptoms are so similar to those of other joint diseases, the condition can be hard to diagnose on the basis of the symptoms alone.

If osteochondritis dissecans is suspected, the doctor will examine the joint and may ask about sports or activities that the patient is involved in. If the bone fragment has come loose it may be possible to spot this on an X-ray (>>319) but an MRI scan (>>297) usually provides a better picture of the position of the fragment. An examination using an arthroscope (>>206) may also be helpful.

What are the treatment options?

Treatment depends on the age of the patient and how far the problem has progressed. If the fragment is still attached and the bone is still growing, it may be possible to treat the disorder by limiting activity or immobilizing the joint. Rarely it may be necessary to fix the fragment in place with pins or screws.

In adults and in more advanced cases, surgery is usually needed to remove the loose body and either reconstruct the bone or graft on replacement tissue. This can often be done using an arthroscope. There is usually some slight loss of joint function following surgery.

OSTEOGENESIS IMPERFECTA

A genetic disease in which the bones are fragile and fracture easily.

Osteogenesis imperfecta affects around 1 in every 20,000 people and around 1 in every 50–60,000 people has a very severe form of the condition. People who suffer from the condition have a problem with the formation of collagen, the tough protein that forms part of bones, cartilage and connective tissue: either there is not enough collagen being produced or the collagen that is produced is abnormal. This causes fragile, easily-fractured bones.

What are the causes?

The condition results from a gene defect which is usually inherited but sometimes occurs spontaneously. As each person has two copies of this particular gene, the child of a parent who has the disease will have a 50 per cent chance of inheriting one normal and one abnormal gene – and therefore inheriting the disease – and a 50 per cent chance of inheriting two normal versions of the gene and being unaffected. There are four recognized types of osteogenesis imperfecta:

- **Type I** is the most common but mildest form of the condition and is usually inherited. It occurs because a reduced amount of collagen is produced. Most bone fractures tend to occur before puberty. As well as fragile bones, people with type I osteogenesis imperfecta often have a blue colouration of the whites of the eyes, a curved spine, thin skin, loose joints and brittle teeth. Hearing problems may develop around the age of 20 or 30.
- **Type II** affects around 10 per cent of sufferers and is the most severe form of the disease. It results from a spontaneous gene mutation that causes the structure of the collagen to develop abnormally so that bones are fragile and deformed. This condition causes breathing problems that are usually fatal soon after birth.
- **Type III** also results from a spontaneous mutation that causes the collagen to have an abnormal structure but is less severe than type II. Fractures occur mostly before puberty and may even occur before birth. Those affected tend to have many of the features of type I and may have small stature, bones that bend as well as fracture and bone deformities. They may also have breathing problems.
- **Type IV** is usually inherited, though it can occasionally result from a spontaneous mutation. It is less severe than type III but more severe than type I. Once again, fractures are most common before puberty and those affected tend to be of short stature.

How is it diagnosed and treated?

The doctor may make the initial diagnosis from an examination. Tests to confirm this include an assessment of the collagen structure and genetic analysis.

There is no cure for the condition at present so treatment aims to relieve the symptoms and keep the bones and muscles as strong as possible. Physiotherapy may be recommended for pain relief and to improve muscle strength. Exercise is important for the same reasons: activities such as swimming and hydrotherapy will help to strengthen the bones and muscles without risking fractures; walking, when possible, is also good exercise. A healthy diet, rich in calcium and vitamin D for bone strength, is also important.

Options for pain management include cold and heat packs, medications and sometimes nerve blocks in which pain-

BOW LEGS AND KNOCK KNEES

Young children are often born with slight bow legs (genu varum), caused when the thigh bones are rotated slightly in the hip sockets. The legs almost always straighten up without treatment, usually by around 18 months of age, and by the time the child is three or four years old, the legs may develop a knock-kneed appearance (genu valgum). Knock knees usually correct themselves by the time the child is five or six. But there is a wide range of variation and the condition may continue into adulthood. They don't normally require treatment, although improperly aligned legs may slightly increase the risk of osteoarthritis of the knee >>228–247.

Occasionally bow legs and knock knees are a sign of a more serious problem. These can include rickets (>>right), Blount's disease (>>280), Paget's disease (>>313) or damage to the growing ends of the long bones in the leg. Warning signs include knock knees that are still present at the age of seven or one leg that appears more curved than the other.

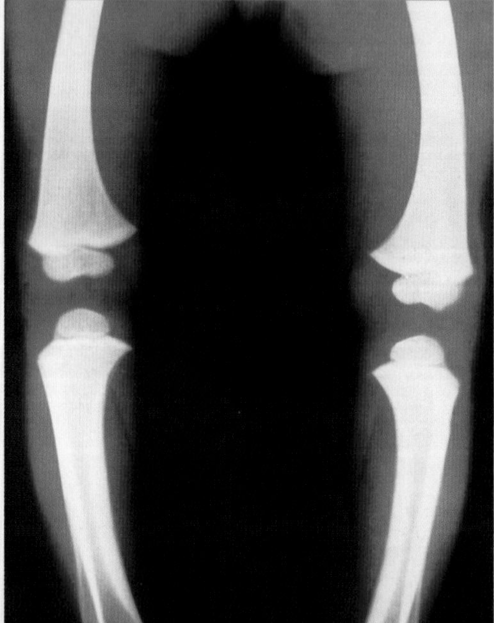

relieving drugs are injected around an affected nerve. Fractures will need to be treated when they occur and in some severe cases metal rods are inserted into the long bones for strength and to prevent deformity.

The outlook for those with the condition varies widely depending on the individual and the type. While babies born with type II osteogenesis imperfecta rarely live long after birth, some people with type I have such mild symptoms that they are never even diagnosed.

OSTEOMALACIA AND RICKETS

Softening of the bones due to a deficiency of vitamin D.

Vitamin D is required by the body in order to absorb calcium effectively from the gut. If there is a deficiency in vitamin D, the body will not absorb enough calcium to build and maintain strong, healthy bones. The vitamin is also vital for muscle function.

In children, a lack of vitamin D can prevent sufficient calcium being laid down as bones form, meaning that bones and teeth fail to develop properly – this condition is called rickets. A deficiency of vitamin D in adults means that calcium is lost from bones that have already formed – in this case the condition is called osteomalacia.

What are the causes?

Vitamin D is produced by the body when the skin is exposed to sunlight. On average, around 90 per cent of the intake comes from this source; the remainder comes from the diet where it is found in foods such as milk, eggs, oily fish, margarine and green vegetables. There are therefore two main causes of deficiency: insufficient sunlight and poor dietary intake.

Certain social groups are at particular risk of developing osteomalacia. Elderly, housebound people may not get much chance to get out in sunlight, for example, while people who avoid exposing skin for cultural or religious reasons are also at risk.

Occasionally a disease affecting the gut may impair the absorption of vitamin D from food and some chronic kidney diseases can also affect calcium and vitamin D absorption. A few cases result from inherited disorders in which vitamin D metabolism is impaired. Certain antiepileptic drugs can also interfere with vitamin D metabolism.

What are the symptoms?

Because children's bones are still developing, rickets will often cause skeletal deformities. Babies who are born with rickets may have a misshapen skull which feels soft to the touch. Older children who develop rickets often have deformities in their leg bones such as bow legs. They may also have deformities of the rib cage, spinal column or pelvis. The tips of the rib bones sometimes enlarge creating a string of lumps known as a rachitic rosary. Bones tend to break more easily than usual so fractures may be common.

Calcium is needed for teeth, so lack of vitamin D may mean teething is delayed or teeth are poorly formed. Insufficient vitamin D also causes muscle weakness and general growth is often impaired.

The signs of osteomalacia in adults are harder to spot – there may not be any obvious symptoms until the condition is fairly well advanced. Bone deformities are uncommon although sufferers often walk with a slightly waddling gait. Bones may ache or be painful and fractures are more likely to occur after minor knocks or falls.

Muscles may feel weak or tender to the touch and sufferers may have problems getting up from chairs or climbing stairs.

How is it diagnosed?

If osteomalacia or rickets is suspected, various blood tests may be arranged including tests to check calcium levels. X-rays can indicate inadequate calcium in the bones but often appear as normal. If blood tests do not clearly confirm the diagnosis, a tiny sample of bone (a biopsy) may be taken from the hip for testing.

Osteomalacia is sometimes detected when testing blood taken from people known to be at risk, for example patients with chronic kidney failure.

What are the treatment options?

Treatment should address the underlying cause wherever possible: if malnutrition or lack of sunlight are responsible, measures should be taken to improve dietary intake or exposure to sunlight. It may also help to take oral vitamin D supplements as well as extra calcium to improve bone strength. People who have problems absorbing vitamin D may need injections of larger doses, in which case calcium levels should be monitored. The symptoms of osteomalacia generally improve rapidly with treatment although the deformities that result from rickets may be irreversible.

OSTEOMYELITIS

An acute or chronic infection of bone which can affect both children and adults.

Acute osteomyelitis is caused by the direct spread of an infection from nearby tissues or by an infection travelling in the bloodstream from elsewhere in the body. The condition sometimes follows an injury to a bone – any bruises that form provide a site for bacteria to live and multiply. Poor nutrition and impaired immunity may play a role.

Chronic osteomyelitis develops when the acute disease is not effectively treated and can persist for years. Thanks to early diagnosis and modern antibiotics, the progression from acute to chronic osteomyelitis is now relatively uncommon in developed countries.

What are the symptoms?

The main symptoms of acute osteomyelitis are bone pain, often severe, and fever.

If the bacteria cannot be successfully treated, a large pus-filled cavity may form. The cavity is connected to the surface of the body by a channel called a sinus, which allows the pus to drain. Again, there may be pain and in some cases associated weight loss. Sometimes pus is released into a joint causing septic arthritis (>>324).

How is it diagnosed?

Blood tests are arranged to check the blood count and look for evidence of infection. X-rays or MRI scans (>>297) may be used to look for the infection site.

What are the treatment options?

Acute osteomyelitis usually requires hospital admission for rest and antibiotics. If the infection is not being brought under control within a few days, the doctors may drill into the bone to allow the pus to drain out. This usually clears up the infection effectively. In a few cases, however, the chronic form of the disease develops.

Chronic osteomyelitis can be treated by surgically removing any irreparably damaged bone and intensive antibiotics. This may be long and difficult as antibiotics are often needed for several months or more. When the infection has cleared, further surgery may be required to replace the infected bone with a healthy bone graft from elsewhere in the body.

What is the outlook?

If the diagnosis of acute osteomyelitis is made quickly and antibiotics are started straight away, the outlook is very good. Delay in starting treatment may mean that the disease becomes chronic, in which case it can be very difficult to treat.

OSTEONECROSIS

Death of bone, usually due to a cut off or restricted blood supply.

Bone is made of living cells, supplied by nerves and blood vessels and undergoing constant repair and regeneration. If the blood supply is cut off the bone cells may die, causing the bone to collapse. The hip is the most commonly affected joint.

DID YOU KNOW?

- **Osteonecrosis can affect any age group but is most common among 30–50 year olds, with the peak age being around 38.**
- **Around 1 in every 10–20,000 people are diagnosed with the condition each year – the chance of a completely healthy person developing the condition is only around 1 in 100,000 but existing health problems, such as arterial disease or hip fractures, greatly increase the risk.**
- **A juvenile form of osteonecrosis, Legg-Calvé-Perthes' disease, sometimes affects children aged around 5–11 years, particularly boys** **>>299****.**

What are the causes?

Osteonecrosis can be divided into post-traumatic and non-traumatic varieties:

- **Post-traumatic** osteonecrosis occurs when a major injury such as a hip fracture or dislocation physically damages the blood vessels leading to an area of bone.

The hip is particularly susceptible because the joint has such a deep socket and wide range of motion. This makes the neck of the thigh bone more difficult to reach and means that the arteries that do supply it are more vulnerable to injury.

- **Non-traumatic** osteonecrosis occurs when there is no trauma. The major risk factors for this type of osteonecrosis are high doses of corticosteroids (>>320) and alcohol abuse. Other possible factors include diseases of the arteries, sickle cell disease, chemotherapy, kidney or liver disease and smoking. Sometimes no cause can be identified.

What are the symptoms?

Initial symptoms include pain and aching during activity – if the hip is affected the pain is usually felt in the groin. Pain and stiffness increase over time and often cause a limp. Arthritis may develop and, if the condition is not effectively treated, the bone will eventually start to collapse.

In its early stages, the disease may be detected on an MRI scan (>>297). As it develops and other symptoms become apparent the damage should also be visible on an X-ray or CT scan (>>301).

What are the treatment options?

Taking weight off the joint may help to delay progression and relieve pain but will not cure the underlying condition, so surgical treatment is usually necessary. Treatment depends on the cause and extent of the necrosis, but options include:

- **A bone graft** It may be possible to replace the dead bone with a graft of live bone taken from elsewhere in the body.
- **A vascularized bone graft** This is a better option if there are still problems with the blood supply to the bone. In this procedure a graft is taken with the blood vessels still attached. These are then linked to the blood vessels around the joint.
- **Joint replacement** If the bone around the hip has started to collapse it may be necessary to replace the head and neck of the femur with an artificial implant that does not require a blood supply >>226-227.

OSTEOPETROSIS

A rare congenital disorder in which the bones become too dense.

Bone renews itself throughout life as cells called osteoclasts break down bone and cells called osteoblasts build new bone. Osteopetrosis is a genetic condition in which the osteoclasts are defective and the bones grow dense and heavy. Despite this density, the bones are usually very weak. There are three distinct forms of osteopetrosis:

Malignant infantile osteopetrosis

This very severe form of the disease is usually apparent at birth.

This form affects bones at an early stage of development. Defective bone tissue tends to replace bone marrow, reducing blood cell production and causing nerve problems. Unless successfully treated, around 30 per cent of children with malignant osteopetrosis die before 10 years of age. Symptoms of malignant osteopetrosis include anaemia, frequent infections due to lack of white blood cells or complete bone marrow failure. The condition also increases pressure in the skull and causes nerve problems that can include blindness or deafness. Other symptoms include failure to thrive and delays in motor development.

Intermediate and adult osteopetrosis

These are much milder forms of the condition that do not affect life expectancy.

Intermediate osteopetrosis occurs in children under the age of 10 and is less severe than the malignant infantile version but more serious than the adult form. It does not restrict life expectancy. Adult-onset osteopetrosis develops in adults aged 20–40 years of age. It is a relatively mild form of the condition.

In the intermediate and adult-onset forms, the symptoms are less obvious than in malignant osteopetrosis but may include frequent fractures and infections. Damage to nerves or blood vessels may cause problems such as blindness or strokes.

What is the treatment?

The only cure for malignant osteopetrosis is a bone marrow transplant to replace the abnormal osteoclasts. However, this process has a high risk of failure with potentially fatal consequences, meaning that it is not suitable for patients with the milder forms of the condition.

Drug treatments that can help to delay the progression of the disease and control the symptoms in all forms of the disease include calcitriol to stimulate the osteoclasts and prednisone to improve blood count. A drug called Interferon gamma-1b (Actimmune) may help to reduce infections and improve bone marrow function in patients with osteopetrosis. Children with osteopetrosis may also benefit from physiotherapy to help them develop normally.

OSTEOPOROSIS >>264–275

PAGET'S DISEASE

A disease affecting middle-aged and elderly people in which the normal process of bone turnover is disrupted.

Bone tissue is constantly being broken down and renewed. In Paget's disease of bone, also known as osteitis deformans, bone turnover is excessive and the bone that replaces the old tissue has an abnormal structure. The new bone is thickened but softer, making it susceptible to deformity and fractures. There is also an increase in blood flow to affected areas.

Paget's disease may affect one bone or several. Common sites include the pelvis, thigh bone, skull and shin bone.

What are the causes?

Why the disease develops is not known; it sometimes runs in families and a gene has been identified that increases the likelihood of Paget's. It has been suggested that a childhood virus, as yet unidentified, may cause Paget's disease later in life.

What are the symptoms?

Often, there are no symptoms at all. If symptoms are present they may include bone pain in the affected area and deformities such as an enlarged skull or bow legs. If the bone ends are involved there may be osteoarthritis and joint pain. In late stages of the disease, the hip joint may become damaged.

Fractures may occur after seemingly trivial injuries. The blood flow to affected areas is increased, which can make them feel warm to the touch. In addition, pumping an increased volume of blood around the body may put the heart under strain. Eventually, heart failure may develop with the main symptom being shortness of breath.

Thickened bone may put pressure on nerves. If the skull presses against the nerves that supply the ear, for example, deafness may follow. Compression of nerves by the bones of the spinal column can cause tingling or weakness in the legs. Very rarely bone tumours can develop.

How is it diagnosed?

A physical examination may be followed by an X-ray, which may reveal features of the disease. A blood test (>>329) can check levels of a substance called acid phosphatase which indicates that bone turnover is taking place, so in Paget's disease the levels are often high due to the excessive breakdown and formation of bone. Acid phosphatase checks are also used to monitor the response to treatment. These tests may be followed by an isotope bone scan (>>281) to identify the site and severity of the disease.

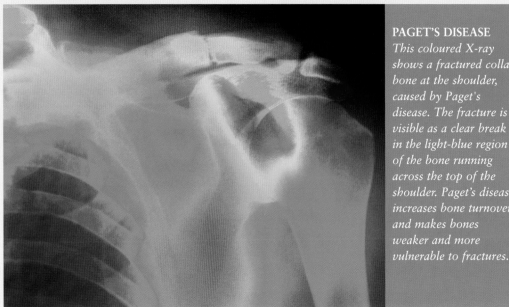

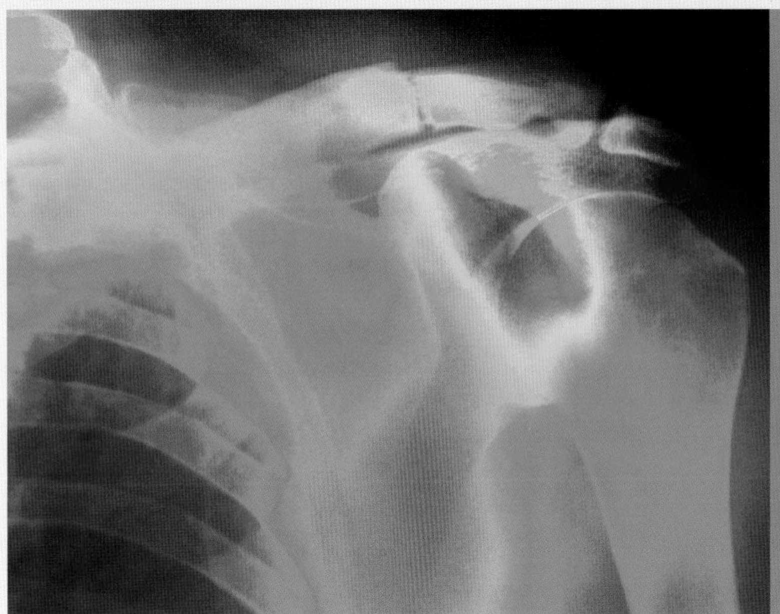

PAGET'S DISEASE
This coloured X-ray shows a fractured collar bone at the shoulder, caused by Paget's disease. The fracture is visible as a clear break in the light-blue region of the bone running across the top of the shoulder. Paget's disease increases bone turnover and makes bones weaker and more vulnerable to fractures.

DID YOU KNOW?

- **Paget's disease usually affects men and women older than 40 years. Around 1 in 20 people over the age of 50 are thought to have the disease but, since it often causes no symptoms, many of them will be unaware of it.**
- **The disease is more common in certain parts of the world. It is particularly prevalent in Europe.**

What are the treatment options?

The disease is usually treated using drugs such as painkillers or anti-inflammatories (NSAIDs >>208) in the first instance. Drugs called bisphosphonates may be prescribed to slow down excessive bone turnover. Bisphosphonates can be given orally or via a drip, either as a one-off infusion or as a series of treatments. In many cases, the pain is relieved in under six months. The treatment is repeated if necessary.

Surgery is sometimes performed to correct deformities, repair fractures or to replace joints affected by osteoarthritis. Taking a bisphosphonate prior to the operation will reduce the blood flow to the affected area and so limit blood loss during or after the surgery.

What is the outlook?

The progress of the disease can be slowed by drugs which means that some problems can be delayed or avoided altogether. Affected bones tend to heal well following fractures. However, existing deformities are usually permanent.

PERTHES' DISEASE

>>Legg-Calvé-Perthes' disease

PLANTAR FASCIITIS

A common condition in which the fibrous tissue supporting the arch of the foot is strained and becomes inflamed.

The plantar fascia is a thick band of tough tissue that extends from the heel bone to the metatarsal bones in the ball of the foot. It acts like a bow string to support the arch of the foot. Repetitive or excessive strain on the tissue stretches it at the point where it attaches to the heel bone causing tiny tears and inflammation. This is the most common cause of pain in the heel.

In around 10–20 per cent of patients both feet are affected. The condition can develop at any age.

What are the causes?

Twisting the foot inwards when walking is a common cause as it puts strain on the plantar fascia. Occasionally, the condition may develop following an injury. Being overweight or wearing poorly cushioned shoes can also be a factor.

Certain activities that put strain on the plantar fascia may aggravate or even cause the condition – these include walking or running for long distances and prolonged periods spent standing, particularly on uneven surfaces. Athletes may be at risk, particularly if they suddenly increase the distances run, wear shoes that are inadequately cushioned or run up steep hills. Dancers may also be at risk due to the repetitive nature of the foot movements.

What are the symptoms?

The condition generally comes on gradually and causes pain, which is usually dull and aching, when the foot is put to the floor. Typically, the pain is worse after periods of rest and is particularly bad on getting up in the morning. If the condition is severe, this pain may persist when the individual is walking. Sometimes the pain can spread along the bottom of the foot.

How is it diagnosed?

In around 70 per cent of cases an X-ray will show small bony outgrowths called heel spurs where the fascia attaches to the bone. However, heel spurs may be present in the absence of any symptoms. X-rays and possibly bone scans can also be used to rule out other possible causes of the symptoms, such as osteomyelitis >>311.

What are the treatment options?

Sometimes no treatment is necessary other than rest from any aggravating activities and possibly painkillers or non-steroidal anti-inflammatory drugs (NSAIDs >>280) to relieve the pain. If being overweight is a factor it may help to lose weight.

If necessary, a podiatrist can advise on appropriate footwear to cushion the foot and support the arch. In more severe cases a corticosteroid drug may be injected directly into the fascia to relieve inflammation, but this procedure is painful and is not necessarily effective.

What is the outlook?

Without treatment the condition may turn into a chronic problem causing long-term pain. Early diagnosis and treatment improves the prognosis but the condition may still take several weeks to improve.

POLYMYALGIA RHEUMATICA

A common condition that tends to affect older people with symptoms of pain and stiffness around the shoulders and hips.

Polymyalgia rheumatica (PMR) almost exclusively affects people over the age of 50, causing pain in muscles and stiffness. Women are affected twice as often as men.

The causes of the condition are not fully understood but it is believed to occur as a result of an abnormal immune response that causes the white blood cells to attack the lining of the joints (synovium). Since the disorder sometimes runs in families, there may well be a genetic link.

What are the symptoms?

The main symptoms are severe pain and stiffness in the shoulders, neck, hips and lower spinal column. The symptoms come on rapidly over a matter of days or a few weeks; in a few cases they seem to develop almost overnight.

Pain and stiffness is usually worse in the morning and episodes of pain can last from 30 minutes to several hours, making it a struggle to get out of bed or get dressed. Prolonged sitting can also bring on a painful episode. Other possible symptoms include fever, weight loss, lack of energy and depression. Less commonly there may be night sweating.

The condition is sometimes associated with giant cell arteritis, an inflammation of the blood vessels in the head and scalp causing severe headaches and scalp tenderness. Left untreated, giant cell arteritis can result in loss of sight, so any symptoms suggestive of the condition, such as headaches, facial pain, scalp pain or visual disturbances should be reported to a doctor immediately.

How is it diagnosed?

The diagnosis may be based on the patient's history but blood tests such as an erythrocyte sedimentation rate (ESR) test or possibly a C-reactive protein (CRP) test will be needed to confirm it (>>329). These tests indicate whether there is inflammation in the body – although they are not specific to polymyalgia rheumatica. In some patients with PMR the results of the tests will be normal or only mildly raised.

Giant cell arteritis can be confirmed by the removal of a small sample of tissue (a biopsy) and an examination of the sample under a microscope to look for the characteristic changes.

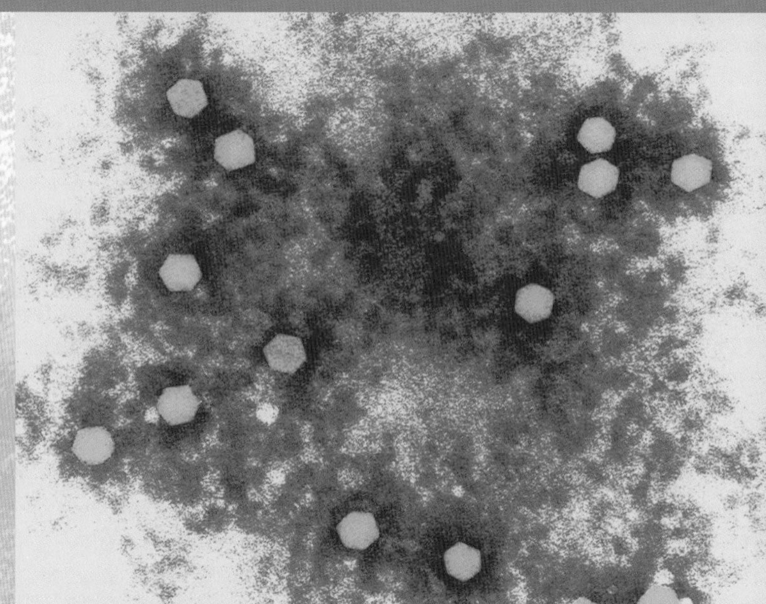

POLIO VIRUS
This coloured transmission electron micrograph shows a cluster of polio virus particles. The polio virus attacks the motor neurons in the brain and spinal cord and can cause severe disability, paralysis and sometimes death.

What are the treatment options?

Oral corticosteroid drugs such as prednisone are the main treatment for polymyalgia rheumatica – steroids usually produce a rapid response within 48 hours. A higher dose may be needed if giant cell arteritis is present. Once the symptoms are brought under control, the dose of steroids is gradually reduced to find the lowest effective dose so as to minimize the side effects. The patient's ESR is checked regularly to ensure that the condition is kept under control.

Normal activities should be resumed once the stiffness has settled. Long-term use of corticosteroids is associated with an increased risk of osteoporosis (>>264–275) so exercise is important to maintain bone strength as well as to improve mobility.

In around 75 per cent of those treated the condition will resolve within three years but in the rest low doses of corticosteroids will need to be continued for many years.

POLIOMYELITIS (POLIO)

A highly infectious disease that damages the nervous system and can result in paralysis.

A potentially disabling and life-threatening disease, poliomyelitis can occur at any age but mainly affects children under five. In over 90 per cent of cases the poliovirus causes no problems but in a small number of people, irreversible paralysis develops. Fortunately, improvements in living conditions together with the development of a polio vaccine in the 1950s mean that the incidence of polio has fallen dramatically over the past half a century.

What are the causes?

The disease is caused by infection with the poliovirus, which enters the body through the mouth and multiplies in the gut. The virus is carried in faeces, so poor sanitation and hygiene are important factors in its transmission. Once inside the body, the

ERADICATING POLIO

The incidence of polio has fallen dramatically with the use of the polio vaccine, which was introduced in the 1950s and 1960s. In 1988, the 'global eradication of polio' programme was launched. The number of reported cases has fallen from 350,000 cases in 1988 to only 1255 in 2004.

In the UK, the polio vaccine is normally given as part of the combined DTP-Polio-Hib vaccine during the routine childhood immunization programme.

virus is carried through the bloodstream to different parts of the nervous system, where it travels along nerves and destroys the cells responsible for controlling muscle contractions. Where this occurs the affected muscles become weak and floppy.

Doctors do not fully understood why some people who are infected with the poliovirus never get any symptoms when others go on to develop paralysis. Susceptibility to polio may be increased by factors such as impaired immunity, injury, pregnancy, exercise in the days following infection or even having tonsils removed.

People who have the infection but suffer no symptoms can pass the virus on unnoticed. And people who have been vaccinated may still pick up the infection and pass it on to others. As a result it is still very important to ensure that children are properly immunized.

What are the symptoms?

Various patterns of symptoms are possible: in many cases there are no symptoms at all and affected individuals are unaware that they have the infection. In others, the duration of the illness may be brief with only general symptoms of viral illness such as sore throat, fever and aching muscles. In less than 1 per cent of infected children and around 1 per cent of infected adults, the severe form with paralysis develops.

In the severe form of polio, general viral symptoms may, after a few days, be joined by muscle pain, particularly in the neck and lower back. There may be neck stiffness, vomiting, headaches and an aversion to bright light. After a few days, paralysis of the upper or lower limbs may start to develop. In a few cases the breathing muscles are affected, which can prove fatal. The muscles of the throat may also be involved, causing problems with swallowing and speech. The acute illness usually lasts for less than two weeks but damage to nerves may be permanent.

How is it diagnosed and treated?

The diagnosis will be made from a description of the symptoms and an examination. Blood tests may be performed to confirm the findings.

There is no cure for polio – treatment focuses on managing the symptoms using bed rest and physiotherapy. Antispasmodic drugs may be given to relax muscle contractions and mechanical ventilation may be required if the muscles involved in breathing are affected.

What is the outlook?

Overall, the vast majority of people affected by polio will have no long-term problems. However, a small but significant number will have persistent paralysis.

POLYMYOSITIS >>myositis

POPLITEAL CYST

A fluid-filled swelling that develops at the back of the knee.

The lining of the knee joint, the synovium, produces fluid that lubricates the joint and helps the bone ends to glide over each other smoothly. A cyst forms when synovial fluid leaks out through the lining to form a swelling. The cysts are most common in children aged 4–7 and adults aged 55–70.

What are the causes?

These swellings are usually associated with an underlying disorder of the knee such as osteoarthritis (>>228–2247), rheumatoid arthritis (>>248–263) or gout (>>294). They may also develop following an injury to the knee such as a torn meniscus (>>303). Sometimes, the cause is not identified.

What are the symptoms?

An uncomfortable swelling develops at the back of the knee which may cause problems when bending the knee or discomfort when walking. Cysts can occur in children as a firm lump in the back of the knee. There may also be pain from the underlying disorder that caused the cyst.

These cysts may go down gradually or they may burst, letting synovial fluid leak into the calf and making it red, hot and tender to the touch.

How is it diagnosed and treated?

The diagnosis is usually made after an examination. Tests, such as X-rays, may be arranged to look for an underlying disorder which will be treated if possible. In many cases, however, no treatment is required for the cyst, which will often disappear by itself. An injection of a steroid solution may encourage the cyst to dry up.

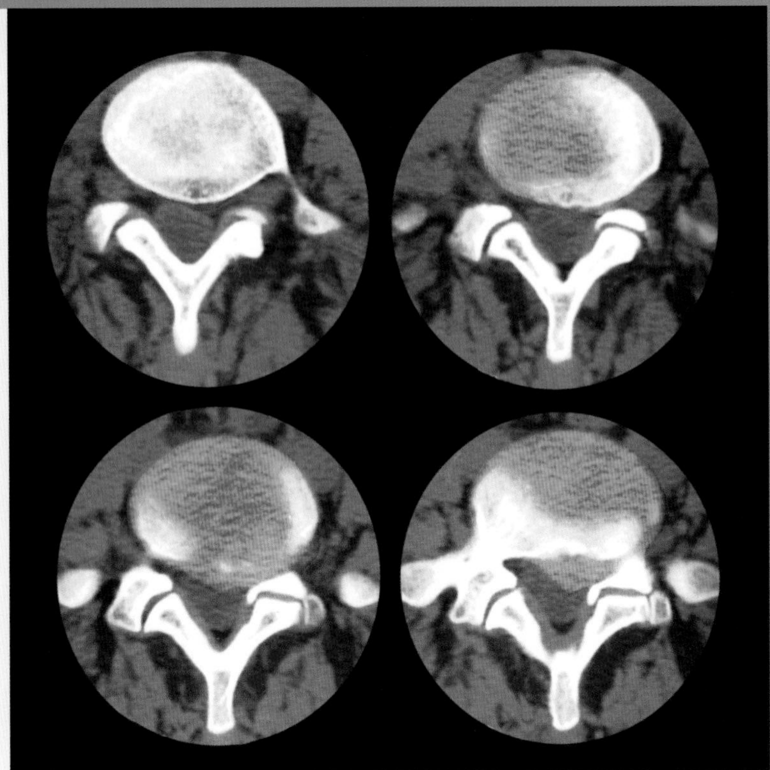

PROLAPSED DISC
These coloured CT scans show four cross-sectional views through an intervertebral disc. In the top left-hand picture the disc (shown in orange) is in the normal position between the spine vertebrae (in white). In subsequent pictures, the jelly-like core of the disc has started to bulge out into the spinal canal where it may be putting pressure on the nerves.

If the cyst ruptures, rest and painkillers are recommended – although a medical assessment may be needed first to exclude other possible causes of the symptoms, in particular a blood clot in one of the veins of the leg. Occasionally, surgery is required to remove the cyst. Cysts may recur unless the underlying cause is treated.

PROLAPSED (SLIPPED) DISC

A common disorder in which one of the discs that lie between the vertebrae of the spinal column bulges backwards.

The intervertebral discs between the vertebrae in the spine act as shock-absorbers. Each disc has a strong outer layer (called the annulus fibrosus) made up of cartilage and fibrous tissue and a softer jelly-like core (the nucleus pulposus).

When a disc prolapses, the soft inner part bulges through a tear in the outer ring, distorting the shape of the disc. The discs themselves have almost no nerve supply, but the distorted bulge and the inflamed tissues surrounding the bulge may put pressure on the spinal cord or on the nerves that branch out from it. In some cases disc herniation may occur, in which case the annulus fibrosus ruptures and leaks its contents into the spinal canal.

The problem most often develops in the lumbar spine because this section of the lower back supports the full weight of the torso and has a greater range of movement than the upper back. Other parts of the spinal column, notably the cervical spine in the neck, can also be affected.

A prolapsed disc is most likely to occur between the ages of 30 and 50: from the age of 30 the annulus fibrosus starts to weaken but after the age 50 the nucleus pulposus begins to harden. Men are affected more often than women.

What are the causes?

A prolapsed disc often occurs following an apparently trivial injury, perhaps a sudden twisting or bending movement of the back; it can also be brought on by lifting a heavy object incorrectly. Particular risk factors for prolapsed discs include obesity, smoking, weight lifting and occupations that involve heavy lifting or prolonged sitting.

What are the symptoms?

The symptoms may come on suddenly or may take weeks to develop. There may be pain in the affected area as well as stiffness and muscle spasm. The pain is often made worse by moving, coughing or sneezing.

If the cervical spine is affected and there is pressure on nerves, there may be pain, weakness, tingling or numbness affecting the arms and hands. Movements of the neck will also be restricted.

If the lumbar spine is affected, any symptoms of pain, weakness, tingling or numbness will affect the legs. Back movements will be restricted with muscle spasm around the affected area of the spine in the lower back.

If herniation of a lumbar disc occurs, fluid leaks into the spinal canal and may damage the cauda equina, a group of nerves that arise from the lower spine. This causes problems with bladder and bowel control; there may also be numbness in the area around the anus or shooting pains down the legs. This requires urgent treatment to avoid irreversible nerve damage.

How is it diagnosed?

The doctor will often make a diagnosis based on symptoms and an examination: the pattern of the symptoms should provide a good indication of the disc affected. Further tests may be arranged, including X-rays (>>box, right), CT scans (>>301), or MRI (>>297), in order to assess the severity of the prolapse and pinpoint its exact site in the spine.

What are the treatment options?

A prolapsed disc will often be treated with rest and painkillers but it is important to get up and about as soon as possible, while avoiding any actions that cause severe pain. Prolonged bed rest is not recommended. In some cases a cervical collar may be worn for a short period to support a prolapsed cervical disc.

Physiotherapy treatment in the acute phase may help to relieve pain and muscle spasm. A physiotherapist can also recommend exercises to build up the strength of the back muscles, which will make a recurrence less likely.

An anaesthetic may be injected into the affected area to relieve pain, possibly in combination with a corticosteroid drug to reduce inflammation in the surrounding tissues. If the pain is severe, an epidural may be given – an injection of anaesthetic into the space around the membranes that cover the spinal cord.

If the cauda equina is damaged, urgent surgery may be required. An operation may also be arranged if the pain is very severe, if the symptoms persist for more than six weeks or if the symptoms get worse despite treatment. The operation involves removal of the affected disc. This may be done by open surgery but increasingly microdiscectomy is used in which the surgeon makes tiny incisions and uses the images from a small camera (an arthroscope >>206) for guidance. Patients usually recover more quickly following these less invasive procedures.

An alternative to surgery is an injection of chymopapaine is (a softening agent) into the disc to relieve symptoms.

What is the outlook?

The condition often settles down with time – the bulge should eventually dry out, taking pressure off the nerve and scar tissue will start to form over the tear. There is a significant chance that the problem will recur at a later point.

Following surgery, there may be some persistence of the pain and a degree of stiffness. There may also be instability of the cervical spine following surgery for a prolapsed cervical disc. Instability can be avoided by fusing the vertebrae together, although this reduces neck mobility.

PSEUDOGOUT

A condition in which the formation of calcium pyrophosphate crystals causes attacks of inflammation inside a joint.

This condition is called pseudogout because although it resembles gout (>>294) it is caused by the formation of calcium crystals in the joints rather than urate crystals. Pseudogout tends to occur in elderly people and women are affected more often than men. It usually attacks the knees but can also affect the joints in the wrists, shoulders, elbows and ankles.

What are the causes?

In most cases it is not known exactly why calcium crystals form inside the joint. Age, genetic factors, thyroid problems and excessive calcium levels in blood (hypercalcaemia) may all be factors. It seems likely, however, that the deposits of calcium build up over time without causing symptoms until eventually even minor stress can trigger the release of the crystals into the joint fluid and subsequent inflammation.

Certain potential triggers have been identified, including joint injuries and generalized illness, particularly if there is a fever or a major physical stress such as an operation or a heart attack. Osteoarthritis (>>228–247) is known to predispose to the condition, particularly in the knee. In most cases the trigger is not known.

What are the symptoms?

Symptoms appear suddenly and the affected joint becomes painful, swollen and tender to the touch. The joint also becomes stiff with pain on movement. The overlying skin may become reddened. The condition will gradually settle over a few weeks but recurrent episodes may occur, sometimes affecting different joints. The attacks usually only involve one joint at a time.

How is it diagnosed?

Although symptoms and an examination may suggest pseudogout, tests are needed to exclude other disorders with similar symptoms, in particular gout (>>294) and septic arthritis (>>324). The doctor may remove a sample of fluid from the joint with a needle and syringe to be tested for the presence of calcium crystals and infective organisms. X-rays may show joint damage, calcification of cartilage and calcium deposits in joints (>>box, right).

WHAT ARE X-RAYS?

X-rays are beams of electromagnetic radiation which, although invisible to the naked eye, will blacken photographic film. If an object such as a human body is placed in between the film and the X-rays, some of the radiation will be absorbed by the body tissues, casting a shadow on the film. The more dense parts of the body, such as bones, absorb more of the radiation and show up lighter on the film. This makes X-rays an excellent way to investigate bone problems such as fractures or dislocations. They are less useful for investigating soft-tissue problems – although certain features, such as gas or air in the tissues, may show up.

Although frequent exposure to X-rays can cause cancer, the amount of radiation needed to capture an image on film is so low that the risk is very small. Techniques have developed greatly since X-rays were first used: the development of more sensitive film, fluorescent tubes that amplify the effect on film, and electronic detectors that measure the intensity of the rays to produce an image on computer, mean that X-rays are now very safe.

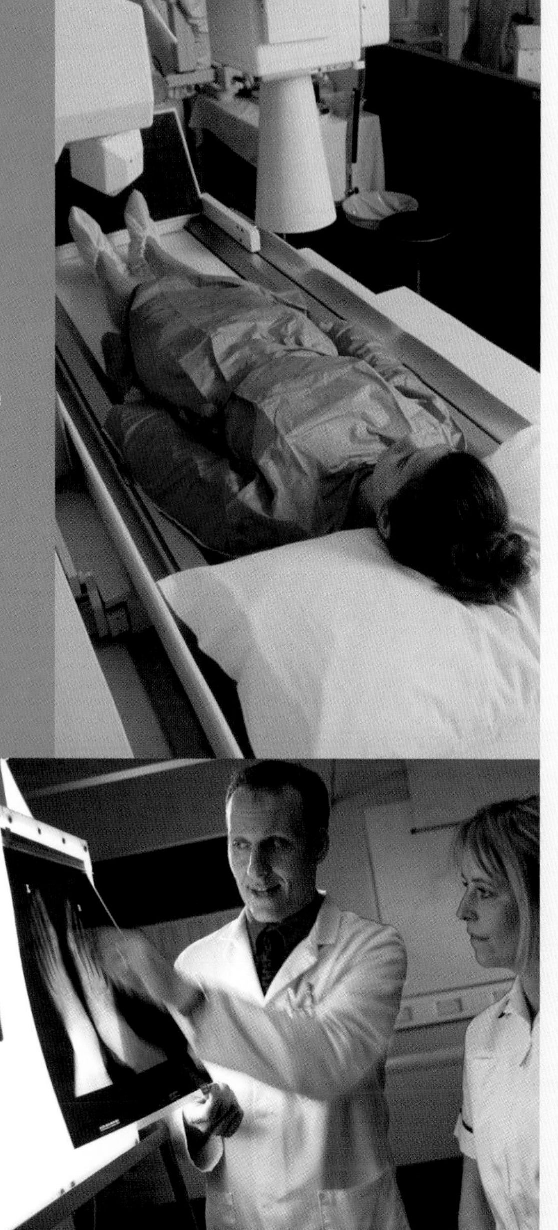

THE X-RAY EXAMINATION

Some types of diagnostic X-ray require the patient to stand; others need the patient to lie down on an X-ray table (above right). After the examination the radiologist will process and check the images (right) and send a report to the doctor who requested the test. In non-emergency cases, the results will usually be available a day or two after the scan.

What are the treatment options?

There is no cure for pseudogout – the aim of treatment is to relieve the symptoms when the flare-ups occur. Episodes may settle down after a few weeks without treatment but as they are often painful, painkillers and non-steroidal anti-inflammatory drugs (NSAIDs >>280) may be prescribed. Other drugs, such as colchicine, may be used for individuals who are unable to take NSAIDs – perhaps because they have impaired kidney function or have previously had a peptic ulcer.

Fluid aspiration may be performed on the joint. This involves drawing fluid out of the joint to relieve the pressure and so reduce the pain. This may be followed by an injection of a corticosteroid (>>320) into the joint to reduce the inflammation.

PSORIATIC ARTHRITIS

Inflammation of the joints in people who also have psoriasis.

Around 1 in 50 people have psoriasis, a condition in which excessive production of new skin cells causes a rough, scaly rash. Of these people, around 1 in 14 patients also develop psoriatic arthritis, a form of joint inflammation specifically associated with the disease. Other forms of arthritis, such as osteoarthritis (>>228–247) or rheumatoid arthritis (>>248–263), may occur independently in people who have psoriasis but are not specifically connected to the disease.

What are the causes?

The underlying cause of psoriasis is not known but it tends to run in families so it is likely that sufferers have some type of genetic predisposition. Among people who have this susceptibility, the condition may be triggered by external factors such as an infection (particularly a throat infection), trauma, stress and certain medications.

In some cases, one of these factors may also trigger the arthritis. In most instances, however, the rash develops first suggesting that it may be bacteria living within the patches of psoriasis that cause the arthritis. No specific infection has been found, so it may be that a variety of different infections can cause the disease.

What are the symptoms?

Psoriasis usually precedes psoriatic arthritis, often by as long as 5–10 years, so most people who have the arthritis will also have symptoms of psoriasis, most notably the patchy red or pink-coloured rash on the elbows, knees or scalp.

The arthritis itself causes painful, stiff or tender joints. Sometimes just one or two joints are affected but it more usually involves several joints, large and small, and on both sides of the body. Any joints in the body can be involved but it is more likely to occur in certain areas.

The finger and toe joints are often very painful, particularly when the nails or the skin over the joints are affected by the rash. This may cause a sausage-like swelling known as dactylitis due to inflammation of joints and tendons. Pain and swelling often also occurs in the knees and ankles. Around a third of sufferers have a stiff, sore back or neck.

Some sufferers find that their arthritis improves when the psoriatic rash improves and gets worse when their skin flares up.

How is it diagnosed?

The doctor is unlikely to diagnose psoriatic arthritis unless psoriasis is also present or the patient has a close relative who has psoriasis. The pattern of joint inflammation will also be considered.

The disease can be hard to distinguish from rheumatoid arthritis (>>248–263), so the doctor may order a blood test to check for rheumatoid factor. However, this antibody is not always present in people with rheumatoid arthritis and it is present in around 10 per cent of people without the disease, so the test is not conclusive.

What are the treatment options?

Non-steroidal anti-inflammatories (NSAIDs) such as ibuprofen can help to relieve pain and stiffness. Disease modifying anti-rheumatic drugs (DMARDs) such as methotrexate or hydroxychloraquine suppress the inflammatory process itself, so can help to slow the rate at which damage occurs. Corticosteroids also help to reduce inflammation and may be injected directly into a particularly painful joint (>>box, left).

All these treatments have side effects, some of which can be serious, so you should balance the advantages of drug treatment against any potential problems and follow your doctor's advice. For more information about these drugs >>256–257.

TAKING CORTICOSTEROIDS

Corticosteroids, often called simply steroids, are powerful drugs related to hormones produced in the adrenal glands – like naturally produced hormones, they prevent the release of chemicals that trigger inflammation. They are used to treat a variety of inflammatory conditions and usually produce a rapid response. Anti-inflammatory corticosteroids should not be confused with anabolic steroids, which are used to build muscle and have many other potentially serious side effects.

Short courses of corticosteroids rarely cause problems but continued on a long-term basis, side effects may develop. The higher the dose and the longer steroids are taken for, the more likely it is that problems will develop. This is why doctors aim to find the lowest effective dose and to stop medication when possible. However steroids should never be stopped suddenly or without medical guidance.

Possible side effects include easy bruising, thinning of the skin, acne, weight increase, indigestion, muscle weakness and mood changes. Long-term use may also cause osteoporosis to develop. Prolonged use of corticosteroids may also cause a rise in blood pressure and, because steroids reduce the activity of the immune system, they may increase the risk of getting infections. Children taking these drugs need to be carefully monitored as growth may be affected.

RICKETS >>Osteomalacia and rickets

REACTIVE ARTHRITIS

Joint inflammation triggered by an infection elsewhere in the body.

This condition is most common between the ages of 20 and 40 years; men are affected more often than women. Reactive arthritis accompanied by urethritis (urinary tract infection) and conjunctivitis (eye infection) is known as Reiter's disease. Arthritis caused by an infection inside the joint is called septic arthritis (>>325).

What are the causes?

Reactive arthritis is usually triggered by a bacterial infection of the gut, such as salmonella, or by an infection of the genital tract such as chlamydia. The bacterial infection streptococcus, which is often responsible for throat infections, is also a common cause of both reactive arthritis and septic arthritis.

What are the symptoms?

The symptoms tend to develop about two weeks after the infection. They usually come on suddenly and often particularly affect the joints of the legs.

Symptoms are likely to include pain and tenderness in the affected joint, joint swelling and redness of the overlying skin. They may be preceded by symptoms of the original infection, perhaps diarrhoea or a discharge from the genital tract. Sometimes the original infection causes no symptoms.

How is it diagnosed and treated?

Samples are taken from the affected area (stool samples, for example, or swabs from the genital area) in order to identify the bacterial cause. If a bacterial infection is still present it will be treated with antibiotics. Blood tests may reveal signs of infection and inflammation. X-rays may also be taken to assess any damage to the affected joints (>>319).

Non-steroidal anti-inflammatory drugs (NSAIDs >>280) will be given to relieve the inflammation and pain. Corticosteroid drugs (>>320) may also be injected directly into the affected joints, once it has been established that no infection is present inside the actual joint. Additional drugs, such as sulfasalazine, may be prescribed for the few people who suffer recurrent attacks of the disease.

What is the outlook?

Around seven in ten people will make a full recovery within six months but the condition may be recurrent in a few cases.

REITER'S DISEASE

>>Reactive arthritis

REPETITIVE STRAIN INJURY (RSI)

A soft tissue injury caused by the repeated movements of an area of the body

The term RSI describes the mechanism of injury rather than the injury itself. Any disorder caused by the repeated motion of a muscle or group of muscles is therefore covered by the term, including tendinitis and carpal tunnel syndrome.

Occupations and pastimes that require the same movements to be performed repeatedly can cause RSI. Production line workers and office employees who spend long periods working at a computer are often vulnerable to RSI, as are those who play an instrument such as a violin or a sport such as tennis.

What are the symptoms?

Symptoms can vary depending on the type of injury caused and the area of the body affected, but typically include pain and aching, tingling, limitation of movement and swelling of tissues. RSI is particularly common in the hand or wrist.

How is it diagnosed and treated?

The diagnosis can usually be made from a description of the symptoms and a description of the activities that bring them on. X-rays may be arranged in some cases to look for underlying disorders.

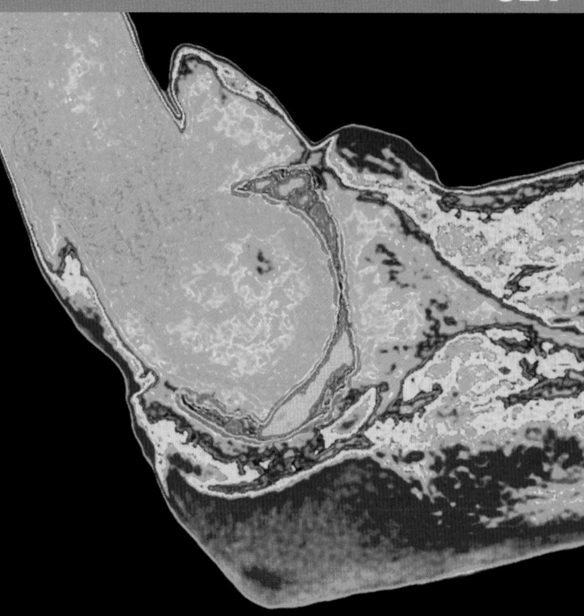

REPETITIVE STRAIN INJURIES
Most repetitive strain injuries are minor but they can be more serious. This coloured X-ray shows the elbow of a construction worker whose use of pneumatic tools has caused repeated shocks to the joint. The space between the joint (shown in orange) reveals how the normally smooth surfaces have grown jagged, causing pain and stiffness.

Treatment may involve adjusting work habits, perhaps by taking more breaks or changing working position in order to put less stress on muscles and tendons. For more details about the measures that you can take to avoid or relieve RSI and some of the ergonomic products available for sufferers >>132–133.

Short-term use of painkillers or mild non-steroidal anti-inflammatories such as ibuprofen may help to relieve the symptoms when they are particularly troublesome. A physiotherapist may be able to recommend exercises to relieve pain and stiffness and strengthen muscles to make them less susceptible to strains. RSI will usually recur unless measures are taken to reduce aggravating factors.

RHEUMATOID ARTHRITIS

>>248–263

RUPTURED TENDON

A tear to one of the tough fibrous bands that connect muscles to bones.

Ruptured tendons usually occur when a sudden muscle contraction jerks sharply on the tendon to which it is attached. In a few cases, a bone fracture or a deep cut may cause a tendon to rupture. Symptoms come on suddenly and may include a snapping sensation followed by pain, swelling and restricted movement.

The Achilles tendon – the tendon that extends from the back of the heel up into the calf – is often affected. Athletes and other sportsmen and women are particularly susceptible to Achilles tendon injuries.

How is it diagnosed and treated?

This condition can usually be diagnosed from the description of the symptoms and an examination of the tendon.

Short-term use of painkillers or non-steroidal anti-inflammatories (NSAIDs >>280) may be recommended to relieve the pain. An operation can also be performed to reattach the severed pieces of tendon.

For an Achilles tendon rupture, treatment may involve holding the tendon in place with a plaster cast. In some cases surgical reattachment may be performed first. The cast will then be replaced every few weeks as the position of the healing tendon is gradually adjusted. Physiotherapy will help to build up the strength of the muscles. It may take some months to get back to normal activity.

Sometimes, the central fibres of the Achilles tendon tear but the outer ones remain intact. In such cases, the problem tends to resolve over 12–18 months.

CAUTION

If you are involved in an accident and can feel the sharp shooting pains associated with sciatica, do not move. Ask for medical help in case there is any damage to your spinal cord.

You should also get immediate medical attention if you experience sciatica together with any bowel or bladder problems or a sensation of numbness around the anus. This may be a sign that you have damaged a group of nerves called the cauda equina, which can cause permanent nerve damage.

SCIATICA

Pain along the course of one or both of the sciatic nerves, the main nerves of the legs.

The sciatic nerve, the largest nerve in the body, runs from the lower back and down the back of each leg. If the nerve is pinched or damaged at the point at which it leaves the spine, it can cause pain or numbness that travels along the entire length of the nerve. Sciatica may be felt in one, or more rarely in both, legs.

What are the causes?

The most common cause of sciatica is a prolapsed disc (>>317) that bulges out into the spinal column and presses against the sciatic nerve. Sometimes sciatica is triggered when an inflamed facet joint or a bony spur pinches the nerve as it leaves the spine. This may be due to osteoarthritic wear and tear on vertebrae or it may result from a condition such as osteoporosis, which can weaken vertebrae and cause fractures and compression. Sciatica may also begin during pregnancy as the mother's posture adjusts to take account of the weight of the foetus. Often no cause can be identified.

This type of pinching might occur only momentarily during strenuous lifting or sudden movements or there may be constant pressure against the nerve. Sometimes the tiny muscles connecting the vertebrae and facet joints go into spasm at the onset of sciatic pain, increasing the pinching effect and exacerbating the pain.

What are the symptoms?

The pain of sciatica can be mild or severe. It extends from the buttock down the leg and may take the form of shooting pains, a tingling sensation or muscle weakness in the affected leg.

The area in which the pain is felt is determined by the site of sciatic nerve compression – it may affect both legs and in some cases pain may extend to the feet and toes. In addition to these symptoms, there may also be pain in the lower back – this is usually less severe than in the legs.

How is it diagnosed and treated?

A description of the symptoms and their distribution will guide the doctor in his diagnosis and help to indicate the site of

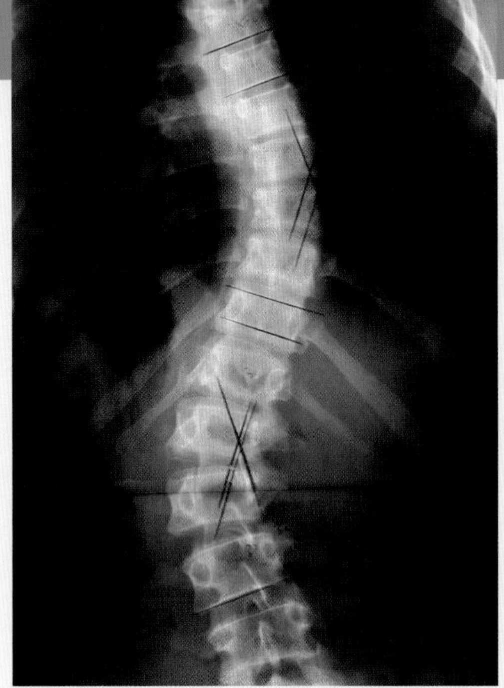

CURVED SPINE

This X-ray shows the pronounced sideways curves typical of scoliosis. In this instance there are two curves, giving an 'S' shape to the spine, but in many cases the spine curves one way only.

the pressure on the sciatic nerve. X-rays or other tests, including MRI (>>297), may be arranged to look for the underlying cause.

Non-steroidal anti-inflammatory drugs (NSAIDs >>208) or other painkillers may be recommended to relieve the symptoms. It is important to remain as active as possible – while being careful not to cause any further injury – in order to maintain mobility and minimize stiffness. Being active also seems to relieve pain and hasten recovery.

An epidural injection of an anaesthetic drug into the space around the membranes covering the spinal cord may be given in cases where there is severe pain. Physiotherapy or back exercises may also be recommended for pain relief.

If the underlying cause of the pain can be identified, it may be helpful to treat this. If the pain is due to a prolapsed disc, for example, corticosteroids may help to relieve inflammation and take pressure off the nerve. It may even be appropriate to perform a miscrodiscectomy in order to surgically remove the portion of the disc pressing against the nerve. In most cases, however, sciatica resolves within around six weeks, so more conservative treatment measures are usually sufficient.

SCOLIOSIS

A sideways curve in the vertebral column.

Scoliosis is visible when looking at the spinal column from the back. Seen from this angle, a normal spine should appear straight. A spine that curves to the left or the right is described as having scoliosis.

The thoracic spine – the portion of the spine that runs down the back of the chest – is the most commonly affected area, but the curve may be present in other sections of the back. In some cases there are two curves, one to the left and one to the right, creating an 'S' shape.

- **Postural scoliosis** is the term used when the structure of the spinal column is normal and the curvature results from a postural problem elsewhere in the body. Possible causes include differences in leg length or habitual poor posture. This type of scoliosis is usually mild and the curve may disappear with movement.
- **Structural scoliosis** describes a curvature of the spine which is there regardless of how the individual moves. Structural scoliosis often develops for no apparent reason – this is known as idiopathic scoliosis. It is relatively common and may arise at any time from infancy to adulthood but most often develops during the growth spurt of adolescence.

Causes of structural scoliosis include deformities of the spinal column that may be present at birth and disorders that affect the muscles around the spine, such as poliomyelitis (>>315).

What are the symptoms

The spinal curve tends to develop slowly. Unequal stresses on the spine are likely to cause back pain and muscular aches. In severe cases the rib cage, shoulders or pelvis may be pulled out of position and there may be problems walking. Osteoarthritis (>>228–247) of the vertebral column may eventually develop as a result of the abnormal stresses placed upon it.

In very severe cases, the abnormal positioning of the rib cage may lead to heart and lung problems in later life.

How is it diagnosed and treated?

The doctor will make the diagnosis by carefully assessing the shape of the vertebral column and checking its alignment when the patient bends forward. X-rays may be taken to complete the assessment.

In many cases, affected individuals are simply monitored for changes – the curve may improve, remain stable or worsen over time. In severe cases, treatments such as bracing or surgery may be considered.

Back braces do not reverse an existing curvature but rather aim to limit any further curving as the child grows. Surgery may involve inserting a metal rod into the back to straighten the spinal column or fusing the vertebrae rigid in the affected area. A brace may be worn for a time following the operation to keep the spinal column in position.

What is the outlook?

Idiopathic scoliosis that develops during infancy often improves as the child grows. However, in a few cases the problem worsens and treatment is needed. Idiopathic scoliosis of adolescence is common and in most cases does not warrant any treatment. In only a few cases does the deformity become severe enough to require surgery.

SEPTIC (INFECTIVE) ARTHRITIS

Inflammation in a joint as a result of an infection, usually bacterial.

Septic arthritis, also known as infectious arthritis or pyogenic arthritis, is caused by an infection in the joint itself: the hips and knees are the joints most often affected. It is a serious condition that requires urgent medical treatment. Arthritis triggered by infection elsewhere in the body is known as reactive arthritis >>320.

What are the causes?

The infection often reaches the joint from sites elsewhere in the body, such as the skin or the respiratory tract. Genital infection with gonococcus is also a possible source of infection. Alternatively, the infection may enter the joint through an open wound – people who have had recent joint injuries or surgery or are receiving medications injected directly into the joint are at particular risk. The most common bacterial cause of infection is Staphylococcus aureus.

Septic arthritis can occur in previously healthy joints, but it is more common in joints affected by disease – particularly those damaged by rheumatoid arthritis (>>248–263). Other risk factors include diabetes mellitus and impaired immunity.

What are the symptoms?

The joint will appear reddened and feel hot. There may be a fever. There will also be swelling and severe pain in the joint. Movements will be limited by the pain and muscle spasm around the joint.

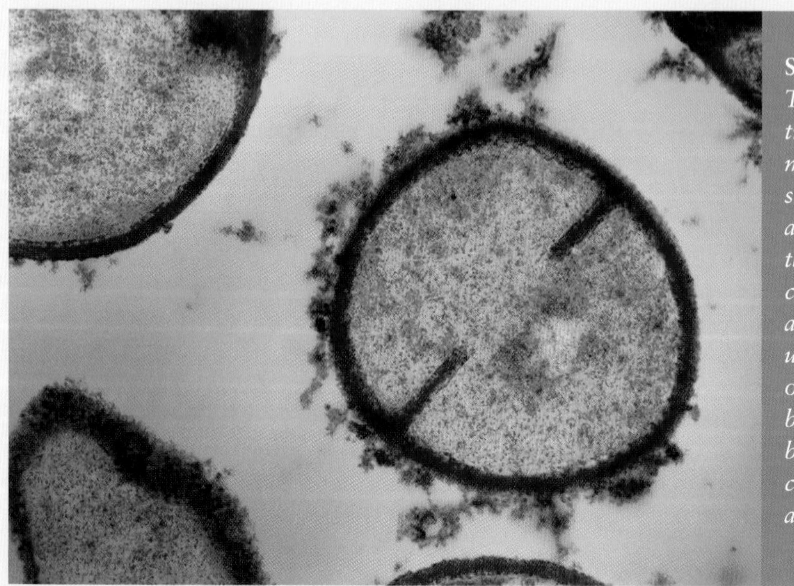

STAPHYLOCOCCUS
This coloured transmission electron micrograph (TEM) shows staphylococcus aureus bacteria, one of the most common causes of septic arthritis. The bacteria usually live harmlessly on skin and in mucus, but if they enter the bloodstream they can cause joint infections and swelling,

How is it diagnosed?

If septic arthritis is suspected from the symptoms and examination, a sample of fluid will be withdrawn from the joint and sent to the laboratory for analysis. In some joints, the fluid may need to be withdrawn using ultrasound scanning to guide the insertion of the needle. Blood tests may be taken to look for evidence of infection.

What are the treatment options?

Septic arthritis requires admission to hospital. Antibiotic treatment is started immediately in order to limit joint damage; the antibiotics may be changed if necessary following the results of tests on the joint fluid. The antibiotics are initially given intravenously and then orally, often for up to three months.

Painkillers will help to control the pain and the affected joint will need to be rested for a brief period. Fluid may be withdrawn regularly to relieve pressure within the joint. In some cases the fluid will be drained surgically. Gentle movement of the joint should start as soon as possible with physiotherapy exercises to maintain muscle strength and avoid stiffness.

What is the outlook?

The prognosis is better the earlier that treatment is started. Without treatment, septic arthritis may go on to cause severe damage to the joint and in a few cases it may be life-threatening. There is also an increased chance that osteoarthritis will develop later in life >>228–247.

SLIPPED DISC >>prolapsed disc

SLIPPED FEMORAL EPIPHYSIS

A condition of childhood and adolescence in which the end of the femur is displaced.

The epiphysis is the name for the end section of a long bone (the tubular bones such as those found in the limbs). It is separated from the shaft of the bone by a plate called the epiphyseal growth plate. During childhood and adolescence this growth plate produces cartilage which is gradually transformed into bone, making the bones grow longer.

During adolescence the growth plate at the upper end of the femur (the thigh bone) sometimes slips (tears) and the epiphysis comes away from the shaft of the femur. In some cases, both legs are affected. More rarely the lower end of the femur can also slip out of position (slipper lower epiphysis), usually as a result of an injury.

What are the causes?

A slipped upper epiphysis may occur suddenly as a result of an injury that causes a fracture or it may develop gradually for no apparent reason. The hormonal changes that take place during adolescence may be a factor. The condition affects more boys than girls and children who are overweight are particularly at risk. The condition can run in families, which suggests that genetic factors may play a role.

What are the symptoms?

Pain is often felt in the knee – this is due to the fact that the same nerves supply both the hip and the knee – but it may also be present in the hip or groin area. The child may have a limp and the leg may be turned outwards. Movement of the hip may be limited. In advanced cases the leg may be unable to support the child's weight.

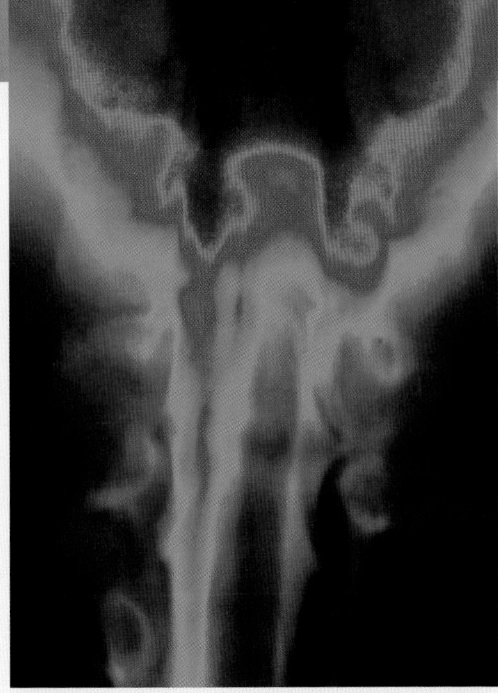

MENINGOCELE SPINA BIFIDA
This coloured myelogram shows the meninges (in green) protruding through a malformed spinal column. The spinal cord itself (shown in red) appears to be undamaged.

How is it diagnosed and treated?

To avoid any permanent hip problems it is important to diagnose and treat the problem as early as possible. If the position of the leg and the age of the patient suggest that a slipped epiphysis may be responsible for the symptoms, an X-ray will be taken to confirm diagnosis and treatment will begin.

The condition is usually treated by fixing the epiphysis in position using pins. In more severe cases, surgery may be needed to re-align the bone and correct any deformity. With early diagnosis the outlook is good and recurrence is uncommon. If the condition is more advanced, there may be a degree of permanent deformity and osteoarthritis may later develop >>228–247.

SPINA BIFIDA

A congenital disorder in which the spinal column fails to close properly causing potentially serious neurological problems.

Spina bifida (SB) occurs when the foetus's spine fails to close properly during the first month of pregnancy. The severity of the spinal deformity varies but usually falls into one of three main categories:

- **Myelomeningocele spina bifida** occurs when the spinal cord and the meninges (the protective cover) protrude out of the spine.
- **Meningocele spina bifida** occurs when the meninges protrude but the spinal cord itself develops normally.
- **Occulta spina bifida** occurs when the spinal cord and meninges develop normally but one or more vertebrae are malformed.

Spina bifida occulta is very common, affecting up to 40 per cent of the population but produces few, if any, symptoms. Only around 1 in every 1000 babies have one of the two more significant types of spina bifida, usually myelomeningocele. Studies suggest that folic acid supplements taken during pregnancy can greatly reduce the risk of neural tube defects such as spina bifida.

What are the symptoms?

Spina bifida occulta does not usually have any symptoms, although it may be possible to see a hairy area, skin lump or birthmark on the lower back. Very occasionally there may be associated problems such as back pain, scoliosis (curved spine), weakness or loss of sensation in the legs, or bowel and bladder problems. In this case it is known as occult spinal dysraphism.

At birth, the most obvious symptom of meningocele or myelomeningocele spina bifida is likely to be a fluid-filled cyst on the spine and possibly a protruding spinal

6 WAYS TO...

Avoid sports injuries

You can never completely avoid the risk of sports injuries but there are a number of measures you can take to make injuries less likely to occur.

1 Take things slowly Most sports injuries are a result of training too long or at too high an intensity: your body needs time to adapt. Build up intensity gradually as your strength and endurance improves.

2 Warm up Warming up before exercise prepares your body for exertion and increases flexibility, preventing strains and sprains.

3 Watch your technique If possible take lessons when starting a new form of exercise to ensure your technique is correct and you know how to avoid common errors. Try to avoid sudden twisting movements.

4 Use the right equipment A good pair of training shoes, in particular, is essential to provide support and absorb shock. For information on choosing trainers >>48–49.

5 Listen to your body Don't push your body too hard and never try to work through pains. If pain persists, get medical attention.

6 Stretch Lack of flexibility increases the risk of sprains and strains. After exercise, always try to stretch the muscles you have just been using to prevent them shortening.

cord or other tissues. In the longer term, the child may have muscle weakness or paralysis below the point in the spine where damage occurred and lack of bowel or bladder control. In 70–90 per cent of children there will be a build up of fluid in the brain (hydrocephalus) that can cause brain damage, seizures or blindness unless treated immediately.

How is it diagnosed and treated?

Prenatal screening for spina bifida is possible using a blood test that helps to predict the risk of neural tube defects. If there is a high risk, the doctors will take a sample of amniotic fluid and examine the foetus using ultrasound. After birth, significant spina bifida is usually obvious at the postnatal physical examination.

A baby with severe spina bifida will require prompt surgery to move the membrane or spinal nerves back into the spine. If the baby has hydrocephalus, a procedure known as shunting will be performed to drain the fluid and release pressure on the brain. The infant may require further surgery through childhood.

Surgery should prevent further nerve damage but will not reverse damage that has already occurred. To manage the symptoms of this damage, the child may require extensive ongoing support from specialists such as physiotherapists, urologists and neurosurgeons.

> ‘Some nutritionists recommend eating fresh pineapple to help heal sports injuries. Pineapple contains the enzyme bromelain which is thought to encourage tissue repair’

SPORTS INJURIES

Damage to soft tissues, bones and joints resulting from sporting activity.

The most common sporting injuries are muscle strains (>>328). More severe but still quite common injuries include muscle ruptures. which occur when some of a muscle's fibres break. Tendons can also be affected, with inflammation of the tendon (tendinitis >>330) being extremely common. Ligaments and cartilage may be damaged; the knee is a common site for such problems (>>197–199). Injuries to bones and joints include fractures (>>291), either due to a sudden injury or to repeated stress, and joint dislocations (>>288).

What are the causes?

Sports injuries may be caused by a sudden injury or they may come on gradually as the result of repeated stresses put on a particular area (overuse injuries). People involved in contact sports such as football and rugby are particularly at risk of acute injuries, including fractures and joint dislocations. Other sportsmen and women are more likely to be affected by injuries that develop gradually such as jogger's knee, stress fractures in the small bones of the feet and plantar fasciitis (>>314).

Risk factors for sports injuries include increasing age, a previous history of injury, poor technique, the lack of a proper warm-up, inadequate equipment, excessive exercise (particularly if it focuses on one particular part of the body), and sudden increases in intensity.

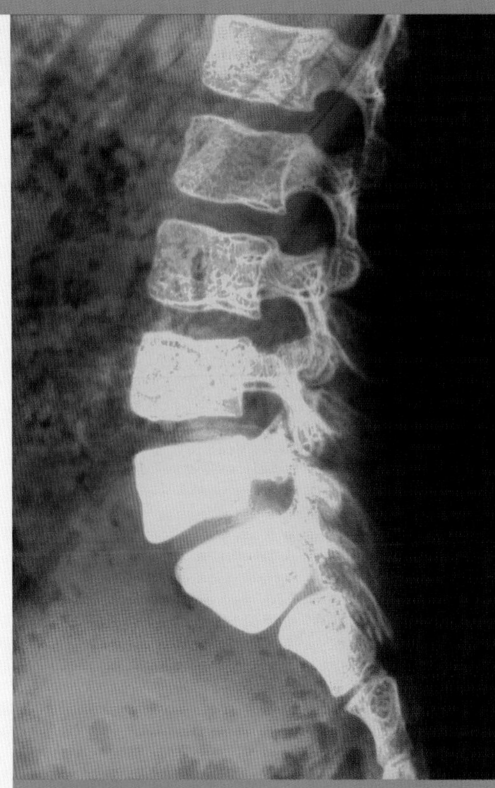

SPONDYLOLISTHESIS
The fifth lumbar vertebra in this coloured X-ray (the sixth bone seen here from the top), has slipped forward over the top of the vertebra underneath, breaking the connecting bone on the right of the vertebral body.

Certain sports are associated with particular injuries: inflammation of the patellar tendon often occurs with sports that require lots of jumping, for example, while anterior ligament sprains are common in sports that involve sudden twisting motions. Both conditions are common in basketball players. For more detailed information on avoiding common sports injuries >>134–135.

What are the treatment options?

Treatment depends on the nature of the injury. Most mild soft tissue injuries such as strains and sprains respond well to RICE treatment (rest, ice, compression, elevation >>204). Warming packs and mild non-steroidal anti-inflammatories (NSAIDs >>280) will also help to reduce swelling and inflammation. Physiotherapy may help to relieve pain, improve mobility and avoid further problems. For more specific details about treatment, see the directory entry for that particular type of injury.

Once the injury has healed, care must be taken to avoid re-injury when resuming exercise – advice from the doctor or physiotherapist may be valuable. For information about avoiding re-injury >>135. For details about exercising with existing injuries or problems >>158–159.

SPONDYLOLISTHESIS

A condition affecting the spinal column in which one of the vertebrae slips forwards on to the vertebra below it.

In children, this type of slippage may result from a congenital malformation of the vertebrae – usually the 5th lumbar vertebra which slips over the 1st sacral vertebra below it. In adults the most common cause is wear and tear on cartilage and vertebrae causing osteoarthritis. This mainly affects women over the age of 60.

Less frequently, the slippage may result from a fracture. Certain sporting activities which involve repeated hyperextension of the spine may lead to stress fractures – examples include javelin throwing and gymnastics. In a few cases, a disease such as osteoporosis (>>264–275), Paget's disease of bone (>>313) or a bone tumour (>>280) may weaken bones in the spine, making them more vulnerable to slippage. The lumbar region is the most commonly affected area of the spine because it supports the full weight of the torso and has a greater range of movement than other regions of the back, making it less stable.

What are the symptoms?

Symptoms of spondylolisthesis may include pain and stiffness in the lower back, tightness in the muscles along the backs of the thighs and sometimes pain in the buttocks and thighs. In some cases there are no symptoms at all.

Spondylolisthesis can cause spasms that stiffen the back and tighten the hamstring muscles, resulting in postural changes. If the slippage is significant, it may begin to compress the nerves as they exit the spine and there may be tingling, weakness or shooting pains in the legs >>322.

How is it diagnosed and treated?

X-rays will be taken to check the alignment of the vertebrae and to see whether any fractures are present. CT scans (>>301) may be arranged to provide a more detailed view of the affected area. The doctor will grade the condition according to how far forward the vertebra has slipped.

Treatment varies depending on the severity of the condition. Strenuous activities should be restricted but exercises to strengthen the muscles that support the vertebral column may be recommended – a physiotherapist can advise on appropriate exercises. A back support may be needed if the back is particularly painful.

If the condition continues to be painful or if the slippage seems to be getting worse, an operation may be needed to fuse the affected vertebra.

SPRAINS >>ligament injury

STILL'S DISEASE >>juvenile arthritis

STRAINS

Muscles and tendon injuries that result from overstretched muscle fibres.

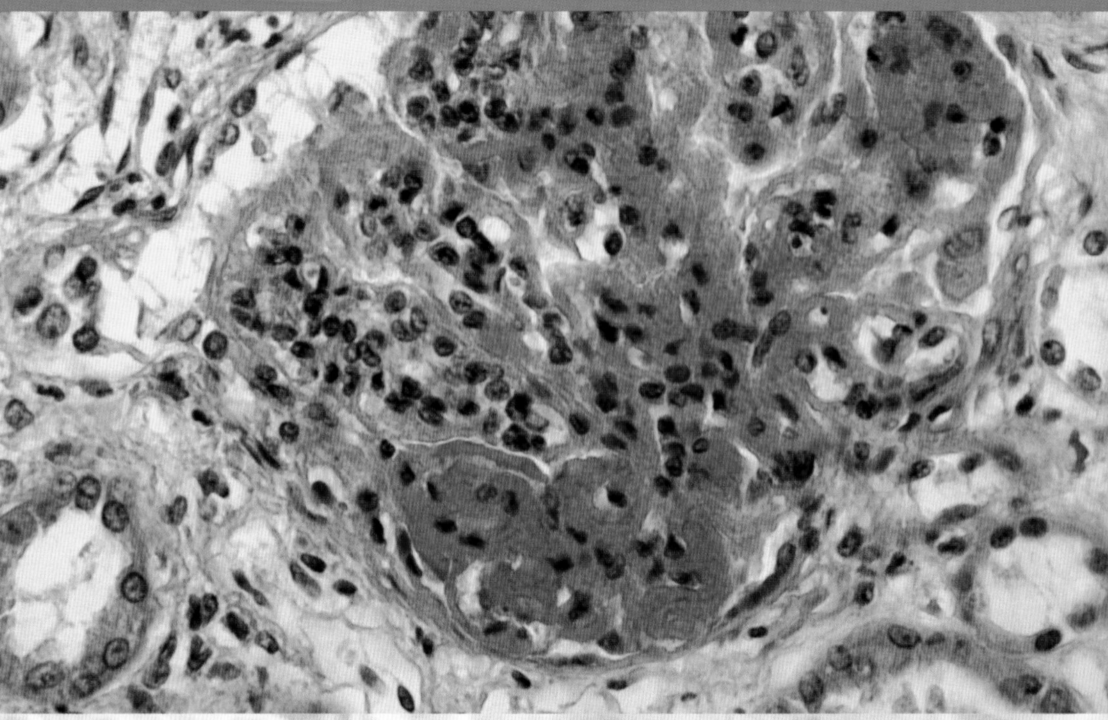

Muscle strains are a common, though usually minor, injury that occur when a muscle is pulled beyond it's normal limits. This can happen during the course of normal activities – when stretching to reach something, for example – but they are frequently brought on by sporting activities. A full warm-up at the start of every session can reduce the risk of strains occurring during exercise.

The muscles of the back, abdominal wall, legs and arms are often affected by strains. Back strains may occur when bending over or when lifting a heavy object awkwardly. Lifting with poor technique can also strain the abdominal muscles. Sometimes the muscle fibres tear (muscle rupture). Ligaments can also be strained – this is known as a sprain >>299.

What are the symptoms?

Muscle strains occur suddenly, sometimes with a popping or snapping sensation. They cause pain, stiffness and restricted movement in the injured area. Bruising or discoloration of the overlying skin may develop over the course of a few hours.

What are the treatment options?

A good guide for treatment is provided by the mnemonic RICE: rest, ice, compression, elevation. Rest is particularly important to give the tissues time to heal – the injured area should be rested for at least 2–3 days and the activity that caused the problem should be avoided until the injury has had time to heal completely. After this initial period, however, exercise is useful in order to maintain muscle condition.

An ice pack or cold compress will help to reduce the swelling and pain. Ice packs should not be placed directly against skin or used for longer than 20–30 minutes at a time. After about 72 hours, when the swelling has subsided, warming packs or hot towels will increase blood flow to the affected area. Compression and elevation (keeping the injured limb raised) can also help to relieve swelling. Non-steroidal anti-inflammatories (NSAIDs >>280) may help to reduce the pain and inflammation.

In most cases, the symptoms should resolve within a few days. If the symptoms persist, medical advice should be sought. In a few cases, an operation may be needed to repair severe muscle ruptures.

SYSTEMIC LUPUS

An autoimmune disorder causing rash and joint pain and mainly affecting pre-menopausal women.

There are two main forms of lupus: discoid lupus, which affects only the skin, and systemic lupus erythematosus (SLE), which also affects the joints and other organs. SLE is usually called just systemic lupus – erythematosus simply means 'red'.

What are the causes?

Systemic lupus is an autoimmune disorder, meaning it occurs when the immune system

SYSTEMIC LUPUS ERYTHEMATOSUS
This light micrograph of a section through an inflamed glomerulus (blood filtration structure) in kidney tissue shows how systemic lupus can irritate tissues around the body.

produces antibodies that bind to the body's own tissues rather than attacking foreign invaders. It is not clear exactly what triggers this response: it is probably caused by a combination of factors including infections, hormones (it is most common in premenopausal women) and genetic factors. Lupus is not inherited.

Systemic lupus primarily affects the skin and joints but it can also involve the hair, kidneys, heart and lungs, brain and occasionally other organs. It also varies considerably in severity. For some people it is only a minor nuisance; in other people it is troublesome or even life-threatening.

What are the symptoms?

Systemic lupus usually begins with joint pain and swelling, especially in the small joints of the hands and feet. The pains may move from one group of joints to another. Unlike rheumatoid arthritis (>>248-263), lupus does not usually cause damage or deformity to joints – although around 5 per cent of sufferers do develop more serious joint problems that can result in permanent damage.

Skin rashes are another characteristic symptom. This rash tends to spread over areas of the body exposed to the sun such as the face and hands. The rash can also affect other areas of the body. If lupus causes circulation problems, the fingers and toes may turn white, blue and red in turn (Reynaud's phenomenon). Recurrent mouth ulcers are also very common.

Other possible symptoms include hair loss (alopecia), inflammation of the kidneys, high-blood pressure, chest pains, migraines, breathlessness and anaemia (a lack of red blood cells). Occasionally lupus affects the heart or lungs directly, causing irritation of the tissues lining the organs.

How is it diagnosed?

Doctors use a range of blood tests (>>box, right) to check for lupus. These tests usually look for the presence of autoantibodies associated with lupus, measure levels of haemoglobin in the blood or test for certain enzymes involved in the immune response. Blood tests may also be used to check bone marrow or kidney function since both can be impaired by lupus. Once lupus has been diagnosed, a variety of other tests may be used to determine which organs are affected, including X-rays, ultrasound scans, MRI scans and CT scans (>>319, 297, 301).

What are the treatment options?

Treatments for lupus focus on controlling symptoms rather than curing the disease. Non-steroidal anti-inflammatories (NSAIDs >>280) and disease-modifying drugs such as hydroxychloraquine can help to relieve swollen, painful joints. Ultraviolet light can cause the skin rash to flare up so avoiding too much exposure to sunlight may help to reduce the rashes.

For more serious complications, steroids (>>320) and other immunosuppressive drugs can help to damp the immune response. All these drugs can have side effects, some of which are potentially serious, so should only be used as directed by a doctor. For the most severe cases doctors may consider intravenous gamma globulin injections or a blood plasma exchange (>>296).

WHAT CAN BLOOD TESTS REVEAL?

Blood contains many different substances. Blood samples, usually taken from a vein near the elbow, may be examined for a range of significant elements or features including:

- **White blood cells** Raised levels of these infection-fighting cells suggest infections or autoimmune disorders. Specific antibodies can often identify a particular condition.
- **Infectious organisms** Viruses and bacteria may enable doctors to identify an infection.
- **C-reactive protein (CRP)** This protein is released in greater quantities in response to injury, infection or inflammation.
- **Haemoglobin** Low haemoglobin in blood cells (anaemia) can occur as a result of conditions including rheumatoid arthritis.
- **Enzymes** Creatine kinase, a muscle enzyme, is raised in many inflammatory conditions; alkaline phosphotase is raised in osteomalacia and Paget's disease.
- **Erythrocyte sedimentation rate (ESR)** This is the rate at which red blood cells settle out of suspension in plasma. A very fast ESR suggests conditions such as rheumatoid arthritis or systemic lupus.
- **Uric acid** High levels may indicate gout.

DID YOU KNOW?

- **Lupus usually affects women of childbearing age. About one in ten cases begins after 50.**
- **It is about nine times more prevalent in women than in men. It is 8–16 times more common among black women living in Europe and America than it is in Caucasian women and is also fairly common in Asian women. However, it is rare in Africa.**

TENDINITIS

Inflammation of a tendon, one of the strong cords that connect muscles to bones.

Tendons frequently become inflamed as a result of being put under repeated or excessive strain – often during sporting activities but also in the course of some occupations. Tendinitis may also be accompanied by tenosynovitis, an inflammation of the tendon sheath >>331. Some tendons are more vulnerable than others to inflammation: the tendon that attaches to the kneecap (the patellar tendon) often becomes inflamed as a result of repeated jumping actions in sports like basketball; the Achilles tendon at the back of the heel may be injured by frequent downhill running. Other common sites for tendon injuries include the ankle, knee, shoulder, elbow and wrist.

Two well-known examples of tendinitis are tennis elbow and golfer's elbow. Another common injury is rotator cuff tendinitis, a condition in which the tendons around the shoulder become inflamed as a result of repeatedly moving the arm above the head. Swimmers, bowlers and tennis players are susceptible to this condition.

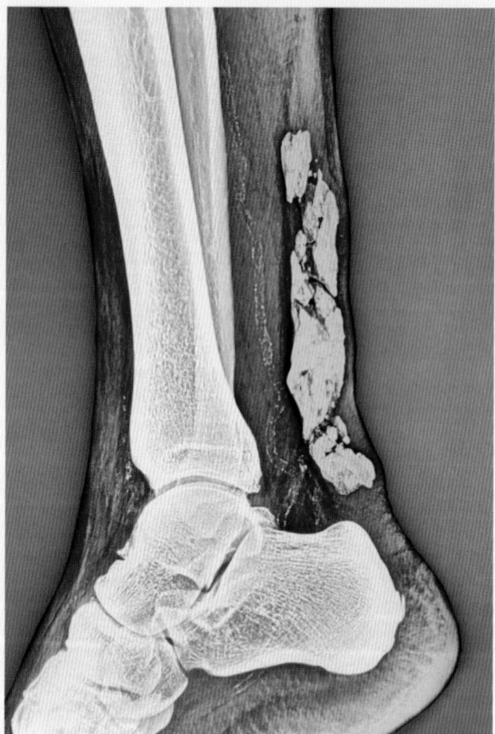

ACHILLES TENDINITIS

In this coloured X-ray, severe inflammation of an Achilles tendon due to tendinitis has led to calcification of the tendon.

What are the symptoms?

Tendinitis causes pain around the tendon. This is often made worse by repeated use of the associated muscle – but pain may also be present at rest. Individuals with patellar tendinitis will experience pain around the kneecap, particularly when exercising. Patients with Achilles tendinitis will often notice the pain when they pull their toes upwards and will feel it when they run. The pain caused by rotator cuff tendinitis may be felt when the arm is brought forwards above the head or across the chest. There may also be mild swelling in the area affected as well as stiffness and limitation of movement.

How is it diagnosed and treated?

The diagnosis is based on the symptoms and an examination of the affected area. The doctor will ask the patient to make certain movements which will indicate whether a particular tendon is involved.

Tendinitis is usually easy to treat: rest and anti-inflammatory drugs (NSAIDs >>280) are generally recommended. If the symptoms are severe or persistent, a steroid may be injected into the sheath covering the tendon. The use of ultrasound therapy in the treatment of tendinitis is currently being evaluated and may prove useful. Daily use of TENS (>>box, right) may help to reduce pain. Sometimes certain exercises will be recommended to build up muscle strength in the affected area.

The outlook is generally good and tendinitis will usually resolve within a few days although it can recur.

TENNIS AND GOLFER'S ELBOW

Two common forms of tendinitis causing inflammation of a tendon where it attaches to the bone at the elbow.

Tennis elbow (lateral epicondylitis) affects the tendon on the outer side of the elbow. Golfer's elbow (medial epicondylitis) is an inflammation of the tendon on the inner side of the elbow. Both tendons are involved in wrist movements – bending the wrist back in the case of the lateral tendon and down in the case of the medial tendon.

- **Tennis elbow** This condition can occur when playing tennis, perhaps as a result of overuse or hitting a ball awkwardly, but it is more common during other activities that require repeated gripping and twisting movements such as plastering and painting, or as a result of a sudden strain caused by lifting. Tennis elbow tends to develop between the ages of 40 and 60 as tendons grow less flexible.
- **Golfer's elbow** This condition may be caused by an acute injury or by repeated strains sustained when playing golf, but it is more commonly associated with other activities such as raquet sports. Like tennis elbow it can develop for no obvious reason.

What are the symptoms?

The affected area will be tender and there may be some mild swelling. Wrist and elbow movements can cause the pain to worsen. In tennis elbow the pain is felt on the bony bump on the outer side of the elbow. The pain of golfer's elbow is felt on the inside of the elbow. In both conditions pain may persist when at rest and, if severe, can cause problems sleeping.

What are the treatment options?

To prevent the inflammation from getting any worse it is important to avoid repetitive movements of the wrist and elbow as well as any other movements that seem to increase the pain. It may help to wear strapping. If the condition is brought on by a particular sporting activity it is important to check technique.

A heat pack or wrapped hot-water bottle held against the elbow can provide relief; alternatively a wrapped ice pack can be applied twice a day for 5–10 minutes. Other options for relieving pain and inflammation include oral or gel-based non-steroidal anti-inflammatories (NSAIDs >>280), physiotherapy, ultrasound and TENS (>>box, right).

If the pain is not relieved by any of these measures, a corticosteroid injection may be given directly into the affected area. The pain sometimes worsens for a day or two after the injection but should then begin to improve.

What is the outlook?

With rest, these conditions usually settle down within a couple of weeks but in a few cases they can persist for a year or more. Occasionally, individuals are referred to orthopaedic surgeons who may perform an operation to release the tendon.

TENOSYNOVITIS

Inflammation of the lining of the sheath that surrounds a tendon.

Tendons are bundles of sinewy, cord-like fibres that connect muscles to bone. To prevent friction as the fibres move over one another, they are surrounded by synovial fluid and contained inside a slippery sheath called the tenosynovium. Tenosynovitis occurs when this sheath becomes irritated. Tenosynovitis often occurs together with inflamed tendons (tendinitis >>330).

What are the causes?

Common causes of inflammation include repeated or excessive stress on the tendon and sheath and acute tendon injuries. It is sometimes caused by rheumatism or arthritis and may be triggered by infection. It also becomes more likely as the tenosynovium starts to thicken with age. Tenosynovitis can affect any tendon in the body but is most common in the tendons around the hands, wrists and feet. Tenosynovitis in a finger is known as trigger finger >>334.

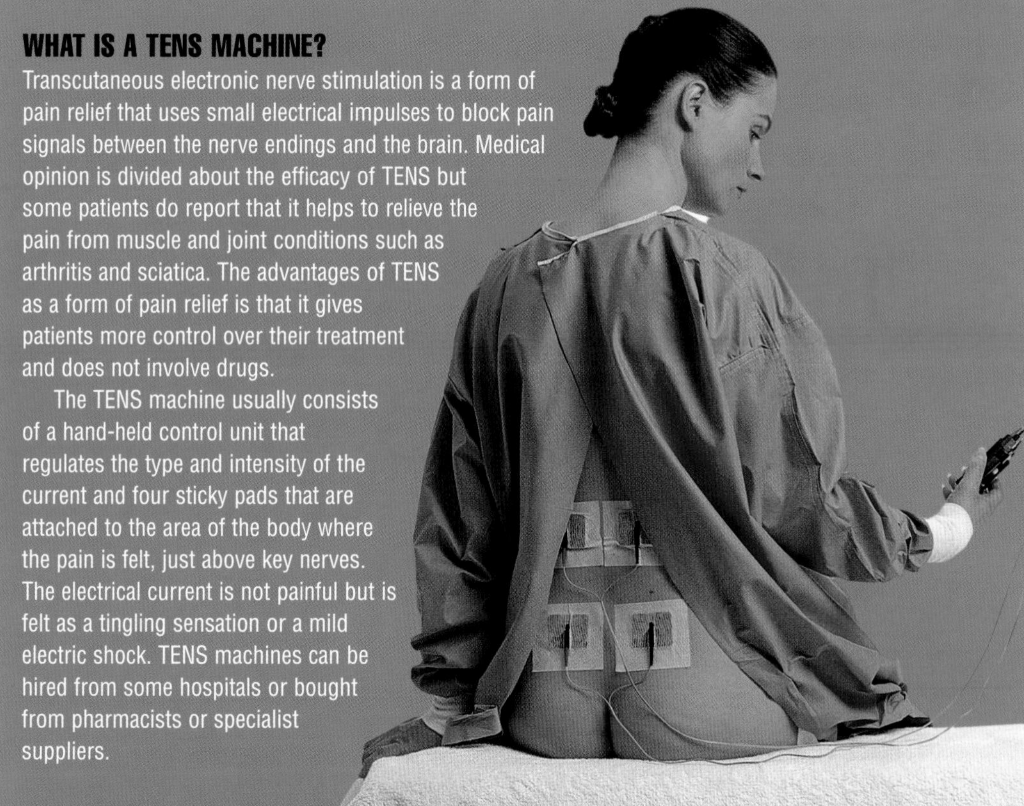

WHAT IS A TENS MACHINE?

Transcutaneous electronic nerve stimulation is a form of pain relief that uses small electrical impulses to block pain signals between the nerve endings and the brain. Medical opinion is divided about the efficacy of TENS but some patients do report that it helps to relieve the pain from muscle and joint conditions such as arthritis and sciatica. The advantages of TENS as a form of pain relief is that it gives patients more control over their treatment and does not involve drugs.

The TENS machine usually consists of a hand-held control unit that regulates the type and intensity of the current and four sticky pads that are attached to the area of the body where the pain is felt, just above key nerves. The electrical current is not painful but is felt as a tingling sensation or a mild electric shock. TENS machines can be hired from some hospitals or bought from pharmacists or specialist suppliers.

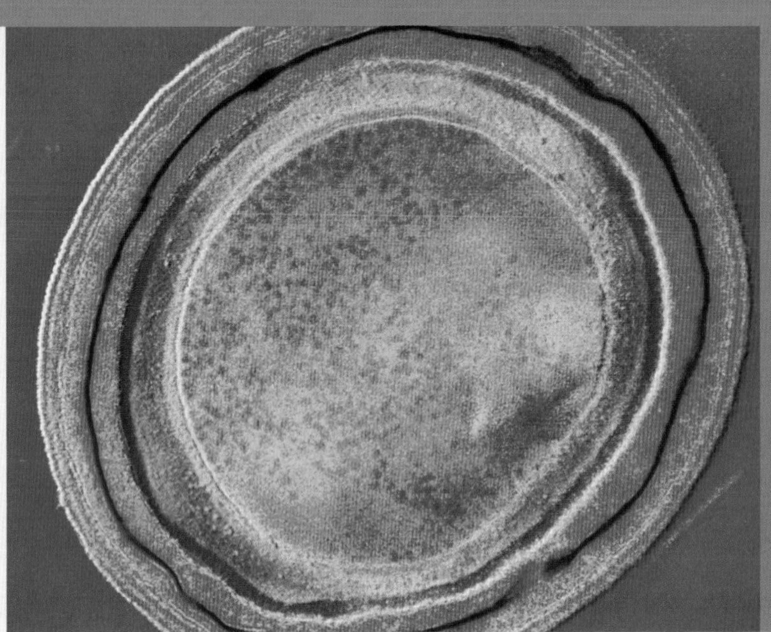

TETANUS SPORE
This false-colour micrograph shows a clostridium tetani spore. The thick membranes surrounding the spore allow it to survive in adverse environments such as soil, intestines or manure. When the spores enter a cut or wound and conditions are more favourable the spore will germinate and may cause tetanus.

What are the symptoms?
Tenosynovitis causes pain, tenderness and swelling of the affected area as well as stiffness in the joint that is moved by the tendon. This may last just a few days but in some cases persists for weeks or months. Sometimes the area feels warmer than the surrounding skin. There may be a slight clicking sensation as the fingers are moved.

What are the treatment options?
Treatment focuses on reducing pain and inflammation. Rest or immobilization, sometimes using a splint or brace, will help to relieve irritation. Mild non-steroidal anti-inflammatories (NSAIDs >>280), heat and cold treatment or steroid injections (>>320) will also reduce inflammation. Once the swelling has gone down, exercises to strengthen the muscles around the affected area will help to prevent recurrence. Repetitive movement or overuse of the tendon should be avoided.

TEMPOROMANDIBULAR JOINT DISORDER

Any disorder of the joint that connects the lower jaw to the upper part of the skull.

The temporomandibular joint (TMJ) is the hinge formed where the mandible (the lower jaw) and the temporal bone of the upper skull meet. The various movements of this joint permit the mouth to open and close and the jaw to move backwards, forwards and from side to side. The term TMJ disorder is an umbrella term for any disorder of this joint or of the structures that move and support it.

What are the causes?
Sometimes the upper and lower teeth do not fit together exactly as they should (malocclusion) causing difficulty or discomfort chewing. TMJ problems can also result from tight jaw muscles or persistent teeth grinding (both of which may be associated with stress) as well as poorly fitting dentures. Temporomandibular function can also be upset by diseases such as osteoarthritis (>>228–247) or by an injury such as a dislocated or broken jaw.

What are the symptoms?
Depending on the cause, symptoms may include a dull, aching pain below the ear, spasm or pain in the jaw muscles or a clicking sensation when the mouth is opened or closed. The pain may extend across the face or cause headaches or earache. The mouth may not open up fully or the teeth may not align properly when the mouth is shut.

How is it diagnosed and treated?
The doctor will make the diagnosis based on the symptoms but may arrange tests, such as X-rays or an MRI (>>319, 297), to pinpoint the cause. Orthodontic treatment may be recommended for a malocclusion and a mouth guard could be fitted over the teeth at night to stop grinding. It may also help to reduce stress where possible.

Treatments to relieve the pain and spasm include heat treatments, ultrasound therapy (>>box, right) and painkillers or non-steroidal anti-inflammatory drugs (NSAIDs >>280). Occasionally, surgery may be recommended to re-align the joint.

TETANUS

A dangerous bacterial infection causing muscle spasm and paralysis.

Also known as lockjaw, tetanus is a serious bacterial infection that affects the nervous system. Tetanus is rare in developed countries as a result of widespread childhood immunization. However newborns, children and adults who have not received the vaccine, as well as adults have not had a booster vaccine within the last 10 years, may be at risk.

What are the causes?

Tetanus is contracted through a cut or wound that becomes infected with the Clostridium tetani bacterium, a type of bacterium widely found in soil, dust and manure. It is possible to contract the disease through minor pricks or scratches but deep cuts, wounds and bites are more susceptible to infection. Tetanus is not spread directly from person to person.

Once inside the body, the bacteria secrete a potent toxin which binds to the motor nerve endings and blocks the release of the neurotransmitters required to check muscle contractions. The result is a state of constant muscle contraction and paralysis, primarily in the neck and jaw muscles.

What are the symptoms?

The toxin affects the peripheral nerves first and moves inwards towards the spine. Spasms and rigidity in the jaw and facial muscles may begin around 7–10 days after infection, although the onset can take anything from three days to three weeks. The spasms are often triggered by touch or noise and may cause headaches, a stiff 'locked' jaw and difficulty swallowing.

From the face, the muscle spasms spread to the hands, arms and legs, back and abdomen. The contractions may be accompanied by fever, sweating and elevated blood pressure or heart rate. If the respiratory muscles are involved, patients may have problems breathing. The muscle contractions last three to four weeks and without treatment are frequently fatal.

How is it diagnosed and treated?

Tetanus is usually diagnosed from the symptoms and can be confirmed using a tissue culture from the site of the wound – although the culture may test negative. The hospital may order a blood test to check for tetanus antibodies as well as other tests to rule out similar diseases.

A patient who develops tetanus will need intensive treatment in hospital. Antibiotics will be used to fight the bacteria and a tetanus antitoxin, such as tetanus immune globulin (TIG), will be used to neutralize any toxin that hasn't yet combined with nerve tissue. The patient will receive medicine to control the muscle

WHAT IS ULTRASOUND THERAPY?

Used to treat a range of musculoskeletal disorders including soft tissue injuries and arthritis, ultrasound waves are sound waves that travel at a frequency above the range at which we can hear. These waves can be applied to the body in two ways: continuous ultrasound waves penetrate deep into the body tissues where they act as a form of heat treatment (diathermy), increasing the blood supply to promote faster healing; pulsed ultrasound travels in short pulses that do not heat the tissue up as much but may reduce swelling and inflammation. Other potential benefits include a pain-killing effect which can reduce muscle spasm. There is, however, little firm evidence that ultrasound helps injured tissues heal faster.

During ultrasound treatment the sound waves are directed into the injured or painful area of the body using the 'head' of a hand-held ultrasound device. A gel is used to help the waves travel into the body rather than reflecting off the skin and the head of the device is moved in small circles. Treatment usually takes a few minutes.

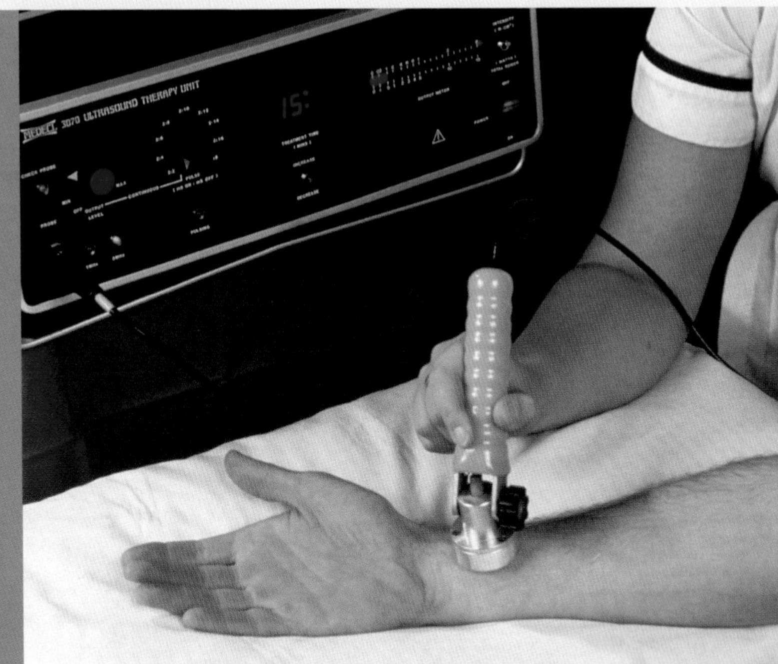

spasms and may need a ventilator to control breathing. Even with treatment, tetanus can prove fatal, particularly in babies and older patients. Recovery is more likely if the disease is caught early.

TORTICOLLIS

Twisting of the neck that causes the head to be held in an abnormal position.

This common condition is usually caused by spasms in the neck muscles, often as a result of sleeping in an awkward position. The muscle spasms may also develop following an injury to the neck.

Torticollis may also occur in childhood, sometimes in babies as a result of damage to the neck muscles during delivery and sometimes in older children due to swollen glands in the neck associated with infection.

What are the symptoms?

A spasm of the muscles on one side of the neck causes the head to be pulled into an abnormal position, usually with the head pulled over to one shoulder and the chin rotated towards the opposite shoulder. The head and neck are often stiff and painful.

What are the treatment options?

Most treatment measures focus on relaxing the muscle spasm. Tense muscles are often a result as well as a cause of the pain, so the short-term use of painkillers is often an effective way to treat the spasm. Heat treatments such as heat pads may provide relief. Massage, physiotherapy and ultrasound therapy may also be used.

The condition usually settles over the course of a few days. Occasionally, when the problem persists, an injection may be given into the muscles to relax them.

TRIGGER FINGER

A problem with the tendon in a finger, causing difficulty straightening the finger.

The tendons of the fingers glide through tendon sheaths which cover and lubricate them as they bend and straighten. In this condition, inflammation or a swelling on the tendon means that it catches as it runs into the sheath, preventing movements.

The reason for this is not fully understood. The condition may be present in one finger or more than one.

What are the symptoms?

Symptoms include a sensation of resistance as the affected finger is straightened or a snapping sensation as the resistance is overcome by the muscles that straighten the finger. The symptoms may be worse after a period of inactivity. Sometimes the finger becomes locked in a bent position and can only be pulled straight using the other hand. In severe cases it may not be possible to straighten the finger at all. In some cases the stiffness is accompanied by pain or discomfort. There may also be a swelling in the palm of the hand.

What are the treatment options?

The condition may resolve itself without treatment. Alternatively, a steroid injection can be given into the tendon sheath to reduce swelling and inflammation, allowing the tendon to glide through the sheath unimpeded. If the problem persists, surgery may be arranged to release the tendon by widening the entrance to the tendon sheath. This operation is usually carried out under local anaesthetic. After a few days the bandage is removed and normal finger movements can be resumed.

MALLET FINGER

Although it's the finger flexor tendons that are responsible for trigger finger, similar problems straightening the finger can be caused by damage to the extensor tendons, the tendons that run along the back of the hand and attach to the muscles in the wrist.

A finger that droops at the end joint because of damage to the extensor tendon is known as mallet finger – a common cause of the injury is a hard blow to the end of the finger. The usual treatment is to place the finger in a splint until it heals.

TUBERCULOSIS OF BONE

A highly infectious bacterial disease that can spread to bone from the lungs.

Tuberculosis usually starts in the lungs but can travel to almost any part of the body including the bones. The most common site of bone infection is the spine when the condition is known as Pott's disease or tuberculosis spondylitis. Tuberculosis can also affect the bones of the hips or knees.

Tuberculosis was once almost eradicated in developed countries but since the 1980s has been making a gradual comeback. This is due to a number of factors including the emergence of more drug-resistant bacteria, the growth in worldwide travel and the rise in HIV infection (which lowers immunity).

What are the symptoms?

The infection usually spreads to bone from another site, such as the lungs. For this reason, bone pain is often accompanied by other symptoms of tuberculosis such as persistent coughing (sometimes with blood in the sputum), fever with sweating, weight loss and chest pain.

Symptoms of the bone infection in the spine (Pott's disease) include back pain and sometimes visible swelling along the vertebral column. If the bacteria infect two adjoining vertebrae it can spread to the intervertebral disc which may then die. As a result, the space between the vertebrae may narrow or collapse, causing kyphosis (an excessive curve of the upper spine) and a hunchback appearance. The collapse of the vertebrae may also compress the spinal cord, causing neurological symptoms such as numbness, tingling or even paralysis of the lower limbs (Pott's paraplegia).

How is it diagnosed?

If tuberculosis is suspected, the doctor may arrange for tests such as urine or sputum analysis to check for evidence of general infection. Other possible tests include the Heaf test, a screening test in which a small amount of tuberculin is deposited on the outer layer of the skin, and the Mantoux test, in which a substance extracted from the TB bacterium is injected just under the skin on the forearm.

An MRI scan or CT scan may show evidence of vertebral compression or disc infection and is usually the best way to look for evidence of spinal infection.

What are the treatment options?

Tuberculosis affecting bone is treated in a similar way to pulmonary tuberculosis with a combination of three (sometimes four) antibiotic drugs. However, it may be necessary to take the medications for a longer period – at least six months and possibly for more than a year.

Surgical immobilization of the spine or vertebral fusion can prevent the problems associated with collapsed vertebrae but will also considerably reduce mobility.

WHIPLASH

A neck injury, often resulting from a car accident, that causes damage to the soft tissues, muscles and ligaments.

This injury most commonly occurs when the head is thrown back and then forwards as a result of a rear impact in a car. About 20 per cent of people involved in rear-end collisions later experience symptoms of whiplash: most of these people recover quickly but a small number develop chronic conditions that can result in severe pain and sometimes disability. The extent of the injuries is not always related to the speed of the impact – significant injuries can occur at speeds as low as 15mph (25kmph).

What are the symptoms?

The main symptoms are pain and stiffness in the neck. There may also be shoulder pain and headaches. The pain from soft tissue injuries such as muscle and ligament sprains and strains may occur immediately after the accident or may take some hours to develop; minor soft tissue injuries will usually persist for a few days or for a few weeks at the most.

Occasionally the sudden flexion and extension can damage the nerves in the neck, in which case there may be shooting pains, tingling or a sensation of heaviness or numbness in the arms or legs. Other symptoms that require urgent medical attention include memory loss, dizziness or periods of unconsciousness.

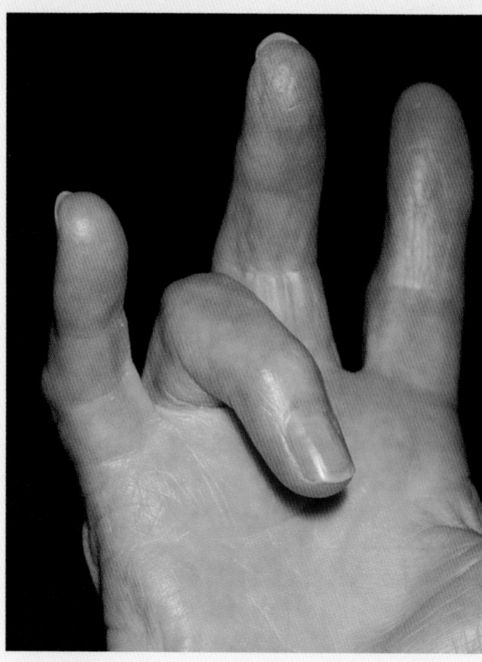

TRIGGER FINGER
This condition arises when the sheath around a tendon in the hand becomes irritated, pinching the tendon and preventing it from moving smoothly. In severe cases such as this one, surgery may be required to release the tendon.

What are the treatment options?

Doctors usually make the diagnosis without any investigations. In a few cases tests are needed to rule out a serious injury, such as a dislocated or fractured vertebra.

Sore muscles and tendons may be treated with painkillers or ice packs and in some cases the short-term use of a soft collar may be helpful for support. More serious injuries, including any evidence of vertebral fractures or neural problems, may require immobilization and further investigation. Physiotherapy may help to reduce stiffness and restore neck movements.

Useful Addresses

MEDICAL

Health and Safety Executive
www.hse.gov.uk
HSE Infoline: 0845 345 0055

National Osteoporosis Society
Camerton
Bath BA2 0PJ
Helpline no. 0845 450 0230
www.nos.org.uk

National Rheumatoid Arthritis Society
Unit B4 Westacott Business Centre
Westacott Way
Maidenhead
Berkshire SL6 3RT
Helpline no. 0845 458 3969
www.rheumatoid.org.uk

Arthritis Research Campaign
Copeman House, St Mary's Court
Chesterfield
Derbyshire S41 7TD
0870 850 5000
www.arc.org.uk

Arthritis Care
18 Stephenson Way
London NW1 2HD
0808 800 4050
www.arthritiscare.org.uk

UK Gout Society
PO Box 527
London WC1V 7YP
www.ukgoutsociety.org

National Ankylosing Spondylitis Society
PO Box 179
Mayfield
East Sussex TN20 6ZL
01435 873 527
www.nass.co.uk

Children's Chronic Arthritis Association
Ground Floor Office
Ambergate
City Walls Road
Worcester WR1 2AH
01905 745 595
www.ccaa.org.uk

National Back Pain Association (BackCare)
16 Elmtree Road
Teddington
Middlesex TW11 8ST
020 8977 5474
www.backcare.org.uk

Muscular Dystrophy Campaign
7–11 Prescott Place
London SW4 6BS
020 7720 8055
www.muscular-dystrophy.org

The Brittle Bone Society
30 Guthrie Street
Dundee DD1 5BS
Helpline no. 08000 282 459
www.brittlebone.org

Fibromyalgia Association UK
PO Box 206
Stourbridge DY9 8YL
Helpline no. 0870 220 1232
www.ukfibromyalgia.com

Lupus UK
St James House
Eastern Road
Romford RM1 3NH
01708 731 251
www.lupusuk.com

Multiple Sclerosis Society
MS National Centre
372 Edgware Road
London NW2 6ND
0808 800 8000
www.mssociety.org.uk

Myositis Support Group
146 Newtown Road
Southampton SO19 9HR
023 8044 9708
www.myositis.org.uk

National Association for the Relief of Paget's Disease
323 Manchester Road
Manchester M28 3HH
0161 799 4646
www.paget.org.uk

Psoriatic Arthritis Alliance
PO Box 111
St Albans
Herts AL2 3JQ
0870 770 3212
www.paalliance.org

Spinal Injuries Association
SIA House
2 Trueman Place
Oldbrook
Milton Keynes MK6 2HH
Helpline no. 0800 980 0501
www.spinal.co.uk

British Rheumatology Centre
Bride House
18–20 Bride Lane
London EC4Y 8EE
020 7842 0901
www.rheumatology.org.uk

Scoliosis Association (UK)
2 Ivebury Court
323-327 Latimer Road
London W10 6RA
Helpline no. 020 8964 1166
www.sauk.org.uk

Association for Spina Bifida and Hydrocephalus
42 Park Road
Peterborough PE1 2UQ
01733 555 988
www.asbah.org

Child Growth Foundation
2 Mayfield Avenue
Chiswick
London W4 1PW
020 8995 0257
www.heightmatters.org.uk

Child Accident Prevention Trust
4th Floor Cloister Court
22–26 Farringdon Lane
London EC1R 3AJ
020 7608 3828
www.capt.org.uk

Pain Concern
PO Box 13256
Haddington EH41 4YD
01620 822572
www.painconcern.org.uk

The British Pain Society
21 Portland Place
London W1B 1PY
0207 631 8870
www.britishpainsociety.org

LIFESTYLE AND WELFARE

ASH (Action on Smoking and Health)
102 Clifton Street
London EC2A 4HW
020 7739 5902
www.ash.org.uk

British Nutrition Foundation
52–54 High Holborn
London WC1V 6RQ
020 7404 6504
www.nutrition.org.uk

British Dietetic Association
5th Floor Charles House
148/9 Great Charles Street
Birmingham B3 3HT
0121 200 8086
www.bda.uk.com

British Association of Nutritional Therapy
27 Old Gloucester Street
London WC1N 3XX
0870 606 1284
www.bant.org.uk

Alcohol Concern
Waterbridge House
32-36 Loman Street
London SE1 0EE
020 7928 7377
www.alcoholconcern.org.uk

Age Concern
Astral House
1268 London Road
London SW16 4ER
0800 009 966
www.ageconcern.org.uk

Help the Aged
207–221 Pentonville Road
London N1 9UZ
020 7278 1144
www.helptheaged.org.uk

EXTEND
22 Maltings Drive
Wheathampstead
Herts AL4 8QJ
01582 832 760
www.extend.org.uk

Ricability
30 Angel Gate
City Road
London EC1V 2PT
www.ricability.org.uk

Disabled Living Foundation
380-384 Harrow Road
London W9 2HU
Helpline no. 0845 130 9177
www.dlf.org.uk

Counsel and Care
Twyman House
16 Bonny Street
London NW1 9PG
0845 300 7585
www.counselandcare.org.uk

THERAPISTS/ COMPLEMENTARY MEDICINE

Health Professions Council
Park House
184 Kennington Park Road
London SE11 4BU
020 7582 0866
www.hpc-uk.org

Chartered Society of Physiotherapy
14 Bedford Row
London WC1R 4ED
020 7306 6666
www.csp.org.uk

College of Occupational Therapists
106–114 Borough High Street
London SE1 1LB
020 7357 6480
www.cot.org.uk

British Complementary Medicine Association
PO Box 5122
Bournemouth BH8 0WG
0845 345 5977
www.bmca.co.uk

Institute for Contemporary Medicine
PO Box 194
London SE16 7QZ
020 7237 5165
www.icmedicine.co.uk

Complementary Medical Association
67 Eagle Heights
The Falcons
Bramlands Close
London SW11 2LJ
0845 129 8434
www.the-cma.org.uk

General Chiropractic Council
344–354 Grey's Inn Road
London WC1X 8BP
0845 601 1796
www.gcc-uk.org

British Chiropractic Association
Blagrave House
17 Blagrave Street
Reading
Berkshire RG1 1QB
0118 950 5950
www.chiropractic-uk.co.uk

General Osteopathic Council
Osteopathy House
176 Tower Bridge Road
London SE1 3LU
020 7357 0011
www.osteopathy.org.uk

Repetitive Strain Injury Association
c/o Keytools Ltd
PO Box 700
Southampton SO17 1LQ
023 8058 4314
rsia@keytools.com

British Acupuncture Council
Park House
63 Jeddo Road
London W12 9HQ
020 8735 0400
www.acupuncture.org.uk

The Society of Teachers of the Alexander Technique
129 Camden Mews
London NW1 9AX
020 7284 3338
www.stat.org.uk

Alexander Works
37 Hope Street
Liverpool
Merseyside L1 9EA
0151 708 6172
www.alexanderworks.org.uk

British Chiropody and Podiatry Association
The New Hall
149 Bath Road
Maidenhead
Berkshire SL6 4LA
01628 632 449
www.bcha-uk.org

The Society of Chiropodists and Podiatrists
1 Fellmonger's Path
Tower Bridge Road
London SE1 3LY
020 7234 8620
www.feetforlife.org

EXERCISE

The Keep Fit Association
Astra House
Suite 1.05
Arklow Road
London SE14 6EB
020 8692 9566
www.keepfit.org.uk

The Ramblers' Association
2nd Floor Camelford House
87–90 Albert Embankment
London SE1 7TW
020 7339 8500
www.ramblers.org

Physical Company
2a Desborough Industrial Park
Desborough Park Road
High Wycombe
Buckinghamshire HP12 3BG
01494 769 222
www.physicalcompany.co.uk

UK Tai Chi Association
PO Box 159
Bromley
Kent BR1 3XX
020 8289 5166
www.tai-chi-assoc.com

Amateur Swimming Association
Harold Fern House
Derby Square
Loughborough
Leicester LE11 5AL
01509 618 700
www.swimming.org

Body Control Pilates
6 Langley Street
London WC2H 9JA
020 7379 3734
www.bodycontrol.co.uk

The Pilates Foundation UK
PO Box 36052
London SW16 1XQ
07071 781 859
www.pilatesfoundation.com

British Yoga Teachers Association
10 Bromley Crescent
Ruislip Gardens
Middlesex HA4 6PG
01895 470 883
www.britishyogateachersassociation.org.uk

British Wheel of Yoga
1 Hamilton Place
Basten Road
Lincolnshire NG34 7ES
01529 306 851
www.bwy.org.uk

Yoga for Health Foundation
Ickewell Bury
Biggleswaide
Bedfordshire SG18 9EF
01767 627 271
www.yogaforhealthfoundation.co.uk

Art of Swimming
27 Greenway Close
London N20 8ES
020 8446 9442
www.artofswimming.com

PRODUCTS AND EQUIPMENT

Promedics (orthopaedic aids)
Moorgate street
Blackburn
Lancashire BB2 4PB
01254 619 000
www.promedics.co.uk

Homecraft AbilityOne
PO Box 5665
Kirkby in Ashfield
Nottinghamshire NG17 7QX
08702 423 305
www.homecraft-rolyan.com

Fellowes Ltd
Yorkshire Way
West Moor Park
Doncaster
South Yorkshire DN3 3FB
01302 836 836
www.fellowes.co.uk

Osmond Ergonomic Workplace Solutions
21 Johnson Road
Ferndown Industrial Estate
Wimborne BH21 7SE
01202 850 423
www.ergonomics.co.uk

Home Working Solutions
500 Chiswick High Road
London W4 5RG
020 8870 2581
www.homeworkingsolutions.co.uk

Keytools
PO Box 700
Southampton SO17 1LQ
023 8058 4314
www.keytools.com

Life Fitness
Queen Adelaide
Ely
Cambridgeshire CB7 4UB
01353 666 017
www.lifefitness.com

Concept 2
Vermont House
Nottingham South & Wilford Ind. Est.
Ruddington Lane
Wilford
Nottinghamshire NG11 7HQ
0115 945 5522
www.concept2.co.uk

INDEX

A

B

C

D

E

F

G

H

I

J

K

L

M

N

O

P

Q

R

S

T

U

V

W

PICTURE CREDITS

1 Digital Vision; **2** (tl) Susumu Nishinaga/SPL; **4** Getty Images; **5** (t) Getty Images; (b) Photodisc; **6** (bl) Punchstock/Stockbyte, (c) Punchstock/Bananastock, (br) Superstock; **7** (l) ©Reader's Digest, (c) Roger Dixon, (r) Punchstock/Creatas; **8/9** Jules Selmes; **10** (t) ©Reader's Digest, (b) Getty Images; **11** (t) Punchstock/IT Stock, (b) Getty Images, (r) BSIP, Cortier/SPL; **12** ©Reader's Digest; **13** (l) Photodisc, (r) Punchstock/IT Stock; **14** (tl) SPL, (br) Montreal Neurological Institute/SPL; **17** (r) GE Healthcare; **25** (cr) GE Healthcare; **27** ©Reader's Digest; **32** (l) Photolibrary; **33** GE Healthcare; **36** SPL; **37** (l) Manfred Kage/SPL, (c) Astrid and Hans-Frieder Michler/SPL, (r) Innerspace Imaging/SPL; **40** M I Walker/SPL; **42/3** Photodisc; **47** (l) Montreal Neurological Institute/SPL, (r) DigitalVision; **48/9** Photolibrary; **50** DigitalVision; **52** Photolibrary; **53** www.feetforlife.org; **54** Jules Selmes; **56/7** Getty Images; **58** (t) Photodisc, (b) DigitalVision; **59** Photodisc; **60** Punchstock/Comstock; **61** ©Reader's Digest; **63** (l) DigitalVision, (r) Jules Selmes; **64/7** v; **68/9** Punchstock/IT Stock; **69** Photodisc; **70/5** Jules Selmes; **77** Punchstock/IT Stock; **78/9** Jules Selmes; **80** www.lifefitness.com except (2nd left) www.concept2.co.uk; **80/1** Punchstock/IT Stock; **82/5** Jules Selmes; **86/7** Superstock; **87** www.artofswimming.co.uk/Zillah Crosby; **88/9** Carroll & Brown; **90/1** Roger Dixon; **92/7** Jules Selmes; **98** (t) Getty Images, (c) ©Reader's Digest, (b) Photodisc; **100** Jules Selmes; **101** (l) Photodisc, (c,r) ©Reader's Digest, (b) Carroll & Brown; **102** ©Reader's Digest; **103/6** Photodisc; **107** Punchstock/Creatas; **108** ©Reader's Digest; **110** Getty Images; **111** Will Heap; **112** Getty Images; **113** (t) RDA/GID, (br) ©Reader's Digest; **114** Punchstock/Comstock; **117** Getty Images; **118** (t) Photolibrary, (bl) Jules Selmes, (br) Punchstock/Bananastock; **120/1** Punchstock/Bananastock; **122** DigitalVision; **123** Punchstock/Photodisc; **124/5** DigitalVision; **126** (l) Photodisc, (r) ©Reader's Digest; **126/7** Punchstock/Bananastock; **127** ©Reader's Digest; **128** Punchstock/Bananstock; **129** Panasonic UK Ltd; **130/1** Punchstock/Digital Vision; **132** www.homeworkingsolutions.co.uk; **132/3** www.ergonomics.co.uk; **133** (l) www.ergonomics.co.uk, (r) Photolibrary; **134** Photodisc; **136/9** Jules Selmes; **141** Superstock; **142** (tl) Jules Selmes, (tr) Punchstock/Comstock; **144/5** Age Concern; **146** Getty Images; **148/9** Robert Harding; **150** (l) Punchstock/Goodshoot, (r) Photodisc; **151** (tl) Photodisc, (tr) Photolibrary, (b) Digital Vision; **152/6** Age Concern; **156/7** SPL; **158** Punchstock/Comstock; **161/3** Jules Selmes; **164** Punchstock/IT Stock; **165/7** Jules Selmes; **168** Punchstock/Imagesource; **169/71** Jules Selmes; **172/5** Roger Dixon/Nick Veasey; **176** Roger Dixon; **177** Jules Selmes; **178** Getty Images; **179** ©Reader's Digest; **180/3** Roger Dixon; **184/5** Punchstock/Imagesource; **187** Photodisc; **189** Michael Donne/SPL; **191** Photodisc; **192** (l) Punchstock/Corbis, (br) www.promedics.co.uk; **196/7** Getty Images; **200** Punchstock/Corbis; **202/3** Jules Selmes; **205** www.promedics.co.uk; **206** CNRI/SPL; **206/7** Brad Nelson/Custom Medical Stock Photo/ SPL; **208/9** all Dr Carlos Widgerowitz except **209** (r, background) BSIP, Cortier/SPL; **210** (l) Getty Images, (tr) SPL, (br) DePuy International; **212** Prof P Motta/Dept of Anatomy/University 'La Sapienza' Rome/SPL; **214** Getty Images/Bongarts; **216** Getty Images; **218** Photodisc; **219** www.promedics.co.uk; **220/1** Roger Dixon; **222** Photodisc; **223** ©Reader's Digest; **224/5** SPL; **226/7** DePuy International; **228** (t,c) Jules Selmes; **230/1** Punchstock/Corbis; **232** (l) Mediscan; **233** CNRI/SPL; **234** Getty Images; **236/7** www.helptheaged.org.uk; **237**(br) www.fellowes.co.uk; **238** Photodisc; **239/41** Jules Selmes; **241**(br) Punchstock/Digital Vision; **243** (t,c) AJ Photo/SPL, (b) CC Studio/SPL; **244** Jules Selmes; **244/5** Getty Images; **247** (t) David Mooney/SPL, (inset) Moredun Animal Health Ltd/SPL, (b) Jules Selmes; **248** (tr, br) Getty Images; **251** Getty Images; **252** (l) Chris Priest/SPL; **253** Dr P Marazzi/SPL; **254** www.artofswimming.com/Zillah Crosby; **255** Punchstock/IT Stock; **256/7** Getty Images; **258** (l) Getty Images, (c) Hattie Young/SPL, (r)Klaus Guldbrandsen/SPL; **259** (l) Getty Images, (c,r) www.promedics.co.uk; **260/1** Robert Francis/South American Pictures; **261** www.medicherb.co.uk; 264 (t) Prof P Motta/Dept of Anatomy/University 'La Sapienza' Rome/SPL, (r) SPL, (b) Jules Selmes; **266** Susumu Nishinaga/SPL; **267** Prof P Motta/Dept of Anatomy/University 'La Sapienza' Rome/SPL; **268** Jules Selmes; **269** Getty Images; **271** Photodisc; **272/3** Jules Selmes; **274** SPL; **279** CNRI/SPL; **281** (t) CNRI/SPL, (b) Josh Sher/SPL; **283** www.thefootandankleclinic.com; **284** Custom Medical Stock Photo/SPL; **289** SPL; **291** www.thefootandankleclinic.com; **292** Sovereign, ISM/SPL; **293** Antonia Reeve/SPL; **295** Arthritis Research Campaign; **296** Dr Ray Clark & Mervyn Goff/SPL; **297/301** GE Healthcare; **303** Eye of Science/SPL; **308** Dr P Marazzi/SPL; **310** Biophoto Associates/SPL; **313** Mehau Kulyk/SPL; **315** Getty Images/Visuals Unlimited; **317** Zephyr/SPL; **319** (t) BSIP Laurent/ H Americain, (b) www.feetforlife.org; **321** Alfred Pasieka/SPL; **323** Mediscan; **324** Dr Kari Lounatmaa/SPL; **325** BSIP, Cavallini James/SPL; **327** Princess Margaret Rose Orthopaedic Hospital/SPL; **328** CNRI/SPL; **330** CNRI/SPL; **331** Carroll & Brown; **332** CNRI/SPL; **333** St Bartholomew's Hospital, London/SPL; **335** Dr P Marazzi/SPL

Front jacket (main photo) Digital Vision; inset(t) Digital Vision; (c) ©Reader's Digest; (b) Photodisc
Back jacket (l) ©Reader's Digest; (c,b) Getty Images

HEALTHY BONES, MUSCLES & JOINTS

was published by The Reader's Digest Association Limited, London

The Reader's Digest Association Limited
11 Westferry Circus, Canary Wharf, London E14 4HE

We are committed to both the quality of our products and the service we provide to our customers. We value your comments, so please feel free to contact us on 08705 113366 or via our website at: www.reader'sdigest.co.uk

If you have any comments or suggestions about the content of our books, email us at: gbeditorial@readersdigest.co.uk

Healthy Bones, Muscles & Joints was created and produced by Carroll & Brown Ltd, London

Origination Colour Systems
Printed and bound in China

Concept code UK1881/IC
Book code 400-221-01
ISBN (10) 0 276 44064 1
ISBN (13) 978 0 276 44064 9
Oracle code 250009716H.00.24

CONTRIBUTORS

Dr Carlos Widgerowitz, MD, PhD, FRCS

Dr Penny Preston, MB, MRCGP

Dr Lesley Hickin, MB BS, BSc, DRCOG, MRCGP

Dr Michael Perring, MS, MB, B.Chir FCP (SA), DPM

Nick Woolley, Neuromuscular Therapist

Fiona Hunter, BSc, Dip, Dietitian

FOR CARROLL & BROWN

Editorial Director Louise Dixon
Art Director Chrissie Lloyd
Project Editors Tom Broder, Ian Wood
Designers Christine Kielty, Emily Cook, Laura de Grasse, Claire Legemah, Vimit Punater
Production Director Karol Davies
IT Management Paul Stradling
Picture Researcher Sandra Schneider
Illustrators Juliet Percival, John Woodcock, Mikki Rain, Nick Veasey
3D Illustration Mirashade, Rajeev Doshi/Medi-mation
Anatomical Reference Joanna Cameron
Special Photography Jules Selmes, Roger Dixon, Will Heap
Photography Assistant David Yems
Index Hilary Bird
Proofreader Geoffrey West

FOR READER'S DIGEST

Project Editor Rachel Warren Chadd
Art Director Nick Clark
Editorial Director Julian Browne
Managing Editor Alastair Holmes
Picture Resource Manager Martin Smith
Pre-press Account Manager Penelope Grose
Product Production Manager Claudette Bramble
Senior Production Controller Deborah Trott

Carroll & Brown would like to thank: Paul Kurring, DePuy International; GE Healthcare (www.gehealthcare.com); The Charteris Sports Centre, London; Steven Shaw, Art of Swimming, London; Help the Aged, London